Tobacco and Public Health: Science and Policy

Tobacco and Public Health: Science and Policy

Edited by

Peter Boyle
Director
Division of Epidemiology and Biostatistics
European Institute of Oncology
Milan, Italy

Nigel Gray
Senior Research Associate
Division of Epidemiology and Biostatistics
European Institute of Oncology
Milan, Italy

Jack Henningfield
Associate Professor of Behavioural Biology
Johns Hopkins School of Medicine
Bethesda, Maryland, USA

John Seffrin
Chief Executive Officer
American Cancer Society
Atlanta, USA

Witold Zatonski
Director
Division of Cancer Epidemiology and Prevention
The Marie-Sklodowska Memorial Cancer Center and
    Institute of Oncology
Warsaw, Poland

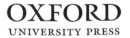

OXFORD
UNIVERSITY PRESS

OXFORD

UNIVERSITY PRESS

Great Clarendon Street, Oxford OX2 6DP

Oxford University Press is a department of the University of Oxford.
It furthers the University's objective of excellence in research, scholarship,
and education by publishing worldwide in

Oxford New York

Auckland Cape Town Dar es Salaam Hong Kong Karachi
Kuala Lumpur Madrid Melbourne Mexico City Nairobi
New Delhi Shanghai Taipei Toronto

With offices in

Argentina Austria Brazil Chile Czech Republic France Greece
Guatemala Hungary Italy Japan South Korea Poland Portugal
Singapore Switzerland Thailand Turkey Ukraine Vietnam

Oxford is a registered trade mark of Oxford University Press
in the UK and in certain other countries

Published in the United States
by Oxford University Press Inc., New York

© Oxford University Press, 2004

British Library Cataloguing in Publication Data

Data available

Library of Congress Cataloging in Publication Data

ISBN 0 19 852687 3

Typeset by Cepha Imaging Pvt Lted., Bangalore, India

Printed in Great Britain
on acid-free paper by Biddles Ltd., King's Lynn, Norfolk

Preface

Tobacco: The public health disaster of the twentieth century

At the dawn of the twentieth century, public health interventions and medical break-throughs were beginning to radically curb many forms of disease and premature death (CDC 1999a). It was also a time in which lung cancer was so rare that surgeons traveled to witness and learn from the few operations performed to save the lives of those afflicted (Kluger 1996; Wynder 1997). It was also a time in which an outgrowth of the cottage tobacco industry was metastasizing into one of the largest companies in the United States (Corti 1931; Taylor 1984; White 1988). That company was the American Tobacco Company, and it came to rival US Steel and Standard Oil as an economic and political powerhouse in the first few two decades of the twentieth century (Taylor 1984; White 1988). In the decades to follow, it would come to be rivaled by no industry and no war in terms of destruction of human life. By the end of the twentieth century, the offspring of this company, which I will collectively refer to as 'Big Tobacco', were selling enough cigarettes to kill more than 400 000 people annually in the United States and 5 million, worldwide (Garrett *et al.* 2002). On current course, the global trajectory will increase to 10 million deaths per year early in the twenty-first century and will cost the lives of nearly one-half of the world's 1.1 billion cigarette smokers (World Bank 1999).

The enormity of that number is almost incomprehensible, but in terms of lives lost to tobacco, it is equal to the Titanic sinking every 27 min for 25 years, or the Vietnam War death toll every day for 25 years.

These statistics can become numbing by their almost inconceivable magnitude. So it becomes important to frame the challenge, and our focus, constructively. When I became the United States' spokesperson for AIDS in the early years of the epidemic, I said we were fighting a disease, not the people who had it. For tobacco use, however, I have to say that we are fighting the diseases produced by tobacco as well as the purveyors of tobacco products, who have knowingly spread disease, disability, and death throughout the world. We should not ostracize those who have been harmed the most, namely tobacco-addicted persons, but rather should work with them to reduce their risk of disease and to prevent the further spread of this deadly affliction. Ostracism should be reserved for those whose greed and duplicity have made Big Tobacco our most loathsome industry.

Insofar as the vector that spreads the disease is Big Tobacco, the major challenge is to isolate and contain it. This will not be easy. Big Tobacco enjoys unparalleled protection from legal recourse, and possesses enormous political influence and economic power that it is willing to use to undermine public health efforts (Orey 1999; Kessler 2000). In addition, it sells a highly addictive product that, ironically, makes many of its most debilitated consumers its strongest supporters (Taylor 1984; Kluger 1996; Givel and Glantz 2001). By way of contrast, there are probably few malaria-afflicted persons who would fight for their 'right' to continue to be exposed to the mosquitoes spreading this disease, nor are HIV-afflicted persons lobbying for the right of other persons to willfully afflict others with the disease, but there is a 'smokers rights' movement, which must be appropriately addressed and hopefully recruited to the side of public health.

The enormity and complexity of the public health assault demands a broad and sophisticated public health response. I would like to take this opportunity to comment briefly on what I believe should be our vision for health, and how we can achieve it. I will begin with a few additional comments on how we got to this place in the epidemic, because an understanding of these issues is crucial in addressing the problem.

Historical perspective

Tobacco use and addiction have existed for centuries, and there surely was resultant death and disease (Corti 1931; US DHHS 1989). However, tobacco-based mass destruction of life on a global scale was only possible with the emergence of multinational companies capable of the daily production and distribution of billions of units of the most destructive of all forms of tobacco—the cigarette. Further, the modern cigarette has extraordinarily toxic and addictive capability: its increasingly smooth and alkaline smoke both enable, and require, inhalation of the toxins deep into the lungs to maximize nicotine absorption. James Albert Bonsack, who invented the modern cigarette machine, also deserves some discredit; however, if he hadn't invented it, someone else would have done so soon enough.

In the early days of the industry's growth, tobacco manufacturing and selling might have appeared to be a legitimate form of consumer product development and marketing. However, there were two important distinctions between legitimate consumer marketing and the tobacco industry that were not generally recognized until decades after the industry was well entrenched in the economic and political framework of many countries, and the fabric of their cultures. The first distinction was clearly appreciated by the first modern cigarette marketers, i.e. following a few occasions of smoking, many cigarette smokers would come to be as addicted to their daily fix of tobacco as other drug addicts become to their form of narcotic. The industry discovered that nicotine was critical to this process (US DHHS 1988; Slade *et al.* 1995; Hurt and Robertson 1998; Kessler 2000). The second distinction was that cigarette smoking carried a substantial risk of lung cancer, as discovered in the pioneering studies of Richard Doll, Alton Ochsner, Ernst Wynder, and others in the 1950s (Wynder 1997).

The cigarette companies hid much of their knowledge of the addiction issue and, until recently, disputed the possibility that cigarette smoking was addictive (Kessler 2000). The industry addressed the lung cancer issue head on in the press, with their *Frank statement to cigarette smokers*, published in major newspapers in 1954. In this statement, Big Tobacco disputed the link between cigarette smoking and lung cancer, accepted an interest in people's health as a basic responsibility, and pledged to cooperate closely with public-health experts, among other promises broken long ago. Such strategies enabled Big Tobacco to buy time, buy influence over politicians, buy exemptions for their products from consumer product laws intended to minimize unnecessary harm from other products, and even to buy questionable science in an effort to undermine, or at least complicate, interpretation of the science that damned their products (Taylor 1984; White 1988; Kluger 1996; Hirschhorn 2000; Hirschhorn *et al.* 2000).

In the 1960s the US Federal Trade Commission (FTC) tried to provide consumers with a means of selecting presumably less toxic products and to provide cigarette companies with an incentive to make such products. The Commission adopted a cigarette testing method originally developed by the American Tobacco Company (Bradford *et al.* 1936) and later recognized as the FTC method for measuring tar and nicotine levels (National Cancer Institute 1996, 2001). Big Tobacco responded by developing creative methods to circumvent the test, in order to enable consumers to continue to expose themselves readily to high levels of tar and nicotine with 'elastic' cigarette designs, and then to thwart efforts to revise constructively the testing methods for greater accuracy (National Cancer Institute 1996, 2001; Wilkenfeld *et al.* 2000). The FTC method was codified internationally as the International Standards Organization (ISO) method and Big Tobacco globally extended its deadly game of consumer deception and obfuscation of efforts to provide meaningful information about the nicotine and toxin deliveries of its products (Bialous and Yach 2001; World Health Organization 2001).

It was not until the 1990s that the American Cancer Society (Thun and Burns 2001) and National Cancer Institute (1996) recognized that the advertised benefits of so-called 'reduced tar' or 'light' cigarettes were virtually nonexistent, and that the marketing of these products may have actually impaired public health by undermining tobacco use prevention and cessation efforts (Stratton *et al.* 2000; Wilkenfeld *et al.* 2000; National Cancer Institute 2001). Many smokers, realizing the scientifically proven health risk to smoking cigarettes, switched to 'reduced tar' or 'lighter' cigarettes, believing they were doing the reasonable thing to reduce risk and improve their health. We can never let history repeat itself. As Big Tobacco, and small tobacco companies, attempt to entice us with the false promises of their new generations of so-called 'reduced risk' products (Fairclough 2000; Slade 2000), we must be at least as skeptical of them as we would be of pharmaceutical and food products sold on the basis of their health claims (explicit or implied). *Scientific proof to the satisfaction of an empowered agency, such as the Food and Drug Administration,* must be the gold standard for 'reduced risk' or other health claims made by the tobacco industry. This standard should apply to claims including those implied through the use of terms such as 'light' or 'low tar'. Meeting the standard should be required *prior* to the marketing of any new brand of cigarettes and any new type of tobacco product making such claims.

My vision for tobacco and health in the twenty-first century

My vision for the future is simple and achievable: To improve global health by drastically reducing the risk of disease and premature death in existing tobacco users and by severing the pipeline of tomorrow's tobacco users. I turn your attention to Fig. 1, developed by the World Bank (1999), projecting mortality from the middle of the twentieth century to 2050 (see above, p. 00). This figure illustrates the grim current course. What gives us hope for the future is the powerful effect of reducing disease by smoking cessation. The benefit would be apparent within a few years, because there is a dramatic reduction in risk of heart disease, evident within 1–2 years of smoking cessation. I believe it is within our reach to do much better than the effect predicted by the World Bank, a decrease in tobacco-related deaths of almost 200 000, but the public-health community will need to marshal powerful political allies to impact that projected figure. We need to make it as easy to get treatment for tobacco addiction as it is to get the disease.

In addition to the dramatic impact of smoking cessation, is the delayed, but powerful, effect of preventing initiation. It will have only a minimal effect by 2050, because the main increase in mortality does not begin until about age 50. Therefore, the effect will be apparent about 30–50 years after prevention, as the generation exposed to prevention reaches the age at which smoking-caused diseases begin to escalate

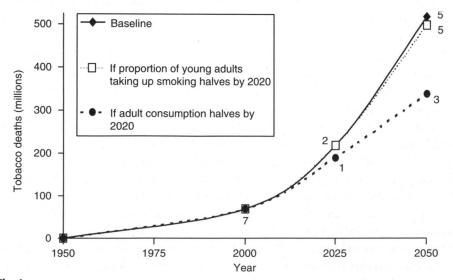

Fig. 1

dramatically. Once more, I am not satisfied with a goal of 50% reduction of initiation, because I think we can do better. If we look at the results of tobacco prevention and cessation efforts in California and Massachusetts during the 1990s, we see that smoking initiation and prevalence can be reduced, and it is reasonable to predict even stronger results if the efforts and expenditures were more commensurate with the magnitude of the health problem caused by tobacco (CDC 1999b, 2000). I would also point out that Fig. 1 shows only premature mortality; it does not include the important, and more rapid, benefits of preventing initiation in terms of projected missed days of school, and lost work productivity due to diseases that may not be life threatening, but can be debilitating and account for unnecessary suffering. Of course, the greatest effect on smoking prevalence in the near and long term would be from the simultaneous reduction of initiation and increase in cessation, which could have synergistic effects (Farkas et al. 1999).

I believe that my vision is possible because we already have the science foundation to support substantial progress. We know enough to predict significant reductions in risk through substantial increases in smoking cessation (US DHHS 1989; World Bank 1999). We have treatments, both behavioral and pharmacological, that can help people quit smoking at far less cost per person and far greater cost benefit than treatment costs of many of the diseases caused by tobacco (Cromwell et al. 1997; World Bank 1999). We know that the prevention of initiation of tobacco use can be accomplished by comprehensive educational programs that increase awareness of the harms inherent in smoking, and by decreased access and increased costs at the point of purchase through increased tobacco taxes (Kessler et al. 1997; Chaloupka et al. 2001; Bachman et al. 2002). We have a solid scientific foundation that will allow us to move forward and make considerable progress in the US and globally (WHO 2001).

Realizing the vision

I have already touched upon some of the elements that will be critical to the realization of my vision for the twenty-first century, and many other potential features are discussed in this volume. At this point, I would like to make some general observations that I think are particularly important for focusing our efforts, so that we may achieve our goals.

First, we have to understand that we are fighting disease and Big Tobacco, not cigarette smokers. We have to isolate and contain Big Tobacco interests in the interest of health. We have to fight for the resources to support the science that is yet needed, and to support the application of its lessons in order to protect those who do not use tobacco products, and to serve those who are addicted and those who will yet become addicted. We need to work to keep our political leaders on the right path, or the powerful interests of Big Tobacco will surely deliberately lead them astray.

As I have written before, we will have to channel outrage to ensure that, from local communities to the global community, we do not become complacent. Our tasks will consume all the energy we can muster (Koop 1998*a*). Consider that on the backs of the approximately 50 million smokers in the United States alone, lawsuit settlements generated a potential monetary pipeline approaching 10 billion US dollars per year for 25 years. But across the nation, the percentage of these funds being used to contain Big Tobacco, to prevent initiation, and to treat the addicted is in the single digits. The decisions to divert the vast majority of those funds have been unconscionably wrong, and I continue to wonder at the relative absence of outrage at this fact (Koop 1998*a, b*). Perhaps I should not be surprised, because, as I have reviewed previously secret documents from Big Tobacco, I have seen that this is not only an evil industry, it is also one that has ensnared its potential political, regulatory, and legal adversaries as tightly as it has the consumers of its products.

Moving forward will require us to build linkages to isolate and contain Big Tobacco. The linkages we need are many and varied. Global, country, community, and organizational linkages are needed to coordinate policy and political efforts. Linkages among research, education, and service sectors are important to maximize their impact.

In addition to linkages, there is much about the process of initiation and maintenance of tobacco addiction that needs to be considered if we are to prevent and treat it more effectively. We need to consider racial, gender, age-related, cultural, and philosophical issues to prevent tobacco use, just as Big Tobacco exploits these same characteristics to initiate the use of its products. We need to appreciate the fact that once exposed to the pernicious effects of tobacco-delivered nicotine, the structure and function of the brain begins to change, so that tobacco use is not a simple adult choice. It is, in part, a behavioral response to deeply entrenched physiological drives created by years of daily exposure to nicotine during the years of adolescent neural plasticity. This means that tobacco users will need education to guide their decisions and, often, treatment support, to act upon them. Addiction to tobacco-delivered nicotine should be considered the primary disease, to which the major causes of morbidity and premature mortality are secondary. We should treat it no less seriously than we treat consequences such as lung cancer and heart disease, because treatment of addiction may help avoid the subsequent need for treatment of lung cancer and heart disease. In fact, such efforts will support prevention because the children of parents who quit smoking are half as likely to initiate, and twice as likely to try quitting if they have already begun (Farkas *et al.* 1999).

Our prevention and containment messages need to move people to action. Decades of research show that perception of harm is a major determinant of use and addiction to drugs, ranging from tobacco to cocaine and marijuana (Bachman *et al.* 2002). Messages that generate emotion convey information about the harms that are meaningful to the targeted populations, and messages that challenge the myths that have been foisted upon the public by Big Tobacco need to become as ubiquitous as Big Tobacco's lies. More than 'tobacco kills', we need consumer-tested messages to ensure that every individual understands that using tobacco does a lot more than simply 'kill', it impairs quality of life for years until the killing is accomplished. Similarly, policy makers should care about reduced productivity and economic viability of the work-force, if not the economics of tobacco-caused disease (Warner 2000).

Our efforts to communicate the relevant reasons for freedom from tobacco will be countered by Big Tobacco, and we must resolve to never again let its false and mislead-ing statements go unanswered. We need a strong voice to ensure that policy makers know the truth about the tobacco products of today and tomorrow. We are beginning to see the twenty-first century version of 'low tar' cigarettes from the tobacco industry— new products with even stronger allusions to reduced risk, with even less precedent upon which to base policy and reaction. We must not forget the lessons of the twentieth-century products and product promotions that were intended, by Big Tobacco, to address smokers' concerns, even as they perpetuated the pipeline of death and disease (Kessler 2000). The release of the tobacco industry documents has been a treasure trove for tobacco-control advocates and policy makers alike. It is tantamount to crack-ing the genetic code of the malaria-carrying mosquito, or the operational plans of an illicit drug smuggling ring. This inside knowledge does not make our course of actions as clear or as easy as we would like, but it provides a sobering view of what we are up against and what kinds of challenges we face.

Getting the message out

I would like to propose a strategy for ensuring that public perceptions will begin to reflect the truth about tobacco. The experience in California and elsewhere has shown that effective public education strategies can mobilize action, and reduce smoking (Balbach and Glantz 1998). However, to be effective *we need to know who the public is, how the public can use our expertise, and what the public should know.*

Who?

The public is a diverse patchwork of cultures, each with special languages, values, norms, and expectations. I propose that at least one-third of our strategic planning and daily endeavors be devoted to understanding cultural diversity, protecting human dignity, and helping each 'public' develop its own means to become free of tobacco disease.

How?

We can take as a starting point the fact that the information and emotions held by con-sumers with respect to tobacco products are derived heavily from explicit advertising, and implicit purchasing of good will, by Big Tobacco, such as its 'philanthropic' efforts to sponsor sporting events, entertainment, charities, and, in some countries, public street signs and traffic signals. Following well-accepted principles of advertising, our message must be simple, consistent, pervasive, repetitious, and delivered through many sources. It must be framed so that it is interesting and relevant to the intended listeners. Although our motivation may be to reverse the course of death and disease, our message should be upbeat and provide hope and opportunity, rather than the promise of death and disease.

We must engage all manner of organizations that provide for society and its well-being. Even as the tobacco industry has attempted to subvert various organizations, we must reclaim them to serve humanity, and to help disseminate messages of freedom from tobacco and its attendant diseases. There can be no place for turf wars or divisive exercises if we are to maximize our effectiveness. Unity should be the watchword, from the level of local community organizations to the World Health Organization. To reach the diverse populations of smokers, we must enlist the support of a diversity of organizations, as measured by culture, ethnicity, and even those with entirely different purposes, ranging from religious organizations to hobby industries, to the entertainment industry.

What?

It is clear that the motivation of Big Tobacco is greed. I believe greed that flourishes at the expense of the destruction of millions of lives a year can only be described as evil; it cannot be reconciled with personal and corporate ethics and morality. Such greed is infectious and pervasive, and in the tobacco industry extends into the realm of financial investment. Those who hold large portfolios such as, colleges, universities, pension plans, etc., by keeping investments in tobacco stock, have convinced themselves that the rules of the marketplace override separation from evil if a profit is to be made. President Reagan called the Soviet Union, 'the evil empire', and President George W. Bush referred to Iraq, Iran, and North Korea, as 'the axis of evil'. Yet these entities to whom evils were attributed have not killed more than 400 000 citizens of the United States, or millions worldwide, each year. The evil empire is Big Tobacco and, unlike military and political enemies who say, 'I intend to kill you if I can', Big Tobacco disguises its evil with the invitation to light up, and become alive with pleasure.

We need more focused themes that can be communicated effectively. The public needs to know that good health and quality of life are taken away by tobacco, and are achieved through its avoidance. The public needs to know that the so-called economic benefits of tobacco to society are naught, and that stronger economic health at the individual and national level is possible without tobacco. The public also needs to know that commercial speech in the form of advertising can be appropriately held to standards of truth and scientific proof, even within the context of freedom of speech. The public needs honest information about the ingredients and design features of their products, presented in a regulated manner, so that, under the guise of full disclosure, the industry is not given new tools to promote their products. Finally, the public needs to know that the tobacco industry does not represent business as usual. Big Tobacco has stepped beyond the bounds of even the most unethical of business practices. This has been made evident through the disclosure of previous secret documents and through litigation by State attorneys general in the United States and elsewhere.

A place for harm reduction?

Much of public health can be viewed as efforts to reduce disease prevalence and severity by reducing exposures to pathogens, and by treating those exposed. In principle, this approach could be applied to reduce the death and disability caused by tobacco in ongoing tobacco users. This has been discussed elsewhere, and in this volume, with respect to tobacco (Food and Drug Law Institute 1998; Warner *et al.* 1998; Stratton *et al.* 2000; Henningfield and Fagerstrom 2001; Warner 2001). It is certainly one of the most controversial elements among potential strategies for reducing the risk of death and disease in tobacco users who, despite our best efforts, will be unable to completely abstain from tobacco. We should not ignore their plight anymore than we should ignore the plight of the person who has contracted a tobacco-caused disease. After all, their volitional control over their tobacco use may be little different than their volitional control over the expression of cancer in their bodies. Furthermore, if we can reduce their risk of disease despite aspects of their behavior that we cannot control, are we not better off, both as a global community and as individuals? Here again, I draw upon my experience with the HIV epidemic in the United States. Before we were even certain that a virus was the etiological culprit, I, as the nation's surgeon general, advocated strategies to reduce the spread of the disease—strategies ranging from the use of condoms to drug abuse measures, including treatment. Despite our best efforts, we could not eliminate risky sex or drug abuse, but we were able to reduce the spread of the disease by reducing the risk of transmission (Bullers 2001).

The problem with harm reduction approaches is that may pose theoretical benefits to a few individuals, along with real and theoretical risks to many others. This was the experience with smokeless tobacco products in the United States, in which relatively few recalcitrant cigarette smokers may have switched from cigarettes to snuff, incurring theoretical (but as yet uncertain) disease reduction, while, at the same time, a new epidemic of smokeless tobacco was observed in young boys, who happened to be athletes (US DHHS 1986). In this domain I concur with the general conclusions of the Institute of Medicine report, which said, in essence, that although there is great potential to reduce disease by harm-reduction methods, none have yet been studied adequately to allow their promotion, and those promoted by tobacco companies, in particular, carry substantial risks of worsening the total public health picture by undermining prevention and cessation (Stratton *et al.* 2000). This is also an area in which our science needs to be substantially expanded, because, at present, the main body of knowledge pertaining to the potential health effects of tobacco product design and ingredient manipulations seems to reside within Big Tobacco. This has been proven an unreliable source of complete and accurate information. In the future we cannot be held hostage to such a state of affairs.

Concluding comments

I have a vision for public health that is optimistic and realistic. In my lifetime, I have seen the rise and fall of epidemics, and I have come to believe that well-intentioned men and women, motivated by a will to serve and guided by science, can control disease and eradicate plagues. Unlike other epidemics, the disease of tobacco addiction and its many life-threatening accompaniments has an important ally in Big Tobacco. But no form of institutionalized evil can perpetuate itself for long when the truth about its intentions and methods becomes known. Therefore, it is realistic to believe that we will turn the tide on this epidemic. We will isolate and contain Big Tobacco, and we will see the decline of tobacco-caused disease and disability. We have the foundation to make tobacco-caused disease history, and the dawn of the next century a time that, once again, will see lung cancer a relative rarity.

There is not unanimity among those in the profession of public health concerning how Big Tobacco should be brought to its knees. Some public-health advocates believe it is possible to have a dialog with Big Tobacco; this implies that it is possible to negotiate morality with Big Tobacco, even though the industry has deliberately spurned such opportunities for many decades, while using their deceitful data to serve the ends of greed rather than health. These folks in public health, in general, are kind, compassionate, and truly believe that the tobacco industry will eventually come around. It is my belief that nothing is further from the truth. I firmly believe that the aforementioned tactic will never work, but with due diligence, the second tactic might work under carefully orchestrated circumstances.

There is another segment of the public-health profession that has quite a different attitude toward Big Tobacco and thinks that the only way it can be brought to its knees is to destroy it as it presently exists. In days of yore, when military combatants protected themselves with suits of armor, combat was at close quarters, and frequently hand-to-hand. You destroyed your enemy by finding the chink in his armor and through it you thrust your spear, shot your arrow, or guided your blade.

Isn't it time that public-health people, united, studied the armor of Big Tobacco carefully, found the chinks therein, and acted accordingly? The tobacco enemy is big, powerful, extraordinarily wealthy, and has learned to practice its deceitful ways over half a century, but the one thing it does not have on its side is righteousness. I do believe that, in the long run, Big Tobacco can be brought to its knees with the combined righteous outrage of the citizens of the world.

Of course, none of this will be easy, and we do not have all the answers to the questions before us. Never has so deadly an epidemic been so well protected by intertwined commercial and political interests. But never has so deadly a commercial empire faced so many assaults on so many fronts. I do believe in the ultimate triumph of right over wrong. The tobacco industry has been blatantly and reprehensibly wrong for much of the twentieth century, and is attempting to extend that record into the twenty-first, but it will not succeed. Now that the truth has leaked out through documents, through research, and through testimony in the courtroom, the clock cannot be turned back and its denials will not hold. Good people will not allow the lies to stand, nor the destructive course to be stayed. Good and dedicated people need to work together, from the voluntary workers in the charitable organizations, to the public-health leaders, and to many leading politicians, who, increasingly, are refusing to take tobacco money and are willing to stand up for public health. The challenge will not be easy, but there is a public-health path, and I predict that many will follow it.

As a doctor, and as the nation's surgeon general, I learned to be guided by scientific truth, even as I was motivated by basic principles of justice and service to humanity. My appraisal of the state of the science confirms that reducing tobacco-caused disease is an achievable goal, and that continued research can be the supportive companion of our public-health efforts. When the history of the twenty-first century is written, I believe it will be observed that its dawn was the beginning of the end for Big Tobacco and its diseases, and that by its end, lung cancer was once again relegated to the status of a rare disease.

Koop Institute, Dartmouth College   C. Everett Koop

References

Bachman, J. G., O'Malley, P. M., Schulenberg, J. E., Johnston, L. D., Bryant, A. L., and Merline, A. C. (2002). *The decline of substance abuse in young adulthood.* Lawrence Erlbaum Associates, Mahwah, New Jersey.

Balbach, E. D., and Glantz, S. A. (1998). Tobacco control advocates must demand high-quality media campaigns: The California experience. *Tobacco Control*, 7, 397–408.

Bialous, S. A., and Yach, D. (2001). Whose standard is it, anyway? How the tobacco industry determines the International Organization for Standardization (ISO) standards for tobacco and tobacco products. *Tobacco Control*, 10, 96–104.

Bradford, J. A., Harlan, W. R., and Hanmer, H. R. (1936). Nature of cigarette smoke. Technic of experimental smoking. *Industrial Engineering and Chemistry*, 28, 836–9.

Bullers, A. C. (2001). Living with AIDS—20 years later. *FDA Consumer*, November–December. Website: www.fda.gov/fdac/features/2001/601_aids.html

Centers for Disease Control and Prevention (1999a). Ten great public health achievements—United States, 1900–1999. *Morbidity and Mortality Weekly Report*, 48(12), 241–3.

Centers for Disease Control and Prevention (1999b). *Best Practices for Comprehensive Tobacco Control Programs*, August.

Centers for Disease Control and Prevention (2000). Declines in lung cancer rates—California, 1988–1997. *Morbidity and Mortality Weekly Report*, 49(47), 1066–9.

Chaloupka, F. J., Wakefield, M., and Czart, C. (2001). Taxing tobacco: The impact of tobacco taxes on cigarette smoking and other tobacco use. In: *Regulating Tobacco*, (ed. R. L. Raabin and S. D. Sugarman), pp. 39–71. Oxford University Press, New York.

Corti, C. (1931). *A history of smoking.* George G. Harrap & Co. Ltd., London.

Cromwell, J., Bartosch, W. J., Fiore, M. C., Hasselblad, V., and Baker, T. (1997). Cost-effectiveness of the clinical practice recommendations in the AHCPR guideline for smoking cessation. *Journal of the American Medical Association,* **278,** 1759–66.

Fairclough, G. (2000). Smoking's next battleground. *Wall Street Journal,* B1 and B4.

Farkas, A. J., Distefan, J. M., Choi, W. S., Gilpin, E. A., and Pierce, J. P. (1999). Does parental smoking cessation discourage adolescent smoking? *Preventive Medicine,* **28,** 213–18.

Food and Drug Law Institute (1998). Special Issue: Tobacco dependence: innovative regulatory approaches to reduce death and disease. *Food and Drug Law Journal,* **53**(Suppl.), 1–137.

Garrett, B. E., Rose, C. A., and Henningfield, J. E. (2001). Tobacco addiction and pharmacological interventions. *Expert Opinion in Pharmacotherapy,* **2,** 1545–55.

Givel, M. S., and Glantz, S. A. (2001). Tobacco lobby political influence on U.S. state legislatures in the 1990s. *Tobacco Control,* **10,** 124–34.

Henningfield, J. E., and Fagerstrom, K. O. (2001). Swedish match company, Swedish snus and public health: a harm reduction experiment in progress? *Tobacco Control,* **10,** 253–7.

Hirschhorn, N. (2000). Shameful science: four decades of the German tobacco industry's hidden research on smoking and health. *Tobacco Control,* **9,** 242–7.

Hirschhorn, N., Bialous, S. A., and Shatenstein, S. (2000). Phillip Morris' new scientific initiative: an analysis. *Tobacco Control,* **10,** 247–52.

Hurt, R. D., and Robertson, C. R. (1998). Prying open the door to the tobacco industry's secrets about nicotine: The Minnesota Tobacco Trial. *Journal of the American Medical Association,* **280,** 1173–81.

Kessler, D. A. (2000). *A question of intent: a great American battle with a deadly industry.* Public Affairs, New York.

Kessler, D. A., Witt, A. M., Barnett, P. S., Zeller, M. R., Natanblut, S. L., Wilkenfeld, J. P., *et al.* (1996). The Food and Drug Administration's regulation of tobacco products. *New England Journal of Medicine,* **335,** 988–94.

Kluger, R. (1996). *Ashes to ashes.* Alfred A. Knopf, New York.

Koop, C. E. (1998*a*). The tobacco scandal: Where is the outrage? *Tobacco Control,* **7,** 393–6.

Koop, C. E. (1998*b*). Don't forget the smokers. *Washington Post,* Sunday 8 March, C7.

National Cancer Institute (1996). *The FTC cigarette test method for determining tar, nicotine, and carbon monoxide yields of U.S. cigarettes: Report of the NCI expert committee. Smoking and tobacco control monograph No. 7.* US Department of Health and Human Services, National Institutes of Health, National Cancer Institute, Bethesda, Maryland.

National Cancer Institute (2001). *Risks associated with smoking cigarettes with low-machine measured yields of tar and nicotine, Smoking and Tobacco Control Monograph, No. 13.* U.S. Department of Health and Human Services, NIH Pub. No. 02–5074, National Institutes of Health, National Cancer Institute, Bethesda, Maryland.

Orey, M. (1999). *Assuming the risk: The mavericks, the lawyers, and the whistle-blowers who beat Big Tobacco.* Little, Brown and Co., New York.

Slade, J. (2000). Innovative nicotine delivery devices from tobacco companies. In: *Nicotine and public health* (ed. R. Ferrence, J. Slade, R. Room, and M. Pope), pp. 209–28. American Public Health Association, Washington.

Slade, J., Bero, L. A., Hanauer, P., Barnes, D. E., and Glantz, S. A. (1995). Nicotine and addiction. The Brown and Williamson documents. *Journal of the American Medical Association,* **274,** 225–33.

Stratton, K., Shetty, P., Wallace, R., and Bondurant, S. (ed.) (2000). *Clearing the smoke: Assessing the science base for tobacco harm reduction*. National Academy Press, Washington.

Taylor, P. (1984). *The smoke ring*. Pantheon Books, New York.

Thun, M. J. and Burns, D. M. (2001). Health impact of 'reduced yield' cigarettes: A critical assessment of the epidemiological evidence. *Tobacco Control*, **10**(Suppl.), i4–11.

US DHHS (US Department of Health and Human Services) (1988). *The health consequences of smoking: nicotine addiction. A report of the Surgeon General*. DHHS Publication No. (CDC) 88–8406, US Department of Health and Human Services, Washington.

US DHHS (US Department of Health and Human Services) (1989). *Reducing the health consequences of smoking: 25 years of progress. A report of the Surgeon General*. DHHS Publication No. (CDC) 89–8411, US Department of Health and Human Services, Washington.

Warner, K. E. (2000). The economics of tobacco: myths and realities. *Tobacco Control*, **9**, 78–89.

Warner, K. E. (2001). Reducing harm to smokers: methods, their effectiveness, and the role of policy. In: *Regulating tobacco* (ed. R. L. Raabin and S. D. Sugarman), pp. 111–42. Oxford University Press, New York.

Warner, K. E., Peck, C. C., Woosley, R. L., Henningfield, J. E. and Slade, J. (1998). Preface to Tobacco dependence: Innovative regulatory approaches to reduce death and disease. *Food and Drug Law Journal*, **53**(Suppl.), 1–16.

Wilkenfeld, J., Henningfield, J. E., Slade, J., Burns, D., and Pinney, J. M. (2000). It's time for a change: cigarette smokers deserve meaningful information about their cigarettes. *Journal of the National Cancer Institute*, **92**, 90–2.

White, L. C. (1988). *Merchants of death*. Beech Tree Books, New York.

World Bank (1999). *Curbing the epidemic: Governments and the economics of tobacco control*. World Bank, Washington.

World Health Organization (2001). *Advancing knowledge on regulating tobacco products*. World Health Organization, Geneva.

Wynder, E. L. (1997). Tobacco as a cause of cancer: Some reflections. *American Journal of Epidemiology*, **146**, 687–94.

Contents

Tobacco and health. Global burden

Tobacco and cancer

Contributors

Amanda Amos
Reader in Health Promotion
Division of Community Health
  Sciences
Medical School
University of Edinburgh
Teviot Place, Edinburgh
EH8 9AG, UK

Michael Bardo
Department of Pharmacology
University of Kentucky
Lexington, Kentucky, USA

Neal L. Benowitz
Professor and Chair
Division of Clinical Pharmacology
University of California
1001 Potrero Avenue Building 30,
Room 3316
San Francisco, CA 941110, USA

Paolo Boffetta
Unit of Analytical Epidemiology
International Agency for Research on
  Cancer
150 cours Albert-Thomas
69372 Lyon cedex 08, France

Ron Borland
Director
Cancer Control Research Institute
100 Drummond Street
Carlton Victoria 3053
Australia

Peter Boyle
Division of Epidemiology and
  Biostatistics
European Institute of Oncology
Via Ripamonti 435, 20141 Milan, Italy

David M. Burns
Professor of Family and Preventive
  Medicine
UCSD School of Medicine
1545 Hotel Circle So., Suite 310
San Diego, CA 92108, USA

Frank J. Chaloupka
Research Associate
Health Economics Program, NBER
850 West Jackson Boulevard
Suite 400, Chicago
IL 60607, USA

Marlo A. Corrao
Program Manager
Tobacco Control Country Profiles
Epidemiology and Surveillance Research
American Cancer Society (ACS)
1599 Clifton Road NE, Atlanta, GA,
30329-4251, USA

Jack Cuzick
Department of Mathematics, Statistics
  and Epidemiology
Cancer Research UK, London, UK

Claire Davey
Research Officer
Centre for Behavioural Research in Cancer,
The Cancer Council Victoria, Australia

Richard A. Daynard
Northeastern University School of Law
400 Huntington Avenue
Boston, MA 02115, USA

Mirjana V. Djordjevic
Bioanalytical Chemist
Behavioral Research Program
Tobacco Research Control Branch
National Cancer Institute
6130 Executive Boulevard, MSC 7337
Executive Plaza North
Bethesda,Maryland 20892, USA

Richard Doll
Clinical Trial Service Unit &
    Epidemiological Studies Unit
Harkness Building, Radcliffe
    Infirmary
Oxford OX2 6HE, UK

Linda Dwoskin
Department of Pharmacology
University of Kentucky
Lexington, Kentucky, USA

Jeff Fowles
Population and Environmental
    Health Group
Institute of Environmental Science and
    Research (ESR), Limited
PO Box 50-348, Porirua
New Zealand

Silvia Franceschi
International Agency for Research on
    Cancer
Unit of Field and Intervention Studies
150 Cours Albert Thomas
69372 Lyon Cedex 08, France

Bridgette E. Garrett
Office on Smoking and Health
National Center for Chronic Disease
    Prevention and Health Promotion

Centers for Disease Control and
    Prevention
Atlanta, GA 30341, USA

Graham G. Giles
Cancer Epidemiology Centre
The Cancer Council Victoria
1 Rathdowne Street, Carlton
Victoria 3053, Australia

Edward Giovannucci
Departments of Nutrition and
    Epidemiology, Harvard School of
    Public Health
Boston, MA 02115, USA

Nigel Gray
Senior Research Associate
Division of Epidemiology and
    Biostatistics
European Institute of Oncology
Milan, Italy

E. Groman
Associate Professor
Institute of Social Medicine
Medical University of Vienna
Rooseveitplatz 3
A 1090 Vienna, Austria

Prakash C. Gupta
Senior Research Scientist
Epidemiology Research Unit
Tata Institute of Fundamental Research
Homi Bhabha Road
Mumbai 400 005, India

Allan Hackshaw
Deputy Director
Cancer Research UK
    and University College London
Cancer Trials Centre
Stephenson House
158-160 North Gower Street
London NW1 2ND, UK

Stephen S. Hecht
University of Minnesota Cancer
  Center
Mayo Mail Code 806, 420 Delaware St SE
Minneapolis MN 55455, USA

Jane Henley
Dept. Epidemiology and Surveillance
  Research
American Cancer Society
1599 Clifton Road
Atlanta, GA 30329-4251, USA

Jack E. Henningfield
Department of Psychiatry and
Behavioral Sciences
Johns Hopkins University School of
  Medicine
Baltimore,Maryland, USA

David Hill
Anti-Cancer Council of Victoria
100 Drummond Street
Carlton Victoria 3053
Australia

Dietrich Hoffmann
American Health Foundation
1 Dana Road
Valhalla, New York, NY 10595, USA

Ilse Hoffmann
American Health Foundation
1 Dana Road
Valhalla, New York, NY 10595, USA

Crystal N. Holick
Department of Epidemiology,
Harvard School of Public Health,
677 Huntington Avenue, Boston,
MA 02115, USA

Yang Honghuan
Professor of Research Center of NCD &
BRFS and Dept. of Epidemiology
Chinese Academy of Medical Science

Peking Union Medical College
5# Dong Dan San Tiao
Beijing 100005, PR China

Konrad Jamrozik
Professor of Primary Care
  Epidemiology
Imperial College of Science, Technology
  and Medicine
Reynolds Building, St Dunstan's Road
London W6 8RP, UK

Prabhat Jha
Canada Research Chair in Health and
  Development,
Centre for Health Development
University of Toronto
30 Bond Street
Toronto, M5B 1W8, Canada

Elaine C. Johnstone
CRUK GPRG
Clinical Pharmacology Radcliffe
  Infirmary,
Oxford OX2 6HE, UK

C. Everett Koop
Koop Institute, Dartmouth College
Hanover, NH 03755-3862, USA

Lynn T. Kozlowski
Department of Biobehavioral Health
Penn State University
University Park, PA 16802, USA

Michael Kunze
Professor of Public Health
Institute of Social Medicine
Medical University of Vienna
Rooseveltplatz 3, A-1090
Vienna, Austria

Areti Lagiou
Department of Hygiene and
  Epidemiology, School of Medicine
University of Athens, Greece

Qing Lan
Division of Epidemiology and
  Genetics
National Cancer Institute, Bethesda
MD 20892, USA

Carlo La Vecchia
Istituto di Ricerche Farmacologiche
"Mario Negri", Via Eritrea 62
20157 Milano, Italy

Fabio Levi
Registres Vaudois et Neuchâtelois des
  Tumeurs
Institut universitaire de médecine
  sociale et préventive
Centre Hospitalier Universitaire Vaudois
Falaises 1, 1011 Lausanne, Switzerland

Alan D. Lopez
World Health Organization
Geneva, Switzerland

Albert B. Lowenfels
Professor of Surgery
New York Medical College
Munger Pavilion
Valhalla, NY, 10595, USA

Judith Mackay
Director
Asian Consultancy on Tobacco
  Control
Riftswood, 9th Milestone
DD 229, Lot 147, Clearwater Bay Road
Kowloon, Hong Kong

Patrick Maisonneuve
Director Clinical Epidemiology
  Program
Division of Epidemiology and
  Biostatistics
European Institute of Oncology
Via Ripamonti 435
20141 Milan, Italy

Michael Murphy
University of Oxford
Department of Paediatrics
Childhood Center Research Group
57 Woodstock Road
Oxford OX2 6HJ, UK

Eva Negri
Istituto di Ricerche Farmacologiche
"Mario Negri"
Via Eritrea 62, 20157 Milano, Italy

Richard J. O'Connor
Department of Biobehavioral Health
Penn State University
University Park, PA 16802, USA

Patricia H. Owens
Department of Epidemiology
  and Public Health
Yale School of Medicine
New Haven, CT, USA

Michael Pertschuk
Co-Director
Advocacy Institute
1629 K Street, NW
Washington DC 20005, USA

Richard Peto
Clinical Trial Service Unit &
  Epidemiological Studies Unit
  (CTSU)
Radcliffe Infirmary,
Oxford, OX2 6HE, UK

John P. Pierce
Sam M.Walton Professor of Cancer
  Research
Associate Director for Cancer Prevention
  and Control
UCSD Cancer Center
9500 Gilman Drive, La Jolla,
California, 92093-0645, USA

Cecily S. Ray
Project Assistant
Epidemiology Research
Tata Memorial Centre
Dr. E. Borges Marg, Parel
Mumbai, 400 012 India

Harvey A. Risch
Department of Epidemiology and
    Public Health,
Yale University School of Medicine,
60 College Street,
PO BOX 208034, New Haven,
CT 06520-8034, USA

Ruth Roemer
Adjunct Professor Emerita
School of Public Health
University of California
Los Angeles, CA 90095-1772, USA

Thomas E. Rohan
Department of Epidemiology and
    Social Medicine
Albert Einstein College of Medicine
1300 Morris Park Avenue, 13th Floor
Bronx, NY 10461, USA

Hana Ross
Associate Director
International Tobacco Evidence Network
850 West Jackson Boulevard, Suite 400
Chicago, Illinois 60607, USA

Yussuf Saloojee
Coordinator, International
Non Governmental Coalition Against
    Tobacco
P O Box 1242, Houghton 2041
South Africa

Jonathan M. Samet
Department of Epidemiology and the
Institute for Global Tobacco Control
Bloomberg School of Public Health

Johns Hopkins University
615 N.Wolfe St., Suite 6041
Baltimore, MD 21205, USA

Dennis Shusterman
Upper Airway Biology Laboratory
1301 So. 46th Street, Bldg. 112
Richmond, CA 94804, USA

Anne Szarewski
Clinical Consultant
Cancer Research
UK Centre for Epidemiology,
Mathematics and Statistics
Wolfson Institute of Preventive Medicine
London ECIM 6BQ, UK

Paul D. Terry
NIEHS, Epidemiology Branch,
PO BOX 12233,
MD A3-05, USA

Michael J. Thun
Dept. of Epidemiology and Surveillance
    Research
American Cancer Society
Atlanta, GA 30329-4251, USA

Dimitrios Trichopoulos
Department of Epidemiology
Harvard School of Public Health
677 Huntington Avenue
Boston, MA 02115, USA

Robert Walton
CRUK GPRG
Clinical Pharmacology
Radcliffe Infirmary
Oxford OX2 6HE, UK

Elisabete Weiderpass
International Agency for Research on
    Cancer
Unit of Field and Intervention Studies
150 Cours Albert Thomas
69372 Lyon Cedex 08, France

Patti White
Public Health Adviser
Health Development Agency
Trevelyan House
30 Great Peter Street
London SWIP 2HW, UK

John Wise
Laboratory of Environmental and
    Genetic Toxicology
Bioscience Research Institute
University of Southern Maine
Portland, ME, USA

David Zaridze
Director
Institute of Carcinogenesis
N.N. Blokhin Russian Cancer Research
    Center, 24 Kashirskoye Shosse
115478,Moscow, Russia

Witold Zato´nski
The Maria Sklodowska - Curie Cancer
    Center and Institute of Oncology

Department of Epidemiology and
    Cancer Prevention
Warsaw, Poland

Bing Zhang
Department of Epidemiology and
Biostatistics,McGill University
Montreal, Canada, H3A 1A2

Yawei Zhang
Department of Epidemiology
    and Public Health
Yale School of Medicine
New Haven, CT, USA

Tongzhang Zheng
Associate Professor
Department of Epidemiology
    and Public Health
Yale School of Medicine
New Haven, CT 06520–8034
USA

Abbreviations

AAA	Abdominal aortic aneurysm	DSM	Diagnostic and statistical manual
AC	Adenocarcinoma	DVT	Deep vein thrombosis
ACO	Adenocarcinoma of the esophages	EPHX1	Epoxide hydrolase
ACS	American Cancer Society	ETS	Environmental tobacco smoke
AMI	Acute myocardial infarction	EU	European Union
APA	The American Psychiatric Association	FCTC	Framework Convention of Tobacco Control
ARCI	Addiction Research Centre Inventory	FDA	Food and Drug Administration
		FISH	Fiter *in situ* hybridization
ASH	Action on Smoking and Health	FSH	Follicle-stimulating hormone
BAT	British America Tobacco	FTC	Federal Trade Commission
BMI	Body mass index	FTND	Fagerström test for tobacco dependence
BPDE	anti-7,8-dihydroxy-9,10-epoxy-7,8,9,10-tetrahydrobenzo[*a*]pyrene	FTQ	Fagerström tolerance questionnaire
BaA	benz(*a*)anthracene	FUBYAS	First usual brand adult smoker
BaP	benzo(*a*)pyrene	GC	Gas chromatography
CDC	Centers for Disease Control	GC-TEA	Gas chromatography with nitrosamine-selective detection
CDCP	Centers for Disease Control and Prevention		
		GC–MS	Gas chromatography–mass spectrometry
CHD	Cardiovascular disease		
CI	Confidence interval	GNP	Gross national product
CIN	Cervical intraepithelial neoplasia	GRAS	Generally regarded as safe
CO	Carbon monoxide	GSTs	Glutathione S-transferases
COLD	Chronic obstructive lung disease	GYTS	Global youth tobacco survey
COMT	Catechol *O*-methyl transferase	HEA	Health Education Authority
COPD	Chronic obstructive pulmonary disease	HIV	Human Immunodeficiency virus
		1-HOP	1-Hydroxypyrene
CORESTA	Centre De Cooperation Pour Les Recherches Scientifiques Relative Au Taba	HPB	4-Hydroxy-1-(3-pyridyl)-1-butanone
		HPLC	High-performance liquid chromatography
COX	cyclooxygenase		
CPP	Conditioned place preference	HPV	Human papillomavirus
CPS	Cancer Prevention Study	HRT	Hormone replacement therapy
CVD	Cardiovascular disease	HSC	Human smoking conditions
CeVD	Cerebrovascular disease	HSV	Herpes simplex virus
DATI	Dopaminergic transporter	Hb	hemoglobin
DBH	Dopamine β-hydroxylase	IARC	International Agency for Research on Cancer
DHEAS	Dehydroepiandrosterone		
DMBA	7,12-dimethylbenz[*a*]anthracene	IC	Intermittent claudication

ICD	The International Classification of Diseases	PAHs	polynuclear aromatic hydrocarbons
IHD	Ischaemic heart disease	PAR	Population attributable risk
ILO	International Labour Organization	PCR	Polymerase chain reaction
IPCS	International programme on clinical safety	PCSS	Perter community stroke study
		PE	Pulmonary embolism
ISO	International Standards Organization	PG	Propylene glycol
		POMS	Profile of mood state
LH	Luteinizing hormone	PREPS	Potential reduced-exposure products
LLETZ	Large Loop Excision of the Transformation Zone	PlCH	Primary intracerebral haemorrhage
MBG	Morphine-Benzedrine group scale		
MMP-1	Matrein metalloproteinase-1 gene	QTL	Quantitative trait loci
MRFIT	Multiple risk factor intervention trial	RR	relative risk
		RT	reconstituted tobacco
MS	Mainstream smoke OR mass spectrometry	s.c.	subcutaneous
		SAH	Subarachnoid haemorrhage
MSA	Master Settlement Agreement	SCC	Squamous cell carcinoma
nAChRs	nicotinic acetylcholine receptors	SHBG	Sex-hormone binding globulin
NATs	N-acetyl transferase	SIDS	sudden infant death syndrome
NHMRC	National Health and Medical Research Council	SS	sidestream smoke
		SSA	sub-Saharan Africa
NNAL	4-(methylnitrosamino)-1-(3-pyridyl)-1-butanol	TAMA	Tobacco Association of Malawi
NNK	4-(methylnitrosamino)-1-(3-pyridyl)-2-butanone	TEAM	Total exposure assessment methodology
NNN	N'-nitrosonornicotine	TIA	Transient cerebral ischaemic attach
NOx	nitrogen oxides (NO, NO$_2$, and N$_2$O)	TPLP	Tobacco products liability project
NPYR	N-Nitrosopyrrolidine	trans-anti-BaP-tetraol	r-7,t-8,9,c-10-tetrahydroxy-7,8,9,10-tetrahydrobenzo[a]pyrene
NRT	Nicotine replacement therapy		
NSDNC	Nocturnal sleep-disturbing nicotine craving	TSNAs	Tobacco-specific N-nitrosamines
OC	Oesophageal cancer	UICC	International union against cancer
OECD	Organization for Economic Collaboration and Development	VAS	Visual analog scale
		VNAs	Volatile N-nitrosamines
2-OEH1	2-hydroxyestrone	WCOO	World tobacco product
16α-OEH1	16-α-hydroxyestrone	WHO	World Health Organization
OTC	Over-the-counter	YAS	Young adult smoker
PAD	Peripheral arterial disease		
PAHs	Polycyclic aromatic hydrocarbons		

Introduction

The publication of this book is timely. Over fifty years after the establishment of the substantial evidence that tobacco caused a great deal of serious disease we are about halfway through the global tobacco epidemic. Declines in consumption and mortality in (some) developed countries are being matched by increases in the developing world, but it seems likely that global tobacco consumption may have reached its peak and be starting to decline.

The severity and social costs of this epidemic are defined clearly now and are covered in the relevant chapters. The reader will probably come to share the editors' wonder that such a controllable man-made epidemic, of complex diseases but simple aetiology, has resisted public health attempts to control it for so long.

The scientific understanding of tobacco, tobacco smoke, and the relationships with disease are now well understood and new factual knowledge in these fields is unlikely to change this greatly. The major toxic and carcinogenic components of smoke are known and the mechanisms by which these substances cause disease is becoming clear. Knowledge exists which, if applied, could reduce the disease-causing potential of tobacco. Although it is clear that no safe cigarette will ever be manufactured, less dangerous variants and other forms of nicotine delivery systems are either here or on the horizon, albeit not at the stage where they can compete with current tobacco products for the global nicotine addiction market.

The chemistry and physiology of nicotine are well documented and the addictive properties of the drug well delineated. The mechanism of addiction is reasonably well understood even though there remains much to learn about methods of treatment and whether there is a substantial genetic contribution towards susceptibility to addiction.

Why, then, is progress against tobacco use and mortality so slow?

The answer lies in the sections devoted to prevalence, policy, and tobacco-related behaviour. A further component of the answer lies in the societal failings of our political systems to deal with the corrupting effects of tobacco industry's behaviour, and to focus on preventing what is preventable about the factors contributing to initiation of the habit. Another failure is the lack of effort committed to stimulating cessation efforts which offer the greatest promise of early (i.e. within one to two decades) mortality decreases, associated with consideration of better sources of competitive nicotine delivery products.

This book sets out to cover the known levers which could be pulled to reduce tobacco's death toll. The information in it will be useful to any student or practitioner of medicine and other health sciences who will gain an understanding of the crucial relationships between science and policy, plus a realistic appraisal of the difficulties which must be overcome before policy is actually applied in the marketplace.

Only when the knowledge we have is used will this most devastating epidemic be brought to a close. This challenge is global.

The authors have been chosen with care for comprehensive knowledge of their topic and global reputation in their fields, and the editors express their thanks for the whole-hearted cooperation received.

Part 1

Tobacco: History

Chapter 1

Evolution of knowledge of the smoking epidemic

Richard Doll

Introduction

Tobacco was grown and used widely in North, Central and South America for two to three millennia before being introduced to Europe at the end of the fifteenth century. Its use was promoted initially for medicinal purposes, for the treatment of a variety of conditions from cough, asthma, and headaches to intestinal worms, open wounds, and malignant tumours, when it was prescribed to be chewed, taken nasally as a powder, or applied locally.

The use of tobacco for pleasure was discouraged by Church and State and it was not until the end of the sixteenth century that it came to be smoked widely in Europe, at first in pipes in Britain, where it was popularized by Sir Walter Raleigh. Here it became so common that by 1614 there are estimated to have been some 7000 retail outlets in London alone (Laufer 1924). Attempts to ban its use for recreational purposes were made in Austria, Germany, Russia, Switzerland, Turkey, India, and Japan, but prohibition was invariably flouted and control by taxation came to be preferred. This eventually proved to be such an important source of revenue that, in 1851, Cardinal Antonelli, Secretary to the Papal States, ordered that the dissemination of anti-tobacco literature was to be punished by imprisonment (Corti 1931).

Gradually, the way in which tobacco was most commonly used changed. By the end of the seventeenth century, its use as nasal snuff had spread from France, largely replacing pipe smoking. This practice remained common until a century later, when it, in turn, began to be replaced by the smoking of cigars, which had long been smoked in a primitive form in Spain and Portugal. By then cigarettes were already being made in South America and their use had spread to Spain, but it was not until after the Crimean War that they began to be at all widely adopted. They were made fashionable in Britain by officers returning from the Crimea, and by the end of the nineteenth century cigarettes had begun to replace cigars. Consumption in this form increased rapidly during the First World War, and by the end of the Second World War cigarettes had largely replaced all other tobacco products in most developed countries.

By this time, smoking had become so much the norm for men that, in Britain, some 80 per cent were regular smokers and some doctors even offered a cigarette to patients who came to consult them, to put them at their ease. Women began to smoke in large numbers much later, except in New Zealand, where, by the end of the nineteenth century, Maori women were commonly smoking pipes. Then, in the 1920s, women began to smoke cigarettes, at first in the USA and then in Britain, where the practice gained popularity during the Second World War, as an increasing proportion of women began to work outside the home and have an independent income. However, in many other developed countries, women have begun to smoke in large numbers only in the past few decades.

The reason for the swing to cigarettes

The important change in the use of tobacco, for its impact on health, was the swing to cigarettes. This was brought about by two industrial developments. The first was a new method of curing tobacco. With the old method, the smoke that had come from pipes and cigars was alkaline, irritating, and difficult to inhale. However, the nicotine in it was predominantly in the form of a free base which could be absorbed across the oral and pharyngeal mucosa. Blood levels of nicotine could consequently be high and addiction was readily produced; but only small amounts of other constituents were absorbed. The new method, called flue-curing, was introduced in North Carolina in the mid-nineteenth century (Tilley 1948). It exposed the leaf to high temperatures and increased its sugar content, which caused the pH of the smoke to be acid. In this environment, the nicotine was predominantly in the form of salts and was dissolved in smoke droplets, which were less irritating than the free base and easier to inhale. With each inhalation there was a rapid rise in the level of nicotine in the blood, which was perceived in the brain, and was particularly satisfying to the addict, but other constituents of the smoke were also absorbed and distributed throughout the body.

The second development was mechanical: namely, the introduction of cigarette-making machines. One was patented in 1880, and was eventually adapted by the Duke family to work so efficiently that 120 000 cigarettes of good quality could be produced every 10 hours by one machine, the equivalent of the production of about 100 unassisted workers. As a result, the price fell and a mass market became feasible.

The impact of tobacco on health

Until cigarette smoking became common, very little evidence of harmful effects was detected—for the good reason that relatively little harm was probably caused. One harmful effect, which was first suggested more than 200 years ago (Sömmering 1795), was the production of cancer of the lip. In the course of the nineteenth century, on the basis of clinical series in France (Bouisson 1859), Germany (Virchow 1863–7), and the United Kingdom (Anon 1890), additional consequences were linked to smoking, such as the production of cancers of the tongue and other parts of the mouth. These findings, are now simply explained because we know that these cancers can be produced at least as easily by the smoking of pipes and cigars as by the smoking of cigarettes.

However, little attention was paid to these effects by clinicians, who characterized cancer of the lip as the result of smoking clay pipes, which was a custom of agricultural workers. When, as a medical student in the mid-1930s, I asked the senior surgeon at my teaching hospital whether he thought pipe smoking or syphilis was a cause of cancer of the tongue, he replied that he didn't know, but that the wise man should certainly avoid the combination of the two.

However, one disease was unequivocally attributed to tobacco, and taught as being so: namely, tobacco amblyopia. It was described by Beer in 1817, and occurred in heavy pipe-smokers in combination with malnutrition. It was probably caused by the cyanide in smoke not being detoxified because of a deficiency of vitamin B_{12} (Heaton *et al.* 1958). The disease is no longer seen, at least in developed countries.

The early impact of cigarette smoking

With the advent of the twentieth century, several new diseases began to be associated with smoking: first, intermittent claudication, which was described by Erb in 1904 and then, in 1908, a rare form of peripheral vascular disease affecting relatively young people, which Buerger called thrombo-angiitis obliterans, and which has subsequently been named after him. It is now recognized that both diseases were made much more common by smoking, with the latter almost limited to smokers, but neither reached the epidemic proportions that two other, relatively new, diseases achieved in the next few decades.

One of these was coronary thrombosis or, as we would now prefer to say, myocardial infarction. It was first described at autopsy in 1876 (Hammer 1878), although it had certainly occurred earlier, and it was not diagnosed in life until 1910, when it was diagnosed by Herrick (1912) in Chicago. Subsequently it was reported progressively more often every year for four or five decades. As early as 1920, Hoffman, an American statistician, linked the increase in coronary thrombosis with the increasing consumption of cigarettes. Several clinical studies of the relationship between the disease and smoking were published, but the findings were confused, and no substantial evidence was obtained until 1940, when English *et al.* reported finding an association in the records of the Mayo Clinic. Their findings led them to conclude that the smoking of tobacco probably had 'a more profound effect on younger individuals owing to the existence of relatively normal cardiovascular systems, influencing perhaps the earlier development of coronary disease'. However, they eschewed reference to causation, because the subject would be controversial, adding perceptively that 'Physicians are not yet ready to agree on this important subject'. That cigarette smoking played a part in the increasing incidence of the disease was eventually clearly demonstrated. The association was not close enough for it to have been the only cause of the increase, or even probably the most important, and, unlike the other disease that burst into medical prominence in the first half of the twentieth century, the full explanation of its rapid increase is still a matter for debate (Doll 1987).

The other disease was, of course, cancer of the lung. Until then it had been thought to be exceptionally rare. A small cluster of cases in tobacco workers in Leipzig had led Rottmann to suggest, in 1898, that the disease might be caused by the inhalation of tobacco dust. The first suggestion that it might be due to smoking was not made until 14 years later, by Adler (1912), who noted that, although the disease was still rare, it appeared to have become somewhat less so in the recent past. Many people were subsequently struck by the parallel increase in the consumption of cigarettes and the incidence of the disease and by the frequency with which patients with lung cancer described themselves as heavy smokers, several even ventured to suggest that the two were related (Tylecote 1927; Lickint 1929; Hoffman 1931; Arkin and Wagner 1936; Fleckseder 1936; Ochsner and de Bakey 1941). However, few believed it. Koch's postulates, which were taught as criteria for determining causality, could not be satisfied, as one required the agent to be present in every case of the disease and cases certainly occurred in non-smokers. Moreover, pathologists generally failed to produce cancer experimentally by the application of tobacco tar to the skin of animals. Only Roffo (1931), in Argentina, succeeded in doing so, and his results were discounted in the United Kingdom and the United States because he had produced the tar by burning the tobacco at unrealistically high temperatures. However, diagnostic methods had certainly improved, notably the widespread use of radiology and bronchoscopy, and the idea that the increase in the incidence of the disease was an artefact of improved diagnosis came to be widely believed.

Three case-control studies that were carried out in Germany and The Netherlands between 1939 and 1948 should have focused attention on smoking, as all three suggested, albeit on rather inadequate grounds (Doll 2001), that smoking was a possible cause of lung cancer. However, the war distracted attention from the German literature (Müller 1939; Schairer and Schöniger 1943), and the Dutch paper (Wassink 1948) was published in Dutch and not noticed widely for several years. Outside Germany, smoking was still commonly regarded as having only minor effects as late as 1950, and inside Germany, where chronic nicotine poisoning had been thought to produce effects in nearly every system, the reaction against the Nazis brought with it a reaction against their antagonism to tobacco—for propaganda against the use of tobacco had been a major plank in the public health policy of the Nazi government (on the grounds that it damaged the national germ plasm and that addiction to it detracted from obedience to the Führer) (Proctor 1999).

The 1950 watershed

Then in 1950, five case-control studies were published in the United Kingdom (Doll and Hill 1950) and the United States (Levin *et al.* 1950; Mills *et al.* 1950; Schrek *et al.* 1950; Wynder and Graham 1950), with much larger numbers of cases and, in some, so refined a technique, that Bradford Hill and I were able to conclude that 'cigarette smoking is a factor, and an important factor, in the production of carcinoma of the lung' (Doll and Hill 1950). The results were given wide publicity, but the conclusion was not widely believed. Medical scientists had as yet to appreciate the power of epidemiology in unravelling the aetiology of non-infectious disease. Statisticians had failed to recognize the implication of such high relative risks as those estimated from the findings, and argued that the association with smoking might be due to confounding with some other factor that was the true cause of the disease. Fisher (1957), of international statistical fame, thought that the lack of an association with inhaling in our first report was a major difficulty, and preferred the idea that some genetic factor caused both the disease and the individual to want to smoke, while Berkson (1955), a leading medical statistician at the Mayo Clinic, argued that the cases and the controls, not being random samples of the population, might have been subject to selection bias. The tobacco industry was consequently able to present the findings as controversial. However, Scientific curiosity had been aroused, a great deal of research was initiated, and government departments were forced to consider the implications of the findings for the practice of public health.

Acceptance of evidence of harm

Further evidence was clearly needed if the scientific world was to accept that cigarette smoking was the cause of the lung cancer epidemic, which was, by then, spreading in all developed countries, and this was rapidly produced. Cohort studies were begun in which people who had provided information about their smoking habits were followed to see the extent to which their habits predicted mortality. One such study obtained information from 34 000 male doctors in the United Kingdom, and showed, within 3 years, that mortality from lung cancer was proportional to the amount smoked—as predicted by the case-control studies—and suggested that there might also be a similar, although less marked, relationship with coronary thrombosis (Doll and Hill 1954). Another study, based on larger numbers in the United States, gave similar results, and found that, under 65 years of age, the mortality from coronary thrombosis among men who smoked 20 or more cigarettes a day was twice that of non-smokers (Hammond and Horn 1954). In the larger study in the United States, the results were much clearer for coronary heart disease than for lung cancer. This was because the switch to cigarette smoking occurred on a mass scale later in North America than it did in the United Kingdom, and it takes several decades of smoking before the risk of cancer is high, whereas less time is required to produce a major risk of coronary disease.

Meanwhile, laboratory workers had shown that tobacco tar, appropriately produced, contained polycyclic aromatic hydrocarbons that were known to be carcinogenic (Cooper and Lindsay 1955), and that the tar could cause cancer on the skin of mice if applied regularly for months on end (Wynder et al. 1953; Doll 1998). As a consequence of these results, in 1957 the Medical Research Council was able to advise the British government that cigarette smoking was the cause of the increased incidence of lung cancer. Similar conclusions were reached, over the next 3 years, by a study group on Smoking and Health (1957) appointed jointly by the US National Cancer and Heart Institute and the US Public Health Service (Burney 1959), and by specially appointed committees in The Netherlands and Sweden, and the World Health Organization (see Doll 1998).

Impact on total mortality

A few years later, when the Royal College of Physicians (1962), in England, and the Surgeon General (1964), in the United States, issued reports on smoking, it had become clear that its total impact was greater than had at first been conceived, and that the incidence of more diseases might be affected. With the passage of time, more and more diseases were found that were linked in some way to smoking. The total number now believed to be caused in part by smoking is at least 35, 22 of which can be recognized in the cohort study of British doctors and in the massive study of a million men and women subsequently undertaken by the American Cancer Society (Table 1.1). Other harmful effects caused in part by smoking are listed in Table 1.2. These are mostly relatively rare and less lethal, and evidence relating to them has often had to be obtained from case-control studies or surveys, or, occasionally, from cohort studies in which special enquiries have been made about the condition of interest. That so many conditions are affected by smoking should not be surprising, as tobacco smoke contains some 4000 different chemicals and many of the diseases are caused by similar mechanisms.

Even the 35 smoking-related diseases mentioned above do not complete the list, because a few others that are primarily associated with smoking through confounding are also probably caused by it in part, including cancer of the liver (Doll 1996) and death from conflagration—two doctors in our study, for example, set fire to themselves by smoking in bed.

Of course, confounding does account for some of the excess mortality from all causes of death. However, detailed investigation has shown that the amount is relatively small and, in some populations, may not exist at all, for confounding can operate in both directions, and certainly does in elderly populations in countries in which there is a high mortality from ischaemic heart disease. Here, confounding with alcohol both causes the excess for cirrhosis of the liver and reduces the mortality from ischaemic heart disease.

It now appears that the excess mortality from smoking is greater than was long suspected, for it has increased with time, as the smoking epidemic has matured and old people have come to be smoking cigarettes throughout their smoking lives. This is shown by the data in Table 1.3 from both the British doctors' study, which has continued for over 40 years with periodic updates on changes in smoking habit, and the studies of the American public carried out by the American Cancer Society over two different periods. Regular cigarette smoking since youth is now seen to double mortality,

Table 1.1 Principal diseases caused in part by smoking

Disease	Ratio of mortality rates in continuing cigarette smokers and lifelong non-smokers		
	British doctors 1951–91[a]	US population 1984–91[b]	
	Men	Men	Women
Cancers of mouth, pharynx, and larynx	24.0	11.4	6.9
Cancers of the oesophagus	7.5	5.6	9.8
Cancers of the lung	14.9	23.9	14.0
Cancers of the pancreas	2.2	2.0	2.3
Cancers of the bladder	2.3	3.9	1.8
Ischaemic heart disease	1.6	1.9	2.0
Hypertension	1.4	2.4	2.6
Myocardial degeneration	2.0		
Pulmonary heart disease	∞[c]	2.1	2.1
Other heart disease	–		
Aortic aneurysm	4.1	6.3	8.2
Peripheral vascular disease	–	9.7	5.7
Arteriosclerosis	1.8	2.7	3.0
Cerebrovascular disease	1.5	1.9	2.2
Chronic bronchitis and emphysema	12.7	17.6	16.2
Pulmonary tuberculosis	2.8	–	–
Asthma[d]	2.2	1.3	1.4
Pneumonia	1.9	2.5	1.7
Other respiratory disease	1.6		
Peptic ulcer	3.0	4.6	4.0
All causes	1.8	2.5	2.1

[a] Doll et al. (1994).

[b] C. Heath Jr and M. Thun, personal communication.

[c] No death was reported in British doctors who were lifelong non-smokers.

[d] Continuing cigarette smokers and ex-cigarette smokers combined, as asthma may cause smokers to stop smoking.

on average, throughout middle and old age, so that 1 in 4 smokers die prematurely as a result of their habit in middle age (now defined as from 35 to 74 years) and 1 in 4 die similarly in old age.

The epidemic that the world is now facing is not, in truth, a smoking epidemic so much as a cigarette epidemic, for the small effect of smoking pipes and cigars that gave rise to so little concern in the nineteenth century has continued to be relatively small.

Table 1.2 Other conditions caused in part by smoking

Cancer of lip	Crohn's disease
Cancer of nose	Osteoporosis
Cancer of stomach	Periodontitis
Cancer of kidney pelvis	Tobacco amblyopia
Cancer of kidney body	Age-related macular degeneration
Myeloid leukaemia	Reduced fecundity
Reduced growth of fetus	

Table 1.3 Cigarette smokers compared with lifelong non-smokers: change in all-cause mortality in men

British doctors[a]	Period	1951–71	1971–91
	Relative risk	1.6	2.1
American Public[b]	Period	1959–65	1982–86
	Relative risk	1.8	2.3

[a] Doll et al. (1994)

[b] Surgeon General (1989).

For example, in our study of British doctors, the mortality of pipe and cigar smokers who had never smoked cigarettes was only 9 per cent greater than that of lifelong non-smokers (Doll and Peto 1976). This represents a material increase in all-cause mortality, certainly, but one qualitatively different from that of cigarette smoking, and it is only the effect of the latter that I shall consider further.

The spread of the epidemic

Two things about the epidemic are clear. First, the number of manufactured cigarettes consumed has increased astronomically, from near zero in 1880 to some 5700 billion a year worldwide in the mid-1990s, since when there has been a very slight decrease (Proctor 2001). Secondly, the increase in cigarette smoking occurred at different rates, at different periods, in each sex, in different countries. Even within developed countries, to which the increase was initially confined, the differences were substantial.

Developed countries

Detailed consumption rates of different tobacco products in 22 developed countries have been brought together by Nicolaides-Bouman et al. (1993) from the time of the earliest record to 1985. The three highest and three lowest rates of consumption of manufactured cigarettes by adults, averaged over the decade 1920–29, are shown in Table 1.4, together with the corresponding age-standardized mortality rates for lung

Table 1.4 Manufactured cigarette consumption in 1920s and lung cancer mortality in 1955

Country	Mean number of cigarettes smoked daily by adults, 1920–29	Lung cancer
Finland	3.6	89
Greece	3.4	57
UK	3.0	109
Sweden	0.8	16
Norway	0.7	11
Portugal	<0.7	11

cancer in 1955, some 30 years later, to allow for a sufficiently long period of exposure to produce an appreciable effect. That lung cancer was more common when manufactured cigarettes were taken up early is clear, but the correlation is not close. This is hardly surprising, because many factors affect the incidence of the disease other than the one examined in Table 1.4: the changes in cigarette consumption over the intervening period, the distribution of consumption by sex and age, the characteristics of the cigarettes, the way they are smoked, the amount of tobacco consumed in hand-rolled cigarettes and in other tobacco products, which are not without hazard, and, it appears, the local diet, which may modify the quantitative effect of a given number of cigarettes (see Darby *et al.* 2001).

In order to determine the extent of the proportion of the total threat to mortality caused by smoking, a method for estimating the mortality attributable to cigarette smoking that is not dependent on statistics for tobacco consumption was suggested by Peto *et al.* (1992). It is worth describing in some detail as so much depends on it. In brief, Peto *et al.* used the excess mortality from lung cancer over that observed in non-smokers in the American Cancer Society's massive second cancer prevention study, as an indication of the extent to which the population had been exposed to tobacco products in the past. This is justified for developed countries because, whenever data are available, the mortality from lung cancer in lifelong non-smokers has been found to be low, approximately the same in each country, and not to have changed over time. However, the same method cannot be used directly to estimate the effects of smoking on mortality from other diseases, as the rates for other diseases in non-smokers vary considerably, and smoking interacts with other causes in a complex way that is nearer multiplicative than additive. Peto *et al.* (1992) consequently divided other causes into eight broad categories (Table 1.5) and used the second cancer prevention study's data as an indication of the *proportional* excess mortality for each broad cause group to be associated with the corresponding *absolute* excess of lung cancer in each 5-year age group. However, to be on the safe side (that is, to under-, rather than to overestimate the mortality attributable to smoking) they excluded all deaths in two categories (cirrhosis and non-medical causes)

Table 1.5 Categories of disease used by Peto *et al.* (1992)

Lung cancer	
Upper aerodigestive cancers	Vascular diseases
Other cancers	Cirrhosis of liver
Chronic obstructive pulmonary disease	Other medical causes
Other respiratory diseases	Non-medical causes

Table 1.6 Trends in per cent mortality attributed to smoking: selected populations

Sex	Country	Year				
		1955	1965	1975	1985	1995
M	UK	27	35	36	34	27
M	USA	14	20	26	28	29
M	OECD	12	19	23	25	25
M	Former socialist	15	22	24	29	32
F	UK	3.0	5.9	9.8	14	17
F	USA	0.3	2.0	7.1	14	22
F	OECD	0.5	1.7	3.9	7.4	12
F	Former socialist	1.3	2.0	3.0	3.7	5.2

and all deaths under 35 years of age in all categories, even though some deaths in both groups were attributable to smoking, and then *halved* the estimated excess proportion for each of the remaining six categories. This last, it should be noted, is not as extreme as halving the number of excess deaths, for it has little effect on the number of deaths attributable to tobacco when the relative risks are high; reducing it, for example, by only 10 per cent if the relative risk is ninefold.

The trends in the proportions of mortality consequently attributed to smoking between 1955 and 1995 are shown in Table 1.6 (the data for 1995 were projected from the trend between 1980 and 1985, but have been found to be generally reliable). They are given separately for men and women, and for the United Kingdom, the United States, and all developed countries, the latter being divided into the Organization for Economic Collaboration and Development (OECD) countries, and former socialist economies. The highest percentage of mortality attributed to smoking was in men in the United Kingdom in 1975; since when the proportion has dropped by a quarter and is now less than that in the United States. The OECD countries, as a group, had slightly lower proportions than the United States and the proportion stabilized after 1985. In the former socialist economy countries, the percentage has increased progressively, and in 1995 was approaching the maximum previously recorded in the United Kingdom. In women the proportions have generally been much lower, but in 1995 were approaching the figures for men, in both the United Kingdom and, most notably, the United States of America. In all four categories the increase in female mortality has been progressive and in the United States and many parts of the United Kingdom lung cancer has now displaced cancer of the breast from its position as the leading cause of death from cancer in women.

Developing countries

For the developing countries there are few quantitative data, apart from those for China, where cigarette consumption per adult increased from about 1 per day in 1952, to 10 per day in 1992. Two studies are particularly revealing. One, a case-control study of a million deaths in men and women in 98 parts of China, both urban and rural, obtained information about the deceased persons' smoking habits and compared those of men and women who died of cancer, respiratory disease, and vascular disease with those of men and women who died of other diseases, postulated not to be due to smoking (Liu *et al.* 1998). The other, a cohort study of a quarter of a million men aged over 40, in 45 selected representative areas, provided mortality rates by smoking habit over a 5–6-year period (Niu *et al.* 1998). Both led to the conclusion that about 12 per cent of deaths in middle-aged and elderly men were attributable to smoking, while the case-control study provided the much lower figure, of 2–3 per cent, in women, few of whom, outside the big towns, had been smoking for long. However, the pattern of mortality was different from that in the developed world, with a much smaller proportion of attributable deaths due to ischaemic heart disease and lung cancer, and a greater proportion due to stroke, chronic obstructive pulmonary disease, and cancers of the oesophagus, stomach, and liver.

Future expectations

What then of the future? For China it is relatively easy to predict, for the prevalence of smoking and attributable mortality are reproducing what was observed in the United States 40 years previously, where cigarette consumption per adult had been 1 per day in 1910 and 10 per day in 1950, and the risk of premature death in smokers, attributable to smoking, increased from 1 in 4 in the early 1960s, to 1 in 2 in the 1980s. For Chinese men who began smoking before they were 20 years old, after the revolution in 1949, the risk is already 1 in 4 and must be expected to become 1 in 2 in 20 years time. Two-thirds of men now become smokers before 25 years of age and, if present patterns continue, about 100 million of the 300 million Chinese males now under 30 years of age will be killed by tobacco. However, the number of female deaths attributable to smoking in the future may be relatively small, as, contrary to what has happened in the West, progressively fewer women have been starting to smoke, and the prevalence for those born between 1950 and 1964 is now only 1–2 per cent.

For the developing world as a whole, Peto and Lopez (1990) estimated that, in the 1990s, there were already likely to have been 1 million deaths per year attributable to tobacco, against approximately 2 million in the developed world. However, in many parts, the prevalence of smoking in men, like that in China, already exceeds 50 per cent, although, again, the female prevalence is relatively low. We also know that in India, for example, where tuberculosis has become a major cause of death, the impact of smoking on that disease is to increase the incidence of clinical cases and double the fatality, as it was in the developed world 40 years ago. However, in many countries there is still major mortality from causes unrelated to tobacco, such as other infectious diseases and trauma, much greater than in the developed world, so that the *proportion* of persistent smokers eventually killed by the habit may be a third, rather than the half suggested by the North American, British, and, indeed, also the Chinese, data. Therefore, perhaps only about 250 million of the 800 million young people who, according to current patterns, will be smokers in early adult life will be killed by the habit. The majority of the deaths will not, of course, occur for some decades, when smoking has been prolonged and the chronic diseases of middle age become common; but in two or three decades the total toll must be expected to be about 10 million deaths a year worldwide, of which some 7 million will be in what are now the developing countries (Peto *et al.* 1996).

The benefit of stopping smoking

If the prevalence of smoking stays as it is, the death toll of tobacco in the first half of the twenty-first century will be tremendous, but it does not have to be. For the prevalence can be reduced and with it, some years later, the mortality from lung cancer and from all other tobacco-related diseases. This is illustrated for lung cancer by the findings in our recent study of the disease in Devon and Cornwall (Peto *et al.* 2000) and in our study of British doctors, in which we found that survival was improved whatever the age at which smoking was stopped. With the numbers we had, survival was indistinguishable from that of lifelong non-smokers when smoking was stopped under 35 years of age (corresponding, in our study, to less than 10 years continued smoking), and longer than that of continuing smokers even if smoking was stopped only after 65 years of age (Doll *et al.* 1994).

I believe, therefore, that with adequate education of the public, for which both doctors and the media must take responsibility, and with the support of government in increasing taxation on tobacco and prohibiting the promotion of the habit, we may see the current predictions materially reduced.

Acknowledgement

I am grateful to the Royal College of Physicians of Edinburgh for permission to reproduce here, under a new title with minor changes and additions, the text of a lecture I gave at the College in October 2001, which has been published in the College Proceedings (*Journal of the Royal College of Physicians of Edinburgh* 2002, **32**, 24–30).

References

Adler, I. (1912). *Primary malignant growths of the lung and bronchi.* Longmans Green and Co., London.

Anon (1890). Cancer and smoking. *British Medical Journal,* 1, 748.

Arkin, A. and Wagner, D. H. (1936). Primary carcinoma of the lung. *Journal of the American Medical Association,* 106, 587–91.

Beer, G. J. (1817). *Lehre von den Augenkrankheiten,* Vol. II, Vienna. (Cited by Duke-Elder, W. S. D. *Textbook of Ophthalmology,* Vol. 3, p. 3009. Henry Kimpton, London.)

Bouisson, E. F. (1859). Du cancer buccal chez les fumeurs. *Montpelier Medical Journal,* 2, 539–99 and 3, 19–41.

Buerger, L. (1908). Thrombo-angiitis obliterans: a study of the vascular lesions leading to presenile spontaneous gangrene. *American Journal of the Medical Sciences,* 136, 567–80.

Cooper, R. L. and Lindsay, A. J. (1955). 3-4 Benzpyrene and other polycyclic hydrocarbons in cigarette smoke. *British Journal of Cancer,* 9, 442–4.

Darby, S., Whitley, E., Doll, R., Key, T., and Silcocks, P. (2001). Diet, smoking and lung cancer: a case-control study of 1000 cases and 1500 controls in South-West England. *British Journal of Cancer,* 84, 728–35.

Doll, R. (1987). Major epidemics of the twentieth century: from coronary thrombosis to AIDS. *Journal of the Royal Statistical Society, Series A,* 150, 373–95.

Doll, R. (1996). Cancers weakly related to smoking. *British Medical Bulletin,* 52, 35–49.

Doll, R. (1998). Uncovering the effects of smoking: historical perspective. *Statistical Methods in Medical Research,* 7, 87–117.

Doll, R. (2001). Commentary: lung cancer and tobacco consumption. *Intertnational Journal of Epidemiology,* 30, 30–1.

Doll, R. and Hill, A. B. (1950). Smoking and carcinoma of the lung. Preliminary report. *British Medical Journal,* 2, 739–48.

Doll, R. and Hill, A. B. (1954). The mortality of doctors in relation to their smoking habits. A preliminary report. *British Medical Journal,* 1, 1451–5.

Doll, R. and Peto, R. (1976). Mortality in relation to smoking: 20 years' observations on male British doctors. *British Medical Journal,* 2, 1525–36.

Doll, R., Peto, R., Hall, E., Wheatley, K., and Gray, R. (1994). Mortality in relation to consumption of alcohol: 13 years' observations on male British doctors. *British Medical Journal,* 309, 911–18.

English, J. P., Willius, F. A., and Berkson, J. (1940). Tobacco and coronary disease. *Journal of the American Medical Association,* 115, 1327–9.

Erb, W. (1904). Ueber dysbasia angiosclerotica ('intermittierendes Hinken'). *Münchener med Woch,* 51, 905–8.

Fleckseder, R. (1936). Ueber den Bronchialkrebs und einiger seiner Entstehungsbedigungen. *Münchener medizin Wochenschr,* 83, 1585–8.

Hammer, A. (1878). Ein fall von thrombotischen Verschlusse einer des Kranzarterien des Herzens. *Wein med Wchnschr,* 28, 97–102.

Hammond, E. C. and Horn, D. (1954). The relationship between human smoking habits and death rates: a follow-up study of 187,766 men. *Journal of the American Medical Association,* 155, 1316–28.

Heaton, J. M., McCormick, A. J. A., and Freeman, A. G. (1958). Tobacco amblyopia. A clinical manifestation of vitamin B_{12} deficiency. *Lancet,* 2, 286–90.

Herrick, J. B. (1912). Clinical features of sudden obstruction of the coronary arteries. *Journal of the American Medical Association,* 59, 2015–20.

Hoffman, F. L. (1920). Recent statistics of heart disease with special reference to its increasing incidence. *Journal of the American Medical Association,* 74, 1364–71.

Hoffman, F. L. (1931). Cancer and smoking habits. *Annals of Surgery*, 50–67.

Laufer, B. (1924). *Introduction of tobacco into Europe*. Field Museum of Natural History, Chicago.

Lickint, F. (1929). Tabak und Tabakrauch als ätiologischer Faktor des Carcinoms. *Zeitschrift für Krebsforsch*, **30**, 349–365

Liu, B. Q., Peto, R., Chen, Z. M., Boreham, J., Wu, Y. P., Li, J. Y., *et al.* (1998). Emerging hazards in China: proportional mortality studies of one million deaths. *British Medical Journal*, **317**, 1411–22.

Medical Research Council (1957). Tobacco smoking and cancer of the lung. *British Medical Journal*, **1**, 1523.

Müller, F. H. (1939). Tabakmissbrauch und lungencarcinoma. *Zeitschrift für Krebsforsch*, **49**, 57–85.

Nicolaides-Bouman, A., Wald, N., Forey, B., and Lee, P. (1993) *International smoking statistics*. Oxford University Press, Oxford.

Niu, S.-R., Yang, G.-H., Chen, Z.-M., Wang, J.-L., Wang, G.-H., He, X.-Z., *et al.* (1998). Emerging tobacco hazards in China: 2. Early mortality results from a prospective study. *British Medical Journal*, **317**, 1423–4.

Ochsner, A. and De Bakey, M. (1941). Carcinoma of the lung. *Archives of Surgery*, **42**, 209–58.

Peto, R. and Lopez, A. D. (1990). Worldwide mortality from current smoking patterns: WHO consultative group on statistical aspects of tobacco-related mortality. In: *Tobacco and health 1990: The global war*, (ed. B. Durston and K. Jamrozik). Proceedings of the 7th World Conference on Tobacco and Health, April, Perth, Western Australia.

Peto, R., Lopez, A., Boreham, J., Thun, M., and Heath, C. (1992). Mortality from tobacco in developed countries: indirect estimation from national vital statistics. *Lancet*, **339**, 1268–78.

Peto, R., Darby, S., Deo, H., Silcocks, P., Whitley, E., and Doll, R. (2000). Smoking, smoking cessation and lung cancer in the UK since 1950: combination of national statistics with two case-control studies. *British Medical Journal*, **321**, 323–9.

Proctor, R. N. (1999). *The Nazi war on cancer*. Princeton University Press, Princeton.

Proctor, R. N. (2001). Tobacco and the global lung cancer epidemic. *Nature Reviews*, **1**, 82–6.

Roffo, A. H. (1931). Durch Tabak beim Kaninchen entwickeltes Carcinom. *Zeitschrift für Krebsforsch*, **33**, 321–32.

Rottmann, H. (1898). *Über primäre lungencarcinoma*. Inaugural dissertation, Universität Würzburg.

Royal College of Physicians of London (1962). *Smoking and health*. Pitman Medical Publishing, London.

Schairer, E. and Schöniger, E. (1943). Lungenkrebs und Tabakverbrauch. *Zeitschrift für Krebsforsch*, **54**, 261–9.

Sömmering, S. T. (1795). De morbis vasorum absorbentium corporis humani. (Cited by Clemmesen, J. (1965). *Statistical studies in malignant neoplasms. I. Review and results*. Munksgaard, Copenhagen.)

Surgeon General (1964). *Smoking and health. Report of the Advisory Committee to the Surgeon General of the Public Health Service*. US Department of Health, Education and Welfare, Public Health Services, US Government Printing Office, Washington, DC.

Surgeon General (1989). *Reducing the health consequences of smoking: 25 years of progress. Report of the Surgeon General, 1989*. US Department of Health and Human Services, Maryland.

Tilley, N. W. (1948). *The Bright-tobacco industry, 1860–1929*. University of North Carolina Press, Chapel Hill.

Tylecote, F. E. (1927). Cancer of the lung. *Lancet*, **2**, 256–7.

Virchow, R. L. (1863~7). *Die krankhaften Geschwülste*. A. Hirschwald, Berlin.

Wassink, W. F. (1948). 'Onstaansvoorwasrden voor Longkanker'. *Ned Tijdschr Geneesk*, **92**, 3732–47.

Wynder, E. L., Graham, E. A., and Croninger, A. B. (1953). Experimental production of carcinoma with cigarette tar. Part I. *Cancer Research*, **13**, 855–64.

Chapter 2

The great studies of smoking and disease in the twentieth century

Michael J. Thun and Jane Henley

Introduction

Much of what is known about the harm caused by tobacco use was learned from large prospective epidemiologic studies conducted during the second half of the twentieth century in the United Kingdom and United States. To understand why these studies were so important in documenting the deleterious effects of smoking, one must appreciate the pervasive grip that tobacco, particularly cigarette smoking, held on the United Kingdom and its former Western colonies at the close of the Second World War. The culture of cigarettes was sustained not only by nicotine addiction and by the political and economic power of the tobacco industry, but also by the symbols and imagery with which advertising had imbued it, and by prevailing social norms. How could an apparently ordinary behavior, practised by so many people with so little evidence of acute toxicity, prove to have such severe chronic effects?

Sir Richard Doll, a pioneer of tobacco epidemiology, has examined the history of scientific and social factors that led ultimately to the recognition of the carcinogenicity and pathogenicity of smoking (Doll 1998b). He notes that, in retrospect, the medical evidence of the adverse health effects of tobacco accumulated for 200 years before it was generally accepted, in the late 1950s, that smoking caused lung cancer and, in the two subsequent decades, that it caused many other diseases as well (Doll 1998b). He cites three factors that contributed to the strength of resistance to the idea that smoking was a major cause of lung cancer: 'the ubiquity of the habit, which was as entrenched among male doctors and scientists as among the rest of the adult male population and had dulled the collective sense that tobacco might be a major threat to health', 'the novelty of the epidemiological techniques, particularly as applied to non-infectious diseases', and 'the primacy given to Koch's postulates in determining causation', since criteria had not yet been developed to assess the causation of chronic diseases such as cancer.

This chapter examines the contributions of several large prospective studies, conducted over the second half of the twentieth century, to our understanding of the health hazards of tobacco use. The designation 'Great Studies' is used to refer to prospective studies that were particularly informative about tobacco during this interval. It does not imply that other studies have not been equally important for understanding health scourges other than tobacco, or that all of the really important questions about tobacco have been answered. There is a continuing need for large cohort studies to understand, and limit, the progression of the tobacco pandemic as it evolves in different cultures with varying background disease profiles, cofactors, and patterns of usage.

Background

Two aspects concerning the historical use of tobacco in Europe help to explain the surprisingly low level of scientific scrutiny regarding its adverse health effects until the mid-twentieth century. First, for approximately 400 years after the introduction of tobacco into Europe by Spanish explorers returning from the New World in the late fifteenth century, most tobacco usage involved pipe or cigar smoking, or use of snuff or chewing tobacco, rather than cigarettes. The historical review by Doll notes that these products were widely used, first for medicinal purposes and then for pleasure (Doll 1998b). Tobacco was denounced periodically by critics such as James VI of Scotland (who later became James I of England), who published the tract entitled 'A Counterblaste to Tobacco' in 1603. Attempts to ban its use in Japan, Russia, Switzerland, and parts of Germany were unsuccessful, and for the most part anti-tobacco movements through the nineteenth century emphasized undesirable moral and social consequences of addiction, rather than documented evidence of adverse health effects (Doll 1998b). Medical concern about carcinogenicity was limited to a few case reports of pipe smokers who developed cancer of the lip, tongue, or oral cavity (Bouisson 1859; Anonymous 1890; Hoffman 1927; Lombard and Doering 1928). However, these were not taken very seriously and, according to Doll, were commonly attributed to the heat of the clay pipe stem rather than to any carcinogenic component of the smoke (Doll 1998b).

Beginning in the late nineteenth century, a series of technological innovations resulted in the rise of manufactured cigarettes and transformation of tobacco use (Slade 1993). The invention of safety matches in the late 1800s made it possible to smoke tobacco more frequently throughout the day in diverse settings. The development of machines to mass-produce and package cigarettes inexpensively allowed the cigarette to displace more expensive or cumbersome products, such as cigars and pipes. New strains of tobacco and new curing processes were patented that produced less-irritating smoke that could be inhaled more deeply than the smoke from traditional tobacco products. Whereas the nicotine released by older products such as cigars, pipes, roll-your own cigarettes, chewing tobacco, and snuff was highly alkaline and could be absorbed in ionized form through the oropharyngeal mucosa, nicotine released from the newer strains of tobacco was un-ionized and had to be inhaled to provide efficient absorption through the trachea and large bronchi. Deeper inhalation increased the surface area exposed to tobacco smoke. These changes in cigarette design were coupled, in the early twentieth century, with mass advertising campaigns to glamorize smoking of particular brands of cigarettes (Slade 1993). Free cigarettes were distributed in military rations to allied soldiers in the First and Second World Wars.

Collectively, these changes caused a large increase in the number of people smoking manufactured cigarettes, greater daily consumption of cigarettes, and a much greater surface area of tissues exposed to the carcinogens in tobacco smoke. A dramatic increase in cigarette smoking occurred first among men in the United Kingdom and United States, and later among women. In Britain, nearly 70 per cent of men and over 40 per cent of women between the ages of 25 and 59 were currently smoking cigarettes by the mid-twentieth century (Peto *et al.* 2000). In the United States, 57 per cent of men, and 28 per cent of women, reported current cigarette smoking in 1955, the time of the first national survey (Haenszel *et al.* 1956). Despite widespread smoking, little scientific attention was paid to the negative health effects of cigarettes before the mid-twentieth century. Rottman had reported a small cluster of lung cancer among tobacco workers in Leipzig in 1898 (Rottmann 1898). Several correlation studies noted the statistical association between the rise in cigarette consumption and the increasing population rates of lung cancer in men (Adler 1912; Tylecote 1927; Lickint 1929; Hoffman 1931; Arkin and Wagner 1936; Fleckseder 1936). Raymond Pearl described reduced longevity in smokers, based on family history records at the Johns Hopkins School of Hygiene (Pearl 1938). Several small case-control studies of smoking and lung cancer published before 1950 found a higher percentage of smokers among patients with lung cancer than with other diseases (Muller 1939; Schairer and Schioninger 1943; Wassink 1948). A series of skin-testing experiments in rabbits were either negative (Leitch 1928; Passey 1929), or demonstrated some increase in skin tumors (Roffo 1931; Cooper *et al.* 1932) after prolonged contact with tar extracts from cigarettes. However, the tumorigenicity of tobacco extracts appeared to be less than that of coal tar, and interpretation of the animal experiments was complicated by controversy about the temperature at which the tar was extracted from tobacco for the animal experiments, compared to the typical burning conditions in a cigarette (Doll 1998*b*). Only in Germany were doctors and the Nazi political authorities concerned about the potential cardiovascular and reproductive toxicity of 'nicotinism', which was not at the time based on sound scientific evidence (Doll 1998*b*).

It was the extraordinary rise in lung cancer that began early in the twentieth century among men in the United Kingdom, later among men in other countries, and subsequently in women, that finally drew serious attention to the hazards of smoking (Doll and Hill 1950; Wynder and Graham 1950). Lung cancer had hitherto been a rare disease. The increase in the age-standardized death rate from lung cancer among men in England and Wales had begun by 1912 and accelerated sharply after the First World War (Doll and Hill 1950). The number of lung cancer deaths recorded per year in England and Wales increased approximately 15-fold over the 25-year period between 1922 and 1947, far in excess of the increase in the size, or longevity of the population. In the United States, where cigarette smoking began later and vital statistics data on mortality did not become available for most of the nation until 1930, the age-adjusted lung cancer death rate increased approximately fivefold from 1930 to the mid-1940s (Thun *et al.* 2000).

For some years it was debated whether the apparent increase in lung cancer incidence and death rates represented a true increase in occurrence, or merely an artifact of improved diagnosis. Skeptics noted that several technologies introduced from the 1920s onwards could have increased recognition of previously undiagnosed disease (Doll 1998*b*). These included the widespread introduction of chest X-rays in the United Kingdom in the 1920s, bronchograms in the 1930s, and bronchoscopy in the 1950s. Open-chest surgery became practicable following improvements in anesthesia during the Second World War (Doll 1998*b*). The introduction of sulfapyridine in 1938 reduced mortality from pneumonia that had previously been lethal in the early stages of lung cancer, allowing cases to live long enough to be diagnosed. Nevertheless, the continued increase in lung cancer over several decades, and its more frequent diagnosis in men than women, made it more and more unlikely that improved diagnosis could explain the entire increase (Doll 1998*b*).

Five case-control studies published in 1950

In 1950 the publication of five case-control studies reporting an association between smoking and lung cancer (Doll and Hill 1950; Levin *et al.* 1950; Mills and Porter 1950; Schrek *et al.* 1950; Wynder and Graham 1950) provoked sudden interest among the medical and scientific communities in the potential health hazards of tobacco use. The two studies that drew the most attention were the British study by Doll and Hill (1950) and an American study by Wynder and Graham (1950). These were considerably larger than were earlier case-control studies of smoking and lung cancer (Muller 1939; Schairer and Schioninger 1943; Wassink 1948), had higher response rates, and defined smoking more precisely. The association between smoking and lung cancer was very strong in the largest case-control studies in Britain [odds ratio (OR) = 14] (Doll and Hill 1950) and the United States (OR = 6.6) (Wynder and Graham 1950); and even the study by Schrek *et al.*, which showed the weakest association, had an odds ratio of 1.8 (Schrek *et al.* 1950).

Although the case-control studies suggested that cigarette smoking was an important cause of lung cancer, the results were viewed as provocative rather than conclusive. Scientists were initially uncertain of the utility of case-control studies for studying chronic conditions such as cancer, since the methods had been developed for infectious diseases (Doll 1998*b*). Some epidemiologists questioned whether smokers with lung cancer were more likely to be hospitalized because of cough, perhaps introducing selection bias (Berkson 1955), or whether the control group might be biased by cultural factors related to smoking (Hammond 1953). Cuyler Hammond, of the American Cancer Society, noted that the studies 'disagree so markedly in their measurement of the size of that relationship' that one could not tell whether the relationship is of 'major clinical interest' or 'of academic interest only' (Hammond and Horn 1952). In retrospect, it seems likely that some of this variation may have arisen from including in the control series patients hospitalized for diseases that later proved to be smoking-attributable. In any case, epidemiologists agreed that sound evidence was essential, given the high prevalence of smoking and the social and economic implications of the results.

The need for cohort studies

Doll and Hill realized that the simplest way to attempt to replicate the findings of the case-control studies, using a different methodology, was to obtain information on the individual smoking habits of a large number of people, and to follow them to determine whether an individual's smoking habits predicted the risk of developing disease (Doll 1998b). Such cohort studies would need to be large so that they could provide a sufficient number of events to be informative within a reasonable time period. They would need to collect questionnaire information on smoking behavior, since such information was not then (and is not now) routinely collected on vital statistics records. In turn, the cohort studies would provide several important advantages over case-control studies. They could examine the relationship between smoking and many different end points, not just a single disease. This was important, because more than 70 per cent of deaths caused by smoking result from diseases other than lung cancer (CDC 2002). The comparison group in cohort studies could be defined as lifelong non-smokers, thus avoiding the problem of including patients with other smoking-attributable diseases in the control group. Finally, cohort studies are intuitively more understandable than case-control studies, because they reflect the desired temporal sequence in which exposure precedes disease.

The earliest cohort studies

The two earliest cohort studies of tobacco use and mortality were the British Doctors Study, which began in the United Kingdom in 1951 (Doll and Hill 1954, 1956), and the Hammond Horn or Nine-State study, initiated by the American Cancer Society (ACS) in 1952 (Hammond 1953, 1954). Both of these were designed to facilitate enrollment and follow-up of large populations. For instance, the physicians who participated in the British Doctors Study were identified from the Medical Register of the United Kingdom and followed through the Registrars General, the British Medical Association, and the General Medical Council (Doll and Hill 1956). The information on clinical diagnoses and cause of death was thought to be more accurate for doctors than for the general population. Similarly, the extensive network of local volunteers for ACS provided an extraordinary human resource to enroll, and help to follow, large prospective epidemiological studies in the United States (Thun *et al.* 2000). Both the ACS cohorts and the British Doctors Study provided effective conduits for disseminating information about the adverse effects of tobacco use. Publicity about the studies caused many doctors in the United Kingdom and United States to stop smoking, well ahead of the general public.

British Doctors Study

In 1951, a questionnaire on smoking habits was sent to all British doctors included in the Medical Register. Of the 41 024 replies received, 40 701 were sufficiently complete to be utilized (Doll and Hill 1954). The 34 494 men and 6207 women included in the follow up comprised 69 per cent and 60 per cent of the men and women, respectively, in the registry. Further questionnaires about changes in smoking habits were sent in 1957 to men, in 1960 to women, and in 1966 and 1972 to all participants. On each occasion, approximately 97 per cent of the doctors responded. The analyses defined lifelong non-smoking as never having smoked as much as one cigarette per day, or $^1/_4$ ounce of other forms of tobacco, for as much as 1 year. A preliminary report was published by Doll and Hill (1954), and a second report in 1956 (Doll and Hill 1956). Results from the 10-year follow-up of male doctors were published in 1964 (Doll and Hill 1964), the 20-year follow-up (through October 1971) for men in 1976 (Doll and Peto 1976), and the 22-year follow-up for women in 1980 (Doll et al. 1980). Results from the 40-year follow-up were published in 1994 (Doll et al. 1994), and the final report of the 50-year follow-up is now being prepared (personal communication, Sir Richard Doll).

Hammond Horn (the nine-state) study

The Hammond Horn study began in October 1952, when over 22 000 ACS volunteers distributed a questionnaire to 10 white men, aged 50–69 years, whom he or she knew well (Hammond 1954). A total of 204 547 men in nine states participated. Patterns of cigarette, cigar, and pipe smoking were similar in the Hammond Horn cohort to those found in a representative survey of American males in 1955 (Haenszel et al. 1956). Study participants were enrolled from among the friends, neighbors, and acquaintances of local volunteers, and thus resembled the socio-demographic characteristics of the volunteers. A higher percentage were graduates of high school or college, and were more affluent, than in the general United States population. After exclusions, a cohort of 187 783 men was followed from 1952 through 1955. A total of 11 783 deaths (6.2 per cent) occurred during an average of 44 months of follow-up, with 1.1 per cent of the cohort being lost to follow-up. Death certificates were collected for all reported deaths and further information was collected from the physician, hospital, or tumor registry whenever cancer was mentioned (Hammond and Horn 1958a). Preliminary results from the first 20 months of follow-up were published in 1954 (Hammond 1954). Final results were published in 1958 for total mortality (Hammond and Horn 1958a), and for specific causes of death (Hammond and Horn 1958b). The Hammond Horn study was terminated after 44 months of follow-up.

Early findings from the British Doctors and Hammond Horn Studies

Preliminary results from both the British Doctors and the Hammond Horn studies were published in 1954. The British cohort demonstrated a statistically significant and steady increase in lung cancer occurrence among smokers, although this was based on only 36 lung cancers. The age standardized rate increased from 0.00 per 1000 among the 3093 non-smokers, to 1.14 per 1000 among the 5203 men recorded as smoking 25 g or more of tobacco daily. A similar, but less steep, rise was seen in mortality from coronary thrombosis (from a rate of 3.89 in non-smokers, to 5.15 in the heaviest smokers). In the Hammond Horn study, men with a history of regular cigarette smoking had a substantially higher death rate from all causes (based on 4854 deaths), from coronary heart disease (1328 deaths), and from lung cancer (167 deaths) than men who had never smoked regularly.

A second report from the British Doctors Study was published in 1956, based on 84 confirmed cases of lung cancer. This, too, demonstrated a steady increase in the annual death rate from lung cancer with increasing amount smoked (Doll and Hill 1956). The annual death rate in men who smoked at least 25 g (approximately 25 cigarettes) per day was 1.66 per 1000, over 20 times the death rate of the non-smokers (0.07 per 1000). Greater cigarette consumption was also associated with higher death rates from chronic bronchitis, peptic ulcer, and pulmonary tuberculosis, although the trend was statistically significant only for chronic bronchitis.

Of interest is that the principal investigators of the earliest cohort studies did not initially expect that cigarette smoking would prove to be the cause of the increasing lung cancer incidence in the United Kingdom and United States. When Doll first began work on the British case-control study in 1948, he suspected that 'motor cars and the tarring of roads' were a more likely explanation than cigarette smoking (Doll 1998a). However, both Doll and Hill were impressed by the results of the case-control study, and in their 1950 publication concluded that 'smoking is a factor, and an important factor, in the production of carcinoma of the lung' (Doll and Hill 1950). Hammond and Horn, both of whom were smokers at the time, remained skeptical of the earlier case-control studies that associated lung cancer with cigarette smoking. When they began the first ACS cohort study, they considered it equally plausible that automotive exhaust, dust from tarred roads, and/or air pollution from coal and oil furnaces might be partly or wholly responsible (Hammond and Horn 1952; Hammond 1953). However, the results of their Nine State Study (Hammond 1954; Hammond and Horn 1958a, b) persuaded Hammond and Horn to stop smoking and to focus ACS attention on tobacco use as an important cause of cancer and other diseases.

Growing scientific consensus

Sufficient scientific evidence had accumulated by the late 1950s that at least six scientific consensus groups concluded that cigarette smokers had higher lung cancer death rates than non-smokers. These expert reviews were convened by health ministries in the United Kingdom (Medical Research Council 1957), United States (Burney 1959), Canada (National Cancer Institute of Canada 1958), Sweden (Swedish Medical Research Council 1958), and The Netherlands (Netherlands Ministry of Social Affairs and Public Health 1957), and by cancer societies in Denmark, Norway, and Finland (United States Public Health Service 1964). The evidence at the time included early reports from the cohort studies (Doll and Hill 1954, 1956; Hammond and Horn 1954, 1958a, b), additional case-control data (Doll and Hill 1952; Kouloumies 1953; Linckint 1953; Gsell 1954; Randig 1954; Kreyberg 1955; Schwartz and Denoix 1957; Segi et al. 1957), and experimental evidence that prolonged application of condensates of tobacco smoke induced skin cancer in rabbits and mice (Wynder et al. 1953, 1955; Sugiura 1956; Engelbreth-Holm and Ahlmann 1957; Guerin and Cuzin 1957; Croninger et al. 1958).

Counterarguments to the idea that smoking caused lung cancer grew increasingly implausible in the face of the evidence that had accumulated by the late 1950s. The hypothesis proposed by R. A. Fisher, that some underlying constitutional factor predisposed smokers to both smoking and lung cancer (Fisher 1957, 1958, 1959) did not explain the temporal increase in lung cancer in the population, nor the decrease in lung cancer in persons who stopped smoking. Berkson's contention that the hospital-based case-control studies were biased by the differential effects of illness on enrollment (Berkson 1955) was countered by the stability of the association between smoking and lung cancer during longer follow-up of the British Doctors Study (Doll and Hill 1956). The lack of specificity whereby smoking was associated with multiple diseases (Berkson 1958) was also not considered strong evidence against causation, because of the complex mixture of chemicals in tobacco smoke (Doll 1998b).

The scientific consensus that tobacco smoking caused lung cancer became even stronger after 1960, with the publication of reports from the World Health Organization (1960), the Royal College of Physicians of London (1962), and the Advisory Committee to the United States Surgeon General (US Public Health Service 1964). In 1962 the Royal College of Physicians concluded, 'Cigarette smoking is a cause of lung cancer and bronchitis and probably contributes to the development of coronary heart disease . . . It delays healing of gastric and duodenal ulcers'. The 1964 Report of the Advisory Group to the Surgeon General in the United States (US Public Health Service 1964) was particularly influential, according to Doll, because of its thoroughness and because its members had been individually vetted by the tobacco industry to exclude those who had publicly expressed views on the topic (Doll 1998b). Based on independent analyses of seven published and unpublished prospective studies, and review of 29 retrospective studies of smoking and health, the report stated, 'Cigarette smoking is associated with a 70 percent increase in the age-specific death rates of males and to a lesser extent with increased death rates of females'. It concluded:

> Cigarette smoking is causally related to lung cancer in men; the magnitude of the effect of cigarette smoking far outweighs all other factors. The data for women, though less extensive, point in the same direction. A relationship exists between cigarette smoking and emphysema, but it has not been established that this relationship is causal: Male cigarette smokers have a higher death rate from coronary artery disease than non-smoking males. Although the causative role of

cigarette smoking in deaths from coronary disease is not proven, the Committee considers it more prudent from the public health viewpoint to assume that the established association has causative meaning than to suspend judgment until no uncertainty remains.

(US Public Health Service 1964)

After 1964 there was no serious scientific controversy about whether smoking caused lung cancer. The official skepticism of the tobacco industry was maintained as a legal and political strategy, rather than a consequence of any genuine scientific debate, as was revealed later through the disclosure of internal documents (Glantz *et al.* 1996). However, many important scientific questions remained concerning other deleterious effects of tobacco use, the magnitude of the problem, and the potential benefits of cessation and other possible interventions.

Additional cohort studies

Among the seven cohort studies considered by the 1964 Report to the Surgeon General (US Public Health Service 1964) were two that, like the British Doctors Study, were of sufficient size and duration to qualify as 'Great Studies'. These were the US Veterans Study, begun by the National Institutes of Health and the US Veterans' Administration in 1954, and Cancer Prevention Study I, a second large cohort study initiated by the American Cancer Society, in 1959 (Auerbach *et al.* 1961).

The US Veterans (Dorn) Study

In September 1954, the US Veterans' Administration contacted 293 958 men who had served in the armed forces at any time between 1917 and 1940, and who held US government life insurance policies (Kahn 1966). Subjects were mainly white men of the middle and upper social classes. A total of 248 195 men (response rate 85 per cent after two mailings) returned a questionnaire on their smoking habits. The vital status of these veterans was followed until death by tracking life insurance claims to the Veterans Administration, or termination of the policy for other reasons. Supplemental information was obtained on deceased persons from certifying physicians or hospitals. Results from the Veterans Study were published in 1958 (Dorn 1958), 1959 (Dorn 1959), 1966 (Kahn 1966), 1990 (Hsing *et al.* 1990), and 1995 (Chow *et al.* 1995). A total of 192 756 deaths occurred during the 26-year follow-up from 1954 to 1980.

Cancer Prevention Study I (CPS-I)

Between October 1959 and February 1960, volunteers for the American Cancer Society in 25 states recruited more than 1 million subjects, from among their friends, neighbors, and acquaintances, to complete a four-page questionnaire (Hammond 1964, 1966). Known as Cancer Prevention Study I (CPS-I) or the 25 State Study, the cohort was substantially larger than the Hammond Horn study, and included women as well as men (Hammond 1964; Garfinkel 1985). Enrollment was by family; all family members over 30 years of age were requested to fill out detailed questionnaires on smoking behavior (Auerbach *et al.* 1961). For the 1 045 087 subjects with usable questionnaire information, vital status was determined annually through the volunteers. Updated information on smoking was obtained every 2 years. Approximately 1 per cent of subjects were lost during the first 6 years of follow-up, through September 1965 (Hammond 1966). Three states were then dropped from the study (Hammond and Seidman 1980) and follow-up in the remainder was 98.49 per cent complete through September 1971, and 92.8 per cent through September 1972 (Garfinkel 1985). Death certificates were obtained from state or local authorities and, when cancer was mentioned, further information was sought from physicians.

Several other large cohort studies initiated after 1960 examined the deleterious effects of tobacco in women and in other geographic regions and time periods. These are described briefly below.

Swedish Study

In 1963, questionnaires about smoking were mailed to a national probability sample of 55 000 Swedish adults, aged 18 through 69 years (Cederlof *et al.* 1975). The response rate was 69 per cent. Information on smoking status was collected in 1963. Mortality follow-up over the ensuing 10 years was conducted through linkage with the national death registry. The results for 10 years of follow-up were published in 1975 (Cederlof *et al.* 1975) and for longer follow-ups in 1987 (Carstensen *et al.* 1987) and 1997 (Nordlund *et al.* 1997).

Japanese Six Prefecture Cohort Study

In late 1965, 142 857 women and 122 261 men, aged 40 years and older, were interviewed in 29 health districts in Japan (Akiba and Hirayama 1990; Hirayama 1990). The study group comprised between 91 and 99 per cent of adults of this age in the districts represented, which were distributed throughout six prefectures. Information on tobacco smoking, diet, alcohol consumption, occupation, and marital status was obtained by interview at enrollment. After 6 years, a second interview of 3728 randomly selected women showed that the percentage of smokers had decreased only slightly (from 10.4 to 9.7 per cent). A record linkage system was established for annual follow-up. During 16 years of follow-up, 51 422 deaths occurred. Until recently, the Hiriyama cohort was unique in being the only large prospective study of smoking and mortality among Asians.

Nurses' Health Study I

A cohort of 121 700 30–55-year-old female nurses was assembled in the United States in 1976. At enrollment, and periodically thereafter, the nurses completed a mailed questionnaire on risk factors for cancer and heart disease. Much of the exposure information concerned nutritional factors, yet the cohort has been very informative about the effects of smoking and smoking cessation on many health end points in women (Kawachi *et al.* 1997; US Department of Health and Human Services 2001).

Kaiser Permanente Study

Between 1979 and 1986, the Kaiser Permanente Medical Care Program obtained baseline information about tobacco smoking from 36 035 women and 24 803 men aged 35 years or older (Friedman *et al.* 1997). Participants in the program made up about 30 per cent of the population in the areas it served. Follow-up through 1987 identified 1098 deaths among all women. The study provides the only published data on premature death associated with cigarette smoking among African-American women.

Cancer Prevention Study II (CPS-II)

The third large prospective study, begun by the American Cancer Society, was called Cancer Prevention Study II (CPS-II). Started in 1982, it is a prospective mortality study of nearly 1.2 million adults, 30 years of age and older, drawn from the entire population of the USA. Like CPS-I, it included more than 50 per cent women. Enrollment into the study was accomplished by completing a brief confidential mailed questionnaire addressing alcohol and tobacco use, diet and other factors affecting mortality. Deaths were ascertained from month of enrollment through 1988 by personal inquiries by American Cancer Society volunteers at 2-year intervals. Follow-up after 1988 has continued through linkage with the National Death Index. Analyses of smoking and mortality have largely been restricted to the first 6 years of follow-up, since information on tobacco use was not updated after enrollment. By 1988, 2 per cent of the cohort were lost to follow-up and 0.2 per cent could not be followed because the personal identifiers provided were insufficient for linkage to the National Death Index. By 1991, 12 per cent of the cohort had died and death certificates were obtained for 98 per cent of the deceased. Participants in CPS-II were more likely to be white (93 per cent), married (81 per cent), middle class, and educated (high school graduates or above, 85.6 per cent) than the general population of the United States of America.

Contributions of later cohort studies

Continuing follow-up of the original cohorts and the initiation of new large cohort studies proved essential to the scientific consensus that smoking caused a multiplicity of diseases besides lung cancer. One advantage of cohort studies was their ability to examine many end points simultaneously. Initially this invoked criticism of the lung cancer hypothesis—Berkson argued that smoking was associated with so many different diseases that none of the associations were interpretable (Berkson 1955, 1958). However, the relative risk for lung cancer was 10.8 among all cigarette smokers, compared to non-smokers, in the seven cohort studies analyzed by the 1964 Advisory Committee to the Surgeon General (US Public Health Service 1964) and was 24 among heavy cigarette smokers in the British Doctors Study (Doll and Hill 1956). While the relative risk (RR) estimates were lower for death from laryngeal cancer (RR = 5.4) and chronic bronchitis (RR = 6.1) than for lung cancer, they nevertheless persuaded the 1964 Advisory Committee to conclude that cigarette smoking caused lung cancer, laryngeal cancer, and chronic bronchitis in men (US Public Health Service 1964).

Early consensus groups were more cautious in interpreting the relationship of smoking with various cardiovascular diseases and other conditions. The 1964 Report to the Surgeon General noted that 'Male cigarette smokers have a higher death rate from coronary artery disease than non-smoking males, but it is not clear that the association has causal significance' (RR = 6.1) (US Public Health Service 1964). The median relative risk for death from coronary heart disease in male smokers compared to non-smokers was 1.7 (range 1.5–2.0) in the cohort studies reviewed in 1964. However, by 1967 a later Surgeon General Report concluded, 'The convergence of many types of evidence—epidemiological, experimental, pathological, and clinical—strongly suggests that cigarette smoking can cause death from coronary heart disease' (US Public Health Service 1967). The language attributing causation became progressively stronger over time, as results from the Framingham Study and other cardiovascular cohorts confirmed that smoking, hypertension, and increased cholesterol were all strong and independent risk factors (Kannell et al. 1966).

With prolonged follow-up, the cohort studies included many more cases and/or deaths from less common conditions, and more detailed analyses of diseases attributable to smoking. By 1989, the US Surgeon General had designated 14 disease categories that contribute to smoking-attributable deaths in the United States (US Department of Health and Human Services 1989). These included coronary heart disease; hypertensive heart disease; cerebrovascular lesions; aortic aneurism (non-syphilitic); ulcer (gastric, duodenal, jejeunal); influenza and pneumonia; bronchitis and emphysema; and cancers of the lip, oral cavity, and pharynx, esophagus, pancreas, larynx, lung, kidney, and bladder and other urinary organs (US Department of Health and Human Services 1989). An updated review by the International Agency for Research on Cancer (IARC) in 2002 refined this list by including cancers of the naso-, oro-, and hypopharynx, nasal cavity, paranasal sinuses, stomach, liver, kidney (parenchyma as well as renal pelvis), ureter, uterine cervix, and bone marrow (myeloid leukemia) (IARC 2002).

Besides contributing to the inventory of diseases officially designated as caused by smoking, the cohort studies also reveal how the epidemic changed, and evolved, over time. This progression is particularly evident in the increase in lung cancer death rates that occurred among women smokers in the two American Cancer Society cohorts, during the past 50 years (Garfinkel and Stellman 1988; Thun et al. 1997), and in the growing disparity in overall survival rates between smokers and non-smokers from the first to the second half of the British Doctors Study (Doll et al. 1994, 2000).

Figure 2.1 illustrates the death rate from lung cancer among women who smoked cigarettes, within 5-year age intervals, for four time periods between 1960 and 1986.

Lung cancer mortality increased enormously in women smokers over the 26-year period. Not shown in Fig. 2.1 is that the death rate from lung cancer remained essentially constant over this interval among women who had never smoked (Garfinkel 1981; Thun *et al.* 1997). Consequently, the relative risk associated with current cigarette smoking in women increased from approximately 2 in 1960–64 to nearly 11 in 1982–86. The protracted increase in lung cancer among women smokers contradicted the hypothesis of the early 1950s, that women might be less susceptible than men to the adverse effects of smoking, and refuted the theory proposed by R. A. Fisher that the absence of increasing lung cancer among women smokers in the 1950s was evidence that smoking did not cause lung cancer (Fisher 1958). Instead, it supported Doll's prediction (Doll *et al.* 1980), that as successive birth cohorts of women smoked more intensively from earlier ages, their lung cancer risk would approach that of male smokers.

An analogous picture of the progression of the epidemic is apparent in the widening gap in overall survival between cigarette smokers and lifelong non-smokers from the first to the second half of the British Doctors Study. Figure 2.2 illustrates the probability of survival to various ages beyond 40 years among male British doctors who never smoked tobacco, or who currently smoked cigarettes during the first or second 20-year interval of follow-up (Doll *et al.* 1994). During both time periods, the percentage surviving was higher among men who had never smoked than among those who smoked regularly. The percentage surviving to age 70 was 58 per cent among current cigarette

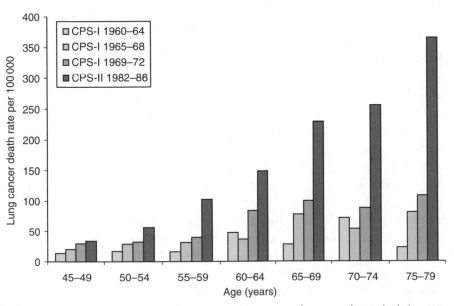

Fig. 2.1 Age-specific lung cancer death rates among women who currently smoked cigarettes when enrolled in CPS-I and CPS-II (from Garfinkel and Stellman 1988).

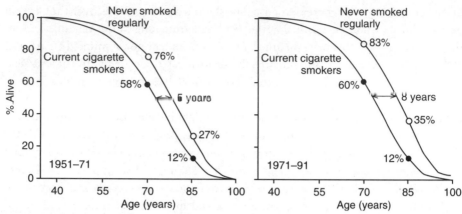

Fig. 2.2 Survival after age 35 among cigarette smokers and non-smokers in the first half (left) and second half (right) of the British Doctors Study. For ages 35–44 years, rates for the whole study are used in both halves, since little information on these is available from the second half. (From Doll *et al.* 1994.)

smokers and 76 per cent among lifelong non-smokers in the interval 1951–71, and 60 per cent and 83 per cent in the follow-up from 1971 to 1991. Furthermore, the median difference in overall survival between smokers and non-smokers widened over time, from 5 years in 1951–71, to 8 years in 1971–91. The difference widened largely because improvements in survival affected never-smokers more than smokers.

Contributing to the increase in lung cancer mortality among female smokers, and to the widening disparity in survival between smokers and non-smokers, was a generational shift towards initiating cigarette smoking at younger ages. Successive birth cohorts of both male and female smokers began smoking regularly earlier in adolescence (Anderson *et al.* 2002). The relationship between an early age of initiation and lung cancer risk is illustrated in Fig. 2.3, showing the lung cancer death rate (per 100 000) among men aged 55–64 years in the US Veterans Study (Kahn 1966). Men who began smoking at an earlier age have higher death rates from lung cancer at a given level of smoking than men who initiated smoking later. The difference in risk is seen for both 'moderate' (10–20 cigarettes per day) and 'heavy' smokers (21–39 cigarettes per day). This analysis cannot differentiate whether the higher lung cancer rate in persons who begin smoking early reflects a longer duration of smoking or greater vulnerability of the immature lung to the carcinogenicity of smoke, since the two factors are inseparably correlated in current smokers of the same age. However, Fig. 2.3 does illustrate that earlier age of initiation is a strong predictor of higher lung cancer risk.

Finally, the cohort studies demonstrate the substantial benefit of smoking cessation in preventing much of the increased mortality caused by continued smoking. Figure 2.4 illustrates the cumulative probability of death from lung cancer, conditional on survival from other conditions, during 7 years of follow-up of CPS-II, in relation to

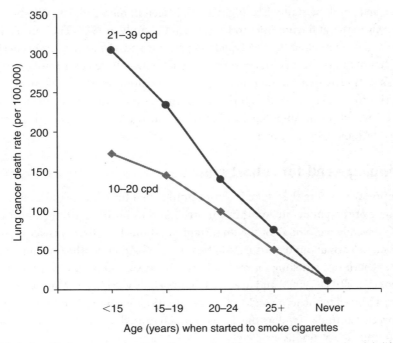

Fig. 2.3 Relationship between age of starting regular cigarette smoking in early adult life and lung cancer death rates at age 55–64 years for US male veterans, 1954–62. Data are presented separately for heavy and moderate smokers. (From Kahn 1966.)

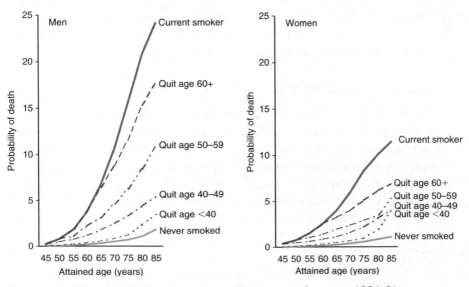

Fig. 2.4 Probability of death from lung cancer: CPS-II men and women, 1984–91.

age, sex, and smoking status. The highest risk is seen in men and women who actively smoked cigarettes at the time of enrollment into the study in 1982. The cumulative risk in men and women older than 85 equals 24 per cent and 11 per cent, respectively. The lowest risk of lung cancer is seen in men and women who have never smoked regularly. The risk is intermediate among men and women who have quit smoking at various ages, prior to enrollment in the study, and decreases most the earlier the age of quitting. Persons who stop smoking avoid much of the dramatic further increase in risk incurred by those who continue.

Continuing need for cohort studies

It is important to note that there is a continuing need for cohort studies to monitor the course of the pandemic in other countries and to improve strategies for ending tobacco dependence. Not all of the important questions have been answered. There is still much to learn about the nature and treatment of addiction, the phenomenon that obligates continued smoking for most adults. This is very important for the 46.5 million Americans (CDC 2002) and over 1.2 billion people worldwide (Corrao *et al.* 2000) who are addicted to tobacco use. Most of the attention of cohort studies in the past has been directed at understanding the disease burden caused by smoking, not at developing or testing interventions.

Furthermore, the diseases that tobacco use causes differ somewhat in different countries, depending on the background risks of contracting diseases that either compete with, or interact with, smoking. For example, much of the disease burden caused by tobacco in the United States and other Western countries involves cardiovascular diseases, because of the high background rate of these conditions. The same is not true in China, where a much higher proportion of the burden involves chronic obstructive pulmonary disease (Liu *et al.* 1998), or in India, where tuberculosis is the most common disease by which smoking causes premature death.

Summary and conclusions

Since the early 1950s, large cohort studies have played a major role in helping to identify the multitude of adverse health effects caused by tobacco use, particularly in manufactured cigarettes. They demonstrated that the harmful effects applied to women as well as men, and that the burden of disease caused by smoking increased over time, as smokers initiated regular cigarette smoking at progressively earlier ages. Large cohort studies will continue to be important for monitoring the course of the epidemic as it evolves in different cultures, and for sustaining the political resolve to end it.

References

Adler, I. (1912). *Primary malignant growths of the lung and bronchi.* Longmans Green, London.
Akiba, S. and Hirayama, T. (1990). *Environmental Health Perspectives,* **87**, 19–26.

Anderson, C. M., Burns, D. M., Major, J.M., Vaughn, J.W., and Shanks, T.G. (2002). In *Changing adolescent smoking prevalence*, Vol. 14 (ed. D. Burns, R. Amacher, and W. Ruppert), pp. 141–55. US Department of Health and Human Services, National Institutes of Health, National Cancer Institute, Bethesda, Maryland.

Anonymous (1890). *British Medical Journal*, **1**, 748.

Arkin, A. and Wagner, D. (1936). *Journal of the American Medical Association*, **106**, 587–91.

Auerbach, O., Stout, A., Hammond, E., and Garfinkel, L. (1961). *New England Journal of Medicine*, **265**, 253–67.

Berkson, J. (1955). *Proceedings of the Staff Meetings of the Mayo Clinic*, **30**, 319–48.

Berkson, J. (1958). *Journal of the American Statistical Association*, **53**, 28–38.

Bouisson, E. (1859). *Montpelier Medical Journal*, **2**, 539–99; **3**, 19–41.

Burney, L. (1959). *Journal of the American Medical Association*, **171**, 1829–37.

Carstensen, J., Pershagen, G., and Eklund, G. (1987). *Journal of Epidemiology and Community Health*, **41**, 166–72.

CDC (2002). *MMWR CDC Surveillance Summaries*, **51**, 300–3.

Cederlof, R., Friberg, L., Hrubec, Z., and Lorich, U. (1975). *The relationship of smoking and some social covariables to mortality and cancer morbidity*. Department of Environmental Hygiene, The Karolinska Institute, Stockholm, Sweden.

Chow, W., McLaughlin, J., Hrubec, Z., and Fraumeni, J. (1995). *British Journal of Cancer*, **72**, 1556–8.

Cooper, E., Lamb, F., Sanders, E., and Hirst, E. (1932). *Journal of Hygiene London*, **32**, 293–300.

Corrao, M., Guindon, G., Sharma, N., and Shokoohi, D. (2000). *Tobacco control: Country profiles*. American Cancer Society, Atlanta, Georgia.

Croninger, A., Graham, E., and Wynder, E. (1958). *Cancer Research*, **18**, 1263–71.

Doll, R. (1998*a*). In *Ashes to ashes: the history of smoking and health* (ed. S. Lock, L. Reynolds, and E. Tansey), pp. 130–42. Clio Medica, Amsterdam/Atlanta, Ga.

Doll, R. (1998*b*). *Statistical Methods in Medical Research*, **7**, 87–117.

Doll, R. and Hill, A. (1950). *British Medical Journal*, **2**, 739–48.

Doll, R. and Hill, A. (1952). *British Medical Journal*, **2**, 1271–86.

Doll, R. and Hill, A. (1954). *British Medical Journal*, **1**, 1451–5.

Doll, R. and Hill, A. (1956). *British Medical Journal*, **2**, 1071–81.

Doll, R. and Hill, A. (1964). *British Medical Journal*, **1**, 1399–410; 1460–7.

Doll, R. and Peto, R. (1976). *British Medical Journal*, **2**, 1525–36.

Doll, R., Gray, R., Hafner, B., and Peto, R. (1980). *British Medical Journal*, **280**, 967–71.

Doll, R., Peto, R., Wheatley, K., Gray, R., and Sutherland, I. (1994). Mortality in relation to smoking: 40 years' observations on male Bristish doctors. *British Medical Journal*, **309**, 901–11.

Doll, R., Peto, R., Boreham, J., and Sutherland, I. (2000). *British Medical Journal*, **320**, 1097–102.

Dorn, H. (1958). *Proceedings of the Society Stat Sect Amer Stat Assn*, 34–71.

Dorn, H. (1959). *Public Health Reports*, **74**, 581–93.

Engelbreth-Holm, J. and Ahlmann, J. (1957). *Acta Pathological Microbiology Scandinavica*, **41**, 267–72.

Fisher, R. (1957). *British Medical Journal*, **2**, 43.

Fisher, R. (1958). *Nature*, **182**, 596.

Fisher, R. (ed.) (1959). *Smoking: the cancer controversy. Some attempts to assess the evidence*. Oliver and Boyd, Edinburgh.

Fleckseder, R. (1936). *Munchener Medizinische Wochenschrift*, **83**, 1585–8.

Friedman, G., Tekawa, I., Sadler, M., and Sidney, S. (1997). *Monographs / National Cancer Institute*, **97**, 477–99.

Garfinkel, L. (1981). *Journal of the National Cancer Institute*, **66**, 1061–6.

Garfinkel, L. (1985). *Monographs / National Cancer Institute*, **67**, 49–52.

Garfinkel, L. and Stellman, S. (1988). Smoking and lung cancer in women: Findings from a prospective study. *Cancer Research*, **48**, 6951–5.

Glantz, S., Slade, J., Bero, L., Hanauer, P., and Barnes, D. (1996). In *The Cigarette Papers* (ed. S. Glantz, J. Slade, L. Bero, P. Hanauer, and D. Barnes), pp. 1–24. University of California Press, Berkeley, California.

Gsell, O. (1954). *Medical Hygiene*, **12**, 429–31.

Guerin, M. and Cuzin, J. (1957). *Bulletin of the Association of France Cancer*, **44**, 387–408.

Haenszel, W., Shimkin, M., and Miller, H. (1956). In *Public Health Monograph Number 45*. PHS Pub. No. 463. Public Health Service. US Government Printing Office, Washington.

Hammond, E. (1953). In *Sixty-Second Annual Meeting of the Association of Life Insurance Medical Directors of America*, pp. 3–7. Press of Recording and Statistical Corporation, New York.

Hammond, E. (1954). *Connecticut State Medical Journal*, **18**, 3–11.

Hammond, E. (1964). *Journal of the National Cancer Institute*, **32**, 1161–88.

Hammond, E. (1966). *Monographs / National Cancer Institute*, **19**, 127–204.

Hammond, E. and Horn, D. (1952). *Proceedings of the 2nd National Cancer Conference*. American Cancer Society, New York, **2**, 871–5.

Hammond, E. and Horn, D. (1954). *Journal of the American Medical Association*, **155**, 1316–28.

Hammond, E. and Horn, D. (1958*a*). *Journal of the American Medical Association*, **166**, 1159–72.

Hammond, E. and Horn, D. (1958*b*). *Journal of the American Medical Association*, **166**, 1294–308.

Hammond, E. and Seidman, H. (1980). *Preventive Medicine*, **9**, 169–73.

Hirayama, T. (1990). In *Contributions to epidemiology and statistics*, Vol. 6. Karger, Basel.

Hoffman, F. (1927). *Cancer and overnutrition*. Prudential Press.

Hoffman, F. (1931). *Annals of Surgery*, **93**, 50–67.

Hsing, A., McLaughlin, J., Hrubec, Z., Blot, W., and Fraumeni, J. (1990). *Cancer Causes and Control*, **1**, 217–21.

IARC (2002). *IARC Monographs on the evaluation of the carcinogenic risk of chemicals to humans: Tobacco smoke and involuntary smoking*. International Agency for Research on Cancer, Lyon.

Kahn, H. (1966). The Dorn study of smoking and mortality among US veterans. Report on eight and one-half years of observation. In *Monograph 19, Epidemiological Study of Cancer and Other Chronic Diseases* (ed. W. Haenszel), pp. 1–126. US Department of Health, Education, and Welfare, Public Health Service, National Cancer Institute, Bethesda, Maryland.

Kannell, W., Dawber, T., and McNamara, P. (1966). *Journal of the Iowa Medical Society*, **56**, 26–34.

Kawachi, I., Colditz, G., Stampfer, M., Willett, W., Manson, J., Rosner, B., *et al.* (1997). In *National Cancer Institute, Smoking and Tobacco Control, Monograph 8: Changes in cigarette-related disease risks and their implication for prevention and control* (ed. D. Burns, L. Garfinkel, and J. Samet), pp. 531–65. National Institute of Health, Washington.

Kouloumies, M. (1953). *Acta Radiologica (Stockholm)*, **30**, 255–60.

Kreyberg, L. (1955). *British Journal of Cancer*, **9**, 495–510.

Leitch, A. (1928). In *Fifth annual report of the British Empire Cancer Campaign*, pp. 26. British Empire Cancer Campaign, London.

Levin, M., Goldstein, H., and Gerhardt, P. (1950). *Journal of the American Medical Association*, **143**, 336–8.

Lickint, F. (1929). *Zeitschrift fur Krebsforschung*, **30**, 349–65.

Lickint, F. (1953). In *Atiologie und Prophylaxe des Lungenkrebses*, pp. 76–102. Theodor Steinkopff, Leipzig.

Liu, B. Q., Peto, R., Chen, Z. M., Boreham, J., Wu, Y. P., Li, J. Y., *et al.* (1998). *British Medical Journal*, **317**, 1411–22.

Lombard, H. and Doering, C. (1928). *New England Journal of Medicine*, **198**, 481–7.

Medical Research Council (1957). *British Medical Journal*, **1**, 1523.

Mills, C. and Porter, M. (1950). *Cancer Research*, **10**, 539–42.

Muller, F. (1939). *Zeitschrift fur Krebsforschung*, **49**, 57–85.

National Cancer Institute of Canada (1958). *Canadian Medical Association Journal*, **79**, 566–8.

Netherlands Ministry of Social Affairs and Public Health (1957). *Nederlands Tijdschrift voor Geneeskunde (Amsterdam)*, **101**, 459–64.

Nordlund, L., Carstensen, J., and Pershagen, G. (1997). *International Journal of Cancer*, **73**, 625–8.

Passey, R. (1929). In *Sixth report of British Empire Cancer Research Campaign*, pp. 85. British Empire Cancer Campaign, London.

Pearl, R. (1938). *Science*, **87**, 216–17.

Peto, R., Darby, S., Deo, H., Silcocks, P., Whitley, E., and Doll, R. (2000). *British Medical Journal*, **321**, 323–9.

Randig, K. (1954). *Off Gesundheitsdienst*, **16**, 305–13.

Roffo, A. (1931). *Zeitschrift fur Krebsforschung*, **33**, 321–2.

Rottmann, H. (1898). Universitat Wurzburg, Wurzburg. *Über primäre lungen carcinoma.* Inaugural dissertation.

Royal College of Physicians of London (1962). *Smoking and health.* Pitman Medical, London.

Schairer, E. and Schioninger, E. (1943). *Zeitschrift fur Krebsforschung*, **54**, 261–9.

Schrek, R., Baker, L., Ballard, G., and Dolgoff, S. (1950). *Cancer Research*, **10**, 49–58.

Schwartz, D. and Denoix, P. (1957). *Semaine des Hopitaux de Paris*, **33**, 3630–43.

Segi, M., Fukushima, L., Fujisako, S., Kurihara, M., Saito, S., Atano, K., *et al.* (1957). *Gann*, **48**, 1–63.

Slade, J. (1993). In *Nicotine addiction, principles and management* (ed. C. Orleans and J. Slade), pp. 3–23. Oxford University Press, New York.

Sugiura, K. (1956). *Gann*, **47**, 243–4.

Swedish Medical Research Council (1958). Statement to the King.

Thun, M., Day-Lally, C., Meyers, D., Calle, E., Flanders, W., Namboodiri, M., *et al.* (1997). In *Monograph 8: Changes in cigarette-related disease risks and their implication for prevention and control* (ed. D. Burns, L. Garfinkel and J. Samet). National Institutes of Health, Bethesda, Maryland.

Thun, M., Calle, E., Rodriguez, C., and Wingo, P. (2000). *Cancer Epidemiology, Biomarkers and Prevention*, **9**, 861–8.

Tylecote, F. (1927). *Lancet*, **2**, 256–7.

US Department of Health and Human Services (1989). *Reducing the health consequences of smoking: 25 years of progress. A Report of the Surgeon General.* US Department of Health and Human Services, Public Health Service, Centers for Disease Control, Center for Chronic Disease Prevention and Health Promotion, Office on Smoking and Health, Rockville, Maryland.

US Department of Health and Human Services (2001). *Women and smoking: A report of the Surgeon General.* US Department of Health and Human Services, Centers for Disease Control and Prevention, National Center for Chronic Disease Prevention and Health Promotion, Office on Smoking and Health, Atlanta, Georgia.

US Public Health Service (1964). *Smoking and health. Report of the Advisory Committee to the Surgeon General of the Public Health Service.* US Department of Health, Education, and Welfare, Public Health Service, Center for Disease Control, Washington.

US Public Health Service (1967). *The health consequences of smoking. A Public Health Review: 1967.* US Department of Health, Education, and Welfare, Public Health Service, Center for Disease Control, Washington.

Wassink, W. (1948). *Nederlands Tijdschrift voor Geneeskunde (Amsterdam)*, **92**, 3732–47.

World Health Organization (1960). *Epidemiology of cancer of the lung.* Report of a study group. WHO Technical Report Series 192. World Health Organization, Geneva.

Wynder, E. and Graham, E. (1950). *Journal of the American Medical Association*, **143**, 329–36.

Wynder, E., Graham, E., and Croninger, A. (1953). *Cancer Research*, **13**, 855–64.

Wynder, E., Graham, E., and Croninger, A. (1955). *Cancer Research*, **15**, 445–8.

Chapter 3

Dealing with health fears: Cigarette advertising in the United States in the twentieth century

Lynn T. Kozlowski and Richard J. O'Connor

Since the beginning of the twentieth century, cigarette advertising in the United States has been largely an effort to deal with the health fears related to smoking. Three main techniques have been used: reassurance, misdirection of attention, and inducements to be brave in the face of fear. Others have also considered the history of cigarette advertising and carried out content analyses (Warner 1985; McCaullife 1988; Pollay 1989; Ringold and Calfee 1989; Cohen 1992). This chapter depends on this earlier work and is an extension of an earlier paper on the topic (Kozlowski 2000). Note that we focus on advertising in the United States—similar themes have been examined in Canadian advertising (see Pollay 2002).

Background

In the 1890s, the leading tobacco companies became organized in a large commercial conglomerate (Heimann 1960). By 1910, the large majority of tobacco products sold in the United States were sold by this group. This monopoly was prosecuted under the Sherman Anti-trust Act and, as a result, was broken up into separate companies in 1911. When the R. J. Reynolds Tobacco Company became a separate company again, as part of this action, it was given no established cigarette brand as part of the settlement (Tilley 1985); Richard Joshua Reynolds responded by creating a new brand. Earlier, he had been successful with a burley-based pipe tobacco blend called Prince Albert, and soon developed a new cigarette brand that made heavy use of burley tobacco in the blend (Heimann 1960). Camel® was introduced in 1913 as a cheaper cigarette with a milder, novel taste. Backed by a national advertising campaign, sales of Camel® cigarettes rose from 1 145 000 cigarettes shipped in the first year, to 2 255 310 000 in 1915, 11 923 640 000 in 1917, and 31 424 218 000 in 1924 (Tilley 1985). It was the leading cigarette of the period. Three national cigarette brands dominated cigarette sales for the first 50 years of the twentieth century: Camel® (R. J. Reynolds), Lucky Strike® (American Tobacco), and Chesterfield® (Liggett and Myers).

The risks of smoking were known

Many smokers at that time were likely to have been aware of health concerns about tobacco. In the late 1800s and early 1900s, the Anti-Cigarette League, under the direction of Lucy Page Gaston, helped spread the word about the dangers of cigarettes (Tate 1999). States had even placed bans on cigarettes. See Tate (1999) for a detailed account of anti-smoking activities, many directed specifically at the dangers to health of cigarette smoking (cf. Robert 1967). There were also widespread concerns in the newspapers about possible impurities, adulterants, and dirty conditions involved in cigarette making (see Young 1917).

President Ulysses S. Grant died a very public death due to throat cancer, and Patterson (1989) has argued that this death of a famous cigar smoker contributed greatly to fear of tobacco-caused cancer in the United States around the turn of the century. A prevailing theory of cancer during the early twentieth century held that cancers were caused by 'irritation' (Patterson 1989). This model proposed that excessive use of tobacco irritated the linings of the throat and mouth, eventually leading to cancerous growths. ('Moderate' tobacco use was viewed as not especially dangerous, even if definitions of moderate and excessive were far from clear—see Young 1917). At this time, cigarettes were a small fraction of the market, and excessive pipe and cigar use were implicated in oral cancers; lung cancer was virtually unheard of at the time (Patterson 1989). Since cigarettes were so mild they could be inhaled, they could be positioned as the obviously safer form of tobacco use (Kozlowski 1982).

During the first few decades of the twentieth century, few laws or guidelines impeded the marketing of cigarettes or the claims that could be made about them. Manufacturers were free to say just about anything they wanted. Once restrictions were enacted, manufacturers could not directly claim safety or healthfulness of their products. Therefore, they had to use alternative routes (within the bounds of the restrictions) to convince customers that smoking was less dangerous than critics claimed. The claims made by manufacturers about cigarettes might be seen both as what was most advantageous for manufacturers to say, and what consumers most desired to hear: cigarettes are safe, and you can continue to smoke. Over the years, the messages have been varied; reassurance, misdirection of attention, and inducements to be brave in the face of fear are three themes that recur repeatedly.

Reassurance

This theme attacks the health issue straight on, offering ways to smoke 'safely'. Various technical 'innovations' over the years have been advertised as 'health protection'. Reassurance marketing began early—consider the text of a 1932 advertisement for Lucky Strike®:

> Do you inhale?
>   What's there to be afraid of? 7 out of 10 inhale knowingly the other 3 do so unknowingly.
> Do you inhale? Lucky Strike meets the vital issue fairly and squarely … for it has solved the vital

problem. Its famous purifying process removes certain impurities that are concealed in even the choicest, mildest tobacco leaves. Luckies created that process. Only Lucky's have it!

(cited in Brecher et al. 1963)

It later proclaims: 'IT'S TOASTED! *Your protection against irritation, against cough*' (as cited in Brecher *et al.* 1963). This advertisement sets Lucky Strike® apart from other cigarettes as purer and safer to inhale. What supposedly sets 'Luckies' apart is their special processing, which removes unspecified impurities (a technical 'innovation'). Other ads at the time touted cigarettes as so healthful athletes could smoke them without affecting their performance (see Lewine 1970).

Filter tips and the 'tar derby'

The introduction of the filter tip, and the concomitant 'tar derby', is one of the best examples of reassurance marketing. Beginning in the 1950s, concern began to appear about the tar content of cigarettes and its relationship to disease (e.g. Wynder and Graham 1950; Doll and Hill 1952). Although manufacturers have argued that the introduction of filter tips was only circumstantially related to health concerns (e.g. Tilley 1985), recently revealed industry documents tell a different story. Ernest Pepples, Vice-President and General Counsel for Brown and Williamson Tobacco, noted in 1976 that 'the manufacturers' marketing strategy has been to overcome and *even to make marketing use of* the smoking/health connection [emphasis added]' (as cited in Glantz *et al.* 1996). Pepples wrote that the smoker had abandoned regular (unfiltered cigarettes) because of health concerns, and that '… the 'tar derby' in the United States resulted from industry efforts to cater to the public's concern and to attract consumers to the new filtered brands' (as cited in Glantz *et al.* 1996).

Filters, although they appeared as early as the 1930s, did not begin to become popular until the 1950s. During this time, filters made of paper, asbestos, and cellulose acetate, among other materials, were attached to cigarettes. Kents® were promoted as the 'greatest health protection in cigarette history' (an ironic claim given the Micronite filter contained asbestos). Other manufacturers were making similar claims regarding the health benefits of their filters (see Table 3.1).

At the height of the tar derby of the late 1950s, the United States Congress held a hearing on false and misleading advertising of filter-tip cigarettes (False and Misleading Advertising 1957), now known as the Blatnik report (Tilley 1985; see Kozlowski 2000 for discussion). During the hearing, the then Federal Trade Commission (FTC) chairman, Sechrest, testified about the Cigarette Advertising Guides developed by his agency (15 September 1955). The Guide specifically prohibited health or physical claims, forbade linking filters to such claims, and eliminated false testimonials. All this seems to have been a legitimate effort to eliminate the most far-fetched health claims. Chairman Sechrest noted that: 'Prior to the issuance of the guides, cigarette advertising generally involved health claims. Since their issuance, the theme of all such advertising,

Table 3.1 Advertising slogans from the tar derby era[a]

Kent® (one of the first lower tar and nicotine cigarettes)	
1952	'No other cigarette approaches such a degree of health protection and taste satisfaction.'
	'Because this filter is exclusive with KENT, it is possible to say that no other cigarette offers smokers such a degree of health protection and taste satisfaction.'
L&M®	
1953	'...Alpha Cellulose. Exclusive to L&M Filters, and entirely pure and harmless to health.'
1954	'L&M Filters are Just What the Doctor Ordered!'
Parliament®	
1952	'...like millions today, you are turning to filter cigarettes for pleasure plus protection ... it's important that you know the Parliament Story.'
Philip Morris	
1954	'The cigarette that takes the FEAR out of smoking!'
Viceroy®	
1951	'*Filtered* cigarette smoke is better for your health.'
1953	'New King-Size Viceroy gives *Double*-Barreled Health Protection ... is safer for throat, safer for lungs than any other king-size cigarette.'

[a]The slogans come from various sources, including: Lewine (1970), Harris (1978), Sobel (1978), Mullen (1979), Glantz *et al.* (1996).

including that of filter tips, has centered around *taste and flavor*' (False and Misleading Advertising 1957, p. 304). This is a key concept, for the FTC's guide stated quite clearly, '...*Nothing contained in these guides is intended to prohibit the use of any representation, claim, or illustration relating solely to taste, flavor, aroma, or enjoyment* [emphasis added]'.

By 1956, the most egregious health claims had vanished, and statements regarding taste and flavor proliferated. In 1960, the industry and the FTC concluded an agreement to eliminate tar information from advertising. In 1964, the Surgeon-General's Report was released (USDHEW 1964), reporting a dose–response relationship between number of cigarettes and disease. This report was seen to encourage using filter cigarettes, as well as those with less tar.

During the 1960s, both the American Cancer Society and *Reader's Digest* criticized the loss of tar information in cigarette advertising. The FTC maintained that any claims had to be supported by objective evidence, and so they began to seek input on devising a standardized test for tar and nicotine content (for a review, see Peeler 1996). FTC Commissioner Sechrest was worried that standardized testing might lead consumers to say, 'I want the one with the least tar' (False and Misleading Advertising 1957, p. 303), which might be a health issue. In 1966, the FTC announced that tar and nicotine statements were not considered health claims, and instituted its cigarette testing program the following year. This opened the door for manufacturers to develop a cigarette that could make health claims implicitly, rather than explicitly: the Light cigarette.

Light cigarettes

Light cigarettes were the natural extension of the tar derby of the 1950s. Since tar was linked to lung cancer, the most dreaded smoking-related disease, smokers would naturally be attracted to products that reduced tar to lower and lower levels. So, lower-tar cigarettes were reassuring, particularly when combined with a consoling name such as 'Light' that implied fewer toxins and purity at the same time (more on this point later).

Several design changes can reduce standard tar and nicotine numbers (for a review, see Kozlowski *et al.* 2001). Probably the most important is filter ventilation (Kozlowski *et al.* 1998a). This introduces air into the mainstream smoke, diluting it and reducing standard machine measurements. However, filter ventilation does not necessarily reduce the amounts of tar and nicotine delivered to smokers, in that smokers are able to compensate for the dilution, primarily by taking bigger puffs, or by blocking the vents with their lips or fingers (Kozlowski and Pillitteri 1996; Kozlowski and O'Connor 2002). For brands with less than 60 per cent ventilation, small increases in puff volume will adequately compensate for the dilution, while for heavily ventilated brands (greater than 60 per cent), vent blocking is more important for compensation.

The Light cigarette increased in popularity in the 1970s, when Light versions of established brands began to appear, and smokers began to switch from 'Full-Flavor' to 'Light' brands (National Cancer Institute 2001). The sales-weighted average tar yield dropped from 21.6 mg in 1968 to 12.0 mg in 1997, a 44.4 per cent decline. See the recent National Cancer Institute (2001) monograph on Lights for a more detailed overview of the product and its epidemiology.

The Light cigarette took full advantage of the allowable advertising claims (Glantz *et al.* 1996). Internal memos from the time show that these products were marketed precisely to keep smokers who were concerned about their health from quitting by offering them a 'safer' smoke. One Brown and Williamson employee wrote:

> All work in this area [communications] should be directed towards providing *consumer reassurance* [emphasis in original] about cigarettes and the smoking habit … by claiming low deliveries, by the perception of low deliveries and by the perception of 'mildness'. Furthermore, the advertising for low delivery or traditional brands should be constructed in ways so as not to provoke anxiety about health, but to alleviate it, and enable the smoker to feel assured about the habit and confident in maintaining it over time.

> (Short 1977)

Amercian Tobacco (Carlton®) and R. J. Reynolds (Now®) competed for the lowest-yield cigarette, and positioned these brands as having the lowest recorded tar and nicotine levels (even though the hard-pack versions that measured the lowest were generally unavailable in stores; Pollay and Dewhirst 2001). Now® was described as a 'break-through' (1980, as cited in Pollay and Dewhirst 2001), while Carlton® advertisements claimed that 'Latest U.S. Gov't Laboratory test confirms, of all cigarettes: Carlton is lowest' (1985, as cited in Pollay and Dewhirst 2001). In 1980, Brown and Williamson introduced Barclay®, a cigarette they promoted as '99 per cent Tar Free' (as cited in Pollay and Dewhirst 2001). However, this cigarette employed a unique ventilation system that was subject to easy compensation, so much so that Brown and Williamson's competitors sued to stop the cigarette's low-tar claim (*FTC* v. *Brown and Williamson* 1985). A campaign for True® cigarettes was explicit about reassurance: 'Considering all I'd heard [presumably about smoking and health], I decided to either quit or smoke True. I smoke True' (as cited in Pollay and Dewhirst 2001). This sort of advertisement allowed smokers to conclude that some cigarettes were a reasonable alternative to quitting, and indeed many smokers were lulled into a false sense of security by Lights (National Cancer Institute 2001).

A secondary effect of ventilation is that it makes the smoke actually taste 'lighter'. That is, even though smokers are very likely not getting less tar and nicotine per cigarette, each puff tastes lighter than a puff of equivalent yield on a regular cigarette (Kozlowski and O'Connor 2002). In national surveys, smokers note that Lights do taste lighter (e.g. Kozlowski *et al.* 1998*b*), and industry studies note that adding ventilation can significantly reduces smokers' ratings of 'irritation', 'impact', and increase ratings of 'mildness' (Anderson 1979; Hirji 1980; Philip Morris 1989).

To sell lower-tar cigarettes to a public used to higher-tar brands, manufacturers had to convince the public that the new cigarettes would offer the same satisfaction or great taste that their old cigarettes did, but still be less dangerous. However, the advertisements also had to deal with issues of lighter taste and satisfaction. Consider a 1972 Vantage® advertisement:

> Anyone who's old enough to smoke is old enough to make up his own mind.
>
> By now, as an adult, you must have read and heard all that's been written and said for and against cigarettes. And come to your own conclusions … if you like to smoke and have decided to continue, we'd like to tell you a few facts about a cigarette you might like to continue with … Vantage gives you real flavor like any high 'tar' and nicotine cigarette you ever smoked, without the high 'tar' and nicotine. And since it is the high 'tar' and nicotine that many critics seem most opposed to, even they should have some kind words for Vantage. We don't want to mislead you. Vantage is not the lowest 'tar' and nicotine cigarette. But, it is the lowest 'tar and nicotine cigarette you'll enjoy smoking. It has only 12 milligrams 'tar' and 0.9 mg nicotine. With anything lower, you'd have to work so hard getting taste through the filter that you'd end up going back to your old brand…
>
> (R. J. Reynolds 1972)

This advertisement promises that the cigarette will: (1) deliver less tar and nicotine (implicitly healthier); and, at the same time, (2) still deliver good taste. This doubly reassures the smoker that he can continue to smoke, with reduced health risk but without losing the taste and pleasure he enjoys. It implies that health advocates who say tar and nicotine are dangerous might have 'kind words' for Vantage®. The 'work so hard' phrase acknowledges that compensatory smoking can require significant effort, but reassures the smoker that Vantage® will not be like that. Other brands have been marketed using similar tactics (see Table 3.2).

Table 3.2 Selected slogans for Light cigarette brands, 1970s to 1990s

Merit®	
1980	Merit Wins Taste Honors. Research establishes low tar MERIT as proven taste alternative to high tar smoking. [20610112428][a]
1992	Merit introduces surprising flavor at only 1 mg tar. [20610071836][a]
1996	(Merit) Yes! Yes, you can switch down from full flavor and still get satisfying taste. [206100073377][a]
True®	
1974	New. True 100's. Lower in both tar and nicotine than 98% of all other 100's sold. [502293758][b]
1974	Is new True 100 lower in tar than your 100? Tests for tar and nicotine by U.S. Gov't Method prove it. New True 100 mm is lowest in both tar and nicotine of all these leading 100 mm cigarettes [lists several brands]. [502293760][b]
Vantage®	
1971	(Vantage). You don't cop out. We don't cop out. You demand good taste. But want low 'tar' and nicotine. Only Vantage gives you both.[c]
Triumph®	
1980	TRIUMPH BEATS MERIT! Triumph, at less than half the tar, preferred over Merit. Taste the UMPH! in Triumph at only 3 mg tar.[c]
Barclay®	
1981	Barclay. 99% Tar Free. The pleasure is back.[c]
Winston Lights®	
1976	Most low 'tar' cigarettes have no taste. A lot of new cigarettes give you low 'tar' and nicotine numbers. But I can't taste numbers. What I can taste is Winston Lights. I get lower 'tar' and nicotine. But I still get real taste. And real pleasure. For me, Winston Lights are for real. [515222693][b]
Kent Golden Lights®	
1976	Kent Golden Lights. As low as you can go and still get good taste and smoking satisfaction ... Kent Golden Lights. Tastes so good, you won't believe the numbers. [500331489][b]

[a] Available at http://www.pmadarchive.com

[b] Available at http://www.rjrtdocs.com

[c] As cited in National Cancer Institute (2001).

Reassurance marketing has not abated, even into a new century. Consider the advertisements for Omni™ that have appeared recently:

> NEW! Omni.™ Reduced Carcinogens. Premium Taste. Introducing the first premium cigarette created to significantly reduce carcinogenic PAH's, nitrosamines, catechols, and organics, which are the major causes of lung cancer in smokers.
>
> (Vector Tobacco 2001)

> What happens to a [picture of cigarette] when you reduce carcinogens? You get a really good tasting smoke. The only cigarette to significantly reduce carcinogens that are among the major causes of lung cancer. The only one to still deliver premium taste. The only one to finally give smokers a real reason to switch. Only Omni.™
>
> (Vector Tobacco 2002)

The advertisements feature disclaimers, in smaller type, noting that reductions in carcinogens are not proven to make a cigarette safer. Still, the offer of 'reduced carcinogens at a premium taste' is likely to be very reassuring to the health-concerned smoker. These advertisements resemble early 'tar derby' ads by making a nearly explicit health claim, small-print disclaimers notwithstanding.

Reassurance marketing took different forms over time, but all of them aimed to keep smokers smoking by encouraging them to believe that smoking was less dangerous. The addition of filters and their aggressive marketing, followed by the introduction of Lights, fostered the notion that cigarettes were getting safer without needing to say so directly. Smokers were doubly reassured that their cigarettes were giving them less deadly tar, but would still taste good enough to keep them satisfied, and the lighter taste of Lights helped convince smokers that Lights were safer for them.

Misdirection of attention

Reassurance marketing can go only so far to convince consumers to keep smoking. Misdirection of attention, as an advertising theme, only indirectly engages the health issue. Instead of directly confronting the health issue with reassurance, advertising simply focuses on other attributes of the product that are consistent with reduced risk. From the earliest days, cigarettes were promoted for their mildness and for their ability to satisfy. Table 3.3 lists slogans from the first decades of the twentieth century. Note the prominence of the 'mild' theme.

To understand how misdirection of attention can work to deflect health concerns, one must understand how words can relate to one another. Kozlowski (2000) has described how 'hyponomy', or the heiarchical organization of words under broader concepts, relates to cigarette advertising. By mentioning 'mild', for example, one can extend its meaning in several directions, following the hyponymic branches. Antonyms such as 'harsh' can come to mind, as well as concepts such as 'good', 'safe', 'not irritating'. Crucial hyponyms of 'good' are 'pleasantness' and 'safety'. Basically, positive terms such

Table 3.3 Selected cigarette advertising slogans, early twentieth century[a]

1929	[Chesterfield] 'MILD … and yet THEY SATISFY'
1929	[Lucky Strike®] '20,679 physicians have confirmed the fact that Lucky Strike is less irritating in the throat than other cigarettes'
1936	[Philip Morris] '… tests proved conclusively that after changing to Philip Morris, every case of irritation due to smoking cleared completely or definitely improved'
1937	[Camel®] 'They're so mild and never make my throat harsh or rough'
1938	[Viceroy®] 'Viceroy's filter neatly checks the throat-irritants in tobacco … Safer smoke for any throat. Inhale without discomfort'
1943	[Viceroy®] '… filtering the flavor and aroma of the world's finest tobaccos into the smoothest of blends and checking OUT resins, tar and throat irritants that can spoil the EVENNESS of smoking enjoyment!'
1946	[Camel®] 'More Doctors Smoke Camels Than Any Other Cigarette'

[a]The slogans come from various sources, including: Lewine (1970), Harris (1978), Sobel (1978), Mullen (1979), Glantz et al. (1996).

as 'pleasantness', 'mildness', 'tastiness', or 'mellowness' evoke 'goodness', which is a hyponym for 'healthful'. If something is 'mild', 'mellow', or 'Light', it is unlikely to be 'unhealthful'. The health issue does not need to be engaged directly, because evoking the semantic networks associated with taste and satisfaction can be enough to influence the consumer's thinking that the cigarette isn't so bad.

Some words or phrases, called tropes, are used in a non-literal way that still carries important meaning (Bloom 1975). In the current case, 'light', 'smooth', 'mild' are all tropes that carry meanings for consumers: less irritating, less risky, less deadly. Those in the industry, and their supporters, often claim that Light labels are justified because Lights actually deliver less tar to machines than 'full-flavors'. However, humans do not smoke like machines. Smokers generally believe that tar numbers reflect what they are inhaling, and that lower-tar cigarettes are safer (see Rickert et al. 1989; Giovino et al. 1996). Surveys of American smokers show that 39 per cent ($n = 360$) of Light and 58 per cent ($n = 218$) of Ultra-light smokers state that *they smoke their brands to reduce the risks of smoking* (Kozlowski et al. 1998b). A Light cigarette, to the consumer, must seem similar to Light ice cream, or Light beer—indicating that they are actually ingesting less of something (fat or calories in the cases of ice cream and beer, tar in the case of cigarettes). The meaning of *Light* as 'lower standard tar yield' is only a 'technical truth' that should not carry assumptions about reduced risk [cf. *P. Lorillard Co.* v. *FTC* (1950)]. *Light* is also a trope referring to 'more pure' and 'not as dangerous' (and literally, 'not heavy'). It makes implicit health and safety claims. Groups in both the United States, and Canada have called for a ban on Light descriptors (National Cancer Institute 2001; Ministerial Advisory Council on Tobacco Control 2002).

Inducements to bravery

A third way advertisers can encourage smokers to keep smoking is to help them identify with being a risk-taker. Without acknowledging the risks of smoking, advertising creates an image of smoking that encompasses bravery, risk taking, and other positive images. The best known, and most successful, of these campaigns has been the cowboy of Philip Morris' Marlboro® brand (the world's best-selling brand).

Marlboro® advertisements generally have little text, but contain strong imagery. Marlboro® print ads often involve obviously dangerous activities, such as bronco-riding or roping horses. By linking smoking with such activites, smoking is acknowledged as dangerous, but possessing similar dangers to those encountered by the Marlboro® cowboy in his life. These images have been extended to Marlboro® Lights (1970s) and Marlboro® Ultra Lights (1990s). Consider an advertisement for Marlboro® Lights (Philip Morris 1976): 'The spirit of Marlboro in a low tar cigarette'. This text is accompanied by a painting of the Marlboro® cowboy riding with horses, seemingly traveling rather quickly. Marlboro® Lights and Ultra Lights might be seen as cigarettes for the cowboy who might be concerned for his health, but not so concerned that he would give up his exciting life style, or his favorite smoke.

R.J. Reynolds has used similar themes to market Camel® Filters and Camel® Lights. In the late 1970s and early 1980s, male smokers were variously seen sitting around campfires with mountains in the background (Pollay Collection, Camel 19.13), canoeing (Pollay Archive, Camel 16.16), whitewater rafting (Pollay Collection, Camel 26.14), driving Jeeps up mountains (Pollay Collection, Camel 34.15), and arm wrestling (Pollay Collection, Camel 10.01) (advertisements available in the Richard W. Pollay 20th Century Tobacco Advertisement Collection at http://roswell.tobaccodocuments.org/pollay/dirdet.cfm). Tag lines proclaimed 'Share a new adventure' and 'Where a man belongs'. During the Joe Camel promotion, Joe was depicted water skiing (Pollay Collection, Camel 20.14), riding motorcycles (Pollay Collection, Camel 35.15), windsailing (Pollay Collection, Camel 20.13), and driving race cars (Pollay Collection, Camel 20.19). He was even seen in a bombadier jacket with fighter jets behind him (Pollay Collection, Camel 27.14). Clearly these images are meant to set the Camel® smoker apart as adventurous and masculine—someone willing to take on the risks of smoking.

Consumer perception and types of persuasion

The *raison d'être* of advertising is to convince consumers to buy and use a particular product, often by convincing them it is the right thing to do (for an overview, see Jones 1998). People generally want to believe the 'right' thing (Cacioppo *et al.* 1996). That is, people do not like to be wrong. Advertisements that present messages aimed at persuading individuals are likely to be consciously processed by consumers. But argument also invites evaluation. Consumers then have the opportunity to consider what is being said, what points are being made, what arguments are being advanced, and who the source is. This is known as the 'central route to persuasion' (cf. Petty *et al.* 1983). Advertisements that rely on reassurance generally follow this route. When a message contains no arguments, however, a 'peripheral route to persuasion' is involved (cf. Petty *et al.* 1983). Little conscious scrutiny is involved: the attractiveness of the images and positive feelings become influential. Ads that rely on misdirection of attention or inducement to bravery involve peripheral persuasion heavily. A claim that a cigarette is Light or Mild or Smooth is not something for which objective evidence can be produced. Similarly, imagery alone is not subject to evaluation in the same way as a claim of 'great taste, less tar'. When an advertisement makes the case that cigarette X is not as dangerous, central processing is engaged. Consumers may or may not be persuaded by the information provided. However, when a cowboy sits alone in the desert smoking a cigarette, the heart and mind process the imagery and are unencumbered by conscious information processing.

An overall effect of the FTC's advertising guidelines, which were enacted to prevent cigarette makers from making specific (unsupportable) claims, was to encourage advertising based on subtle implications and symbolism related to taste and satisfaction (Kozlowski 2002). However, since 'health protection' messages may remind the consumer that their health needed protection (i.e. cigarettes are dangerous), eliminating health claims may have benefited manufacturers. Making use of semantic networks allows manufacturers to imply safety without ever having to say the word. This also has the added benefit of not needing objective evidence—for example, the smokers' own judgement, that the cigarette tastes lighter, can be enough to substantiate the claim. By using the peripheral route of persuasion, manufacturers run less risk of consumers rejecting the message by evaluation, because the Marlboro® cowboy is unevaluable—he simply is. Consumers can accept or reject new charcoal filters, exclusive blends, and even claims about better taste, but Joe Camel the fighter pilot, and the name Merit Ultra Light are much harder to dismiss.

Advertising since the Master Settlement Agreement

The Master Settlement Agreement, entered into by 47 states' attorneys general and the major cigarette manufacturers, set new guidelines for advertising, primarily aimed at reducing appeals to children. Billboards, product placements, and advertisements in magazines with large youth readership were banned (National Association of Attorneys General 2002). However, the agreement did not address the crucial advertising issues discussed in this chapter (National Association of Attorneys General 2002). The Marlboro® cowboy is alive and well. Omni® implies that its cigarettes are safer. Only recently have counter-marketing efforts begun to correct consumers' misapprehensions surrounding Light cigarettes (e.g. Kozlowski *et al.* 1999, 2000; Shiffman *et al.* 2001*a, b*). Both Brown and Williamson and Philip Morris, perhaps responding to such countermarketing, have added disclaimers to their listings of

FTC test results in advertising: Brown and Williamson: 'Actual deliveries will vary based on how you hold and smoke your cigarette'; Philip Morris: 'The amount of 'tar' and nicotine you inhale will vary depending on how you smoke the cigarette'.

Because the MSA made no provisions for the advertising themes discussed in this chapter, manufacturers remain free to use health fears to market their products.

Conclusions

Cigarette advertising in the United States since the beginning of the 20th century has been an enterprise in reducing health fears around smoking. Advertisements have relied on three basic themes. Some ads reassure smokers that (1) new developments are making cigarettes safer, and (2) these developments will not remove the flavor and enjoyment from smoking. Others use tropes and semantic networks to imply safety without actually making explicit health claims. A third class of ads uses imagery to convince smokers that smoking might be risky, but is worth the risk. By allowing imagery and claims based on taste, regulators opened the door for manufacturers to subtly suggest that cigarettes were becoming less dangerous and that consumers could continue to smoke.

References

Anderson, P. (1979). HTI test of production Marlboro 85 versus Marlboro 85, Model '1' with 10% dilution and no reduction in tar delivery. Philip Morris. Available at http://www.pmdocs.com (Bates Number 2040077052).

Bloom, H. (1975). *A map of misreading.* Oxford University Press, Oxford.

Brecher, R., Brecher, E., Herzog, A., Goodman, W., and Walker, G. (ed.) (1963). *The consumers union report on smoking and public interest.* Consumers Union, Mount Vernon, New York.

Cacioppo, J. T., Petty, R. E., Feinstien, J. A., Blair, W., and Jarvis, G. (1996). Dispositional differences in cognitive motivation: The life and times of individuals varying in need for cognition. *Psychological Bulletin,* **119**, 197–253.

Cohen, J. B. (1992). Research and policy issues in Ringold and Calfee's treatment of cigarette health claims. *Journal of Public Policy and Marketing,* **11**, 82–6.

Doll, R. and Hill, A. B. (1952). A study of the aetiology of carcinoma of the lung. *British Medical Journal,* 1271–82.

False and Misleading Advertising (Filter-tip cigarettes) (1957). Hearings before a subcommittee of the Committee on Government Operations, House of Representatives, 85th Congress, First Session, (18–26 July). John A. Blatnik, chair.

FTC v. Brown and Williamson Tobacco Corporation (1985). 580. SUPP 981 (D.C.C., 1983), 778F.2d 35 (D.C.CIR. 1985).

Giovino, G. A., Tomar, S. L., Reddy, M. N., Peddicord, J. P., Zhu, B. P., Escobedo, L. G., *et al.* (1996). Attitudes, knowledge and beliefs about low-yield cigarettes among adolescents and adults. In: *The FTC cigarette test method for determining tar, nicotine, and carbon monoxide yields of U.S. cigarettes: report of the NCI Expert Committee,* pp. 39–57. National Cancer Institute, US Department of Health and Human Services, Bethesda, Maryland.

Glantz, S. A., Slade, J., Bero, L. A., Hanauer, P., and Barnes, D. E. (1996). *The cigarette papers.* University of California Press, Berkeley.

Harris, R. W. (1978). *How to keep on smoking and live.* St. Martin's Press, New York.

Heimann, R. K. (1960). *Tobacco and Americans.* McGraw-Hill, New York.

Hirji, T. (1980). Effects of paper permeability, filtration, and tip ventilation on deliveries, impact, and irritation. British American Tobacco. Available at http://www.bw.aalatg.com (Bates Number 650331009).

Jones, J. P. (ed.) (1998). *How advertising works: the role of research.* Sage, Thousand Oaks, California.

Kozlowski, L. T. (1982). The determinants of tobacco use: Cigarettes in the context of other forms of tobacco use. *Canadian Journal of Public Health,* **73**, 236–41.

Kozlowski, L. T. and O'Connor, R. J. (2002). Filter ventilation is a defective design because of lighter taste, bigger puffs, and blocked vents. *Tobacco Control,* **11**(Suppl. 1), i40–i50.

Kozlowski, L. T. and Pillitteri, J. L. (1996). Compensation for nicotine by smokers of lower yield cigarettes. In *The FTC cigarette test method for determining tar, nicotine, and carbon monoxide yields of U.S. cigarettes: report of the NCI Expert Committee.* National Cancer Institute, US Department of Health and Human Services, Bethesda, Maryland.

Kozlowski, L. T., Mehta, N. Y., Sweeney, C. T., Schwartz, S. S., Vogler, G. P., Jarvis, M. J., *et al.* (1998*a*). Filter ventilation and nicotine content of tobacco in cigarettes from Canada, the United Kingdom, and the United States. *Tobacco Control,* **7**(4), 369–75.

Kozlowski, L. T., Goldberg, M. E., Yost, B. A., White, E. L., Sweeney, C. T., and Pillitteri, J. L. (1998*b*). Smokers' misperceptions of light and ultra-light cigarettes may keep them smoking. *American Journal of Preventive Medicine,* **15**, 9–16.

Kozlowski, L. T., Goldberg, M. E., Sweeney, C. T., Palmer, R. F., Pillitteri, J. L., Yost, B. A., *et al.* (1999). Smoker reactions to a 'radio message' that light cigarettes are as dangerous as regular cigarettes. *Nicotine and Tobacco Research,* **1**, 67–76.

Kozlowski, L. T., Yost, B., Stine, M. M., and Celebucki, C. (2000). Massachusetts' advertising against light cigarettes appears to change beliefs and behavior. *American Journal of Preventive Medicine,* **18**(4), 339–42.

Kozlowski, L. T. (2000). Some lessons from the history of American tobacco advertising and its regulations in the 20th century. In: R. Ferrence, J. Slade, R. Room, and M. Pope, *Nicotine and Public Health.* Washington DC: American Public Health Association.

Kozlowski, L. T., O'Connor, R. J., and Sweeney, C. T. (2001). Cigarette design. In: *Risks associated with smoking cigarettes having low machine-measured levels of tar and nicotine.* Smoking and Tobacco Control Monograph, No. 13. US Department of Health and Human Services, National Institutes of Health, National Cancer Institute, Bethesda, Maryland.

Lewine, H. (1970). *Good-bye to all that.* McGraw-Hill, New York.

P. Lorillard Co. v. FTC (1950). 6140, US Court of Appeals, 4th Circuit, 29 December, pp. 52–9.

McCaullife, R. (1988). The FTC and the effectiveness of cigarette advertising regulations. *Journal of Public Policy and Marketing,* **7**, 49–64.

Ministerial Advisory Council on Tobacco Control (2002). *Putting an End to the Deception: Proceedings of the International Expert Panel on Cigarette Descriptors.* Ottawa, ON: Canadian Council for Tobacco Control.

Mullen, C. (1979). *Cigarette pack art.* Totem Books, Toronto.

National Association of Attorneys General (2002). Multistate settlement with the tobacco industry. Available at: http://www.tobacco.neu.edu/Extra/multistate_settlement.htm.

National Cancer Institute (2001). *Risks associated with smoking cigarettes having low machine-measured levels of tar and nicotine.* Smoking and Tobacco Control Monograph, No. 13. US Department of Health and Human Services, National Institutes of Health, National Cancer Institute, Bethesda, Maryland.

Patterson, J. T. (1989). *The dread disease: Cancer and modern American culture.* Harvard University Press, Cambridge, Massachusetts.

Peeler, C. E. (1996). *Cigarette testing and the Federal Trade Commission: a historical overview. The FTC cigarette test method for determining tar, nicotine, and carbon monoxide yields of U.S. cigarettes.* Smoking and Tobacco Control Monograph, No. 7. National Cancer Institute, Bethesda, Maryland.

Petty, R. E., Cacioppo, J. T., and Schumann, D. (1983). Central and peripheral routes to advertising effectiveness: The moderating role of involvement. *Journal of Consumer Research*, **10**, 135–46.

Philip Morris (1976). Advertisement for Marlboro Lights cigarettes. Available at http://www.pmadarchive.com (Bates Number 2061015726).

Philip Morris (1989). Korea product tests. Philip Morris. Available at http://www.pmdocs.com (Bates Number 2504034439).

Pollay, R. W. (1989). Filters, flavor . . . flim-flam, too! On 'health information' and policy implications in cigarette advertising. *Journal of Public Policy and Marketing*, **8**, 30–9.

Pollay, R. W. and Dewhirst, T. (2001). Marketing cigarettes with low machine measured yields. In: National Cancer Institute, Risks Associated with Smoking Cigarettes with Low Machine-Measured Yields of Tar and Nicotine. Bethesda, MD: National Cancer Institute.

Pollay, R. W. (2002). *How cigarette advertising works: Rich imagery and poor information.* Tobacco Research Unit, Special Report Series, June 2002, Toronto, Ontario .

R. J. Reynolds (1972). Advertisement for Vantage cigarettes. Available at http://www.rjrtdocs.com (Bates Number 502612052).

Rickert, W. S., Robinson, J. C., and Lawless, E. (1989). Limitations to potential uses for data based on the machine smoking of cigarettes: Cigarette smoke contents. In: *Nicotine, smoking and the low tar programme* (ed. N. Wald and P. Froggatt), pp. 85–99. Oxford University Press, New York.

Ringold, D. J. and Calfee, J. E. (1989). The informational content of cigarette advertising: 1926–1986. *Journal of Public Policy and Marketing*, **8**, 1–23.

Robert, J. C. (1967). *The story of tobacco in America.* The University of North Carolina Press, Chapel Hill.

Shiffman, S., Pillitteri, J. L., Burton, S. L., Rohay, J. M., and Gitchell, J. G. (2001*a*). Effect of health messages about 'Light' and 'Ultra Light' cigarettes on beliefs and quitting intent. *Tobacco Control*, **10**(Suppl 1), i24–i32.

Shiffman, S., Burton, S. L., Pillitteri, J. L., Gitchell, J. G., Di Marino, M. E., Sweeney, C. T., *et al.* (2001*b*). Test of 'Light' cigarette counter-advertising using a standard test of advertising effectiveness. *Tobacco Control*, **10**(Suppl 1), i33–i40.

Short, P. L. (1977). *Smoking and health item 7: The effect on marketing.* BATCO, April 14. (Minnesota Exhibit 030).

Sobel, R. (1978). *They satisfy: The cigarette in American life.* Doubleday, New York.

Tate, C. (1999). *Cigarette Wars: The Triumph of the Little White Slaves.* Oxford: Oxford University Press.

Tilley, N.M. (1985). *The R.J. Reynolds Tobacco Company.* The University of North Carolina Press, Chapel Hill.

US Department of Health, Education, and Welfare (1964). *Smoking and health: Report of the advisory committee to the Surgeon General of the Public Health Service, 1964.* Public Health Publication, No. 1103. US Public Health Service, Washington DC.

Vector Tobacco (2001). Advertisement for Omni cigarettes. *Parade*, 23 December.

Vector Tobacco (2002). Advertisement for Omni cigarettes. *Playboy*, June.

Warner, K. E. (1985). Tobacco industry response to public health concern: A content analysis of cigarette ads. *Health Education Quarterly*, **12**, 115–27.

Wynder, E. L. and Graham, E. (1950). Tobacco smoking as a possible etiologic factor in bronchiogenic carcinoma: a study of 684 proven cases. *Journal of the American Medical Association*, 143, 329–36.

Yang, W. W. (1917). *The Story of the Cigarette.* New York: D. Appleton & Company.

Part 2

Tobacco: Composition

Chapter 4

The changing cigarette: Chemical studies and bioassays

Ilse Hoffmann and Dietrich Hoffmann

Introduction

In 1950, the first large-scale epidemiological studies on smoking and lung cancer (by Wynder and Graham in the United States and by Doll and Hill in the United Kingdom) strongly supported the concept of a dose response between the number of cigarettes smoked, and the risk for cancer of the lung (Doll and Hill 1950; Wynder and Graham 1950).

In 1953 the first successful induction of cancer in a laboratory animal with a tobacco product was reported, with the application of cigarette tar to mouse skin (Wynder *et al.* 1953). (Throughout this chapter, the term 'tar' is used as a descriptive noun only.) The particulate matter of cigarette smoke generated by an automatic smoking machine was suspended in acetone (1:1) and painted on to the shaven backs of mice three times weekly for up to 24 months. A clear dose response was observed between the amount of tar applied to the skin of mice and the percentage of animals in the test group bearing skin papillomas and carcinomas (Wynder *et al.* 1957). Since then, mouse skin has been widely used as the primary bioassay method for estimating the carcinogenic potency of tobacco tar and its fractions, as well as for particulate matters of other combustion products (Wynder and Hoffmann 1962, 1967; Hoffmann and Wynder 1977; National Cancer Institute 1977*a*, *b*, *c*, 1980; International Agency for Research on Cancer 1986*a*). Intratracheal instillation on rats of the polynuclear aromatic hydrocarbon (PAH)-containing neutral subfraction of cigarette tar led to squamous cell carcinoma of the trachea and lung (Davis *et al.* 1975). A cigarette tar suspension in acetone painted on to the inner ear of rabbits led to carcinoma, with metastasis in thoracic organs (Graham *et al.* 1957).

Dontenwill *et al.* (1973) developed a method whereby Syrian golden hamsters were placed, individually, into plastic tubes and exposed twice daily, 5 days a week, for up to 24 months to cigarette smoke diluted with air (1:15). The method led to lesions, primarily in the epithelial tissue of the outer larynx. Using an inbred strain of Syrian golden hamsters with increased susceptibility of the respiratory tract to carcinogens, long-term exposure to cigarette smoke produced a high tumor yield in the larynx

(Bernfeld *et al.* 1974). A dose response was recorded between the amount of smoke exposure and the induction of benign and malignant tumors in the larynges of the hamsters.

In general, inhalation studies with tobacco smoke have not led to squamous cell carcinoma of the lung (Wynder and Hoffmann 1967; Mohr and Reznik 1978; International Agency for Research on Cancer 1986*a*, *b*). Dalbey *et al.*, from the National Laboratory in Oak Ridge, Tennessee, exposed female F344 rats to diluted smoke of up to seven cigarettes daily, five times a week for up to 2.5 years. A high percentage of the smoke-exposed rats developed hyperplasia and metaplasia in the epithelium of the nasal turbinates and in the larynx, and also some hyperplasia in the trachea. The sham-treated rats developed a small number of lesions in nasal and laryngeal epithelia, but none in the trachea. Ten tumors of the respiratory system were observed in 7 out of 80 smoke-exposed rats. These were: 1 adenocarcinoma, 1 squamous cell carcinoma in the nasal cavity, 5 adenomas of the lung, 2 alveologenic carcinomas, and 1 squamous cell carcinoma of the lung (Dalbey *et al.* 1980). In the control group of 93 sham-exposed rats, one developed an alveologenic carcinoma (Dalbey *et al.* 1980). In 1952, Essenberg reported that cigarette smoke induces an excessive number of pulmonary adenomas, whereas the sham-exposed mice, as well as the untreated mice, developed significantly lower rates of pulmonary tumors. In the following years, the Leuchtenbergers repeatedly confirmed the findings by Essenberg. They also demonstrated that even the gas phase, as such, increased the occurrence of pulmonary tumors in mice (Leuchtenberger *et al.* 1958; Leuchtenberger and Leuchtenberger 1970). Several additional studies demonstrated the induction of pulmonary tumors in several strains of mice exposed to diluted cigarette smoke (Mühlbock 1955; Wynder and Hoffmann 1967; Mohr and Reznik 1978; International Agency for Research on Cancer 1986*a*, *b*). Otto (1963) exposed mice to diluted cigarette smoke for 60 min daily, for up to 24 months. Of 30 exposed mice, 4 developed lung adenomas, and 1, an epidermoid carcinoma of the lung. In the untreated control group, 3 of 60 mice developed lung adenomas.

Identification of carcinogens and tumor promoters in tobacco smoke

Green and Rodgman estimated that there were about 4800 compounds in tobacco smoke. In addition, several additives out of a list of 599 compounds disclosed by tobacco companies (Doull *et al.* 1994) may be added to cigarette tobacco during the manufacturing process in the United States (Doull *et al.* 1994; Green and Rodgman 1996). Tables 4.1 and 4.2 list the major constituents of the vapor phase (Table 4.1) and the particulate phase (Table 4.2), and their concentrations in the mainstream smoke (MS) of non-filter cigarettes (Ishiguro and Sugawara 1980; Hoffmann and Hecht 1990). Agricultural chemicals and pesticides, as well as their specific thermic degradation products, are omitted from the two tables because of the many variations in the nature and amounts of these agents in tobacco from country to country, and from year to year (Wittekindt 1985). Table 4.3 lists the major toxic components in the MS of cigarettes (Hoffmann and Hoffmann 1995).

Table 4.1 Major constituents of the vapor phase of the mainstream smoke of nonfilter cigarettes

Compound[a]	Concentration/cigarette (% of total effluent)
Nitrogen	280–320 mg (56–64%)
Oxygen	50–70 mg (11–14%)
Carbon dioxide	45–65 mg (9–13%)
Carbon monoxide	14–23 mg (2.8–4.6%)
Water	7–12 mg (1.4–2.4%)
Argon	5 mg (1.0%)
Hydrogen	0.5–1.0 mg
Ammonia	10–130 μg
Nitrogen oxides (NO_x)	100–600 μg
Hydrogen cyanide	400–500 μg
Hydrogen sulfide	20–90 μg
Methane	1.0–2.0 mg
Other volatile alkanes (20)	1.0–1.6 mg[b]
Volatile alkenes (16)	0.4–0.5 mg
Isoprene	0.2–0.4 mg
Butadiene	25–40 μg
Acetylene	20–35 μg
Benzene	12–50 μg
Toluene	20–60 μg
Styrene	10 μg
Other volatile aromatic hydrocarbons (29)	15–30 μg
Formic acid	200–600 μg
Acetic acid	300–1700 μg
Propionic acid	100–300 μg
Methyl formate	20–30 μg
Other volatile acids (6)	5–10 μg
Formaldehyde	20–100 μg

Table 4.1 (continued) Major constituents of the vapor phase of the mainstream smoke of nonfilter cigarettes

Compound[a]	Concentration/cigarette (% of total effluent)
Acetaldehyde	400–1400 µg
Acrolein	60–140 µg
Other volatile aldehydes (6)	80–140 µg
Acetone	100–650 µg
Other volatile ketones (3)	50–100 µg
Methanol	80–180 µg
Other volatile alcohols (7)	10–30 µg
Acetonitrile	100–150 µg
Other volatile nitriles (10)	50–80 µg[b]
Furan	20–40 µg
Other volatile furans (4)	45–125 µg[b]
Pyndine	20–200 µg
Picolines (3)	15–80 µg
3-Vinylpyridine	10–30 µg
Other volatile pyridines (25)	20–50 µg[b]
Pyrrole	0.1–10 µg
Pyrrolidine	10–18 µg
N-Methylpyrrolidine	2.0–3.0 µg
Volatile pyrazines (18)	3.0–8.0 µg
Methylamine	4–10 µg
Other aliphatic amines (32)	3–10 µg

[a]Numbers in parentheses represent the individual compounds identified in a given group.
[b]Estimate.

Table 4.2 Major constituents of the particulate matter of the mainstream smoke of nonfilter cigarettes

Compound[a]	µg/cigarette[b]
Nicotine	1000–3000
Nornicotine	50–150
Anatabine	5–15
Anabasine	5–12
Other tobacco alkaloids (17)	na
Bipyridyls (4)	10–30

Table 4.2 (continued) Major constituents of the particulate matter of the mainstream smoke of nonfilter cigarettes

Compound[a]	μg/cigarette[b]
n-Hentriacontane (n-$C_{31}H_{64}$)[c]	100
Total nonvolatile hydrocarbons (45)[c]	300–400[c]
Naphthalene	2–4
Naphthalenes (23)	3–6[c]
Phenanthrenes (7)	0.2–0.4[c]
Anthracenes (5)	0.05–0.1[c]
Fluorenes (7)	0.6–1.0[c]
Pyrenes (6)	0.3–0.5[c]
Fluoranthenes (5)	0.3–0.45[c]
Carcinogenic polynuclear aromatic hydrocarbons (11)[b]	0.1–0.25
Phenol	80–160
Other phenols (45)[c]	60–180[c]
Catechol	200–400
Other catechols (4)	100–200[c]
Other dihydroxybenzenes (10)	200–400[c]
Scopoletin	15–30
Other polyphenols (8)[c]	na
Cyclotenes (10)[c]	40–70[c]
Quinones (7)	0.50
Solanesol	600–1000
Neophytadienes (4)	200–350
Limonene	30–60
Other terpenes (200–250)[c]	na
Palmitic acid	100–150
Stearic acid	50–75
Oleic acid	40–110
Linoleic acid	150–250
Linolenic acid	150–250
Lactic acid	60–80
Indole	10–15
Skatole	12–16
Other indoles (13)	na
Quinolines (7)	2–4
Other aza-arenes (55)	na

Table 4.2 (continued) Major constituents of the particulate matter of the mainstream smoke of nonfilter cigarettes

Compound[a]	μg/cigarette[b]
Benzofurans (4)	200–300
Other O heterocyclic compounds (42)	na
Stigmasterol	40–70
Sitosterol	30–40
Campesterol	20–30
Cholesterol	10–20
Aniline	0.36
Toluidines	0.23
Other aromatic amines (12)	0.25
Tobacco-specific N-nitrosamines (6)	0.34–2.7
Glycerol	120

[a]Numbers in parentheses represent individual compounds identified.
[b]For details, see Table 4.4.
[c]Estimate.
na, Not available.

Table 4.3 Major toxic agents in cigarette smoke[a] (from Hoffmann *et al.* 1998)

Agent	Concentration/ nonfilter cigarette	Toxicity
Carbon monoxide	10–23 mg	Binds to hemoglobin, inhibits respiration
Ammonia	10–130 μg	Irritation of respiratory tract
Nitrogen oxide (NO_x)	100–600 μg	Inflammation of the lung
Hydrogen cyanide	400–500 μg	Highly ciliatoxic, inhibits lung clearance
Hydrogen sulfide	10–90 μg	Irritation of respiratory tract
Acrolein	60–140 μg	Ciliatoxic, inhibits lung clearance
Methanol	100–250 μg	Toxic upon inhalation and ingestion
Pyridine	16–40 μg	Irritates respiratory tract
Nicotine[b]	1.0–3.0 mg	Induces dependence, affects cardiovascular and endocrine systems
Phenol	80–160 μg	Tumor promoter in laboratory animals
Catechol	200–400 μg	Cocarcinogen in laboratory animals
Aniline	360–655 μg	Forms methemoglobin, and this affects respiration
Maleic hydrazide	1.16 μg	Mutagenic agent

[a]This is an incomplete list.
[b]Toxicity: oral/rat, LD_{50} free nicotine 50 mg/kg, nicotine bitartrate 65 mg/kg.

Development of highly sensitive analytical methods, as well as reproducible short-term and long-term assays, has led to the identification of 69 carcinogens in cigarette smoke (Table 4.4). Of these, 11 are known human carcinogens (Group I), 7 are probably carcinogenic in humans (Group 2A), and 49 of the animal carcinogens are possibly carcinogenic to humans (Group 2B). This classification of the carcinogens is according to the International Agency for Research on Cancer (IARC) (1983, 1984, 1986b, 1988, 1990, 1991, 1992, 1994a, b, c, d, 1995a, b, 1996, 1999a, b). Two suspected carcinogens have, so far, not been evaluated by the IARC.

Table 4.4 Carcinogens in cigarette smoke

Agent	Conc./nonfilter cigarette	IARC evaluation of carcinogenicity		
		in lab animals	in humans	Group [a]
PAH				
Benz(*a*)anthracene	20–70 ng	Sufficient		2A
Benzo(*b*)fluoranthene	4–22 ng	Sufficient		2B
Benzo(*j*)fluoranthene	6–21 ng	Sufficient		2B
Benzo(*k*)fluoranthene	6–12 ng	Sufficient		2B
Benzo(*a*)pyrene	20–40 ng	Sufficient	Probable	2A
Dibenz(*a,h*)anthracene	4 ng	Sufficient		2A
Dibenzo(*a,l*)pyrene	1.7–3.2 ng	Sufficient		2B
Dibenzo(*a,e*)pyrene	Present	Sufficient		2B
Indeno(1,2,3-*cd*)pyrene	4–20 ng	Sufficient		2B
5-Methylchrysene	0.6 ng	Sufficient		2B
Heterocyclic compounds				
Quinoline [b]	1–2 ng			
Dibenz(*a,h*)acridine	0.1 ng	Sufficient		2B
Dibenz(*a,j*)acridine	3–10 ng	Sufficient		2B
Dibenzo(*c,g*)carbazole	0.7 ng	Sufficient		2B
Benzo(*b*)furan	Present	Sufficient		2B
Furan	18–37 ng	Sufficient		2B
***N*-Nitrosamines**				
N-Nitrosodimethylamine	2–180 ng	Sufficient		2A
N-Nitrosoethylmethylamine	3–13 ng	Sufficient		2B
N-Nitrosodiethylamine	ND–2.8 ng	Sufficient		2A
N-Nitroso-di-*n*-propylamine	ND–1.0 ng	Sufficient		2B

Table 4.4 (continued) Carcinogens in cigarette smoke

Agent	Conc./nonfilter cigarette	IARC evaluation of carcinogenicity		
		in lab animals	in humans	Group[a]
N-Nitroso-di-n-butylamine	ND–30 ng	Sufficient		2B
N-Nitrosopyrrolidine	3–110 ng	Sufficient		2B
N-Nitrosopiperidine	ND–9 ng	Sufficient		2B
N-Nitrosodiethanolamine	ND–68 ng	Sufficient		2B
N-Nitrosonornicotine	120–3700 ng	Sufficient		2B
4-(Methylnitrosamino)-1-(3-pyridyl)-1-butanone	80–770 ng	Sufficient		2B
Aromatic amines				
2-Toluidine	30–337 ng	Sufficient		2B
2,6-Dimethylaniline	4–50 µg	Sufficient		2B
2-Naphthylamine	1–334 ng	Sufficient	Sufficient	1
4-Aminobiphenyl	2–5.6 ng	Sufficient	Sufficient	1
N-Heterocyclic amines				
AaC	25–260 ng	Sufficient		2B
IQ	0.3 ng	Sufficient		2B
Trp-P-1	0.3–0.5 ng	Sufficient		2B
Trp-P-2	0.8–1.1 ng	Sufficient		2B
Glu-P-1	0.37–0.89 ng	Sufficient		2B
Glu-P-2	0.25–0.88 ng	Sufficient		2B
PhIP	11–23 ng	Sufficient	Possible	2A
Aldehydes				
Formaldehyde	70–100 µg	Sufficient	Limited	2A
Acetaldehyde	500–1400 µg	Sufficient	Insufficient	2B
Volatile hydrocarbons				
1,3-Butadiene	20–75 µg	Sufficient	Insufficient	2B
Isoprene	450–1000 µg	Sufficient		2B
Benzene	20–70 µg	Sufficient	Sufficient	1
Styrene	10 µg	Limited		2B
Misc. organic compounds[c]				
Acetamide	38–56 µg	Sufficient		2B
Acrylamide	Present	Sufficient		2B

Table 4.4 (continued) Carcinogens in cigarette smoke

Agent	Conc./nonfilter cigarette	IARC evaluation of carcinogenicity		
		in lab animals	in humans	Group[a]
Acrylonitrile	3–15 µg	Sufficient	Limited	2A
Vinyl chloride	11–15 ng	Sufficient	Sufficient	1
DDT	800–1200 µg	Sufficient	Probable	2B
DDE	200–370 µg	Sufficient		2B
Catechol	100–360 µg	Sufficient		2B
Caffeic acid	< 3 µg	Sufficient		2B
1,1-Dimethylhydrazine	Present	Sufficient		2B
Nitromethane	0.3–0.6 µg	Sufficient		2B
2-Nitropropane	0.7–1.2 µg	Sufficient		2B
Nitrobenzene	25 µg	Sufficient		2B
Ethyl carbamate	20–38 µg	Sufficient		2B
Ethylene oxide	7 µg	Sufficient	Sufficient	1
Propylene oxide	12–100 ng	Sufficient		2B
Methyleugenol	20 ng			
Inorganic compounds				
Hydrazine	24–43 ng	Sufficient	Inadequate	2B
Arsenic	40–120 µg	Inadequate	Sufficient	1
Beryllium	0.5 ng	Sufficient	Sufficient	1
Nickel	ND–600 ng	Sufficient	Sufficient	1
Chromium (only hexavalent)	4–70 ng	Sufficient	Sufficient	1
Cadmium	7–350 ng	Sufficient	Sufficient	1
Cobalt	0.13–0.2 ng	Sufficient	Inadequate	2B
Lead	34–85 ng	Sufficient	Inadequate	2B
Polonium-210	0.03–1.0 pCi	Sufficient	Sufficient	1

ND, not detected; PAH, polynuclear aromatic hydrocarbons; AaC, 2-amino-9H-pyrido[2,3-b]indole; IQ, 2-amino-3-methylimidazo[4,5-b]quinoline; Trp-P-1, 3-amino-1,4-dimethyl-5H-pyrido[4,3-b]indole; Trp-2, 3-amino-1-methyl-5H-pyrido[4,3-b]indole; Glu-P-1, 2-amino-6-methyldipyrido[1,2-a:3′,2″-d]imidazole; Glu-P-2, 2-aminodipyrido[1,2-a:3′,2″-d]imidazole; PhIP, 2-amino-1-methyl-6-phenylimidazo[4,5-b]pyridine.

[a]*IARC Monographs on the Evaluation of Carcinogenic Risks*. Volume 1 and Supplements 1–8, 1972–1999. (1) Human carcinogens; (2A) probably carcinogenic in humans; (2B) possibly carcinogenic to humans; (3) not classifiable as to their carcinogenicity to humans.

[b]Unassigned carcinogenicity status by IARC at this time.

Smoking conditions

In 1936, the American Tobacco Company began using standard machine-smoking conditions, which reflected, to some extent, the smoking habits of cigarette smokers at that time. The estimated sales-weighted average nicotine yields of the cigarettes smoked at that time were around 2.8 mg (Bradford *et al.* 1936). In 1969, in agreement with the United States tobacco industry, the Federal Trade Commission (FTC) adapted the standard method of 1936 with only slight modifications. Since then, machine-smoking conditions have been 1 puff/minute, with a volume of 35 ml drawn during 2 seconds, leaving a butt length of 23 mm for a non-filter (plain) cigarette and length of the filter plus overwrap, plus 3 mm for filter cigarettes (Pillsbury *et al.* 1969). In Canada and the United Kingdom, the standard smoking conditions of the International Standards Organization (ISO) have been accepted since 1991 (ISO 1991). In other European countries, the standard smoking conditions for cigarettes are those developed by CORESTA (Centre De Cooperation Pour Les Recherches Scientifiques Relative Au Tabac), which are similar to the FTC standard smoking conditions (CORESTA 1991). In Japan, the FTC standard smoking conditions are employed for machine smoking of cigarettes (Pillsbury *et al.* 1969). The FTC method defines tar as smoke particulates minus water and nicotine, whereas CORESTA defines tar as total particular minus water (Pillsbury *et al.* 1969; CORESTA 1991; ISO 1991). The standard conditions for machine smoking of tobacco products used by the different testing protocols are presented in Table 4.5. Using the FTC method, the sales-weighted average tar and nicotine yields of United States cigarettes decreased from about 37 mg and 2.7 mg, respectively, in 1954, to 12 mg and 0.85 mg in 1993 (Fig. 4.1).

More than 20 years ago, M. A. H. Russell in the United Kingdom and N. L. Benowitz in the United States reported that long-term smokers of cigarettes with lower nicotine yields took more than one puff per minute, drew puff volumes exceeding 35 ml, and inhaled the smoke more deeply than smokers of higher yield cigarettes (Russell 1976 1980; Benowitz *et al.* 1983).

Table 4.6 presents the smoking characteristics of 56 volunteer smokers who regularly consumed low-yield cigarettes (≤0.8 mg nicotine/cigarette according to the FTC machine-smoking method) and of 77 volunteer smokers regularly consuming medium-nicotine cigarettes (FTC, 0.9–1.2 mg nicotine/cigarette). These two ranges of nicotine yield constituted more than 73.4 per cent of all cigarettes smoked in the United States in 1993 (Federal Trade Commission 1995). The results of this study clearly indicate that the majority of smokers in the United States smoke their cigarettes much more intensely to satisfy their acquired need for nicotine. Comparing the yields of the same cigarettes smoked under FTC standard machine-smoking conditions with the smoke inhaled by the consumers of cigarettes with low- and medium-nicotine content, reveals that smokers inhale 2.5 and 2.2 times more nicotine/cigarette, 2.6 and 1.9 times more tar, 1.8 and 1.5 times more carbon monoxide, 1.8 and 1.6 times more

Table 4.5 Standard conditions for machine smoking of tobacco products

Parameters	Cigarettes		Bidis	Little cigars	Small cigars	Cigars	Premium	Pipes*
	FTC	CORESTA		FTC	CORESTA	CORESTA	CORESTA	CORESTA
Weight (g)	0.8–1.1	0.8–1.1	0.55–0.80	0.9–1.3	1.3–2.5	5–17	6–20	
Puff								
Frequency (s)	60.0	60.0	30.0	60.0	40.0	40.0	40.0	20.0
Duration (s)	2.0	2.0	2.0	2.0	1.5	1.5	1.5	2.0
Volume (ml)	35.0	35.0	35.0	35.0	40.0	40.0	40.0	50.0
Butt length (mm)								
Non-filter	23.0	23.0	23.0	23.0	33.0	33.0	33.0	
Filtered	F and OW + 3	F + 8	F and OW + 3					

FTC, Federal Trade Commission method; CORESTA, Centre De Cooperation Pour Les Recherches Scientifiques Relative Au Tabac method; F, filter tip; OW, overwrap.

*One gram of pipe tobacco smoked.

Sources: [a]Hoffmann et al. (1974); [b]International Committee for Cigar Smoking (1974); [c]Miller (1963).

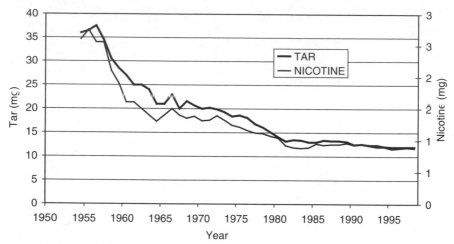

Fig. 4.1 Sales-weighted tar and nicotine values for US cigarettes as measured by machine using the FTC method 1954–1998. Values before 1968 are estimated from available data (D. Hoffmann, personal communication).

benzo(a)pyrene (BaP), and 1.7 and 1.7 times more 4-(methylnitrosamino)-1-(3-pyridyl)-2-butanone (NNK) than is generated by the FTC machine-smoking method (Table 4.6, Djordjevic *et al.* 2000).

The discrepancy in exposure assessment between recent measurements and former interpretations of machine-smoking data has led to criticism of the FTC standard machine-smoking method for consumer guidance. The suggestion that there is a meaningful quantitative relationship between the FTC-measured yields and actual intake (by the cigarette smoker) is misleading (Benowitz 1996). In view of these concerns, it appears 'that the time has come for meaningful information on the yields of cigarettes' (Wilkenfeld *et al.* 2000*a*, *b*). The FTC agrees, in principle, that a better and more comprehensive test program for cigarettes is needed (Peeler and Butters 2000).

Changes in cigarette smoke composition with various design changes

Filter tips

In 1959, Haag *et al.* reported the selective reduction of volatile smoke constituents by filtration through charcoal filter tips (Haag *et al.* 1959). Several of the compounds that are selectively removed from mainstream smoke (MS) in this fashion are major cilia-toxic agents, such as hydrogen cyanide, formaldehyde, acrolein, and acetaldehyde. Charcoal filters reduce the MS levels of these agents by up to 66 per cent (Kensler and

Table 4.6 A comparison of smoke data for two low-yield US filter cigarettes smoked according to the FTC method and by smokers (from Djordjevic et al. 2000)

Parameters	FTC machine smoking	Cigarette smokers	
		FTC 0.6–0.8 nicotine	FTC 0.9–1.2 nicotine
Puff			
Volume (ml)	35.0	48.6 (45.2–52.3)[a]	44.1 (40.8–46.8)[b]
Interval (s)	58.0	21.3 (19.0–23.8)[a]	18.5 (16.5–20.6)[b]
Duration (s)	2.0	1.5 (1.4–1.7)[a]	1.5 (1.4–1.6)[b]
Nicotine (mg/cigarette)	0.7 (0.6–0.8) 0.1 (1.09–1.13)	1.74 (1.54–1.98)[c]	2.39 (2.20–2.60)[d]
Tar (mg/cigarette)	8.5 (7.7–9.5) 15.4 (14.2–14.9)	22.3 (18.8–26.5)[e]	29.0 (25.8–32.5)[f]
CO (mg/cigarette)	9.7 (9.0–10.4) 14.6 (14.2–14.9)	17.3 (15.0–20.1)[g]	22.5 (20.3–25.0)[h]
BaP (ng/cigarette)	10 (8.2–12.3) 14 (10.1–19.4)	17.9 (15.3–20.9)[i]	21.4 (19.2–23.7)[j]
NNK (ng/cigarette)	112.9 (96.6–113.0) 146.2 (132.5–165.5)	186.5 (158.3–219.7)[i]	250.9 (222.7–282.7)[j]

Test Groups: [a]56 smokers; [b]71 smokers; [c]30 smokers; [d]42 smokers; [e]18 smokers; [f]19 smokers; [g]15 smokers; [h]16 smokers; [i]6 smokers; [j]3 smokers.

BaP, benzo(a)pyrene; CO, carbon monoxide; NNK, 4-(methylnitrosamino)-1-(3-pyridyl)-2-butanone.

Battista 1966; Battista 1976; Tiggelbeck 1976). However, for tar reduction, charcoal filters are less efficient than cellulose acetate filters. Several types of combination filters are in use. The early charcoal-activated dual and triple filter tips were cellulose acetate filters with embedded charcoal powder, or granulated charcoal sandwiched between cellulose acetate segments. These filters have been improved by innovative filter designs, incorporating cellulose acetate, charcoal, and cigarette filter paper (Shepherd 1994). However, in the United States, cigarettes with charcoal filters have accounted for only about 1 per cent of all cigarette sales over the past 15 years. In most developed countries charcoal-filter cigarettes have had, at most, a few per cent of the open cigarette market. Exceptions are Japan, South Korea, Venezuela, and Hungary, where at least 90 per cent of the cigarettes have charcoal filter tips (John 1996; Fisher 2000).

Cellulose acetate filter cigarettes first became popular during the early 1950s in Switzerland and soon thereafter in Germany, then in the United States, later in the United Kingdom and Japan, and, finally, in France. In 1956, the market share of filter cigarettes in Switzerland, Germany, and the United States was 57.2 per cent, 16.7 per cent, and 29.6 per cent, respectively, with only a few per cent in Japan, England, and France. By 1965, the filter cigarette market share in these countries had risen to about

82 per cent (Switzerland), 80 per cent (Germany), 63 per cent (United States of America), 50 per cent (Japan), 52 per cent (England), and 21 per cent (France). At the present time, cellulose acetate filter cigarettes account for at least 95 per cent of the cigarette markets in all of the developed countries, except in France, where filter cigarettes remain at 85 per cent of all cigarette sales (Waltz and Häusermann 1963; Wynder and Hoffmann 1994; Hoffmann and Hoffmann 1997).

In the early 1960s, investigators found that cellulose acetate filter tips retained up to 80 per cent of the volatile phenols from the smoke. Reduction of the emissions of volatile phenols from cigarettes was desirable because their tumor-promoting activity had been demonstrated in carcinogenesis assays (Roe *et al.* 1959; Wynder and Hoffmann 1961; Hoffmann and Wynder 1971). When tested on a gram-for-gram basis, the tar from cellulose acetate-filtered smoke is somewhat more toxic, but less carcinogenic, than tars obtained from charcoal-filtered smoke, or from the smoke of non-filter cigarettes (Wynder and Mann 1957; Bock *et al.* 1962; Hoffmann and Wynder 1963; Spears 1963; National Cancer Institute 1977c). Cellulose acetate filter tips also selectively remove up to 75 per cent of the carcinogenic, volatile *N*-nitrosamines (VNAs) from the smoke; whereas charcoal filter tips are much less effective in removing VNA (Brunnemann *et al.* 1977). Exposure of Syrian golden hamsters to the diluted smoke from two different cellulose acetate filter cigarettes, twice daily for 5 days per week, over 60 weeks, elicited a significantly lower incidence of carcinoma of the larynx than exposure to the diluted smoke from the non-filter cigarette ($p < 0.01$). In contrast, the incidence rate of carcinoma of the larynx of hamsters exposed to diluted smoke from charcoal filter cigarettes did not differ significantly from that of larynx carcinoma in hamsters exposed to diluted smoke from the non-filter cigarette (Dontenwill *et al.* 1973).

Filter perforation allows air dilution of the smoke during puff drawing. The velocity of the airflow through the burning cones of cigarettes with perforated filters is slowed down. This is because the negative pressure generated by drawing a puff is reduced by drawing air through the filter perforations, and the pressure drop across the tobacco rod is reduced, thus slowing the flow of smoke through the rod. This results in less incomplete (more complete) combustion of the tobacco, and a higher retention of particulate matter by the cellulose acetate in the filter tip (Baker 1984; Durocher 1984; Norman *et al.* 1984; Hoffmann and Hoffmann 1997). Presently, more than 50 per cent of all cigarettes have perforated filter tips. Table 4.7 compares smoke yields of cigarettes without filter tips, cigarettes with cellulose acetate filter tips, and cigarettes with cellulose acetate filter tips that are perforated. The filling tobaccos of these experimental cigarettes were made of an identical blend. The conventional filter tip of cellulose acetate retains more tar, nicotine, and phenol but releases more CO and the ciliatoxic agents, hydrogen cyanide, acetaldehyde, and acrolein, into the smoke than does the cigarette with the perforated filter tip (National Cancer Institute 1976). In mouse skin assays, the tars from both types of filter cigarettes have comparable tumorigenic activity. However, one needs to bear in mind: (1) that these comparative data are generated

Table 4.7 Comparison of experimental cigarettes (yield/cigarette) [a],[b] (from National Cancer Institute 1977c)

Smoke components	Unit of measurement	Non-filter cigarette	Cellulose acetate filter cigarette	Cellulose acetate filter w/perforation	Cellulose acetate filter w/perforation and highly porous paper
Carbon monoxide	ml	16.2	19.2	8.62	6.66
Hydrogen cyanide	µg	368	296	201	109
Nitrogen oxides—NO_x	µg	406	438	364	224
Formaldehyde	µg	36.0	20.9	31.7	21.4
Acetaldehyde	µg	1040	1290	608	550
Acrolein	µg	105	104	58.6	48.6
Tar	mg	27.0	14.7	19.2	19.5
Nicotine	mg	1.8	0.94	1.31	1.5
Phenol	µg	161	61.7	122	129
Benz(a)anthracene	µg	40.6 [1.40]	35.3 [2.25]	38.5 [1.88]	40.1 [1.91]
Benzo(a)pyrene	ng	29.9 [1.09]	19.6 [1.25]	29.2 [1.13]	23.9 [1.14]

[a]The composition of the cigarette tobacco is identical in all four experimental cigarettes.
[b]Numbers in square brackets = µg/dry tar.

with tars obtained by the standardized machine-smoking method, with a 35-ml puff, taken once a minute over 2 s; (2) that more than 60 per cent of today's smokers in the United States and in many developed countries smoke cigarettes with nicotine yields of only 1.2 mg or less (according to FTC standards of smoking); and (3) that most of these smokers compensate for the low nicotine delivery.

Compensation and greater smoke intake is governed by the smokers' acquired need for nicotine and, in essence, negates the intended benefits of reducing smoke yields by technical means (Russell 1976, 1980; Schultz and Seehofer 1978; Moody 1980; Herning *et al.* 1981; Benowitz *et al.* 1983; Gritz *et al.* 1983; Nil *et al.* 1986; Benowitz and Henningfield 1994; Djordjevic *et al.* 1995, 2000).

Paper porosity

Since about 1960, higher cigarette paper porosity and treatment of paper with citrate has significantly contributed to the reduction of smoke yields of several smoke components. During and in between puff drawing, porous paper enhances the outward diffusion through the paper of hydrogen, NO, CO, CO_2, methane, ethane, and ethylene. On the other hand, it accelerates the diffusion of O_2 and N_2 into the tobacco column; this, in turn, causes more rapid smoldering during puff intervals (Hoffmann and Hoffmann 1997; Owens 1998). Porous cigarette paper causes a significant decrease of smoke yields of CO, hydrogen cyanide, nitrogen oxides, volatile aldehydes, yet it hardly changes the yields of tar, nicotine, benz(*a*)anthracene (BaA), and BaP. Importantly, the significant reduction of nitrogen oxides in the smoke of these cigarettes reduces the formation and, thus, significantly lowers the yields of volatile and tobacco-specific *N*-nitrosamines (TSNAs) (Brunnemann *et al.* 1994; Owens 1998).

Cigarette construction

Smoke yields of cigarettes are also dependent on physical parameters, such as length and circumference of the cigarette, and the width of the cut (number of cuts per inch) of the tobacco filler. Extending the cigarette length from 50 mm to 130 mm produces an increase in the level of oxygen in the mainstream smoke, while the absolute levels of hydrogen, carbon monoxide, methane, ethane, and ethylene decrease. The major reason for this lies in the diffusion of oxygen through the paper into the smoke stream (Terrell and Schmeltz 1970). This phenomenon is also reflected in an increased CO delivery with ascending number of puffs, because the available surface area of the paper diminishes as the cigarette is smoked. With increasing length of the cigarette, the overall yields of tar, nicotine, PAH, and other particulate components increase (DeBardeleben *et al.* 1978). A circumference of cigarettes smaller than the regular 24.8–25.5 mm, e.g. 23 mm or less, translates into less tobacco being burned but a greater volume of oxygen available during combustion. Thus, the smoke yields of tar, nicotine, and other particulate components are lowered (DeBardeleben *et al.* 1978; Lewis 1992; Brunnemann *et al.* 1994; Hoffmann and Hoffmann 1997). Cigarettes with a small circumference also have a lower ignition propensity toward inflammable materials than cigarettes that have a 24.8–25.5 mm circumference. In 1990, almost 5200 residents of the United States died in fires, an estimated 1200 of these deaths occurred in fires started by cigarettes (US Consumer Product Safety Commission 1993).

The number of cuts per inch (width of tobacco strands) applied to the filler tobacco of cigarettes has an impact on smoke yields and/or on the carcinogenicity of the tars. The first investigation on the importance of tobacco cuts per inch, with regard to smoke yields and tumorigenicity of the resulting tars, was published in 1965. It compared the smoke yields of tar and BaP when 8, 30, 50, and 60 cuts per inch of leaf were applied. Tar yields per cigarette decreased from 29.1 to 23.0 mg and BaP from 37 to 21 ng. The tumorigenicities of tars derived from cigarettes made with 8, 30, or 50 cuts per inch of tobacco declined from 27 per cent to 16 per cent and 13 per cent of tumor-bearing mice. In a large-scale study of cigarettes filled with an identical blend, cut 20 and 60 times per inch, the smoke yields per cigarette of tar, nicotine, volatile aldehydes, BaA, and BaP were significantly reduced for the fine-cut tobacco. However, hydrogen cyanide was insignificantly increased. Gram-for-gram comparison of tumorigenicities of both tars on mouse skin revealed statistically insignificant differences (National Cancer Institute 1977*a*). As the large-scale bioassay was repeated twice, one has to conclude that in terms of mouse-skin carcinogenicity, activities of tars obtained from coarse-cut and fine-cut tobaccos are comparable.

Tobacco types

The botanical genus *Nicotiana* has two major subgenera: *N. rustica* and *N. tabacum*. *Nicotiana rustica* is grown primarily in Russia, the Ukraine, and other East European countries, including Georgia, Moldavia, and Poland. It is also grown in South America and, to a limited extent, in India. In the rest of the world, *N. tabacum* is grown as the major tobacco crop; it is classified into *flue-cured type* (often called bright, blond, or Virginia tobacco), *air-cured type* (often called burley tobacco; light air-cured tobacco grown in Kentucky, and dark air-cured type grown in parts of Tennessee and Kentucky, South America, Italy, and France), and *sun-cured* (often called oriental tobacco; primarily grown in Greece and Turkey). In addition, there are special classes of air-cured tobaccos for cigars, chewing tobacco, and snuff (Tso 1990).

Prior to the past two decades, flue-cured tobaccos were used exclusively for cigarettes in the United Kingdom and in Finland; they were also the predominate type used in Canada, Japan, China, and Australia. Air-cured tobaccos are preferred for cigarettes in France, southern Italy, some parts of Switzerland and Germany, and South America; cigarettes made exclusively from sun-cured tobaccos are popular in Greece and Turkey. In the rest of western Europe and in the United States, cigarettes contain blends of flue-cured and air-cured tobaccos as major components. Today, in many countries, such as the United Kingdom, France, and other developed nations, the US blended cigarette is gaining market share. In the United States, the composition of the cigarette blend has undergone gradual changes. In the 1960s and early 1970s, 45–50 per cent of the cigarette blend comprised flue-cured (Virginia) tobaccos; 35 per cent, air-cured (burley) tobaccos; and a few per cent were Maryland air-cured and oriental tobaccos. By 1980, the average blend was composed of 38 per cent flue-cured, 33 per cent air-cured, and a few per cent each of Maryland and oriental tobaccos. In the early 1990s, these proportions were about 35 per cent, 30 per cent, and, again, a few per cent of Maryland and oriental tobaccos (Spears and Jones 1981; Hoffmann and Hoffmann 1997). The blended cigarette is preferred in many countries, in part because each of the three major *N. tabacum* types adds a certain aroma to the smoke. Some isoprenoids, and a relatively high number of agents with carboxyl content, are associated with the aroma of flue-cured tobacco. Other isoprenoids, and especially the composition of the acidic fraction, are related to the special aroma of air-cured tobaccos (Roberts and Rowland 1962; Enzell 1976; Spears and Jones 1981; Tso 1990). 3-Methylbutanoic acid (isovaleric acid) is considered to impart the most important flavor characteristic to oriental tobacco (Stedman *et al.* 1963; Schumacher 1970).

However, in regard to the toxicity and carcinogenicity of tobacco and tobacco smoke, the difference in the nitrate content of the tobaccos is of primary significance. Flue-cured tobacco can contain up to 0.9 per cent of nitrate; yet, as it is used for regular cigarettes, it contains <0.5 per cent of NO_3. In oriental tobaccos one finds up to 0.6 per cent of NO_3, in air-cured tobaccos between 0.9 per cent and 5.0 per cent, but generally below 3 per cent in commercial cigarettes. The highest concentration of nitrate is present in the ribs, and the lowest concentration is in the laminae, especially in the laminae harvested from the top stalk positions of the tobacco plant (Neurath and Ehmke 1964; Tso *et al.* 1982). With the utilization of a greater proportion of air-cured tobacco in the American cigarette tobacco blend, the nitrate content of the blended US cigarette tobacco has risen from about 0.5 per cent in the 1950s to 1.2–1.5 per cent in the late 1980s (US DHHS 1989).

The concentrations of nitrogen oxides (NO_x) and methyl nitrite in smoke depend primarily on the nitrate concentrations in the tobacco, even though a portion of the nitrogen oxides is also formed during smoking from amino acids and certain proteins (Philippe and Hackney 1959; Sims *et al.* 1975; Norman *et al.* 1983). Cigarettes made with flue-cured tobaccos deliver up to 200 µg of NO_x, and 20 µg methyl nitrite in the smoke. Smoking US blended cigarettes produces up to 500 µg NO_2 and 200 µg methyl nitrite, and the smoke of air-cured tobacco cigarettes contains up to 700 µg NO_x and 400 µg methyl nitrite. The major source of nitrate is air-cured tobacco and, thus, the major source of NO_x in its smoke is nitrogen fertilizer (Sims *et al.* 1975). The stems of air-cured tobaccos are especially rich in nitrate ($\leq$6.8 per cent). Consequently, stems, as components of expanded and reconstituted tobaccos, contribute in a major way to NO_x in the smoke (Brunnemann *et al.* 1983).

Freshly generated smoke, as it leaves the mouthpiece of a cigarette, contains NO_x virtually only in the form of nitric oxide (NO), and contains practically no nitrogen dioxide (NO_2). However, nitrogen dioxide is quickly formed upon aging of the smoke. It has been estimated that, within 500 seconds half of the NO in undiluted smoke is oxidized to NO_2 (Neurath 1972). Of major importance is the high reactivity of NO_x upon its formation in the burning cone and in the hot zones of a cigarette. The thermically activated nitrogen oxides serve as scavengers of C,H- radicals, whereby they inhibit the pyrosynthesis of carcinogenic polynuclear aromatic hydrocarbons. Table 4.8 presents data on the smoke yields of tar, nicotine, phenol, and BaP and the tumorigenicities of the tars on mouse skin (Wynder and Hoffmann 1963).

Freshly generated nitrogen oxides also react with secondary and tertiary amines to form volatile N-nitrosamines (VNAs) and several N-nitrosamines from amino acids, as well as from additives. The NO_x also form tobacco-specific N-nitrosamines (TSNAs) by N-nitrosation of nicotine and of the minor tobacco alkaloids (Brunnemann *et al.* 1977; Brunnemann and Hoffmann 1981; Tsuda and Kurashima 1991; Hoffmann *et al.* 1994). BaP declined while NNK increased in the smoke of a leading US non-filter cigarette between 1974 and 1997. Both trends are correlated with the use of tobaccos with higher nitrate content. Recently, it was suggested (Peel *et al.* 1999) that the formation of tobacco-specific nitrosamines in flue-cured tobacco in the United States is, in part, due to the use of propane gas heaters in the curing process. Oxides of nitrogen generated during the burning of the liquid propane react with nicotine in the tobacco leaf to form TSNA. This change in the curing method, introduced in the mid-1960s, is a likely contributor to the increase of TSNA levels in cigarette tobacco. Other important factors are the proportionally greater use of air-cured tobacco and the use of reconstituted

Table 4.8 Smoke yields and tumorigenicity of the tars from the four major *N. tabacum* varieties (from Wynder and Hoffmann 1963)

Factors	Flue-cured tobacco	Sun-cured tobacco	Air-cured tobacco Kentucky[a]	Maryland
Yields/cigarette				
Tar (mg)	33.4	31.5	25.6	21.2
Nicotine (mg)	2.4	1.9	1.2	1.1
Phenol (µg)	95	120	60	43
Benzo(a)pyrene (ng)	53 (1.6)[b]	44 (1.4)[b]	24 (0.94)[b]	18 (0.85)[b]
Tumorigenicity[c]				
Percentage of mice with skin tumors	34	35	23	18

[a]Low-nicotine, air-cured tobacco (Kentucky).

[b]Number in parentheses: µg BaP/g dry tar.

[c]Bioassayed on a gram-for-gram basis of tar.

tobaccos in the cigarette tobacco blend (Neurath and Ehmke 1964; Brunnemann *et al.* 1983; Peel *et al.* 1999). Increased amounts of TSNAs in tobacco compound the carcinogenic potency of the resulting cigarette smoke (Hoffmann *et al.* 1994) and are considered to contribute to the rise of adenocarcinoma, which has become the dominant form of lung cancer in both male and female smokers during the past three decades (Vincent *et al.* 1977; Cox and Yesner 1979; El-Torkey *et al.* 1990; Devesa *et al.* 1991; Stellman *et al.* 1997). Increasing concentrations of nitrate in tobacco have also led to an increase in cigarette smoke of the human bladder carcinogens 2-naphthylamine and 4-aminobiphenyl, and of other aromatic amines (Patrianakos and Hoffmann 1979; Grimmer *et al.* 1995).

An important aspect relative to the toxicology of cigarette smoke is the correlation between the nitrate content of tobacco and the pH of cigarette smoke. Even though the different processes used to flue-cure and air-cure tobaccos have a significant impact on the smoke composition of the major types of tobacco, the role of nitrate is of major importance in determining the pH of the smoke. Whereas flue-cured tobacco and US cigarette tobacco blends deliver weakly acidic smoke (pH 5.8–6.3), the smoke of cigarettes made from air-cured tobacco delivers neutral to weakly alkaline smoke (pH 6.5–7.5). A major reason for the range of pH values encountered in the smoke of the two major tobacco types is the concentration of ammonia in the smoke, which is tied directly to the concentration of nitrate in the tobacco. When pH levels of the smoke rise above 6.0, the percentage of free, unprotonated nicotine increases to about 30 per cent at pH 7.4 and to about 60 per cent at pH 7.8 (Brunnemann and Hoffmann 1974). Protonated nicotine is only slowly absorbed in the oral cavity; yet, unprotonated nicotine, which is partially present in the vapor phase of the smoke, is quickly absorbed through the mucosal membranes of the mouth (Armitage and Turner 1970). The pH of cigar smoke rises with increasing puff numbers from pH 6.5 to 8.5; consequently, the rapid oral absorption of the free nicotine in the vapor phase gives a primary cigar smoker immediate nicotine stimulation so that he has no need for inhaling the smoke. Similarly, the smoker of black, air-cured cigarettes tends to inhale the smoke not at all, or only minimally (Armitage and Turner 1970; National Cancer Institute 1998).

In 1963, the first comparative study on the tumorigenicity on mouse skin of tars from the four major types of *N. tabacum* revealed the highest activity for tars from flue-cured and sun-cured tobaccos, and the lowest for the two varieties of air-cured tobaccos (Table 4.8; Wynder and Hoffmann 1963). The concentration of BaP, as an indicator of the concentrations of all carcinogenic PAHs, is correlated with the tumor initiation potential of the tars. Upon topical application to mouse skin and human epithelia, carcinogenic PAHs induce papilloma and carcinoma. In inhalation studies with Syrian golden hamsters, the smoke of a cigarette, made with a particular tobacco blend, was significantly more active in inducing carcinoma of the larynx than was the smoke of a cigarette with air-cured (black) tobacco (Dontenwill *et al.* 1973).

To verify whether a reduction of carcinogenic PAHs in the smoke due to the presence of high levels of nitrate in tobacco leads to reduced mouse skin tumorigenicity of the tar, sodium nitrate (8.3 per cent) was added to the standard tobacco blend. On a gram-for-gram basis, the tar from the cigarette with added nitrate (0.6 μg BaP/gram tar) induced skin tumors in only 2 of 50 mice, whereas the tar from the control cigarette (without the addition of nitrate; 1.05 μg BaP/gram tar) induced skin tumors in 25 of 100 mice (Hoffmann and Wynder 1967). In inhalation experiments with Syrian golden hamsters, smoke from the control cigarette plus 8.0 per cent of sodium nitrate induced laryngeal carcinomas in only 25 of 160 animals (15.6 per cent) compared to this type of neoplasm in 60 of 200 animals (30 per cent) in assays with the control cigarette (Dontenwill et al. 1973). Thus, all of these bioassays on the skin of mice and the inhalation studies with hamsters support the concept that increased nitrate content of the tobacco inhibits the pyrosynthesis of the carcinogenic PAHs and that the tars of these cigarettes, and their smoke as a whole, have a reduced potential for inducing benign and malignant tumors in epithelial tissues when compared to the tar or whole smoke of cigarettes with tobacco that is low in nitrate.

Reconstituted tobacco and expanded tobacco

In the early 1940s, the technology for making reconstituted tobacco (RT) was developed. Manufacturing RT enables the utilization of tobacco fines, ribs, and stems in cigarette tobacco blends (Halter and Ito 1979). Prior to this technology, tobacco fines and stems had been wasted. With the utilization of RT as part of the tobacco blend, less top-quality tobacco is needed, and thereby the cost of making cigarette has been reduced. Laboratory studies have shown that cigarettes made entirely of RT deliver a smoke with significantly reduced levels of tar, nicotine, volatile phenols, and carcinogenic PAHs.

The two major technologies for making RT for cigarettes are the slurry process and the paper process. Either process leads to RT with low density. The advantage of RT lies in the creation of a high degree of aeration of the tobacco, which enhances combustibility. Most of the tested tars from reconstituted tobaccos had significantly reduced carcinogenic activity on mouse skin (Wynder and Hoffmann 1965; National Cancer Institute 1977a). In inhalation assays with Syrian golden hamsters, diluted smoke from cigarettes made of reconstituted tobacco induced significantly fewer carcinomas in the larynx (19/160) than the diluted smoke from control cigarettes (60/200). The cigarette with RT gave, per cigarette, only 7 puffs and yielded 20.8 mg tar and 16 ng of BaP, compared to 10 puffs, 33.7 mg tar, and 35.4 ng BaP for the control cigarette (Dontenwill et al. 1973). This result supports the concept that, at least in the experimental setting, the carcinogenic PAHs, with BaP as a surrogate, are correlated with the induction of papilloma and carcinoma in epithelial tissues. The procarcinogenic TSNAs, on the other hand, are not activated by enzymes to their reactive species in epithelial tissues; thus, they induce few, if any, tumors in such tissues. Tobacco ribs and stems, the major components of RT, are richer in nitrate (and this applies especially to the ribs and stems of air-cured tobaccos) than the laminae of tobacco (Neurath and Ehmke 1964; Brunnemann *et al.* 1983; Brunnemann and Hoffmann 1991; Burton *et al.* 1992). Therefore, in general, the nitrate content of today's blended US cigarette, which may contain 20–30 per cent RT, is—at 1.2–1.5 per cent—much higher than the nitrate level in cigarettes during the 1950s and 1960s, when it was ≤0.5 per cent (Spears 1974; US DHHS 1989). Cigarettes with RT emit in their smoke significantly greater amounts of TSNAs than cigarettes of the past. These TSNAs include the adenocarcinoma-inducing NNK, which is metabolically activated to carcinogenic species in target tissues such as the lungs (Hoffmann *et al.* 1994). One major US cigarette manufacturer was awarded a patent in December of 1978 for developing a process that reduces more than 90 per cent of the nitrate content of the RT made from ribs and stems (Gellatly and Uhl 1978; Kite *et al.* 1978). It is unclear to what extent this patented method has been applied to RT manufacture for US commercial cigarettes.

There are at least three methods for expanding tobacco by freeze-drying (National Cancer Institute 1977*b*). As a result of freeze-drying, expanded tobacco has greater filling power than natural tobacco, meaning that less tobacco is needed to fill a cigarette. An 85-mm filter cigarette, filled entirely with expanded tobacco, requires 630 mg tobacco; while a regular non-filter control cigarette of the same dimensions requires 920 mg tobacco. The tar yields in the smoke of both types of cigarettes amounted to 12.4 mg and 22.1 mg, respectively (National Cancer Institute 1977*b*, 1980). In 1982, incorporation of all possible modifications in the make-up of the cigarette required only 785 mg leaf tobacco; in contrast, in 1950, the blended US cigarette required 1230 mg leaf tobacco (Spears 1974). Table 4.9 presents analytical data for the smoke of experimental cigarettes

Table 4.9 Smoke analyses of cigarettes made from puffed, expanded, and freeze-dried tobacco and from a control cigarette (from National Cancer Institute 1980)

Smoke component	Puffed tobacco	Expanded tobacco	Freeze-dried tobacco	Expanded stems	Control
CO (mg)	9.33	11.8	12.3	23.1	18.0
Nitrogen oxides (μg)	247.0	293.0	235.0	349.0	269.0
HCN (μg)	199.0	287.0	234.0	248.0	413.0
Formaldehyde (μg)	20.7	21.7	33.4	58.0	31.7
Acetaldehyde (μg)	814.0	720.0	968.0	803.0	986.0
Acrolein (μg)	105.0	87.7	92.4	93.0	128.0
Tar (mg)	16	18	16	23	37
Nicotine (mg)	0.8	0.7	0.8	0.4	2.6
BaA (ng)	13.7	11.8	15.3	19.5	37.1
BaP (ng)	11.8	8.2	9.2	16.2	28.7

CO, carbon monoxide; HCN, hydrogen cyanide; BaA, benz(a)anthracene; BaP, benzo(a)pyrene.

filled with puffed tobacco, expanded or freeze-dried tobacco, and a control cigarette. Levels of most components measured in the smoke of cigarettes with puffed tobacco, expanded tobacco, or freeze-dried tobacco were reduced, compared with data for the control cigarette (National Cancer Institute 1977*b*, 1980).

The changes that have occurred between 1950 and 1995 in the make-up of US cigarettes, have significantly altered smoke composition. Table 4.10 compares data for individual components in the smoke of US blended cigarettes of the 1950s with corresponding data for the cigarette smoke composition profiles that have been established between 1988 and 1995. All of these cigarettes were smoked with the FTC method (Pillsbury *et al.* 1969).

Table 4.10 The changing cigarette: changes in the yields of selected toxic agents in the smoke of US cigarettes (FTC smoking conditions; Pillsbury *et al.* 1969)

Smoke component	Earlier cigarettes[a]		Current cigarettes[a]	
	Year	Concentration	Year	Concentration
Carbon monoxide (CO)	1953	33–38 mg (NF)	1994	11 mg (F)
Nitrogen oxides (HNO$_x$)	1965	330 µg (NF)	1994	500 µg (NF)
Benzene	1962	30 µg (NF)	1988	48 µg (NF)
	1962	25–30 µg (F)	1990	42 µg (F)
Acetaldehyde	1960	1000 µg (NF)	1992	400 µg (F)
NDMA	1976	43 ng (NF)	1989	65 ng (NF)
Tar	1953	38 mg (NF)	1994	12 mg (F)
Nicotine	1953	2.7 mg (NF)	1994	0.85 mg (F)
	1959	1.7 mg (F)	1994	1.1 mg (F)
Phenol	1960	100 µg (NF)	1994	70 µg (NF)
	1960	46 µg (F)	1994	35 µg (F)
Catechol	1965	390 µg (NF)	1994	
	1976	790 µg (F)	1994	140 µg (F)
2-Naphthylamine	1968	22 ng (NF)	1985	35 ng (F)
BaP	1959	50 ng (NF)	1995	19 ng (NF)
	1959	27 ng (F)	1995	8 ng (F)
NNN	1978	220 ng (NF)	1995	300 ng (NF)
	1978	240 ng (F)	1995	280 ng (F)
NNK	1978	110 ng (NF)	1995	190 ng (NF)
	1978	100 ng (F)	1995	144 ng (F)

[a]NF, non-filter; F, filter.

NDMA, *N*-nitrosodimethylamine; BaP, benzo(a)pyrene; NNN, *N'*-nitrosonornicotine; NNK, 4-(methylnitrosamino)-1-(3-pyridyl)-1-butanone.

Additives

Humectants

Humectants serve to retain moisture and plasticity in cigarette and pipe tobaccos. They prevent the drying of tobacco, which would lead to a harsh-tasting smoke; importantly, they also preserve those compounds that impart flavor to the smoke. Today, the principal humectants in cigarette tobacco are glycerol (propane-1,2,3-triol) and propylene glycol (PG; propane-1,2-diol); of lesser importance are diethylene glycol (2,2'-di[hydroxyethyl]ether) and sorbitol (Voges 1984). In the past, ethylene glycol (ethane-1,2-diol) has been used as a humectant for cigarette tobacco. However, because this compound leads to the formation of ethylene oxide, which is carcinogenic to both animals and humans, its use has been prohibited (IARC 1994a). In 1972, Binder and Lindner reported the presence of 20 µg ethylene oxide per cigarette in the smoke of the untreated tobacco of one cigarette brand (Binder and Lindner 1972). In this context, it is noteworthy that Törnqvist et al. (1986) found significant levels of the N-hydroxyethylvaline moiety of hemoglobin in the blood of smokers (ranging between 217 and 690 pmol/g Hb, averaging 389 ± 138 pmol/g); while levels in the blood of nonsmokers ranged between 27 and 106 pmol/g Hb and averaged 58 ± 25 pmol/g Hb. The authors suggest that most of the ethylene oxide in the hemoglobin adduct is derived from endogenous oxidation of ethene in cigarette smoke (50–250 µg/cigarette).

Humectants may comprise up to 5 per cent of the weight of cigarette tobacco. In a 1964 study, 18 US cigarette tobacco blends that were analysed for humectants contained between 1.7 and 3.15 per cent of glycerol, which is, to some extent, decomposed to the ciliatoxic acrolein, and between 0.46 and 2.24 per cent of PG (Cundiff et al. 1964). The smoke of four American cigarettes contained between 0.34 and 0.96 mg/cigarette of PG (Lyerly 1967). However, PG may thermically degrade to yield propylene oxide. This would be of concern, because propylene oxide is regarded as possibly carcinogenic to humans (IARC 1994b). Four US cigarettes contained between 0.34 and 0.96 mg/cigarette (Lyerly 1967). In 1999, between 12 and 100 ng of propylene oxide were detected in the smoke of cigarettes filled with PG-treated tobacco. Several commercial samples of PG, used as a humectant for cigarette tobacco, already contained traces of propylene oxide (Kagan et al. 1999).

Flavor additives

Natural tobacco is composed of a wide spectrum of components that, upon heating, release agents that contribute to the flavor of the smoke. These include tobacco-specific terpenoids, pyrroles, and pyrazines, among others (Roberts and Rowland 1962; Gutcho 1972; Senkus 1976; Leffingwell 1987; Roberts 1988). The effective reduction of smoke yields by filter tips and by the incorporation of reconstituted tobacco also brought about a reduction of flavor components in the smoke. To counteract this loss of smoke flavor, the tobacco blends are treated with additives that are essentially precursors to smoke flavors. They include natural agents contributing to minty, spicy, woody, fruity, and flowery flavors. In some instances, such additives also include synthetic agents as flavor enhancers. While most of the flavor enhancers are chosen indiscriminately, it is realized that some of them may contribute to toxicity or carcinogenicity of cigarette smoke. A case in point was the cessation of the use of deer tongue extract which contained several per cent of the animal carcinogen coumarin (Voges 1984).

In 1993 and 1994, the tobacco industry convened an expert panel of toxicologists to screen agents that were in use, or considered for use, as tobacco additives. The panel established a list of 599 agents that were generally regarded as safe (GRAS), whereby the term 'safe' applied to each of the additives as such without consideration of the fate and reactivity of these agents during and after combustion (Doull *et al.* 1994). An exception was menthol, which was known to transfer into the smoke without yielding appreciable amounts of carcinogenic hydrocarbons (Jenkins *et al.* 1970). A recent toxicologic evaluation of flavor ingredients dealt with 170 such agents that are commonly used in the manufacture of American blended cigarettes, and examined their effects in four sub-chronic, nose-only smoke inhalation studies in rats compared to effects of the smoke of tobacco blends without additives. Control animals were exposed to filtered air (Gaworski *et al.* 1998). Smoke exposure was monitored with internal dose markers, including carboxyhemoglobin, serum nicotine, and serum cotinine. The mainstream smoke (MS) of flavored and nonflavored cigarette types caused essentially the same responses in the respiratory tracts of the rats; specifically hyperplasia and metaplasia in the nose and larynx. As this study involved maximally 65 h of exposure (while induction of tumors would not be expected until animals reach half their life span), one cannot deduce with certainty that the addition of these flavoring agents to tobacco blends has no impact on the development of tumors.

New types of cigarettes

The tobacco companies have undertaken a substantial research effort to develop new types of nicotine delivery devices. These devices were intended to generate an aerosol with nicotine in the range of the levels present in conventional cigarettes but with very low emissions of tar and other toxic agents. Toward the end of the 1980s, the first prototype of these new types of cigarettes was on the test market, a product named 'Premier'. It was a cigarette that 'heats rather than burns tobacco' (R. J. Reynolds Tobacco Co. 1988; Borgerding *et al.* 1990a, b, 1997; DeBethizy *et al.* 1990). This 80-mm cigarette is comprised of three sections. The first 40-mm section of this cigarette is made with compressed charcoal, which is immediately linked to an inner aluminum tube containing tobacco, flavor additives, and glycerol. This tube is embedded in tobacco. Section 2 (~10 mm) is a cellulose acetate filter dusted with charcoal powder. The third section (~30 mm) is a cellulose acetate filter tip. Under FTC standard machine-smoking conditions, the 'Premier' delivers smoke containing 0.3 mg nicotine, 6.3 mg water,

4.6 mg glycerol, 0.4 mg propylene glycol, and 0.7 mg tar. Compared with the reference (conventional) cigarette, and disregarding nicotine, the majority of the known toxic and carcinogenic agents in the smoke are reduced by more than 90 per cent. Known exceptions are carbon monoxide (CO) (+3.5 per cent), ammonia (−5.6 per cent), formaldehyde (−35.3 per cent), resorcinol (−73.3 per cent), quinoline (−56.6 per cent), and acetamide (−18.2 per cent). This new type of cigarette did not gain consumer acceptance; possibly because of difficulty in igniting the 'Premier', the need for frequent puffing to ensure continuous burning, the lack of flavor, and the low nicotine delivery (0.3 mg/cigarette). Nicotine emission was below the level that would satisfy most smokers' acquired need for this agent, even with compensatory smoking.

In 1996, a modified 'Premier' came on the market. In the United States it is known as 'Eclipse', in Germany it is called 'HiQ', and in Sweden it goes by the name 'Inside'. The 'Eclipse' consists of four sections. Section 1, the heat source, is a specially prepared charcoal; section 2 consists of tobacco plus glycerol; section 3 contains finely shredded tobacco; and section 4 is a filter tip. Upon ignition, the special charcoal heats the air stream during puff drawing. The heated airstream enters the tobacco sections and vaporizes glycerol, as well as the volatile and semi-volatile tobacco components, including nicotine. Under FTC smoking conditions, the 'Eclipse' delivers 8 mg CO (low-tar filter cigarette: 6–12 mg), 150 μg acetaldehyde (700 μg), 30 μg NO_x (200–300 μg), 180 μg hydrogen cyanide (300–400 μg), 5.1 mg tar (11–12 mg), and 0.2–0.4 mg nicotine (0.7–1.0 mg). The remainder of the smoke particulates consists of 33 per cent water, 47 per cent glycerol, and 17 per cent of various other compounds. The concentrations of the major carcinogens, such as BaP, 2-aminonaphthalene, 4-aminobiphenyl, and the TSNAs are lowered by 85–95 per cent (Rose and Levin 1996; Smith et al. 1996). Currently, the 'Eclipse' is being test marketed and it appears that response is somewhat more favorable than it was to its predecessor, the 'Premier'. The products labeled, 'Eclipse Full Flavor', 'Eclipse Mild', and 'Eclipse Menthol' produce FTC-standardized smoke yields of 0.2, 0.1, and 0.2 mg nicotine and of 3, 2, and 3 mg tar per cigarette. Regular cigarette smokers were asked to switch for 2 weeks to 'Eclipse'. There were four study groups, each composed of 26–30 volunteers, for a total of 109 smokers. Smoking of 'Eclipse' resulted in about a 30 per cent larger puff volume, about 50 per cent more puffs, which added up to a total puff volume per cigarette that was more than twice that of the total volume drawn from the control cigarettes (Stiles et al. 1999). These data suggest that the volunteers smoked 'Eclipse' more intensely than their non-filter cigarettes. This observation is also supported in the uptake of nicotine (Benowitz et al. 1997). The mutagenic activities of the urine of smokers of four types of 'Eclipse' were assayed on two bacterial strains and were reduced by 72–100 per cent, compared with the mutagenic activities of the urine of the same volunteers after smoking their regular cigarettes (Smith et al. 1996).

An Expert Committee from the Institute of Medicine of the National Academy of Sciences studied the scientific basis for a possible reduction of the 'harm' induced by

'Eclipse' relative to the 'harm' induced by smoking conventional cigarettes. On the basis of the available data, the committee came to the following conclusions: 'Eclipse' offers the committed smoker an option that is currently not available. 'Eclipse' does not add to the inherent biological activity of smoke from the range of cigarettes currently on the market. The elevated COHb levels should be regarded as a potential risk factor for cardiovascular diseases. The magnitude of this risk remains to be determined (Gardner 2000).

The high concentration of glycerol in the 'Eclipse' aerosol led to bioassays of glycerol in 2-week (1.0, 1.93, and 3.91 mg/l) and in 13-week (0.033, 0.167, and 0.662 mg/l) in 'nose only' inhalation studies with Sprague–Dawley rats, testing for toxicity and especially for irritating effects. The investigators detected metaplasia of the lining of the epiglottis (Gardner 2000). The 13-week inhalation studies with rats and hamsters had also resulted in some early histopathological changes in the upper respiratory tract in both laboratory animals. These observations signal the need for lifetime inhalation assays with the smoke of 'Eclipse' in rats, preferably Fisher 344 rats, or better yet, in Syrian golden hamsters, possibly with an inbred strain of hamsters susceptible to carcinogens in the respiratory tract (Bernfeld et al. 1974). Pauly et al., from the Roswell Park Cancer Institute, Buffalo, New York, caution that harmful glass fibers have been found to migrate into the filter tip of the 'Eclipse' and may be inhaled during puffing (Pauly et al. 2000).

The Health Department of Massachusetts and the Society for Research on Nicotine and Tobacco disputed the claims made for 'Eclipse.' They requested that the FTC and the Food and Drug Administration (FDA) institute regulatory procedures to ensure that insufficiently documented health claims are not made for tobacco products. Declaring 'Eclipse' the 'next best choice,' or calling TSNA-reduced tobacco products 'safer tobacco' (Anonymous 2000; Society for Research on Nicotine and Tobacco 2000) is deceiving.

In 1998, Philip Morris USA released a new type of cigarette (EHC) that is heated electrically to release an aerosol. On the basis of chemical analyses and short-term bioassays, it has significantly lower toxicity and mutagenicity than the smoke of the Kentucky reference filter cigarette, 1R4F. The prototype, containing a tobacco filler wrapped in a tobacco mat, is kept in constant contact with eight electrical heater blades in a microprocessor-controlled lighter. This cigarette contains about half the amount of the tobacco of a conventional cigarette. Under FTC-standardized smoking conditions, the cigarette delivers, with an average of eight puffs, about 1 mg of nicotine, whereas all other smoke constituents analysed were significantly lower than those in the smoke of the low-yield Kentucky reference cigarette, 1R4F (Terpstra et al. 1998). However, formaldehyde yields were significantly higher in the smoke of the EHC and emissions of glycerol and 2-nitropropane were comparable to those recorded in the smoke of the 1R4F cigarette. Per gram of tar, the smoke of the EHC had significantly lower mutagenic activity than the smoke of the 1R4F reference cigarette in TA98 and TA100 tester strains with metabolic activation (Terpstra et al. 1998).

Observations on cigarette smokers

In mice, rats, and hamsters, NNK induces adenomas and adenocarcinomas (AC) in the peripheral lung. This effect is independent of route and form of application (Hoffmann *et al.* 1994). NNK is metabolically activated primarily to the unstable 4-(hydroxymethylnitrosamino)-1-(3-pyridyl)-1-butanone and to 4-(α-hydroxymethylene)-1-(3-pyridyl)-1-butanol, which decomposes into methane diazohydroxide and 4-keto-4-(3-pyridyl)butane diazohydroxide, respectively. The diazohydroxides react with DNA bases to form 7-methyl guanine, O^6-methyl guanine, and O^4-methyl thymidine, respectively, and also form a pyridyloxobutyl adduct of presently unknown structure. Upon acid hydrolysis, this adduct releases 4-hydroxy-1-(3-pyridyl)-1-butanone. These adducts have been found in the lungs of mice and rats following treatment with NNK, and they have also been identified in human lungs. The origin of 7-methyl guanine in DNA from human lungs is unclear; conceivably, in addition to TSNA, nitroso compounds such as N-nitrosodimethylamine may also have been a source for this DNA methylation. However, it is clear that higher levels of 7-methyl guanine have been found in the lung of smokers than in the lung of nonsmokers, thus strengthening the evidence that NNK is a major contributor to the methylation of the lung DNA of smokers (Hecht 1998).

PAHs induce squamous cell carcinoma of the lung in laboratory animals and in workers with exposures to aerosols that are high in PAH. NNK metabolites induce primarily AC of the lung in laboratory animals. Reactive PAH metabolites bind to DNA in epithelial tissues. In laboratory animals, metabolically activated forms of NNK react with the DNA of Clara cells in the peripheral lung (Belinsky *et al.* 1990) to form methylguanine and methylthymidine, as well as pyridyloxobutylated adducts. 7-Methylguanine has been found in smokers' lungs at higher levels than in the lungs of nonsmokers.

Additional support for the observation that adenocarcinoma of the lung, among cigarette smokers, has increased relative to squamous cell carcinoma during the past 25 years, and for the concept that the lung cancer risk of smokers of low-nicotine filter cigarettes is similar to that of smokers of non-filter cigarettes, comes from biochemical studies. In the mouse, the O^6-methylguanine pathway of metabolically activated NNK is clearly the major route for induction of lung tumors; this conclusion is consistent with the high percentage of GGT→GAT mutations in the K-*ras* oncogene induced by NNK (Singer and Essigmann 1991; Hecht 1998). A study from The Netherlands has shown that mutations on codon 12 of the K-*ras* oncogene are present in 24–50 per cent of human primary adenocarcinoma. These mutations occur more frequently in AC of the lung in smokers than in nonsmokers. Twenty per cent of the mutations in codon 12 involve GGT→GAT conversions, which supports the concept that NNK plays a role in the induction of AC of the lung in smokers. Histochemical examination of human lung cancer showed cyclooxygenase (COX)-2 expression in 70 per cent of invasive carcinoma cases (Hida *et al.* 1998). COX-2 expression was also identified in adenocarcinoma of the lung in rats treated with NNK (El-Bayoumy *et al.* 1999). It is anticipated that future studies in molecular biology will fully elucidate the significance of TSNAs, especially of NNK, and of the carcinogenic PAHs in the induction of lung cancer in tobacco smokers.

Summary

Major modifications in the make-up of the commercial cigarette have been introduced between 1950 and 1975. Since then, there have been no substantive changes toward a further reduction of the toxic and carcinogenic potential of cigarette smoke, beyond reducing MS yields of tar, nicotine, and carbon monoxide. Some of these modifications have also resulted in diminished yields of several toxic and carcinogenic smoke constituents.

Cigarettes with charcoal filter tips deliver MS with significantly lower concentrations of the major ciliatoxic agents, such as hydrogen cyanide and volatile aldehydes. However, except in Japan, South Korea, Venezuela, and Hungary, cigarettes with charcoal filter tips account for less than 1 per cent (USA), and at most for a few per cent, of all cigarettes sold worldwide (Fisher 2000).

Cellulose acetate filters, with or without perforation, have the capacity for selective reduction of smoke yields of volatile *N*-nitrosamines and semi-volatile phenols. The latter are major tumor promoters in cigarette tar. In contrast to cigarettes manufactured in the 1950s, most of the cigarettes on the market today use a highly porous wrapper of paper treated with agents that enhance burning, thus contributing to the reduction of machine-measured yields of carbon monoxide, hydrogen cyanide, volatile aldehydes, volatile *N*-nitrosamines, PAH, and TSNA.

Reconstituted tobacco and expanded tobacco today amount to between 25 and 30 per cent of the cigarette tobacco blend. Reconstituted tobacco reduces the yields of smoke components such as tar and CO. The tar from cigarettes made entirely of reconstituted tobacco is less carcinogenic on mouse skin, and the smoke of these cigarettes reduces significantly the induction of carcinoma in the larynx of hamsters, compared to the smoke of reference cigarettes made of natural tobacco. Reconstituted tobaccos and expanded tobaccos have a significantly greater filling power than natural tobacco. An 85-mm filter cigarette that is filled entirely with expanded tobacco requires 363 mg tobacco while a regular filter-tipped cigarette requires 667 mg tobacco. The smoke of cigarettes made of expanded tobacco has significantly lower MS yields of tar, nicotine, CO, hydrogen cyanide, PAH, and TSNA. On the basis of weight-to-weight comparisons, the tar from these cigarettes is significantly less tumorigenic on mouse skin than the tar of a reference cigarette made of the corresponding natural tobacco.

Since 1959, each year the levels of tar, nicotine, and benzo(*a*)pyrene in the mainstream smoke of a leading US non-filter cigarette have been monitored. Beginning in 1977, the MS was also analysed for NNK and, in 1981, determinations of CO in the mainstream smoke were added. For all of these analyses, the MS was generated with the standardized machine smoking parameters that are mandated by the Federal Trade Commission.

Table 4.11 documents the decline of tar levels, from 29.8 mg to 24.3 mg in the years between 1959 and 1984, while nicotine levels fell from 2.4 mg to 1.6 mg between 1959 and 1977. Since then, the smoke yields of tar and nicotine for this non-filter brand have not changed. Carbon monoxide has remained stable at 16–18 mg/cigarette since it was first reported in 1981. By 1997, it was clear that significant changes in the smoke yields of the major lung carcinogens BaP and NNK have occurred since 1977, in that BaP levels declined from 49 ng to 19 ng but NNK increased from 120 ng to 195 ng/non-filter cigarette.

It is important to note that we are lacking analytical data regarding the levels of these major carcinogens and toxins in the MS of leading cellulose acetate filter-tipped cigarettes with and without filter perforation, as well as in the MS of charcoal filter cigarettes. These cellulose acetate filter cigarettes were actually the ones dominating the US cigarette market as the use of cigarettes faded over the years and charcoal-filter cigarettes had only a modest market share. Most importantly, we are also lacking data on biological activities of the tars of leading brands of filter cigarettes produced since the 1960s, because tumorigenicity and carcinogenicity of tars have not been monitored on a regular basis. There is now also an urgent need for analytical profiles of the toxic and carcinogenic MS constituents that are generated under conditions reflecting the puff drawing profiles actually exhibited by humans who smoke these cigarettes with lower yields as per FTC measurements. Such analytical data would have to be established for major US cigarette brands manufactured since 1960. They would

Table 4.11 Tar, nicotine, CO, BaP, and NNK in the mainstream smoke of a leading US non-filter cigarette, 1959–1997[a]

Year	Tar (mg)	Nicotine (mg)	Carbon monoxide[b] (mg)	BaP (ng)	NNK[b] (ng)
1959	29.8	2.4		40	
1967	27.2	1.6		49	
1971	29.0	1.8		22	
1977	26.0	1.59		19	120
1981	24.3	1.52	16.7	19	130
1988	24	1.5	16	19	140
1991	25	1.7	16	18	190
1997	26	1.7	18	19	195

CO, carbon monoxide; NNK, 4-(methylnitrosamino)-1-(3-pyridyl)-1-butanone; BaP, benzo(a)pyrene.

[a]The analytical data were generated by smoking the leading US non-filter cigarette according to the FTC-mandated standard machine smoking method (Pillsbury *et al.* 1969).

[b]The open fields document the lack of analytical data for the years 1959, 1967, 1971, and 1977 for CO and for 1959, 1967, and 1971 for NNK.

From Wynder and Hoffmann (1960), Federal Trade Commission (1971, 1977, 1981, 1988, 1991, 1997), Hoffmann and Hoffmann (1997).

serve as the scientific basis in support of epidemiological observations regarding the risk of cancer of the lung and upper aerodigestive tract for smokers who have exclusively smoked filter-tipped brands, as compared to the risk for smokers who used non-filter cigarettes.

Changes in the agricultural, curing, and manufacturing processes of cigarettes have resulted in an increase in tobacco-specific nitrosamines in cigarette smoke that may have contributed to the increase in adenocarcinoma of the lung observed over the past several decades.

Conclusions

1. Major modifications in the make-up of the commercial cigarette were introduced between 1950 and 1975, but since that time there have been few substantive changes toward a further reduction of the toxic and carcinogenic potential of cigarette smoke.

2. A variety of changes in cigarette design and filtration have resulted in chemical changes in cigarette smoke, some of which have also demonstrated decreased toxicity in animal assays. Toxicity or carcinogenicity in animal assays has not been monitored to allow evaluation of changes over time that have occurred for cigarette smoke produced by commercial brands of cigarettes.

3. Changes in the agricultural, curing, and manufacturing processes of cigarettes have resulted in an increase over the past several decades in the amounts of tobacco-specific nitrosamines in cigarette smoke. These changes are considered to have contributed to the increase in adenocarcinoma of the lung observed over the past several decades.

4. On the basis of the standard machine-smoking method for cigarettes that has been mandated by the FTC, the sales-weighted average nicotine yields of US cigarettes decreased gradually from 2.7 mg/cigarette in 1953 to 0.85 mg by the mid-1990s. Today, the smoker of filter cigarettes will greatly increase his/her smoking intensity to satisfy an acquired need for nicotine. Thus, the inhaled smoke of one cigarette contains 2–3 times the amount of tar, nicotine, and carbon monoxide, and 1.6–1.8 times the level of biomarkers for the major lung carcinogens BaP and NNK, compared to amounts in the smoke generated by the FTC method.

References

Anonymous (2000). Massachusetts disputes claims about Eclipse cigarettes. *Tobacco Reporter,* **127** (11), 11–13.

Armitage, A. K. and Turner, D. H. (1970). Absorption of nicotine in cigarette and cigar smoke through the oral mucosa. *Nature (London),* **226**, 1231–2.

Baker, R. R. (1984). The effect of ventilation on cigarette combustion mechanisms. *Recent Advances in Tobacco Science,* **10**, 88–150.

Battista, S. P. (1976). Ciliatoxic components in cigarette smoke. In: *Proceedings of the Third World Conference on Smoking and Health, New York, 2–5 June 1975. Vol. 1. Modifying the risk for the smoker* (ed. E. L. Wynder, D. Hoffmann, and G. B. Gori). US Department of Health, Education, and Welfare, Public Health Service, National Institutes of Health, National Cancer Institute.

Belinsky, S. A., Foley, J. F., White, C. M., Anderson, M. W., and Maronpot, R. (1990). Dose–response relationship between O^6-methylguanine formation in Clara cells and induction of pulmonary neoplasia in the rat with 4-(methylnitrosamino)-1-(3-pyridyl)-1-butanone. *Cancer Research,* **50** (12), 3772–80.

Benowitz, N. L. (1996). Biomarkers of cigarette smoking. *The FTC Cigarette Test Method for Determining Tar, Nicotine, and Carbon Monoxide Yields of U.S. Cigarettes. Report of the NCI Expert Committee.* Smoking and Tobacco Control Monograph No. 7. US Department of Health and Human services, National Institutes of Health, National Cancer Institute.

Benowitz, N. L. and Henningfield, J. E. (1994). Establishing a nicotine threshold for addiction. The implications for tobacco regulation. *New England Journal of Medicine,* **331** (2), 123–5.

Benowitz, N. L., Hall, S. M., Herning, S. I., Jacob, P. III, Jones, R. T., and Osman, A.-L.(1983). Smokers of low yield cigarettes do not consume less nicotine during cigarette smoking. *New England Journal of Medicine,* **309** (3), 139–42.

Benowitz, N. L., Jacob, P. J., Slade, J., and Yu, L. (1997). Nicotine content of the Eclipse nicotine delivery device. *American Journal of Public Health,* **87** (11), 1865–6.

Bernfeld, P., Homberger, F., and Russfield, A. B. (1974). Strain differences in the response of inbred Syrian hamsters to cigarette smoke inhalation. *Journal of the National Cancer Institute,* **53** (4), 1141–57.

Binder, H. and Lindner, W. (1972). Determination of ethylene oxide in the smoke of untreated cigarettes [in German]. *Fachliche Mitteilungen Austria Tabakwerke,* **13**, 215–20.

Bock, F. G., Moore, G. E., Dowd, J. E. and Clark, P. C. (1962). Carcinogenic activity of cigarette smoke condensate. *Journal of the American Medical Association,* **181**, 668–73.

Borgerding, M. F., Bodnar, J. A., Chung, H. L., Mangan, P. P., Morrison, C. C., Risner, C. H., *et al.* (1998). Chemical and biological studies of a new cigarette that primarily heats tobacco. Part 1. Chemical composition of mainstream smoke. *Food and Chemical Toxicology,* **36** (7), 169–82.

Borgerding, M. F., Hicks, R. D., Bodnar, J. E., Riggs, D. M., Nanni, E. J., Fulp, G. W. Jr, *et al.* (1990*a*). Cigarette smoke composition. Part 1. Limitations of FTC method when applied to cigarettes that heat instead of burn tobacco. *Journal of the Association of Official Analytical Chemists,* **73** (4), 605–9.

Borgerding, M. F., Milhous, L. A., Hicks, R. D., and Giles, J. A. (1990*b*). Cigarette smoke composition. Part 2. Method for determining major components in smoke of cigarettes that heat instead of burn tobacco. *Journal of the Association of Official Analytical Chemists,* **73** (4), 610–15.

Bradford, J. A., Harlan, W. R., and Hanmer, H. R. (1936). Nature of cigarette smoke; technique of cigarette smoking. *Industrial Engineering and Chemistry,* **28**, 836–9.

Brunnemann, K. D. and Hoffmann, D. (1974). Chemical studies on tobacco smoke. XXV. The pH of tobacco smoke. *Food and Cosmetics Toxicology,* **12** (1), 115–24.

Brunnemann, K. D., Hoffmann, D. (1981). Chemical studies on tobacco smoke. LXIX. Assessment of the carcinogenic *N*-nitrosodiethanolamine in tobacco products and tobacco smoke. *Carcinogenesis,* **2** (11), 1123–7.

Brunnemann, K. D. and Hoffmann, D. (1991). Analytical studies on *N*-nitrosamines in tobacco and tobacco smoke. *Recent Advances in Tobacco Science,* **17**, 71–112.

Brunnemann, K. D., Yu, L., and Hoffmann, D. (1977). Chemical studies on tobacco smoke XVII. Assessment of carcinogenic volatile *N*-nitrosamines in mainstream and sidestream smoke from cigarettes. *Cancer Research,* **37** (9), 3218–22.

Brunnemann, K. D., Masaryk, J., and Hoffmann, D. (1983). The role of tobacco stems in the formation of *N*-nitrosamines in tobacco and cigarette mainstream and sidestream smoke. *Journal of Agricultural and Food Chemistry*, **31**, 1221–4.

Brunnemann, K. D., Hoffmann, D., Gairola, C. G., and Lee, B. C. (1994). Low ignition propensity cigarettes: smoke analysis for carcinogens and testing for mutagenic activity of the smoke particulate matter. *Food and Chemical Toxicology*, **32** (10), 917–22.

Burton, H. R., Dye, N. K., and Bush, L. P. (1992). Distribution of tobacco constituents in tobacco leaf tissue. I. Tobacco-specific nitrosamines, nitrate, nitrite, and alkaloids. *Journal of Agricultural and Food Chemistry*, **40**, 1050–5.

CORESTA (1991). Standard Smoking Methods 23: Determination of total and nicotine-free dry particulate matter using a routine analytical cigarette-smoking machine. Determination of total particulate matter and preparation for water and nicotine measurements. *CORESTA Information Bulletin*, **1991–3**, 141–51.

Cox, J. D. and Yesner, R. A. (1979). Adenocarcinoma of the lung. Recent results from the Veterans Administration lung group. *American Review of Respiratory Disease*, **120** (5), 1025–9.

Cundiff, R. H., Greene, G. H., and Laurene, A. H. (1964). Column elution of humectants from tobacco and determination by vapor chromatography. *Tobacco Science*, **8**, 163–70.

Dalbey, W. E., Nettesheim, P., Griesemer, R., Caton, J. E., and Guerin, M. R. (1980). Chronic inhalation of cigarette smoke by F344 rats. *Journal of the National Cancer Institute*, **64** (2), 383–90.

Davis, B. R., Whitehead, J. K., Gill, M. E., Lee, P. N., Butterworth, A. D., and Roe, F. J. (1975). Response of rat lung to tobacco smoke condensate or fractions derived from it ministered repeatedly by intratracheal installation. *British Journal of Cancer*, **31** (4), 453–61.

DeBardeleben, M. Z., Claflin, W. E., and Gannon, W. F. (1978). Role of cigarette physical characteristics on smoke composition. *Recent Advances in Tobacco Science*, **4**, 85–111.

DeBethizy, J. D., Borgerding, M. F., Doolittle, D. J., Robinson, J. H., McManus, K. T., Rahn, C. A., *et al.* (1990). Chemical and biological studies of a cigarette that heats rather than burns tobacco. *Journal of Clinical Pharmacology*, **30** (8), 755–63.

Devesa, S. S., Shaw, G. L., and Blot, W. J. (1991). Changing patterns of lung cancer incidence by histologic type. *Cancer Epidemiology Biomarkers and Prevention*, **1** (1), 29–34.

Djordjevic, M.V., Fan, J., Ferguson, S., and Hoffmann, D. (1995). Self-regulation of smoking intensity, smoke yields of low-nicotine, low 'tar' cigarettes. *Carcinogenesis*, **16** (9), 2015–21.

Djordjevic, M. V., Stellman, S. D., and Zang, E. (2000). Doses of nicotine and lung carcinogens delivered to cigarette smokers. *Journal of the National Cancer Institute*, **92** (2), 106–11.

Doll, R. and Hill, A. B. (1950). Smoking and carcinoma of the lung. Preliminary report. *British Medical Journal*, **2**, 739–48.

Dontenwill, W., Chevalier, H. J., Harke, H.-P., Lafrenz, U., Reckzeh, G., and Schneider, B. (1973). Investigations on the effects of chronic cigarette smoke inhalation in Syrian golden hamsters. *Journal of the National Cancer Institute*, **51** (6), 1781–832.

Doull, J., Frawley, J. P., and George, W. (1994). List of ingredients added to tobacco in the manufacture of cigarettes by six major American cigarette companies. Covington and Burling, Washington, DC. [Reprinted: *Tobacco Journal International*, **196**, 32–9.]

Durocher, D. F. (1984). The choice of paper components for low-tar cigarettes. *Recent Advances in Tobacco Science*, **10**, 52–71.

El-Bayoumy, K., Iatropoulos, M., Amin, S., Hoffmann, D., and Wynder, E. L. (1999). Increased expression of cyclooxygenase-2 in rat lung tumors induced by the tobacco-specific nitrosamine 4-(methylnitrosamine)-4-(3-pyridyl)-4-(3-pyridyl)-butanone: Impact of a high-fat diet. *Cancer Research*, **59** (7), 1400–3.

el-Torkey, M., el-Zeky, F., and Hall, J. C. (1990). Significant changes in the distribution of histologic types of lung cancer. A review of 4,928 cases. *Cancer,* **65** (10), 2361–7.

Enzell, C. R. (1976). Terpenoid components of leaf and their relationship to smoking quality and aroma. *Recent Advances in Tobacco Science,* **2**, 32–60.

Essenberg, J. M. (1952). Cigarette smoke and the incidence of primary neoplasm of the lung in the albino mouse. *Science,* **116**, 561–2.

Federal Trade Commission (1971). *Report of 'Tar' and Nicotine Content of the Smoke of 121 Varieties of Cigarettes.* Federal Trade Commission, Washington, DC.

Federal Trade Commission (1977). *Report of 'Tar' and Nicotine Content of the Smoke of 166 Varieties of Cigarettes.* Federal Trade Commission, Washington, DC.

Federal Trade Commission (1981). *Report of 'Tar', Nicotine and Carbon Monoxide of the Smoke of 187 Varieties of Cigarettes.* Federal Trade Commission, Washington, DC.

Federal Trade Commission (1988). *Report of 'Tar', Nicotine and Carbon Monoxide of the Smoke of 272 Varieties of Domestic Cigarettes.* Federal Trade Commission, Washington, DC.

Federal Trade Commission (1991). *Tar, Nicotine, and Carbon Monoxide of the Smoke of 475 Varieties of Domestic Cigarettes.* Federal Trade Commission, Washington, DC.

Federal Trade Commission (1995). *Tar, Nicotine, and Carbon Monoxide of the Smoke of 1,107 Varieties of Domestic Cigarettes.* Federal Trade Commission, Washington, DC.

Federal Trade Commission (1997). *Tar, Nicotine, and Carbon Monoxide of the Smoke of 1,206 Varieties of Domestic Cigarettes.* Federal Trade Commission, Washington, DC.

Fisher, B. (2000). Filtering new technology. *Tobacco Reporter,* **127** (12), 46–7.

Gardner, D. E. (ed.) (2000). A safer cigarette? *Inhalation Toxicology,* **12** (suppl. 5), 1–58.

Gaworski, C. L., Dozier, M. M., Heck, J. D., Gerhard, J. M. Rajendran, N., David, R. M., *et al.* (1998). Toxicological evaluation of flavor ingredients added to cigarette tobacco: 13-week inhalation exposures in rats. *Inhalation Toxicology,* **10**, 357–81.

Gellatly, G., and Uhl, R. G. (1978). Method for removal of potassium nitrate from tobacco extracts. US Patent 4,131,118, December 26, 1978.

Graham, E. A., Croninger, A. B., and Wynder, E. L. (1957). Experimental production of carcinoma with cigarette tar. IV. Successful experiments with rabbits. *Cancer Research,* **17**, 1058–66.

Green, C. R. and Rodgman, A. (1996). The Tobacco Chemists' Research Conference. A half-century of advances in analytical methodology of tobacco and its products. *Recent Advances in Tobacco Science,* **22**, 131–304.

Grimmer, G., Schneider, D., Naujack, K.-W., Dettbarn, G., and Jacob, J. (1995). Intercept-reactant method for the determination of aromatic amines in mainstream tobacco smoke. *Beitrage zur Tabakforschung International,* **16**, 141–56.

Gritz, E. R., Rose, J. E., and Jarvik, M. E. (1983). Regulation of tobacco smoke intake with paced cigarette presentation. *Pharmacology, Biochemistry, and Behavior,* **18**, 457–62.

Gutcho, S. (1972). *Tobacco flavoring substances and methods.* Noyes Data Corporation, Park Ridge, NJ.

Haag, H. B., Larson, P. S., and Finnegan, J. K. (1959). Effect of filtration on the chemical and irritating properties of cigarette smoke. *AMA Archives of Otolaryngology,* **69**, 261–5.

Halter, H. M. and Ito, T. I. (1979). Effect of reconstitution and expansion processes on smoke composition. *Recent Advances in Tobacco Science,* **4**, 113–32.

Hecht, S. S. (1998). Biochemistry, biology, and carcinogenicity of tobacco-specific N-nitrosamines. *Chemical Research in Toxicology,* **11** (6), 559–603.

Herning, R .I., Jones, R. T., Bachman, G., and Mines, A. H. (1981). Puff volume increases when low-nicotine cigarettes are smoked. *British Medical Journal (Clin Res Ed),* **283** (6285), 187–9.

Hida, T., Yatabe, Y., Achiwa, H., Muramatsu, H., Kozaki, K-I., Makamura, S., *et al.* (1998). Increased expression of cyclooxygenase-2 occurs frequently in human lung cancers, especially in adenocarcinoma. *Cancer Research*, **58** (17), 3761–4.

Hoffmann, D. and Hecht, S. S. (1989). Advances in tobacco carcinogenesis. In: *Handbook of experimental pharmacology* (ed. C. S. Cooper and P. L. Grover). Springer Publications, New York.

Hoffmann, D. and Hoffmann, I. (1997). The changing cigarette, 1950–1995. *Journal of Toxicology and Environmental Health*, **50** (4), 307–64.

Hoffmann, D. and Wynder, E. L. (1963). Filtration of phenols from cigarette smoke. *Journal of the National Cancer Institute*, **30**, 67–84.

Hoffmann, D. and Wynder, E. L. (1967). The reduction in the tumorigenicity of cigarette smoke condensate by addition of sodium nitrate to tobacco. *Cancer Research*, **27** (1), 172–4.

Hoffmann, D. and Wynder, E. L. (1971). A study of tobacco carcinogenesis. XI. Tumor initiation, tumor acceleration, and tumor promoting activity of condensate fraction. *Cancer*, **27** (4), 848–64.

Hoffmann, D. and Wynder, E. L. (1977). Chemical analysis and carcinogenic bioassays of organic particulate pollutants. In: *Air pollution* (ed. A. L. Stern), pp. 361–455. Academic Press, New York.

Hoffmann, D., Sanghvi, L. D., and Wynder, E. L. (1974). Comparative chemical analysis of India bidi and American cigarette smoke. *International Journal of Cancer*, **14** (1), 49–53.

Hoffmann, D., Brunnemann, K. D., Prokopczyk, B., and Djordjevic, M. V. (1994). Tobacco-specific *N*-nitrosamines and *Areca*-derived *N*-nitrosamines. Chemistry, biochemistry, carcinogenicity, and relevance to humans. *Journal of Toxicology and Environmental Health*, **41** (1), 1–52.

Hoffmann, D., Hoffmann, I., and Wynder, E. L. (1998). The changing cigarette: 1950–1997: facts and expectations. In *Report of Canada's Expert Committee on Cigarette Toxicity Reduction*, (ed. W. S. Rickert). Health Canada, Toronto, Ontario, Canada.

International Agency for Research on Cancer (1982). Di(2-ethylhexyl)phthalate. *Some industrial chemicals and dyestuffs.* IARC Monographs on the Evaluation of Carcinogenic Risk of Chemicals to Humans 29, pp. 257–80. IARC, Lyon, France.

International Agency for Research on Cancer (1983). *Polynuclear aromatic compounds. Part 1. Chemical, environmental and experimental data.* IARC Monographs on the Evaluation of the Carcinogenic Risk of Chemicals to Humans 33. IARC, Lyon, France.

International Agency for Research on Cancer (1984). Coke production. *Polynuclear aromatic compounds, Part 3: Industrial exposure in aluminum production, coal gasification, coke production, and iron and steel founding.* IARC Monographs on the Evaluation of the Carcinogenic Risk of Chemicals to Humans 34, pp. 101–31. IARC, Lyon, France.

International Agency for Research on Cancer (1986*a*). *Tobacco smoking.* IARC Monographs on the Evaluation of Carcinogenic Risks to Humans 38. IARC, Lyon, France.

International Agency for Research on Cancer (1986*b*). Amino acid pyrolysis products in food. *Some naturally occurring and synthetic food components, furocoumarins, and ultraviolet radiation.* IARC Monographs on the Evaluation of Carcinogenic Risks to Humans 40, pp. 233–80. IARC, Lyon, France.

International Agency for Research on Cancer (1987). *Overall evaluation of carcinogenicity: An updating of IARC monographs 1 to 42.* IARC Monographs on the Evaluation of Carcinogenic Risks to Humans Suppl. 7. IARC, Lyon, France.

International Agency for Research on Cancer (1988). Radon. *Man-made mineral fibres and radon.* IARC Monographs on the Evaluation of Carcinogenic Risks to Humans 43, pp. 173–254. IARC, Lyon, France.

International Agency for Research on Cancer (1991). DDT and associated compounds. *Occupational exposures in insecticide application, and some pesticides.* IARC Monographs on the Evaluation of Carcinogenic Risks to Humans 53, pp. 179–249. IARC, Lyon, France.

International Agency for Research on Cancer (1992). 1,3-Butadiene. *Occupational exposures to mists and vapours from strong inorganic acids; and other industrial chemicals.* IARC Monographs on the Evaluation of Carcinogenic Risks to Humans 54, pp. 237–85. IARC, Lyon, France.

International Agency for Research on Cancer (1994*a*). Ethylene oxide. *Some industrial chemicals.* IARC Monographs on the Evaluation of Carcinogenic Risks to Humans 60, pp. 73–159. IARC, Lyon, France.

International Agency for Research on Cancer (1994*b*). Propylene oxide. *Some industrial chemicals.* IARC Monographs on the Evaluation of the Carcinogenic Risks of Chemicals to Humans 60, pp. 181–213. IARC, Lyon, France.

International Agency for Research on Cancer (1994*c*). Isoprene. *Some industrial chemicals.* IARC Monographs on the Evaluation of Carcinogenic Risks to Humans 60, pp. 215–32. IARC, Lyon, France.

International Agency for Research on Cancer (1994*d*). Styrene. *Some industrial chemicals.* IARC Monographs on the Evaluation of Carcinogenic Risks to Humans 60, pp. 233–320. IARC, Lyon, France.

International Agency for Research on Cancer (1994*e*) Acrylamide. *Some industrial chemicals.* IARC Monographs on the Evaluation of Carcinogenic Risks to Humans 60, pp. 389–433. IARC, Lyon, France.

International Agency for Research on Cancer (1995*a*). Furan. *Dry cleaning, some chlorinated solvents and other industrial chemicals.* IARC Monographs on the Evaluation of the Carcinogenic Risks to Humans 63, pp. 393–407. IARC, Lyon, France.

International Agency for Research on Cancer (1995*b*). Benzofuran. *Dry cleaning, some chlorinated solvents and other industrial chemicals.* IARC Monographs on the Evaluation of the Carcinogenic Risks to Humans 63, pp. 431–441. IARC, Lyon, France.

International Agency for Research on Cancer (1996). Nitrobenzene. *Printing processes and printing inks, carbon black and some nitro compounds.* IARC Monographs on the Evaluation of the Carcinogenic Risks to Humans 65, pp. 381–408. IARC, Lyon, France.

International Agency for Research on Cancer (1999*a*). 1,3-Butadiene. *Re-evaluation of some organic chemicals, hydrazine, and hydrogen peroxide.* IARC Monographs on the Evaluation of the Carcinogenic Risks to Humans 71, pp. 109–225. IARC, Lyon, France.

International Agency for Research on Cancer. Acetaldehyde (1999*b*). *Re-evaluation of some organic chemicals, hydrazine, and hydrogen peroxide.* IARC Monographs on the Evaluation of the Carcinogenic Risks to Humans 71, pp. 319–44. IARC, Lyon, France.

International Agency for Research on Cancer (2000). Di(2-ethylhexyl)phthalate. *Some industrial chemicals.* IARC Monographs on the Evaluation of Carcinogenic Risk of Chemicals to Humans 77, pp. 41–148. IARC, Lyon, France.

International Committee for Cigar Smoking Study (1974). Machine smoking of cigars. *CORESTA Information Bulletin,* 1, 31–4.

International Standards Organization (1991). *Routine analytical cigarette smoking machine: Part I. Specifications and standard conditions.* ISO, Geneva, Switzerland.

Ishiguro, S. and Sugawara, S. (1980). The Chemistry of Tobacco Smoke [in Japanese; English translation 1981]. Central Institute, Japanese Tobacco Monopoly Corporation, Yokohama, Japan.

Jenkins, R. W. J., Neroman, P. H., and Charms, M. D. (1970). Cigarette smoke formation. II. Smoke distribution and mainstream pyrolytic composition of added ^{14}C-menthol (U). *Beitrage zur Tabakforschung International,* 5, 299–301.

John, A. L. (1996). Japan. Always something new. *Tobacco International,* August, 30–5.

Kagan, M. R., Cunningham, J. A., and Hoffmann, D. (1999). Propylene glycol. A precursor of propylene oxide in cigarette smoke. *53rd Tobacco Science Research Conference*, Abstract Nos 41 and 42.

Kensler, C. J. and Battista, S. P. (1966). Chemical and physical factors affecting mammalian ciliary activity. *American Review of Respiratory Disease*, **93** (3), 93–102.

Kite, G. F., Gellatly, G., and Uhl, R. G. (1978). Method for removal of potassium nitrate from tobacco extracts. US Patent 4,131,117, December 26.

Leffingwell, J. C. (ed.). (1987). Chemical and sensory aspects of tobacco flavor. *Recent Advances in Tobacco Science*, **14**, 1–218.

Leuchtenberger, C. and Leuchtenberger, R. (1970). Effects of chronic inhalation of whole fresh cigarette smoke and of its gas phase on pulmonary tumorigenesis in Snell's mice. In: *Morphology of experimental respiratory carcinogenesis. Proceedings of a Biology Division, Oak Ridge National Laboratory, Conference, Gatlinburg, Tennesee, 13–16 May* (ed. P. Nettesheim, M. G. Hanna Jr, and J. W. Deatherage Jr), pp. 329–46. US Atomic Energy Commission, Washington, DC.

Leuchtenberger, C., Leuchtenberger, R., and Doolin, P. T. (1958). A correlated histological, cytological, and cytochemical study of tracheobronchial tree and lungs of mice exposed to cigarette smoke. *Cancer*, **11**, 490–506, 1958.

Lewis, C. I. (1992). The effect of cigarette construction parameters on smoke generation and yield. *Recent Advances in Tobacco Science*, **16**, 73–101.

Lyerly, L. A. (1967). Direct vapor chromatographic determination of menthol, propylene glycol, nicotine and triacetin in cigarette smoke. *Tobacco Science*, **11**, 49–51.

Miller, J. E. (1963). Determination of the components of pipe tobacco smoke by means of a new pipe smoking machine. *Proceedings of the 3rd World Tobacco Congress, Salisbury, Rhodesia, CORESTA*, February, p. 11.

Mohr, U. and Reznik, G. (1978). Tobacco carcinogenesis. In *Pathogenesis and therapy of lung cancer*, (ed. C. C. Harris), pp. 263–361. Marcel Dekker, New York.

Moody, P. M. (1980). The relationships of qualified human smoking behavior and demographic variables. *Social Science and Medicine*, **14A**, 49–54.

Mühlbock, O. (1958). Carcinogenicity of cigarette smoke in mice (Dutch). Nederlands Tijdschrift voor Geneeskunde 99: 2276–8, 1958.

National Cancer Institute (1977*a*). *Tar and less hazardous cigarettes. First set of experimental cigarettes.* Smoking and Health Program. DHEW Publ. No. (NIH) 76–905.

National Cancer Institute (1977*b*). *Toward less hazardous cigarettes. Second set of experimental cigarettes.* Smoking and Health Program. DHEW Publ. No. (NIH) 76–111.

National Cancer Institute, Smoking and Health Program (1977*c*). *Toward less hazardous cigarettes. Third set of experimental cigarettes.* DHEW Publ. No. (NIH) 77–1280.

National Cancer Institute (1980). *Toward less hazardous cigarette. Fourth set of experimental cigarettes.* Smoking and Health Program. DHEW Publ. No. (NIH) 80.

National Cancer Institute (1998). Cigars: health effects and trends. In *Smoking and tobacco control monograph 9* (ed. D. M. Burns, D. Hoffmann, and K. M. Cummings). US DHHS, Public Health Service, NIH-NCI. NIH Publ. No. 98–1302, Bethesda, MD.

Neurath, G. B. (1972). Nitrosamine formation from precursors in tobacco smoke. In: N-*Nitroso compounds. Analysis and formation* (ed. P. Bogovski, R. Preussmann, and E. A. Walker). IARC Sci. Publ. 3, pp. 134–6. International Agency for Research on Cancer, Lyon, France.

Neurath, G. and Ehmke, H. (1964). Studies on the nitrate content of tobacco [in German]. *Beiträge zur Tabakforschung International*, **2**, 333–44.

Nil, R., Buzzi, R., and Bättig, K. (1986). Effect of different cigarette smoke yields on puffing and inhalation. Is the measurement of inhalation volumes relevant for smoke absorption? *Pharmacology, Biochemistry, and Behavior,* 24 (3), 587–95.

Norman, V., Ihrig, A. M., Larson, T. M., and Moss, B. L. (1983). The effect of nitrogenous blend components on NO/NO_x and HCN levels in mainstream and sidestream smoke. *Beiträge zur Tabakforschung International,* 12, 55–62.

Norman, V., Ihrig, A. M., Shoffner, R. A., and Ireland, M. S. (1984). The effect of tip dilution on the filtration efficiency of upstream and downstream segments of cigarette filters. *Beiträge zur Tabakforschung International,* 12, 178–85.

Otto, H. (1963). Inhalation studies with mice exposed passively to cigarette smoke [in German]. *Frankfurter Zeitschrift für Pathologie,* 73, 10–23.

Owens, W.R., Jr. (1998). Effect of cigarette paper on smoke yield and composition. *Recent Advances in Tobacco Science,* 4, 3–24.

Patrianakos, C. and Hoffmann, D. (1979). Chemical studies on tobacco smoke. LXIV. On the analysis of aromatic amines in cigarette smoke. *Journal of Analytical Toxicology,* 3, 150–4.

Pauly, J. L., Lee, H. J., Hurley, E. L., Cummings, K. M., Lesser, J. D., and Streck, R. J. (1998). Glass fiber contamination of cigarette filters: an additional health risk to the smoker? *Cancer Epidemiology, Biomarkers and Prevention,* 7 (11), 967–79.

Peel, D. M., Riddick, M. G., Edwards, M. E., Gentry, J. S., and Nestor, T. B. (1999). Formation of tobacco specific nitrosamines in flue-cured tobacco. Presented at the 53rd Tobacco Science Research Conference. Montreal, Quebec, Canada, 12–15 September.

Peeler, C. L. and Butters, G. R. (2000). Correspondence re: 'It's time for a change: cigarette smokers deserve meaningful information about their cigarettes'. *Journal of the National Cancer Institute,* 92 (10), 842.

Philippe, R. J. and Hackney, E. (1959). The presence of nitrous oxide and methyl nitrite in cigarette smoke and tobacco pyrolysis gases. *Tobacco Science,* 3, 139–43.

Pillsbury, H. C., Bright, C. C., O'Connor, K. J., and Irish, F. W. (1969). Tar and nicotine in cigarette smoke. *Journal of the Association of Official Analytical Chemists,* 52, 458–62.

R. J. Reynolds Tobacco Company (1988). *New cigarette prototypes that heat instead of burn tobacco. Chemical and biological studies.* Reynolds Tobacco Co., Winston-Salem, NC.

Roberts, D. L. Natural tobacco flavor. *Recent Advances in Tobacco Science,* 14, 49–81, 1988.

Roberts, D. L. and Rowland, R. L. (1962). Macrocyclic diterpenes, α- and β-4,8,13-duvatriene-1,3-diol from tobacco. *Journal of Organic Chemistry,* 27, 3989–95.

Roe, J. F. C., Salaman, M. H. Cohen, J., and Burgan, J. C. (1959). Incomplete carcinogens in cigarette smoke condensate. Tumor promotion by phenolic fraction. *British Journal of Cancer,* 13, 623–33.

Rose, J. E. and Levin, E. D. (ed.) (1996). *Eclipse and the harm reduction strategy for smoking.* Conference, Duke University, Bryan Center, Durham, NC, 23 August.

Russell, M. A. H. (1976). Low-tar, medium nicotine cigarettes: A new approach to safer smoking. *British Medical Journal,* 6023, 1430–3.

Russell, M. A. H. (1980). The case for medium-nicotine, low-tar, low-carbon monoxide cigarettes. *Banbury Report 3,* pp. 297–310. Cold Spring Harbor, Cold Spring Harbor Laboratory, NY.

Schultz, W. and Seehofer, F. (1978). Smoking behavior in Germany. The analysis of cigarette butts. In: *Smoking behavior, physiological and psychological influences,* (ed. R. E. Thornton), pp. 259–76. Churchill Livingston, Edinburgh.

Schumacher, J. N. (1970). The isolation of 6-*O*-acetyl-2,3,4-tri-*O*-[(+)-3 methylvaleryl]-β-D-glucopyranose from tobacco. *Carbohydrate Research,* 13, 1–8.

Senkus, M. (ed.) (1976). Leaf composition and physical properties in relation to smoking quality and aroma. *Recent Advances in Tobacco Science*, **2**, 1–135.

Shepherd, R. J. K. (1994). New charcoal filters. *Tobacco Reporter*, **121** (2), 10–14.

Sims, J. L., Atkinson, W. D., and Benner, P. (1975). Nitrogen fertilization and genotype effects of selected constituents from all-burley cigarettes. *Tobacco Science*, **23**, 11–13.

Singer, B. and Essigmann, J. M. (1991). Site-specific mutagenesis: Retrospective and prospective. *Carcinogenesis*, **12** (6), 945–55.

Smith, C. J., McCarns, S. C., Davis, R. A., Livingston, S. D., Bombick, B. R., Avolos, J. T., *et al.* (1996). Human urine mutagenicity study comparing cigarettes which burn or primarily heat tobacco. *Mutation Research*, **361** (1), 1–9.

Society for Research on Nicotine and Tobacco (2000). Policy committee urges regulation on Eclipse. *SRNT Newsletter*, **6** (2–3), 21–2.

Spears, A. W. (1974). Effect of manufacturing variables in cigarette smoke composition. *CORESTA Bulletin* Montreux, Switzerland, Symp. p. 6.

Spears, A.W. (1963). Selective filtration of volatile phenolic compounds from cigarette smoke. *Tobacco Science*, **7**, 76–80.

Spears, A. W. and Jones, S. T. (1981). Chemical and physical criteria for tobacco leaf of modern day cigarettes. *Recent Advances in Tobacco Science*, **7**, 19–39.

Stedman, R. L., Burdick, D., and Schmeltz, I. (1963). Composition studies on tobacco. XVII. Steam-smoke, volatile acid fraction of cigarette. *Tobacco Science*, **7**, 166–9.

Stellman, S. D., Muscat, J. E., Thompson, S., Hoffmann, D., and Wynder, E. L. (1997). Risk of squamous cell carcinoma and adenocarcinoma of the lung in relation to lifetime filter cigarette smoking. *Cancer*, **80** (3), 362–8.

Stiles, M. F., Guy, T. D., Morgen, W. T., Edwards, D. W., Davis, R. W., and Robinson, J. H. (1999). Human smoking behavior study. ECLIPSE cigarette compared to usual brand. *Toxicologist*, **48**, 119–20.

Terpstra, P. M., Renninghaus, W., and Solana, R. P. (1998). Evaluation of the electrically heated cigarette. S.O.T. 1998 Annual Meeting, *The Toxicologist*. *Toxicological Sciences*, **42** (1S), 295; Abstract 1452.

Terrell, J. H. and Schmeltz, I. (1970). Alteration of cigarette smoke composition. II. Influence of cigarette design. *Tobacco Science*, **14**, 82–5.

Tiggelbeck, D. (1976). Vapor phase modification. An under-utilized technology. *Proceedings of the 3rd World Conference on Smoking and Health*. Vol. 1, *Modifying the Risk for the Smoker*. DHEW Publ. No. (NIH) 76–1221, pp. 507–14.

Törnqvist, M., Osterman-Golkar, S., Kautiainen, A., Jensen, S., Farmer, P. B., and Ehrenberg, L. (1986). Tissue doses of ethylene oxide in cigarette smokers determined from adduct levels in hemoglobin. *Carcinogenesis*, **7** (9), 1519–21.

Tso, T. C. (1990). *Production, physiology and biochemistry of tobacco Plant*. Ideals, Beltsville, MD.

Tso, T. C., Chaplin, J. P., Adams, J. D., and Hoffmann, D. (1982). Simple correlation and multiple regression among leaf and smoke characteristics of burley tobaccos. *Beiträge zur Tabakforschung International*, **11**, 141–50.

Tsuda, M. and Kurashima, Y. (1991). Tobacco smoking, chewing and snuff dipping. Factors contributing to the endogenous formation of *N*-nitroso compounds. *Critical Reviews in Toxicology*, **21** (4), 243–53.

US Consumer Product Safety Commission (1993). *Practicability of developing a performance standard to reduce cigarette ignition propensity*, Vol. 1. USCPSC, Washington, DC.

US Department of Health and Human Services (1989). *Reducing the health consequences of smoking. 25 Years of progress.* A Report of the Surgeon General of the Public Health Service, Rockville, MD. DHHS Publ. No. (CDC) 89–8411.

Vincent, R. G., Pickren, J. W., Lane, W. W., Bross, I., Takita, H., Haten, L., *et al.* (1977). The changing histopathology of lung cancer. *Cancer,* **39** (4), 1647–55.

Voges, E. (1984). *Tobacco encyclopedia.* Tobacco Journal International, Mainz, Germany.

Waltz, P. and Häusermann, M. (1963). Modern cigarettes and their effects on the smoking habits and on the composition of cigarette smoke [in German]. *Zeitschrift fur Präventivmedizin,* **8**, 3–98.

Wilkenfeld, J., Henningfield, J., Slade, J., Burns, D., Pinney, J. (2000*a*). It's time for a change: cigarette smokers deserve meaningful information about their cigarettes. *Journal of the National Cancer Institute,* **92** (2), 90–2.

Wilkenfeld, J., Henningfield, J., Slade, J., Burns, D., and Pinney, J. (2000*b*). Response to correspondence re: 'It's time for a change: cigarette smokers deserve meaningful information about their cigarettes'. *Journal of the National Cancer Institute,* **92** (2), 842–3.

Wittekindt, W. (1985). Changes in recommended plant protection agents for tobacco. *Tobacco Journal International,* **5**, 390–4.

Wynder, E. L. and Graham, E. A. (1950). Tobacco smoking as a possible etiologic factor in bronchiogenic carcinoma. A study of six hundred and eighty-four proved cases. *Journal of the American Medical Association,* **143**, 329–36 [reprinted in *Journal of the American Medical Association,* **253** (20), 2986–94].

Wynder, E. L., Graham, E. A., and Croninger, A. G. (1953). Experimental production of carcinoma with cigarette tar. *Cancer Research,* **13**, 855–64.

Wynder, E. L. and Hoffmann, D. (1960). Some practical aspects of the smoking—cancer problem. *New England Journal of Medicine,* **262**, 540–5.

Wynder, E. L. and Hoffmann, D. (1961). A study of tobacco carcinogenesis. VIII. The role of acidic fractions as promoters. *Cancer,* **14**, 1306–15.

Wynder, E. L. and Hoffmann, D. (1962). A study of air pollution carcinogenesis. III. Carcinogenic activity of gasoline engine exhaust. *Cancer,* **152**, 103–8.

Wynder, E. L. and Hoffmann, D. (1963). A contribution to experimental tobacco carcinogenesis [in German]. *Deut. Med. Wochenschr.,* **88**, 623–8.

Wynder, E.L. and Hoffmann, D. (1965). Reduction of tumorigenicity of tobacco smoke. An experimental approach. *Journal of the American Medical Association,* **192**, 85–94.

Wynder, E. L. and Hoffmann, D. (1967). *Tobacco and tobacco smoke. Studies in experimental carcinogenesis.* Academic Press, New York.

Wynder, E. L. and Hoffmann, D. (1994). Smoking and lung cancer: scientific challenges and opportunities. *Cancer Research,* **54** (20), 5284–95.

Wynder, E. L. and Mann, J. (1957). A study of tobacco carcinogenesis III. Filtered cigarettes. *Cancer,* **10**, 1201–5.

Wynder, E. L., Kopf, P., and Ziegler, H. (1957). A study of tobacco carcinogenesis. II. Dose–response studies. *Cancer,* **10**, 1193–200.

Chapter 5

Tobacco smoke carcinogens: Human uptake and DNA interactions

Stephen S. Hecht

Introduction

Tobacco products cause approximately 30 per cent of all cancer death in developed countries (Peto *et al.* 1996; World Health Organization 1997). In spite of this, there are over 1 billion smokers in the world (World Health Organization 1997). Exposure to environmental tobacco smoke (ETS) is also a recognized cause of cancer (National Cancer Institute 1999). Mortality from cancers caused by tobacco products—lung, larynx, oral cavity, esophagus, pancreas, kidney, liver, bladder, stomach, and colon—will continue to be significant in the foreseeable future (International Agency for Research on Cancer 1986*b*; Doll 1996; Chao *et al.* 2000). We need to achieve a better understanding of mechanisms of tobacco-induced cancer in humans in order to develop new cancer prevention strategies.

Carcinogens form the link between nicotine addiction and lung cancer (Fig. 5.1) (Hecht 1999). Nicotine is the reason people continue to smoke in spite of the well-known adverse health effects of this habit. Nicotine is not a carcinogen. However, the cigarette is a disastrous nicotine-delivery device because carcinogens accompany nicotine in each puff. Although the dose of each carcinogen per cigarette is quite small, the cumulative dose in a lifetime of smoking can be considerable. Carcinogens are responsible for cancer induction by tobacco products.

In most cases, tobacco carcinogens require enzymatic processing (metabolic activation) to reactive forms (electrophiles) that bind to DNA, forming covalent binding products called DNA adducts (Fig. 5.1). There are competing detoxification processes which are protective. DNA adducts are absolutely central to the carcinogenic process. They can be removed by cellular repair mechanisms. But if they persist, miscoding can occur during DNA replication, leading to permanent mutations. If the mutations occur in critical regions of genes involved in regulation of growth, such as oncogenes or tumor suppressor genes, normal cellular growth control mechanisms can be lost and, ultimately, cancer can develop. The carcinogen dose depends on the amount of a tobacco product that an individual may use, and the way in which he or she uses it. Individuals differ in the extent to which they activate tobacco carcinogens metabolically

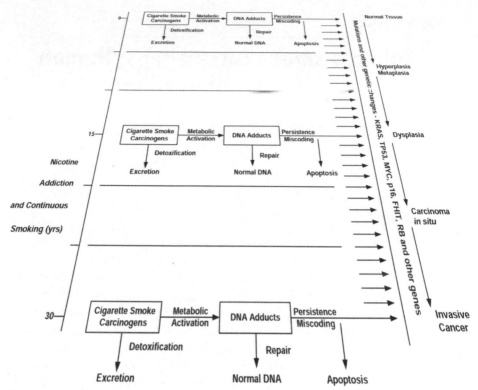

Fig. 5.1 Scheme illustrating the central role of carcinogens and their DNA adducts as causes of the multiple genetic changes observed in lung cancer after years of nicotine addiction and cigarette smoking.

and in the ways that they process DNA adducts. These and other factors may determine cancer susceptibility. Figure 5.1 illustrates the way in which chronic exposure to the multiple carcinogens in cigarette smoke results in multiple genetic changes in critical genes and to lung cancer. The same scheme can be applied to other tobacco-related cancers, although the details may differ somewhat. This chapter will discuss some important aspects of cancer induction as related to inhaled tobacco carcinogens: the role of particular carcinogens as causes of tobacco-induced cancers; quantifying carcinogen uptake in humans by measurement of urinary carcinogen metabolites; and DNA adducts of tobacco carcinogens.

Tobacco smoke carcinogens and cancer

The potential role of tobacco smoke carcinogens in smoking-associated cancers can be evaluated by various means, but it is important to consider levels of the compounds in cigarette smoke and their ability to induce tumors in laboratory animals. In the following, these factors are discussed with respect to cancers of the lung, oral cavity, esophagus, pancreas, and bladder.

Established pulmonary carcinogens in cigarette smoke include polycyclic aromatic hydrocarbons (PAH), aza-arenes, tobacco-specific nitrosamines, e.g. 4-(methylnitrosamino)-1-(3-pyridyl)-1-butanone (NNK), 1,3-butadiene, ethyl carbamate, ethylene oxide, nickel, chromium, cadmium, polonium-210, arsenic, and hydrazine. These compounds convincingly induce lung tumors in at least one animal species and have been positively identified in cigarette smoke.

Among the PAH, benzo(a)pyrene (BaP) (see Fig. 5.2 for structures) is the most extensively studied compound and its ability to induce lung tumors upon local administration or inhalation has been established convincingly (International Agency for Research on Cancer 1972a, 1983; Hecht 1999). Lung tumors were not observed when BaP was administered in the diet to B6C3F1 mice (Culp *et al.* 1998). In studies of lung tumor induction by implantation in rats, BaP is more carcinogenic than the benzo-fluoranthenes or indeno[1,2,3-cd]pyrene (Deutsch-Wenzel *et al.* 1983). Extensive analytical data convincingly demonstrate the presence of BaP in cigarette smoke. Its sales-weighted concentration in current 'full-flavored' cigarettes is about 9 ng/cigarette (Chepiga *et al.* 2000). The abundant literature on BaP tends to diminish attention to other PAH such as dibenz[a,h]-anthracene, 5-methylchrysene (5-MeC), and dibenzo-[a,i]pyrene, which are substantially stronger lung tumorigens than BaP in mice or hamsters, but occur in lower concentrations in cigarette smoke than does BaP (Sellakumar and Shubik 1974; Nesnow *et al.* 1995).

Among the N-nitrosamines, N-nitrosodiethylamine is an effective pulmonary carcinogen in the hamster, but not the rat (International Agency for Research on Cancer 1978; Reznik-Shuller 1983). Its levels in cigarette smoke (up to 3 ng/cigarette) are low compared to those of other carcinogens. The tobacco-specific N-nitrosamine, NNK, is a potent lung carcinogen in rodents (Hecht 1998). Its activity is particularly impressive in rats, where total doses as low as 6 mg/kg, administered by subcutaneous (s.c.) injection, or 35 mg/kg administered in the drinking water, produced significant lung tumor incidences. Even lower doses induced lung tumors when considered in dose–response trend analyses (Hecht 1998). It is the only compound in cigarette smoke known to induce lung tumors systemically in all three commonly used rodent models. NNK has remarkable affinity for the lung, causing mainly adenoma and adenocarcinoma, independent of the route of administration (Hecht 1998). NNK is the most abundant systemic lung carcinogen in cigarette smoke. Multiple international studies definitively document the presence of NNK in cigarette smoke; its sales-weighted concentration in current 'full-flavored cigarettes' is 131 ng/cigarette (Hecht and Hoffmann 1988; Spiegelhalder and Bartsch 1996; Chepiga *et al.* 2000). NNK is tobacco specific because it is a chemical relative of nicotine. It is only found in tobacco products or tobacco-related materials.

The lung is one of the multiple sites of tumorigenesis by 1,3-butadiene in mice, but is not a target in the rat (International Agency for Research on Cancer 1992). B6C3F1 mice develop lung tumors at exposure concentrations that are three orders of

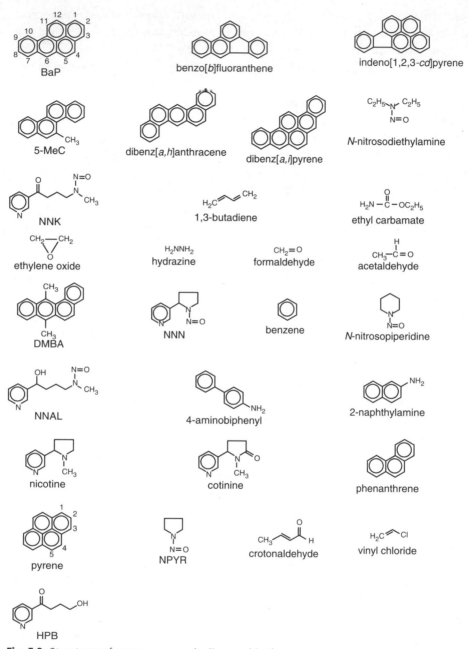

Fig. 5.2 Structures of some compounds discussed in the text.

magnitude lower than those that cause cancer in Sprague–Dawley rats (Owen *et al.* 1987; National Toxicology Program 1993). These interspecies differences are likely due to differences in metabolism of 1,3-butadiene. Mice convert a higher portion of the parent compound to highly carcinogenic 1,2,3,4-diepoxybutane, while the detoxification pathway via conjugation with glutathione is more prominent in rats (Thornton-Manning *et al.* 1995). Ethyl carbamate is a well-established pulmonary carcinogen in mice but not in other species (International Agency for Research on Cancer 1974*a*). Ethylene oxide induces pulmonary tumors in mice, but not in rats (International Agency for Research on Cancer 1986*a*). Nickel, chromium, cadmium, and arsenic are all present in tobacco, and a percentage of each is transferred to mainstream smoke (Hoffmann *et al.* 2001). Levels of polonium-210 in tobacco smoke are insufficient to have a significant impact on lung cancer initiation in smokers (Harley *et al.* 1980). Hydrazine is an effective lung carcinogen in mice and has been detected in cigarette smoke (International Agency for Research on Cancer 1973). Formaldehyde and acetaldehyde induce nasal tumors in rats when administered by inhalation (Swenberg *et al.* 1980; International Agency for Research on Cancer 1982, 1985, 1999). Although they are not lung carcinogens, their concentrations in cigarette smoke are so high that they may nevertheless play a significant role. There is approximately 100 000 times more acetaldehyde than BaP in a cigarette (Chepiga *et al.* 2000).

Collectively, the available data indicate that PAH and NNK are important lung carcinogens in cigarette smoke, and are most likely to be involved in lung cancer initiation in smokers. Their potent carcinogenic activities compensate for their relatively low concentrations in tobacco smoke. Other carcinogens mentioned here, as well as tumor promoters and co-carcinogens, may also play a role as causes of lung cancer in smokers.

The potent PAH carcinogen 7,12-dimethylbenz[*a*]anthracene (DMBA) is used routinely for induction of oral tumors in the hamster (Solt *et al.* 1987). However, DMBA is not present in cigarette smoke. Other PAHs have been less frequently tested in this model. A mixture of NNK and *N'*-nitrosonornicotine (NNN) induced oral tumors in rats treated repetitively by oral swabbing (Hecht *et al.* 1986). The rat oral cavity is one target of benzene carcinogenicity (National Toxicology Program 1986). The risk for oral cancer is markedly enhanced by alcohol consumption in smokers, perhaps due in part to enhancement of carcinogen metabolic activation by ethanol (McCoy and Wynder 1979; Melikian *et al.* 1990).

Numerous *N*-nitrosamines are potent esophageal carcinogens in rats (Preussmann and Stewart 1984). Among these, NNN, a tobacco-specific *N*-nitrosamine, is by far the most prevalent in cigarette smoke. *N*-Nitrosodiethylamine and *N*-nitrosopiperidine are two other smoke constituents that could be involved in esophageal tumor induction in smokers. BaP induces some esophageal tumors when administered to mice in the diet (Culp *et al.* 1998). The risk for esophageal cancer in humans is also enhanced by alcohol consumption (McCoy and Wynder 1979).

NNK and its major metabolite 4-(methylnitrosamino)-1-(3-pyridyl)-1-butanol (NNAL) are the only known pancreatic carcinogens in cigarette smoke (Rivenson *et al.* 1988). Low doses of these *N*-nitrosamines induce pancreatic tumors in rats, in addition to lung tumors (Hecht 1998). Pancreatic tumors are also observed in the offspring of pregnant rats treated with NNK, and this effect is markedly enhanced by ethanol (Schüller *et al.* 1993).

4-Aminobiphenyl and 2-naphthylamine are known human bladder carcinogens (International Agency for Research on Cancer 1972*b*, 1974*b*). Both are present in cigarette smoke. Hemoglobin adducts of 4-aminobiphenyl and other aromatic amines have been used as dosimeters of 4-aminobiphenyl uptake in humans, and their levels are associated with bladder cancer induction in smokers (Castelao *et al.* 2001). The evidence is strong that aromatic amines play a significant role as causes of bladder cancer in smokers (Vineis *et al.* 2001).

Cigarette smoke contains free radicals and induces oxidative damage (Pryor 1997; Arora *et al.* 2001). The gas phase of freshly generated cigarette smoke has large amounts of nitric oxide and other unstable oxidants (Hecht 1999). The particulate phase is postulated to contain long-lived radicals that may undergo quinone–hydroquinone redox cycling (Pryor 1997). The presence of such free radicals and oxidants can lead to oxidative DNA damage. However, the role of oxidative damage in cancer induced by cigarette smoke is unclear.

Urinary metabolites as biomarkers of tobacco carcinogen uptake in humans

It is important to understand the carcinogen dose in smokers. Carcinogen-related biomarkers, such as metabolites or adducts, have been used to quantify carcinogen uptake in humans. DNA adduct measurements give direct information on the extent of carcinogen reactions with DNA (Bartsch 1996; Phillips 1996; Poirier and Weston 1996; Kriek *et al.* 1998). If measured in target tissues or cells, DNA adduct levels could relate directly to risk, because DNA adducts are central to the carcinogenic process. There are technical problems associated with the measurement of specific DNA adducts, but nevertheless some valuable information is available. Tobacco carcinogen-DNA adducts are discussed later in this chapter. Protein adducts have frequently been used as surrogates for DNA adducts because the two parameters tend to be correlated, and protein, such as hemoglobin or albumin, is relatively easy to obtain in large quantities (Ehrenberg and Osterman-Golkar 1976; Skipper and Tannenbaum 1990). There are no known repair processes for protein adducts and they accumulate over the lifetime of the protein in which they are formed, potentially providing an integrated measure of exposure. A third type of carcinogen biomarker is urinary metabolites, which will be the focus of human tobacco carcinogen uptake studies discussed here. Urinary metabolites have certain advantages. Important among these is their quantity, which is generally great enough that, with the use of modern analytical methods, reliable data can almost always be obtained. This is frequently not the case when one is measuring DNA or protein adducts. A potential disadvantage of urinary biomarkers is their transitory nature. However, this is mitigated by the chronic use of tobacco products, which provides a consistent level of urinary biomarkers.

The major use of urinary compound measurements to date has been to estimate carcinogen dose. This is presently a particularly relevant question in the area of tobacco and cancer. At this time, new products are being introduced by the tobacco industry. Advertisements for these new products claim substantially reduced levels of well-known tobacco carcinogens, such as PAH and tobacco-specific *N*-nitrosamines. These products have been termed 'potential reduced-exposure products' (PREPS) by the Institute of Medicine in their 2001 report *Clearing the smoke*, which assesses the science base for tobacco harm reduction (Institute of Medicine 2001). Constituents of PREPS have been determined by the industry using standardized machine methods. However, such methods clearly do not reflect actual human use patterns for tobacco products, because smokers may change the way they use the new products (smokers' compensation) (Djordjevic *et al.* 1995, 2000). Therefore, we do not know whether, in fact, carcinogen uptake by users of PREPS will be reduced. Urinary biomarkers can determine, in a straightforward way, whether carcinogen exposure has actually been altered in people who use PREPS. This would be the essential first step in evaluating the potential reduced risk of these products. The evaluation of such products is mandatory in view of the findings of the recent report *Risks associated with smoking cigarettes with low machine-measured yields of tar and nicotine*, which demonstrates that smokers of 'light' cigarettes marketed over the past several decades are not protected, and that the popularity of these brands resulted in a sustained increase in lung cancer among older smokers (National Cancer Institute 2001).

Cotinine and its further transformation products, major metabolites of nicotine, have been used extensively as biomarkers of nicotine uptake from tobacco products (Benowitz *et al.* 1994; Benowitz 1996). However, cotinine and nicotine are not carcinogenic and, although cotinine measurements do provide a measure of nicotine exposure, they say little about potential carcinogenicity.

This chapter will present two examples—metabolites of PAH and NNK—as urinary biomarkers of tobacco carcinogen uptake in humans. Among the PAHs, metabolites of phenanthrene are one group of urinary biomarkers that have been used to monitor uptake. Phenanthrene is the simplest nonlinear PAH and is a reasonable model for metabolism studies of carcinogenic PAH molecules (International Agency for Research on Cancer 1986*b*; Hoffmann and Hecht 1990; Hecht 1999). However, phenanthrene is inactive as a carcinogen (LaVoie and Rice 1988). Concentrations of phenanthrene in mainstream smoke are 85–620 ng/cigarette (International Agency for Research on Cancer 1986*b*). Hydroxyphenanthrenes and phenanthrene dihydrodiols have been quantified in human urine. Heudorf and Angerer (2001), using high performance liquid chromatography (HPLC) with fluorescence detection, reported highly significant differences between smokers and nonsmokers, and in dose–response relationships to cigarettes smoked/day, in levels of 2-, 3-, and 4-hydroxyphenanthrene, but not 1-hydroxyphenanthrene. There are important sources of phenanthrene exposure other than smoking. This has been well documented in environmental and occupational settings with high PAH exposure (Heudorf and Angerer 2001). Phenanthrene metabolites appear to have considerable promise for probing human PAH metabolism.

Pyrene is a noncarcinogenic component of all PAH mixtures. Its concentration in mainstream cigarette smoke is 50–270 ng/cigarette (International Agency for Research on Cancer 1986b). The major urinary metabolite of pyrene is 1-hydroxypyrene (1-HOP), excreted as a glucuronide conjugate. Jongeneelen pioneered the development of a method for measurement of 1-HOP in urine (Jongeneelen et al. 1985). After enzymatic hydrolysis, the released 1-HOP is enriched by reverse-phase chromatography and quantified by HPLC with fluorescence detection. Variations of this method have been described. 1-HOP has been measured in hundreds of studies of occupational and environmental PAH exposure. Data on the effects of smoking have been reviewed by Jongeneelen (1994, 2001), van Rooj et al. (1994), Heudorf and Angerer (2001), and Levin (1995). Most studies find significantly higher levels of 1-HOP in smokers than in nonsmokers. Some representative data from recent investigations of urinary 1-HOP are summarized in Table 5.1. These data are from non-occupationally exposed individuals. Levels in the urine of nonsmokers vary considerably and are likely to be influenced by environmental pollution and diet. In most studies, 1-HOP levels in smokers' urine are about twice as great as in nonsmokers, although greater differences have been reported. Levels may be influenced by genetic polymorphisms in carcinogen-metabolizing enzymes (Alexandrie et al. 2000; Nerurkar et al. 2000; Nan et al. 2001; van Delft et al. 2001).

Measurement of BaP metabolites in the urine of smokers could potentially provide a direct assessment of carcinogen dose. However, unlike the lower molecular weight PAH considered above, the concentrations of BaP in cigarette smoke are quite low, and in laboratory animals its metabolites are excreted mainly in the feces. Therefore, BaP metabolites are difficult to quantify in smokers' urine.

3-HydroxyBaP is a major metabolite of BaP *in vitro* and is excreted in urine as its glucuronide. Methods for quantitation of 3-hydroxyBaP in human urine have been described (Grimmer et al. 1997; Gundel and Angerer 2000; Simon et al. 2000). These methods are based on HPLC with fluorescence detection or gas chromatography–mass spectrometry (GC–MS). Reported levels are quite low, ranging from about 1 to 14 ng/l in exposed workers. Limited data are available on smokers.

r-7,t-8,9,c-10-Tetrahydroxy-7,8,9,10-tetrahydrobenzo[a]pyrene (*trans-anti-*BaP-tetraol) is a hydrolysis product of *anti*-7,8-dihydroxy-9,10-epoxy-7,8,9,10-tetrahydrobenzo[a]pyrene (BPDE), the major established DNA-reactive metabolite of BaP. This metabolite has been quantified in human urine by GC-negative ion chemical

Table 5.1 1-Hydroxypyrene in the urine of smokers and nonsmokers: representative recent studies

1-Hydroxypyrene level[a]		Fold Increase	Significant Difference?	Reference
Nonsmoker	**Smoker**			
0.12 µmol/mol C[b]	0.21 µmol/mol C	1.8	Yes	(Roggi et al. 1997)
0.55 nmol/l	1.04 nmol/l	1.9	Yes	(Sithisarankul et al. 1997)
0.089 µmol/mol C	0.176 µmol/mol C (<15 cig/day)	2.0	Yes	(Merlo et al. 1998)
	0.226 µmol/mol C (>15 cig/day)	2.5	Yes	(Merlo et al. 1998)
0.784 nmol/24h	1.59 nmol/24h	2.0	Yes	(Scherer et al. 2000)
1.10 nmol/l	2.47 nmol/l	2.2	Yes	(Pastorelli et al. 1999)
1.0 nmol/24h	2.77 nmol/24h	2.8	Yes	(Jacob et al. 1999)
0.04 µmol/mol C	0.20 µmol/mol C: light	5.0	Yes	(Li et al. 2000)
	0.46 µmol/mol C: medium	11.5	Yes	(Li et al.2000)
	1.16 µmol/mol C: heavy	29	Yes	(Li et al. 2000)
0.27 nmol/12h	0.51 nmol/12h	1.9	Yes	(Nerurkar et al. 2000)
0.03 µmol/mol C[c]	0.04 µmol/mol C[c]	1.3	Yes	(Dor et al. 2000)
0.10 µmol/mol C	0.17 µmol/mol C	1.7	Yes	(Alexandrie et al. 2001)
0.04 µmol/mol C[d]	0.05 µmol/mol C[d]	1.3	No	(Nan et al. 2001)
0.27 µmol/mol C	0.70 µmol/mol C	2.6	Yes	(van Delft et al. 2001)
0.03 µmol/mol C	0.05 µmol/mol C	1.7	Yes	(Kim et al. 2001)
0.11 µmol/mol C	0.57 µmol/mol C	5.2	Yes	(Szaniszlo and Ungvary, 2001)

[a]Arithmetic mean unless noted otherwise.
[b]C, creatinine.
[c]Median.
[d]Geometric mean.

ionization–MS (Simpson et al. 2000). The method was applied to psoriasis patients treated with a coal tar ointment, coke oven workers, and smokers. Levels of *trans-anti-*BaP-tetraol in the urine of smokers were lower than in the other two groups, ranging from not detected to 0.2 fmol/µmol creatinine. It was not detectable in urine samples from 12 of 21 smokers (Simpson et al. 2000). Immunoaffinity-synchronous fluorescence spectroscopy methods for quantitation of BaP-tetraols in human urine have also been reported, but they have not been applied to smokers' urine (Weston *et al.* 1993; Bowman *et al.* 1997; Bentsen-Farmen *et al.*, 1999).

BaP metabolites can be converted to BaP by treatment with hydrogen iodide (HI). This reaction has been employed as the basis for a technique to determine urinary metabolites of BaP and several other PAHs (Becher and Bjorseth 1983; Becher *et al.* 1984; Venier *et al.* 1985; Haugen *et al.* 1986; Buckley *et al.* 1995). In occupationally non-exposed individuals, levels of BaP determined by this method ranged from 4 to 19 ng/mmol creatinine in nonsmokers ($N = 5$) and 18 to 102 ng/mmol creatinine in smokers ($N = 4$) (Becher *et al.* 1984). Problems with this method include different conversions for various metabolites and low analytical recoveries (Buckley *et al.* 1995).

An unstable BaP–DNA adduct, 7-(benzo[*a*]pyren-6-yl)adenine, has been reported in the urine of 3 of 7 smokers, and, in one, its quantity was estimated as 0.6 fmol/mg creatinine (Casale *et al.* 2001).

Several studies have reported the presence of other PAH metabolites in urine, including hydroxychrysenes and chrysene dihydrodiols (Grimmer *et al.* 1997), 3-hydroxybenz[*a*]anthracene (Gundel and Angerer 2000), and—under high-exposure conditions—3-hydroxyfluoranthene, 6-hydroxychrysene, and 6-hydroxyindeno-[1,2,3-*cd*]pyrene (Mumford *et al.* 1995). None of these studies investigated the relationship of these metabolites to smoking. In addition, several PAHs have been reported in urine treated with HI, as described above (Becher and Bjorseth 1983; Becher *et al.* 1984; Haugen *et al.* 1986). These include fluorene, phenanthrene, anthracene, fluoranthene, benz[*a*]anthracene, chrysene and benzo[*e*]pyrene, but there are insufficient data to evaluate the utility of this methodology as a biomarker of PAH uptake in smokers.

NNAL and its glucuronides are quantitatively significant metabolites of NNK in rodents and humans (Hecht 1998). NNAL, like NNK, is a pulmonary carcinogen with particularly strong activity in the rat (Hecht 1998). Glucuronidation of NNAL at the pyridine nitrogen gives NNAL-*N*-Gluc while conjugation at the carbinol oxygen yields NNAL-*O*-Gluc. Both NNAL-*N*-Gluc and NNAL-*O*-Gluc exist as a mixture of two diastereomers, and each diastereomer is a mixture of *E*- and *Z*-rotamers (Upadhyaya *et al.* 2001). The NNAL glucuronides are collectively referred to as NNAL-Gluc. (*R*)-NNAL-*O*-Gluc is inactive as a tumorigen in mice (Upadhyaya *et al.* 1999).

NNAL and NNAL-Gluc can be determined readily in urine by gas chromatography with nitrosamine-selective detection (GC-TEA) (Carmella *et al.* 1993, 1995; Hecht *et al.* 1999). The presence of these metabolites in human urine has also been established by MS methods, but, at present, these are less convenient and sensitive than GC-TEA (Carmella *et al.* 1993, 1999; Parsons *et al.* 1998; Lackmann *et al.* 1999; Hecht *et al.* 2001). Typical levels are about 1 nmol/24 h NNAL and 2.2 nmol/24 h NNAL-Gluc; unchanged NNK is not detected. Investigations of NNAL and NNAL-Gluc in human urine are summarized in Table 5.2. Several points are noteworthy. In studies to date, this biomarker is absolutely specific to tobacco exposure. It has not been detected

Table 5.2 NNAL and its glucuronides (NNAL-Gluc) in urine: biomarkers of NNK uptake

Study group	Main conclusions	Reference
A. Smokers		
1. 11 smokers (9F)[a] 7 nonsmokers	NNAL and 2 diastereomers of NNAL-O-Gluc identified in smokers' urine, but not in non-smokers' urine. NNK not detected	(Carmella et al. 1993)
2. 74 smokers (41F)	NNAL + NNAL-Gluc: levels stable day to day in smokers' urine; NNAL-Gluc:NNAL ratios fairly stable; Range of NNAL-Gluc:NNAL ratios 0.7–10.8	(Carmella et al. 1995)
3. 11 smokers (6F)	NNAL + NNAL-Gluc increased by 33.5% (P<0.01) on days when watercress was consumed compared to baseline and follow-up periods	(Hecht et al. 1995)
4. 61 smokers (31F)	NNAL-Gluc:NNAL ratio higher in Caucasians than African-Americans	(Richie et al. 1997)
5. 19 smokers	NNAL-Gluc: NNAL ratio and NNAL plus NNAL-Gluc fairly stable over a two year period in one individual	(Meger et al. 1996)
6. 13 smokers (F)	Indole-3-carbinol caused significant decreases in levels of NNAL and NNAL plus NNAL-Gluc and increased NNAL-Gluc: NNAL ratio	(Taioli et al. 1997)
7. 27 smokers (13F)	NNAL and NNAL-Gluc highly persistent after smoking cessation; 34.5% of baseline amount remained after 1 week, 15.3% after 3 weeks. No effect of nicotine patch use on levels or persistence of NNAL or NNAL-Gluc	(Hecht et al. 1999)
8. 30 smokers (18F)	Enantiomeric distribution of NNAL, 54%(S); diastereomeric distribution of NNAL-Gluc, 68%(S)	(Carmella et al. 1999)
9. 23 smokers (13F)	Reduction in smoking caused a significant decrease in NNAL-Gluc but not NNAL	(Hurt et al. 2000)
10. 20 smokers (M)	Levels of NNAL and NNAL-Gluc were (mean ± S.D.) 1494 ± 1090 and 1724 ± 946 pmol/day, respectively	(Meger et al. 2000)
11. 10 smokers	NNAL-N-Gluc identified in urine, comprises 50 ± 25% of total NNAL-Gluc	(Carmella et al. 2002)
B. Smokeless tobacco users		
1. 7 toombak users (M)	Exceptionally high levels of NNAL and NNAL-Gluc (0.12–0.44 mg) excreted daily. (S)-NNAL-O-Gluc:(R)-NNAL-O-Gluc ratio, 1.9	(Murphy et al. 1994)

Table 5.2 (continued) NNAL and its glucuronides (NNAL-Gluc) in urine: biomarkers of NNK uptake

Study group	Main conclusions	Reference
2. 47 smokeless tobacco users (chewers and snuff-dippers) (M)	NNAL and NNAL-Gluc levels similar to those in smokers. Significant association between total NNAL + NNAL-Gluc and oral leukoplakia	(Kresty et al. 1996)
3. 13 smokeless tobacco users (M)	Distribution half-lives of NNAL and NNAL-Gluc significantly shorter in smokeless tobacco users than smokers. Ratios of (S)-NNAL:(R)-NNAL and (S)-NNAL-Gluc:(R)-NNAL-Gluc significantly higher 7 days after cessation than at baseline, suggesting receptor site for (S)-NNAL	(Hecht et al. 2002)
4. 10 smokeless tobacco users and 4 toombak users	NNAL-N-Gluc identified in urine, comprises 24 ± 12% of total NNAL-Gluc	(Carmella et al. 2002)
C. ETS and transplacental exposure		
1. 5 men exposed to ETS	Significantly increased levels of NNAL plus NNAL-Gluc after exposure to ETS in a chamber: mean ± S.D. after exposure, approx 0.16 ± 0.10 pmol/ml	(Hecht et al. 1993)
2. 5M, 4F exposed to ETS, 5 controls unexposed	Significantly increased levels of NNAL-Gluc in workers exposed to ETS compared to negative controls: mean ± S.D. in exposed workers, 0.059 ± 0.028 pmol/ml	(Parsons et al. 1998)
3. 30 non-smokers (13F)	NNAL + NNAL-Gluc levels correlated with nicotine levels on personal samplers. NNAL, 20.3 ± 21.8 pmol/day, NNAL-Gluc, 22.9 ± 28.6 pmol/day in exposed non-smokers	(Meger et al. 2000)
4. 45 non-smoking women, 23 exposed to ETS in the home, 22 non-exposed	NNAL and NNAL-Gluc significantly higher in exposed than in non-exposed women. NNAL + NNAL-Gluc in exposed women, 0.050 ± 0.068 pmol/ml	(Anderson et al. 2001)
5. 204 non-smoking elementary school-aged children	34% with total cotinine ≥ 5 ng/ml; 52/54 of these samples had detectable NNAL or NNAL-Gluc, 93-fold range. Mean ± S.D., NNAL + NNAL-Gluc 0.056 ± 0.076 pmol/ml	(Hecht et al. 2001)
6. 31 newborns of mothers who smoked; 17 newborns of mothers who did not smoke	NNAL-Gluc detected in 71% of urines of newborns of smokers, NNAL in 13%; neither detected in urines of newborns of non-smokers, a significant difference; NNAL + NNAL-Gluc in urine of newborns of smoking mothers, 0.13 ± 0.15 pmol/ml	(Lackmann et al. 1999)

Table 5.2 (continued) NNAL and its glucuronides (NNAL-Gluc) in urine: biomarkers of NNK uptake

Study group	Main conclusions	Reference
7. 21 smokers and 30 non-smokers	NNAL detected in amniotic fluid of 52.4% of smokers and 6.7% of non-smokers, a significant difference. NNAL levels in amniotic fluid of smokers, 0.025 ± 0.029 pmol/ml	(Milunsky et al. 2000)
8. 12 smokers and 10 non-smokers	NNAL and NNAL-Gluc not detected in follicular fluid	(Matthews et al. 2002)

[a]Number and letter in parentheses represent number and gender of subjects.

ETS, environmental tobacco smoke.

in the urine of non-tobacco users unless they were exposed to ETS. Since NNAL is not present in cigarette smoke, the origin of NNAL and NNAL-Gluc in urine is metabolism of NNK. Most investigations to date demonstrate a correlation between NNAL plus NNAL-Gluc and cotinine, indicating that NNAL plus NNAL-Gluc is an effective biomarker of lung carcinogen (NNK) uptake, whereas cotinine is an effective biomarker of nicotine uptake. The NNAL-Gluc:NNAL ratio varies at least tenfold in smokers and, since NNAL-Gluc is a detoxification product whereas NNAL is carcinogenic, this ratio could be a potential indicator of cancer risk (Carmella et al. 1995; Richie et al. 1997). In human urine, (S)-NNAL-O-Gluc is the predominant diastereomer of NNAL-O-Gluc, while (S)-NNAL is slightly in excess over (R)-NNAL (Carmella et al. 1999). (S)-NNAL is the more tumorigenic enantiomer of NNAL in A/J mouse lung (Upadhyaya et al. 1999). NNAL and NNAL-Gluc are only slowly released from the human body after smoking cessation, and this has been linked to particularly strong retention of (S)-NNAL, possibly at a receptor site (Hecht et al. 1999).

Human uptake of carcinogens from ETS has been reviewed (Scherer and Richter 1997). Levels of 1-HOP and hydroxyphenanthrenes in urine are not consistently increased by exposure to ETS, although small effects have been seen under some high-exposure conditions (Hoepfner et al. 1987; Scherer et al. 1992, 2000; van Rooij et al. 1994; Siwinska et al. 1999). All studies reported to date show significantly higher amounts of NNAL plus NNAL-Gluc, or NNAL-Gluc, in the urine of ETS-exposed humans than in unexposed controls (Table 5.2C, entries 1–5). In one study, uptake of NNK was over six times higher in women who lived with smokers compared to women who lived with nonsmokers (Anderson et al. 2001). In another investigation, widespread uptake of NNK was demonstrated in a group of economically disadvantaged schoolchildren (Hecht et al. 2001). As in smokers, a correlation between levels of cotinine and NNAL plus NNAL-Gluc in urine has been consistently observed in ETS-exposed nonsmokers. The assay for NNAL and NNAL-Gluc in urine is ideally suited to investigations of ETS exposure, for two reasons. First, it has the required sensitivity to measure relatively low levels (typically about 0.05 pmol/ml urine). Secondly, since

NNK is a tobacco-specific compound, detection of NNAL and NNAL-Gluc in urine specifically signals ETS exposure. The uptake of NNK by nonsmokers exposed to ETS provides a biochemical link between ETS exposure and lung cancer.

NNAL-Gluc has been detected in the urine of newborns of women who smoked, indicating that NNK, a transplacental carcinogen, crosses the placental barrier and is taken up by the fetus (Lackmann *et al.* 1999). Consistent with these results, NNAL was detected in amniotic fluid of pregnant smokers (Milunsky *et al.* 2000). However, neither NNAL nor NNAL-Gluc could be detected in follicular fluid (Matthews *et al.* 2002).

DNA adducts: Structures, detection, and mutation induction

Table 5.3 summarizes information on structures of some DNA adducts that are formed from representative tobacco smoke carcinogens and related compounds. Available data on the detection of these adducts in lung DNA from smokers, and some likely mutations that may result from their presence, are also summarized.

Adduct structures

Bay region diol epoxides are among the principal PAH metabolites involved in DNA adduct formation (Conney 1982; Szeliga and Dipple 1998). A bay region is an angular region of a PAH molecule, such as the 10–11 positions of BaP (Fig. 5.2). Each diol epoxide metabolite has four stereoisomeric forms. Each of the four diol epoxides reacts with DNA to differing extents, either at the exocyclic amino group of deoxyguanosine (N^2-) or deoxyadenosine (N^6-) (Szeliga and Dipple 1998). Each reaction of the exocyclic amino group results in either *trans-* or *cis-* ring opening of the epoxide ring. Therefore, there are 16 possible adducts of this type from each PAH diol epoxide metabolite (Szeliga and Dipple 1998). All adducts have been thoroughly characterized for multiple PAH molecules. Table 5.3 illustrates only one adduct from each of two PAHs in tobacco smoke: BaP and 5-MeC. This is quantitatively the major one in each case, but it should be noted that 15 other adducts are formed from BPDE and from 5-MeC-1,2-diol-3,4-epoxide. In addition, another set of 16 adducts can be formed from 5-MeC-7,8-diol-9,10-epoxide (Melikian *et al.* 1988). The diol epoxide pathway is not the only mechanism for adduct formation from PAH. Depurinating adducts have been detected as a result of one-electron oxidation, and adducts resulting from quinone formation have also been characterized (Penning *et al.* 1999; Casale *et al.* 2001). Adducts are also formed via 9-hydroxy-BaP-4,5-oxide (Ross and Nesnow 1999).

N-Nitrosamines are metabolized to intermediates that alkylate various positions of the DNA bases (Preussmann and Stewart 1984). The most thoroughly investigated are 7-alkylguanines and O^6-alkylguanines, shown for *N*-nitrosodimethylamine and NNK in Table 5.3. Other products include *N*-1, *N*-3, and N^2-deoxyguanosines, *N*-1, *N*-7, *N*-3, and N^6-deoxyadenosines, O^2-, O^4-, and *N*-3 thymidines, O^2-, *N*-3, and *N*-4 deoxycytidines, and phosphotriesters (Singer and Grunberger 1983). NNK and NNN are metabolized to intermediates that pyridyloxobutylate deoxyguanosine (Hecht 1998).

Table 5.3 Representative DNA adducts of some cigarette smoke carcinogens and related compounds. Occurrence and likely consequent mutations

Carcinogen[a]	DNA base	Adduct[b]	Detected in smokers' lung? (type of evidence)[c]	Likely mutations	Reference
BaP	G		Yes (2)	GC→TA	(Kozack et al. 2000; Seo et al. 2000)
5-MeC	G		No	GC→TA GC→CG	(Misra et al. 1998)
NDMA NNK	G	7–CH$_3$	Yes (1)	d	(Zhao et al. 1999)
		O^6–CH$_3$	Yes (1)	GC→AT	(Loechler et al. 1984; Wilson et al. 1989)
NNK, NNN	G		Yes (2)	GC→TA, GC→AT	(Foiles et al. 1991; Ronai et al. 1993)
NPYR	G		No		(Wang et al. 2001b)
Ethylene oxide	G	7–CH$_2$CH$_2$OH	Yes (1)	d	(Zhao et al. 1999)

Table 5.3 (continued) Representative DNA adducts of some cigarette smoke carcinogens and related compounds. Occurrence and likely consequent mutations

Carcinogen[a]	DNA base	Adduct[b]	Detected in smokers' lung? (type of evidence)[c]	Likely mutations	Reference
1,3-Butadiene	G	$7-CH_2CHCH{=}CH_2$ OH	No	d	(Koc et al. 1999; Tretyakova et al. 1997)
	G	$7-CHCH{=}CH_2$ CH_2OH	No	d	(Koc et al. 1999; Tretyakova et al. 1997)
	A	$1-CH_2CHCH{=}CH_2$ OH	No		(Tretyakova et al. 1997)
	A	$1-CHCH{=}CH_2$ CH_2OH	No		(Tretyakova et al. 1997)
	G	$7-CH_2CHCHCH_2OH$ OH OH	No	d	(Koc et al. 1999; Koivisto et al. 1999)
	A	$1-CH_2CHCHCH_2OH$ OH OH	No		(Zhao et al. 2000)
	G	$N^2-CH_2CHCHCH_2OH$ OH OH	No	GC→TA>GC→ AT>GC→CG	(Carmical et al. 2000)
Acetaldehyde	G	$N^2{=}CHCH_3$	No	GC→AT, AT→TA	(Noori and Hou 2001; Wang et al. 2000a)
	G		No		
Crotonaldehyde	G		No		(Chung et al. 1999)

	Base	Structure	Hotspot	Mutation	Reference
	G	N^2=CHCH$_2$CHCH$_3$ OH	No		(Wang et al. 2001a)
4-Aminobiphenyl	G	C8—NH—(biphenyl)	Yes (1,2)	GC→TA, GC→CG	(Culp et al. 1997; Lin et al. 1994; Melchior et al. 1994)
Vinyl chloride	G	7—CH$_2$CHO	No	d	(Swenberg et al. 1999)
Vinyl chloride	G	(etheno-G structure)	No	GC→AT	(Nair et al. 1999)
Vinyl chloride, Ethyl carbamate	A	(etheno-A structure)	No	AT→GC AT→TA AT→CG	(Guengerich and Kim, 1991; Nair et al. 1999)
2-nitropropane	G	8—NH$_2$ N^2—NH$_2$	No		(Sodum and Fiala, 1998)
Oxidants	G	8—OXO	Yes (3)	GC→TA	(Asami et al. 1997; Moriya, 1993)
Nitric oxide	G	(oxanosine structure)	No		(Burney et al. 1999)

Table 5.3 (continued) Representative DNA adducts of some cigarette smoke carcinogens and related compounds. Occurrence and likely consequent mutations

Carcinogen[a]	DNA base	Adduct[b]	Detected in smokers' lung? (type of evidence)[c]	Likely mutations	Reference
Peroxynitrite	8-oxo-G		No	GC→TA	(Henderson et al., 2002)
			No	GC→TA	
			No	GC→TA	

[a]Abbreviations: BaP, benz[a]pyrene; 5-MeC, 5-methylchrysene; NDMA, N-nitrosodimethylamine; NNK, 4-(methylnitrosamino)-1-(3-pyridyl)-1-butanone; NNN, N'-r itrosonornicotine; NIPYR, N-nitrosopyrrolodine

[b]Adduct structures show the position of attachment to the base (e.g. $N2$-, $O6$-, or 7- of G) and the organic moiety derived from the carcinogen.

[c]Type of evidence

1. detection of nucleoside or base by relatively non-specific method (e.g. ^{32}P-post-labelling or immunoassay)

2. detection of released adducting moiety by specific method

3. detection of nucleoside or base by specific method (e.g. MS, HPLC-fluorescence, or HPLC-electrochemical detection)

[d]Likely to give GC→TA transversions via depurination to an apurinic site

N-Nitrosopyrrolidine (NPYR), a cyclic N-nitrosamine, displays alkylation chemistry that is somewhat different from that of acyclic nitrosamines because the alkylating intermediate is tethered to an aldehyde. A complex mixture of deoxyguanosine adducts is produced, among which the N^2-tetrahydrofuranyl structure shown in Table 5.3 predominates (Wang et al. 2001b).

Ethylene oxide behaves like a typical alkylating agent, reacting primarily at N-7 of deoxyguanosine, as shown in Table 5.3, but also at other positions (Zhao et al. 1999). 1,3-Butadiene is metabolized to 3,4-epoxy-1-butene, 3,4-epoxy-1,2-butanediol, and 1,2,3,4-diepoxybutane (Tretyakova et al. 1997; Koc et al. 1999; Koivisto et al. 1999; Zhao et al. 2000). Most of the DNA adducts arise from the reactions of the diol epoxide at the N-7 position of guanine, N-3 adenine, and N^6-adenine (Table 5.1). Multiple stereoisomers are formed.

Acetaldehyde reacts with the exocyclic amino group of deoxyguanosine to give a Schiff base as the major adduct (Wang et al. 2000a). Several other adducts, including a G–G crosslink, shown in Table 5.3, have also been identified. Crotonaldehyde produces cyclic 1,N^2-deoxyguanosine adducts by Michael addition, and Schiff base adducts by reaction of the aldehyde group with the exocyclic amino group of deoxyguanosine (Chung et al. 1999; Wang et al. 2001a). Other adducts are formed, with multiple stereoisomers, by dimers of 3-hydroxybutanal, produced by hydration of crotonaldehyde (Wang et al. 2000b).

Aromatic amines such as 4-aminobiphenyl and heterocyclic aromatic amines react with DNA mainly at C-8 of deoxyguanosine via their N-hydroxy-metabolites (Delclos and Kadlubar 1997). Adducts have also been observed at N^2- of deoxyguanosine, O^6- of deoxyguanosine, and N^6- of deoxyadenosine.

Vinyl chloride is metabolized to chloroethylene oxide, which reacts with DNA giving 7-oxoethyldeoxyguanosine as a major product along with 'etheno' adducts such as 3,N^2-ethenodeoxyguanosine and 1,N^6-ethenodeoxyadenosine, as shown in Table 5.3 (Nair et al. 1999; Swenberg et al. 1999). Ethyl carbamate is metabolized to vinyl carbamate which similarly reacts giving 1,N^6-ethenodeoxyadenosine (Guengerich and Kim 1991).

2-Nitropropane is metabolized to intermediates that aminate deoxyguanosine at the C-8 and N^2- positions (Sodum and Fiala 1998). Radical oxidants in cigarette smoke are believed to give rise to 8-oxodeoxyguanosine, while nitric oxide yields deoxyoxanosine (shown in Table 5.3) along with other products (Asami et al. 1997; Burney et al. 1999). Recent studies demonstrate that 8-oxodeoxyguanosine is further oxidized by peroxynitrite to a variety of products, including those illustrated in Table 5.3 (Henderson et al. 2002).

Adduct detection

Table 5.3 summarizes information on the detection of specific adducts in lung DNA from smokers. The BaP adduct shown in Table 5.3, BPDE-N^2-dG, has been the subject of numerous studies. Convincing evidence, obtained by HPLC with fluorescence detection of BaP-tetraols released upon acid hydrolysis, clearly demonstrates the presence of BPDE-N^2-dG in some samples of human pulmonary DNA (Kriek *et al.* 1998; Rojas *et al.* 1998). However, the intact nucleoside adduct has never been identified conclusively in human lung DNA. Methods such as ^{32}P-postlabeling and immunoassay have reported the presence of 'PAH–DNA adducts' or 'aromatic DNA adducts' in human lung, but these are mainly uncharacterized (Kriek *et al.* 1998; Santella 1999). It is not certain that they are in fact derived from PAH. Gupta *et al.* (1999) have reported that adducts detected by ^{32}P-postlabeling in lung DNA of cigarette smoke-exposed rats were endogenous adducts enhanced by cigarette smoke. No other specific PAH adducts have been detected with certainty in human lung.

7-Methylguanine and 7-hydroxyethylguanine have been detected in human lung DNA by ^{32}P-postlabeling (Zhao *et al.*, 1999). Levels of 7-methylguanine are higher in smokers than in nonsmokers in some, but not all, studies (Hecht and Tricker 1999). Evidence has also been presented for O^6-methyl- and O^6-ethyldeoxyguanosine in human lung DNA, but confirmation by other methods is lacking (Wilson *et al.* 1989). GC–MS analysis of released 4-hydroxy-1-(3-pyridyl)-1-butanone (HPB) establishes the presence of NNK- or NNN-derived pyridyloxobutyl DNA adducts in human lung (Foiles *et al.* 1991). These adducts, which are produced in part by reaction with deoxyguanosine, are higher in lung DNA from smokers than nonsmokers, as expected, based on the specificity of NNK and NNN to tobacco products.

GC–MS analysis of 4-aminobiphenyl released from human lung DNA provides evidence in support of the presence of the C-8 adduct, as also indicated by ^{32}P-postlabeling and immunoassay (Lin *et al.* 1994; Culp *et al.* 1997). Levels of this adduct were not related to smoking. One study demonstrated the presence of 8-oxodeoxyguanosine in human lung DNA using HPLC with electrochemical detection (Asami *et al.* 1997). Levels were higher in smokers than in nonsmokers.

Collectively, the available data provide convincing evidence for the presence of certain adducts, listed in Table 5.3, in human lung DNA. It is very likely that many of the other adducts are also present, but the available methodology is not sensitive or specific enough to detect them, or has not yet been applied. Adducts are also present in tissues other than lung.

Likely mutations

Table 5.3 summarizes data obtained mainly, although not exclusively, from site-specific mutagenesis studies designed to determine the types of mutations that could be formed during replication of DNA containing the adducts. The major adduct of BaP illustrated in Table 5.3 produces GC→TA mutations (Kozack *et al.* 2000; Seo *et al.* 2000). However, this is sequence dependent. This adduct induced >95 per cent G→T mutations in one sequence context (5′-TGC) and approximately 95% G→A mutations in another context (5′-AGA). This may result from conformational complexities

(Kozack *et al.* 2000; Seo *et al.* 2000). Some PAH diol epoxides, such as those derived from benzo[*c*]phenanthrene, react extensively at deoxyadenosine in DNA and consequently produce significant levels of A mutations (Bigger *et al.* 1992; Szeliga and Dipple 1998).

7-Alkyldeoxyguanosines, such as those derived from *N*-nitrosodimethylamine, NNK, ethylene oxide, 1,3-butadiene, and vinyl chloride, readily depurinate, giving rise to abasic sites. Replication past abasic sites results predominantly in GC→TA mutations (Kunkel 1984). Therefore, these cigarette smoke constituents can be expected to produce GC→TA mutations in pulmonary DNA. Pyridyloxobutylation of DNA gives both GC→TA and GC→AT mutations, as demonstrated by analysis of *ras* mutations in lung DNA of mice treated with a model pyridyloxobutylating compound, NNKOAc (Ronai *et al.* 1993).

Site-specific mutagenesis experiments in human embryonic kidney cells have shown that the mispairing characteristics of O^6-pyridyloxobutyldeoxyguanosine are comparable to those of O^6-methyldeoxyguanosine, with a high number of G→A transitions and smaller amounts of G→T transversions and other mutations observed (Pauly *et al.* 2002).

GC→TA mutations are also the predominant ones observed in studies of mutagenesis by N^2-deoxyguanosine adducts of 1,3-butadiene (Carmical *et al.* 2000), adducts of 4-aminobiphenyl (Melchior *et al.* 1994), and 8-oxodeoxyguanosine (Moriya 1993). Other studies of butadiene mutagenesis demonstrate the occurrence of GC→AT, AT→TA, and GC→TA mutations (Recio *et al.* 2000). Products of the further oxidation of 8-oxodeoxyguanosine by peroxynitrite are highly efficient in producing GC→TA mutations (Henderson *et al.* 2002).

Collectively, the available data indicate that many DNA adducts associated with cigarette smoke exposure produce GC→TA mutations. A number of other types of mutations are also produced. It is easy to see how tobacco carcinogens can produce multiple mutations in smokers' DNA.

Effects of tobacco smoke carcinogens on the *p53* and K-*ras* genes

The preceding sections provide definitive evidence that tobacco smoke carcinogens are taken up by smokers and metabolically activated to forms that react with DNA. The resulting DNA adducts can cause mutations. If these mutations occur in critical genes such as the *p53* tumor suppressor gene and the K-*ras* oncogene, cancer can result because the normal role of these genes in the delicate growth control processes of the cell is subverted. Extensive studies have examined mutations in the *p53* gene in lung tumors (Hecht 1999; Pfeifer *et al.* 2002). Mutations in the *p53* gene are found in approximately 40 per cent of human lung cancers and are more common in smokers than in nonsmokers. G→T mutations in *p53* occur in 30 per cent of lung cancers from smokers, and in 12 per cent of those from nonsmokers, a significant difference. G→A mutations in *p53* occur in 29 per cent of lung cancers from smokers and in 47 per cent of those from nonsmokers. Other studies show a positive relationship between lifetime cigarette consumption and the frequency of *p53* mutations and G→T mutations on the nontranscribed (slowly repaired) DNA strand. These observations are generally consistent with the fact that most activated carcinogens react predominantly at G in DNA, as outlined in Table 5.3 and that many of the adducts so formed cause G→T or G→A mutations. It has been hypothesized that G→T mutations, in particular, are characteristic of lung cancer and result from interactions of the *p53* gene with metabolically activated cigarette smoke carcinogens (Pfeifer *et al.* 2002).

Mutations in the *p53* gene in lung cancer frequently occur at codons 157, 158, 245, 248, and 273, and are commonly G→T mutations (Pfeifer *et al.* 2002). These mutations have been called 'lung cancer hotspots'. Reactions of PAH diol epoxide metabolites with the *p53* gene *in vitro* result in frequent adduct formation at codons 156, 157, 158, 245, 248, and 273, leading to the hypothesis that PAHs such as BaP are the responsible agents in cigarette smoke for the observed mutations. Apparently there is enhanced adduct formation when a 5-methyldeoxycytidine nucleotide is adjacent to the modified deoxyguanosine (CpG dinucleotide sequence). In the *p53* gene of lung cancer, five major G→T mutation sites (codons 157, 158, 245, 248, and 273) have methylated CpG sequences. However, it should be noted that a number of different activated carcinogens, such as those summarized in Table 5.3, can react at these positions. Because of the complexity of DNA adduct formation by cigarette smoke carcinogens, it is unlikely that the observed mutations result from reactions only with metabolically activated PAH. Nevertheless, in aggregate, the common occurrence of G mutations in lung cancer is consistent with the higher reactivity of G than other DNA bases with metabolically activated carcinogens.

Mutations in codon 12 of the K-*ras* oncogene are found in 24–50 per cent of human adenocarcinoma of the lung (Hecht 1999). They are more common in smokers than in nonsmokers. The most common mutation is from the normal GGT sequence to TGT, a G→T mutation. This accounts for about 60 per cent of the observed mutations in codon 12. GGT→GAT mutations are observed in 20 per cent and GGT→GTT mutations in 15 per cent. This pattern is quite similar to that observed in lung tumors from mice treated with PAHs. Other tobacco smoke carcinogens may also produce this pattern of mutations.

Summary

There is a wealth of data generally consistent with the mechanistic framework presented in Fig. 5.1. Over 60 carcinogens have been identified in cigarette smoke, and their abilities to induce tumors at specific sites associated with tobacco-induced cancer in humans are, in many cases, well established. There is convincing evidence that smokers and people exposed to ETS take up and metabolize these carcinogens. In some cases, the DNA adducts resulting from tobacco carcinogen exposure have been characterized in tissues from smokers. Other studies demonstrate convincingly that some of these DNA adducts cause mutations during DNA replication. The observed mutations are frequently similar to those seen in oncogenes and tumor suppressor genes isolated from human lung cancers. Mutations in these genes lead to cancer by disrupting normal cellular signaling processes that control growth. The studies summarized here therefore demonstrate how cigarette smoke carcinogens—through human uptake, metabolic activation, and induction of mutations—firmly link nicotine addiction to cancer in smokers.

Acknowledgements

Research on tobacco and cancer in the author's laboratory is supported by grants from the US National Institutes of Health (CA-81301, CA-92025, CA-46535, ES-11297, DA-13333) and the American Cancer Society (RP-00–138).

References

Alexandrie, A. K., Warholm, M., Carstensen, U., Axmon, A., Hagmar, L., Levin, J. O., *et al.* (2000). CYP1A1 and GSTM1 polymorphisms affect urinary 1-hydroxypyrene levels after PAH exposure. *Carcinogenesis*, **21**, 669–76.

Anderson, K. E., Carmella, S. G., Ye, M., Bliss, R., Le, C., Murphy, L., *et al.* (2001). Metabolites of a tobacco-specific lung carcinogen in the urine of nonsmoking women exposed to environmental tobacco smoke in their homes. *Journal of the National Cancer Institute*, **93**, 378–81.

Arora, A., Willhite, C. A., and Liebler, D. C. (2001). Interactions of beta-carotene and cigarette smoke in human bronchial epithelial cells. *Carcinogenesis*, **22**, 1173–8.

Asami, S., Manabe, H., Miyake, J., Tsurudome, Y., Hirano, T., Yamaguchi, R., *et al.* (1997). Cigarette smoking induces an increase in oxidative DNA damage, 8-hydroxydeoxyguanosine, in a central site of the human lung. *Carcinogenesis*, **18**, 1763–6.

Bartsch, H. (1996). DNA adducts in human carcinogenesis: etiological relevance and structure–activity relationship. *Mutation Research*, **340**, 67–79.

Becher, G. and Bjorseth, A. (1983). Determination of exposure to polycyclic aromatic hydrocarbons by analysis of human urine. *Cancer Letters*, **17**, 301–11.

Becher, G., Haugen, A., and Bjorseth, A. (1984). Multimethod determination of occupational exposure to polycyclic aromatic hydrocarbons in an aluminum plant. *Carcinogenesis*, **5**, 647–51.

Benowitz, N. L. (1996). Cotinine as a biomarker of environmental tobacco smoke exposure. *Epidemiologic Reviews*, **18**, 188–204.

Benowitz, N. L., Jacob, P., Fong, I., and Gupta, S. (1994). Nicotine metabolic profile in man: comparison of cigarette smoking and transdermal nicotine. *Journal of Pharmacology and Experimental Therapeutics*, **268**, 296–303.

Bentsen-Farmen, R. K., Botnen, I. V., Noto, H., Jacob, J., and Ovrebo, S. (1999). Detection of polycyclic aromatic hydrocarbon metabolites by high-pressure liquid chromatography after purification on immunoaffinity columns in urine from occupationally exposed workers. *International Archives of Occupational and Environmental Health*, **72**, 161–8.

Bigger, C. A. H., St. John, J., Yagi, H., Jerina, D. M., and Dipple, A. (1992). Mutagenic specificities of four stereoisomeric benzo[c]phenanthrene dihydrodiol epoxides. *Proceedings of the Nationall Academy of Sciences, USA*, **89**, 368–72.

Bowman, E. D., Rothman, N., Hackl, C., Santella, R. M., and Weston, A. (1997). Interindividual variation in the levels of certain urinary polycyclic aromatic hydrocarbon metabolites following medicinal exposure to coal tar ointment. *Biomarkers*, **2**, 321–7.

Buckley, T. J., Waldman, J. M., Dhara, R., Greenberg, A., Ouyang, Z., and Lioy, P. J. (1995). An assessment of a urinary biomarker for total human environmental exposure to benzo[a]pyrene. *International Archives of Occupational and Environmental Health*, 67, 257 66.

Burney, S., Caulfield, J. L., Niles, J. C., Wishnok, J. S., and Tannenbaum, S. R. (1999). The chemistry of DNA damage from nitric oxide and peroxynitrite. *Mutation Research*, **424**, 37–49.

Carmella, S. G., Akerkar, S., and Hecht, S. S. (1993). Metabolites of the tobacco-specific nitrosamine 4-(methylnitrosamino)-1-(3-pyridyl)-1-butanone in smokers' urine. *Cancer Research*, **53**, 721–4.

Carmella, S. G., Akerkar, S., Richie, J. P. Jr, and Hecht, S. S. (1995). Intraindividual and interindividual differences in metabolites of the tobacco-specific lung carcinogen 4-(methylnitrosamino)-1-(3-pyridyl)-1-butanone (NNK) in smokers' urine. *Cancer Epidemiology, Biomarkers and Prevention*, **4**, 635–42.

Carmella, S. G., Ye, M., Upadhyaya, P., and Hecht, S. S. (1999). Stereochemistry of metabolites of a tobacco-specific lung carcinogen in smokers' urine. *Cancer Research*, **59**, 3602–5.

Carmella, S. G., Le Ka, K. A., Upadhyaya, P., and Hecht, S. S. (2002). Analysis of N- and O-glucuronides of 4-(methylnitrosamino)-1-(3- pyridyl)-1-butanol (NNAL) in human urine. *Chemical Research in Toxicology*, **15**, 545–50.

Carmical, J. R., Zhang, M., Nechev, L., Harris, C. M., Harris, T. M., and Lloyd, R. S. (2000). Mutagenic potential of guanine N^2 adducts of butadiene mono- and diolepoxide. *Chemical Research in Toxicology*, **13**, 18–25.

Casale, G. P., Singhal, M., Bhattacharya, S., Ramanathan, R., Roberts, K. P., Barbacci, D. C., et al. (2001). Detection and quantification of depurinated benzo[a]pyrene-adducted DNA bases in the urine of cigarette smokers and women exposed to household coal smoke. *Chemical Research in Toxicology*, **14**, 192–201.

Castelao, J. E., Yuan, J. M., Skipper, P. L., Tannenbaum, S. R., Gago-Dominguez, M., Crowder, J. S., et al. (2001). Gender- and smoking-related bladder cancer risk. *Journal of the National Cancer Institute*, **93**, 538–45.

Chao, A., Thun, M. J., Jacobs, E. J., Henley, S. J., Rodriguez, C., and Calle, E. E. (2000). Cigarette smoking and colorectal cancer mortality in the cancer prevention study II. *Journal of the National Cancer Institute*, **92**, 1888–96.

Chepiga, T. A., Morton, M. J., Murphy, P. A., Avalos, J. T., Bombick, B. R., Doolittle, D. J., et al. (2000). A comparison of the mainstream smoke chemistry and mutagenicity of a representative sample of the U.S. cigarette market with two Kentucky reference cigarettes (K1R4F and K1R5F). *Food and Chemical Toxicology*, **38**, 949–62.

Chung, F. L., Zhang, L., Ocando, J. E., and Nath, R. G. (1999). Role of 1,N^2-propanodeoxyguanosine adducts as endogenous DNA lesions in rodents and humans. In: *Exocyclic DNA adducts in mutagenesis and carcinogenesis* (ed. B. Singer and H. Bartsch), pp. 45–54. International Agency for Research on Cancer, Lyon, France.

Conney, A. H. (1982). Induction of microsomal enzymes by foreign chemicals and carcinogenesis by polycyclic aromatic hydrocarbons: G.H.A. Clowes Memorial Lecture. *Cancer Research*, **42**, 4875–917.

Culp, S. J., Roberts, D. W., Talaska, G., Lang, N. P., Fu, P. P., Lay, J. O. Jr, et al. (1997). Immunochemical, ^{32}P-postlabeling, and GC/MS detection of 4-aminobiphenyl-DNA adducts in human peripheral lung in relation to metabolic activation pathways involving pulmonary N-oxidation, conjugation, and peroxidation. *Mutation Research*, **378**, 97–112.

Culp, S. J., Gaylor, D. W., Sheldon, W. G., Goldstein, L. S., and Beland, F. A. (1998). A comparison of the tumors induced by coal tar and benzo[a]pyrene in a two-year bioassay. *Carcinogenesis*, **19**, 117–24.

Delclos, K. B. and Kadlubar, F. F. (1997). Carcinogenic aromatic amines and amides. In: *Comprehensive toxicology: Chemical carcinogens and anticarcinogens* (ed. G. T. Bowden and S. M. Fischer), pp. 141–70.

Deutsch-Wenzel, R. P., Brune, H., Grimmer, G., Dettbarn, G., and Misfield, J. (1983). Experimental studies in rat lung on the carcinogenicity and dose response relationships of eight frequently occurring enviromental polycyclic aromatic hydrocarbons. *Journal of the National Cancer Institute*, **71**, 539–43.

Djordjevic, M. V., Fan, J., Ferguson, S., and Hoffmann, D. (1995). Self-regulation of smoking intensity. Smoke yields of the low-nicotine, low-'tar' cigarettes. *Carcinogenesis*, **16**, 2015–21.

Djordjevic, M. V., Stellman, S. D., and Zang, E. (2000). Doses of nicotine and lung carcinogens delivered to cigarette smokers. *Journal of the National Cancer Institute*, **92**, 106–11.

Doll, R. (1996). Cancers weakly related to smoking. *British Medical Journal*, **52**, 35–49.

Dor, F., Haguenoer, J. M., Zmirou, D., Empereur-Bissonnet, P., Jongeneelen, F. J., Nedellec, V., *et al.* (2000). Urinary 1-hydroxypyrene as a biomarker of polycyclic aromatic hydrocarbons exposure of workers on a contaminated site: influence of exposure conditions. *Journal of Occupational and Environmental Medicine*, **42**, 391–7.

Ehrenberg, L. and Osterman-Golkar, S. (1976). Alkylation of macromolecules for detecting mutagenic agents. *Teratogenesis, Carcinogenesis, and Mutagenesis*, **1**, 105–27.

Foiles, P. G., Akerkar, S. A., Carmella, S. G., Kagan, M., Stoner, G. D., Resau, J. H., *et al.* (1991). Mass spectrometric analysis of tobacco-specific nitrosamine-DNA adducts in smokers and nonsmokers. *Chemical Research in Toxicology*, **4**, 364–8.

Grimmer, G., Jacob, J., Dettbarn, G. and Naujack, K. W. (1997). Determination of urinary metabolites of polycyclic aromatic hydrocarbons (PAH) for the risk assessment of PAH-exposed workers. *International Archives of Occupational and Environmental Health*, **69**, 231–9.

Guengerich, F. P. and Kim, D. H. (1991). Enzymatic oxidation of ethyl carbamate to vinyl carbamate and its role as an intermediate in the formation of $1,N^6$-ethenoadenosine. *Chemical Research in Toxicology*, **4**, 413–21.

Gundel, J. and Angerer, J. (2000). High-performance liquid chromatographic method with fluorescence detection for the determination of 3-hydroxybenzo[a]pyrene and 3-hydroxybenz[a]anthracene in the urine of polycyclic aromatic hydrocarbon-exposed workers. *Journal of Chromatography. B, Biomedical Applications*, **738**, 47–55.

Gupta, R. C., Arif, J. M. and Gairola, C. G. (1999). Enhancement of pre-existing DNA adducts in rodents exposed to cigarette smoke. *Mutation Research*, **424**, 195–205.

Harley, N. B., Cohen, B. S., and Tso, T. C. (1980). Polonium-210: a questionable risk factor in smoking related carcinogenesis. In: *Banbury Report 3: A Safe Cigarette?* (ed. G. B. Gori and F. G. Beck), pp. 93–104. Cold Spring Harbor Laboratory.

Haugen, A., Becher, G., Benestad, C., Vahakangas, K., Trivers, G. E., Newman, M. J., *et al.* (1986). Determination of polycyclic aromatic hydrocarbons in the urine, benzo[a]pyrene diol epoxide-DNA adducts in lymphocyte DNA, and antibodies to the adducts in sera from coke oven workers. *Cancer Research*, **46**, 4178–83.

Hecht, S. S. (1998). Biochemistry, biology, and carcinogenicity of tobacco-specific *N*-nitrosamines. *Chemical Research in Toxicology*, **11**, 559–603.

Hecht, S. S. (1999). Tobacco smoke carcinogens and lung cancer. *Journal of the National Cancer Institute*, **91**, 1194–210.

Hecht, S. S. and Hoffmann, D. (1988). Tobacco-specific nitrosamines, an important group of carcinogens in tobacco and tobacco smoke. *Carcinogenesis*, **9**, 875–84.

Hecht, S. S. and Tricker, A. R. (1999). Nitrosamines derived from nicotine and other tobacco alkaloids. In: *Analytical determination of nicotine and related compounds and their metabolites* (ed. J. W. Gorrod and P. Jacob, III), pp. 421–88. Elsevier Science, Amsterdam.

Hecht, S. S., Rivenson, A., Braley, J., DiBello, J., Adams, J. D., and Hoffmann, D. (1986). Induction of oral cavity tumors in F344 rats by tobacco-specific nitrosamines and snuff. *Cancer Research*, **46**, 4162–6.

Hecht, S. S., Carmella, S. G., Murphy, S. E., Akerkar, S., Brunnemann, K. D., and Hoffmann, D. (1993). A tobacco-specific lung carcinogen in the urine of men exposed to cigarette smoke. *New England Journal of Medicine*, **329**, 1543–6.

Hecht, S. S., Chung, F. L., Richie, J. P. Jr, Akerkar, S. A., Borukhova, A., Skowronski, L., *et al.* (1995). Effects of watercress consumption on metabolism of a tobacco-specific lung carcinogen in smokers. *Cancer Epidemiology, Biomarkers and Prevention*, **4**, 877–84.

Hecht, S. S., Carmella, S. G., Chen, M., Koch, J. F. D., Miller, A. T., Murphy, S. E., *et al.* (1999). Quantitation of urinary metabolites of a tobacco-specific lung carcinogen after smoking cessation. *Cancer Research*, **59**, 590–6.

Hecht, S. S., Ye, M., Carmella, S. G., Fredrickson, A., Adgate, J. L., Greaves, I. A., *et al.* (2001). Metabolites of a tobacco-specific lung carcinogen in the urine of elementary school-aged children. *Cancer Epidemiology, Biomarkers and Prevention*, **10**, 1109–16.

Hecht, S. S., Carmella, S. G., Ye, M., Le, K., Jensen, J. A., Zimmerman, C. L., *et al.* (2002). Quantitation of metabolites of 4-(methylnitrosamino)-1-(3-pyridyl)-1-butanone after cessation of smokeless tobacco use. *Cancer Research*, **62**, 129–34.

Henderson, P. T., Delaney, J. C., Gu, F., Tannenbaum, S. R., and Essigmann, J. M. (2002). Oxidation of 7,8-dihydro-8-oxoguanine affords lesions that are potent sources of replication errors in vivo. *Biochemistry*, **41**, 914–21.

Heudorf, U. and Angerer, J. (2001). Urinary monohydroxylated phenanthrenes and hydroxypyrene— the effects of smoking habits and changes induced by smoking on monooxygenase-mediated metabolism. *International Archives of Occupational and Environmental Health*, **74**, 177–83.

Hoepfner, I., Dettbarn, G., Scherer, G., Grimmer, G., and Adlkofer, F. (1987). Hydroxy-phenanthrenes in the urine of nonsmokers and smokers. *Toxicology Letters*, **35**, 67–71.

Hoffmann, D. and Hecht, S. S. (1990). Advances in tobacco carcinogenesis. In: *Handbook of experimental pharmacology* (ed. C. S. Cooper and P. L. Grover), pp. 63–102. Springer-Verlag, Heidelberg.

Hoffmann, D., Hoffmann, I., and El Bayoumy, K. (2001). The less harmful cigarette: a controversial issue. A tribute to Ernst L. Wynder. *Chemical Research in Toxicology*, **14**, 767–90.

Hurt, R. D., Croghan, G. A., Wolter, T. D., Croghan, I. T., Offord, K. P., Williams, G. M., *et al.* (2000). Does smoking reduction result in reduction of biomarkers associated with harm? A pilot study using a nicotine inhaler. *Nicotine and Tobacco Research*, **2**, 327–36.

Institute of Medicine (2001). Executive Summary. In: *Clearing the smoke: The science base for tobacco harm reduction* (ed. K. Stratton, P. Shetty, R. Wallace, and S. Bondurant), pp. 1–18. National Academy Press, Washington, DC.

International Agency for Research on Cancer (1972*a*). *Certain polycyclic aromatic hydrocarbons and heterocyclic compounds.* IARC Monographs on the Evaluation of the Carcinogenic Risks of Chemicals to Man, Vol. 3, pp. 45–268. IARC, Lyon, France.

International Agency for Research on Cancer (1972*b*). *Some inorganic substances, chlorinated hydrocarbons, aromatic amines, N-nitroso compounds, and natural products.* IARC Monographs on the Evaluation of the Carcinogenic Risk of Chemicals to Man, Vol. 1. IARC, Lyon, France.

International Agency for Research on Cancer (1973). *Some aromatic amines, hydrazine and related substances, N-nitroso compounds and miscellaneous alkylating agents*. IARC Monographs on the Carcinogenic Risk of Chemicals to Man, Vol. 4, pp. 127–36. IARC, Lyon, France.

International Agency for Research on Cancer (1974*a*). *Some anti-thyroid and related substances, nitrofurans and industrial chemicals*. IARC Monographs on the Carcinogenic Risk of Chemicals to Man, Vol. 7, pp. 111–40. IARC, Lyon, France.

International Agency for Research on Cancer (1974*b*). *Some aromatic amines, hydrazine and related substances, N-nitroso compounds and miscellaneous alkylating agents*. IARC Monographs on the Evaluation of the Carcinogenic Risk of Chemicals to Humans, Vol. 4, pp. 97–111. IARC, Lyon, France.

International Agency for Research on Cancer (1978). *Some N-nitroso compounds*. IARC Monographs on the Evaluation of the Carcinogenic Risk of Chemicals to Humans, Vol. 17, pp. 83–124. IARC, Lyon, France.

International Agency for Research on Cancer (1982). *Some industrial chemicals and dyestuffs*. IARC Monographs on the Evaluation of the Carcinogenic Risk of Chemicals to Humans, Vol. 29, pp. 93–148. IARC, Lyon, France.

International Agency for Research on Cancer (1983). *Polynuclear aromatic compounds, part 1, chemical, environmental, and experimental data*. IARC Monographs on the Evaluation of the Carcinogenic Risk of Chemicals to Humans, Vol. 32, pp. 211–24. IARC, Lyon, France.

International Agency for Research on Cancer (1985). *Allyl compounds, aldehydes, epoxides and peroxides*. IARC Monographs on the Evaluation of the Carcinogenic Risk of Chemicals to Humans, Vol. 36, pp. 101–132. IARC, Lyon, France.

International Agency for Research on Cancer (1986*a*). *Some industrial chemicals*. IARC Monographs on the Evaluation of the Carcinogenic Risk of Chemicals to Humans, Vol. 60, pp. 73–159. IARC, Lyon, France.

International Agency for Research on Cancer (1986*b*). *Tobacco smoking*. IARC Monographs on the Evaluation of the Carcinogenic Risk of Chemicals to Humans, Vol. 38, pp. 37–375. IARC, Lyon, France.

International Agency for Research on Cancer (1992). *Occupational exposures to mists and vapours from strong inorganic acids; and some other industrial chemicals*. IARC Monographs on the Evaluation of the Carcinogenic Risk of Chemicals to Humans, Vol. 54, pp. 237–85. IARC, Lyon, France.

International Agency for Research on Cancer (1999). *Re-evaluation of some organic chemicals, hydrazine and hydrogen peroxide (part one)*. IARC Monographs on the Evaluation of Carcinogenic Risks to Humans, Vol. 71, pp. 109–225. IARC, Lyon, France.

Jacob, J., Grimmer, G., and Dettbarn, G. (1999). Profile of urinary phenanthrene metabolites in smokers and non-smokers. *Biomarkers*, **4**, 319–27.

Jongeneelen, F. J. (1994). Biological monitoring of environmental exposure to polycyclic aromatic hydrocarbons; 1-hydroxypyrene in urine of people. *Toxicology Letters*. **72**, 205–11.

Jongeneelen, F. J. (2001). Benchmark guideline for urinary 1-hydroxypyrene as biomarker of occupational exposure to polycyclic aromatic hydrocarbons. *Annals of Occupational Hygiene*, **45**, 3–13.

Jongeneelen, F. J., Anzion, R. B. M., Leijdekkers, C. H. M., Bos, R. P., and Henderson, P. T. (1985). 1-Hydroxypyrene in human urine after exposure to coal tar and a coal tar derived product. *International Archives of Occupational and Environmental Health*, **57**, 47–55.

Kim, H., Cho, S. H., Kang, J. W., Kim, Y. D., Nan, H. M., Lee, C. H., *et al.* (2001). Urinary 1-hydroxypyrene and 2-naphthol concentrations in male Koreans. *International Archives of Occupational and Environmental Health*, **74**, 59–62.

Koc, H., Tretyakova, N. Y., Walker, V. E., Henderson, R. F., and Swenberg, J. A. (1999). Molecular dosimetry of N-7 guanine adduct formation in mice and rats exposed to 1,3-butadiene. *Chemical Research in Toxicology,* 12, 566–74.

Koivisto, P., Kilpelainen, I., Rasanen, I., Adler, I. D., Pacchierotti, F., and Peltonen, K. (1999). Butadiene diolepoxide- and diepoxybutane-derived DNA adducts at N7- guanine: a high occurrence of diolepoxide-derived adducts in mouse lung after 1,3-butadiene exposure. *Carcinogenesis,* 20, 1253–9.

Kozack, R., Seo, K. Y., Jelinsky, S. A., and Loechler, E. L. (2000). Toward an understanding of the role of DNA adduct conformation in defining mutagenic mechanism based on studies of the major adduct (formed at N(2)-dG) of the potent environmental carcinogen, benzo[a]pyrene. *Mutation Research,* 450, 41–59.

Kresty, L. A., Carmella, S. G., Borukhova, A., Akerkar, S. A., Gopalakrishnan, R., Harris, R. E., *et al.* (1996). Metabolites of a tobacco-specific nitrosamine, 4-(methylnitrosamino)-1-(3-pyridyl)-1-butanone (NNK), in the urine of smokeless tobacco users: relationship of urinary biomarkers and oral leukoplakia. *Cancer Epidemiology, Biomarkers and Prevention,* 5, 521–5.

Kriek, E., Rojas, M., Alexandrov, K., and Bartsch, H. (1998). Polycyclic aromatic hydrocarbon-DNA adducts in humans: relevance as biomarkers for exposure and cancer risk. *Mutation Research,* 400, 215–31.

Kunkel, T. A. (1984). Mutational specificity of depurination. *Proceedings of the National Academy of Sciences of the United States of America,* 81, 1494–8.

Lackmann, G. M., Salzberger, U., Tollner, U., Chen, M., Carmella, S. G., and Hecht, S. S. (1999). Metabolites of a tobacco-specific carcinogen in the urine of newborns. *Journal of the National Cancer Institute,* 91, 459–65.

LaVoie, E. J. and Rice, J. E. (1988). Structure-activity relationships among tricyclic polynuclear aromatic hydrocarbons. In: *Polycyclic aromatic hydrocarbon carcinogenesis: Structure–activity relationships* (ed. S. K. Yang and B. D. Silverman), pp. 151. CRC Press, Boca Raton, Florida.

Levin, J. O. (1995). First international workshop on hydroxypyrene as a biomarker for PAH exposure in man—summary and conclusions. *Science of the Total Environment,* 163, 165–8.

Li, H., Krieger, R. I., and Li, Q. X. (2000). Improved HPLC method for analysis of 1-hydroxypyrene in human urine specimens of cigarette smokers. *Science of the Total Environment,* 257, 147–53.

Lin, D., Lay, J. O. Jr, Bryant, M. S., Malaveille, C., Friesen, M., Bartsch, H., *et al.* (1994). Analysis of 4-aminobiphenyl-DNA adducts in human urinary bladder and lung by alkaline hydrolysis and negative ion gas chromatography-mass spectrometry. *Environmental Health Perspectives,* 102 (Suppl. 6), 11–16.

Loechler, E. L., Green, C. L., and Essigmann, J. M. (1984). In vivo mutagenesis by O^6-methylguanine built into a unique site in a viral genome. *Proceedings of the National Academy of Sciences of the United States of America,* 81, 6271–5.

Matthews, S. J., Hecht, S. S., Picton, H. M., Ye, M., Carmella, S. G., Shires, S., *et al.* (2002). No association between smoking and the presence of tobacco-specific nitrosamine metabolites in ovarian follicular fluid. *Cancer Epidemiology, Biomarkers and Prevention,* 11, 321–2.

McCoy, G. D. and Wynder, E. L. (1979). Etiological and preventive implications in alcohol carcinogenesis. *Cancer Research,* 39, 2844–50.

Meger, M., Meger-Kossien, I., Dietrich, M., Tricker, A. R., Scherer, G., and Adlkofer, F. (1996). Metabolites of 4-(N-methylnitrosamino)-1-(3-pyridyl)-1-butanone in urine of smokers. *European Journal of Cancer Prevention,* 5 (Suppl. 1), 121–4.

Meger, M., Meger-Kossien, I., Riedel, K., and Scherer, G. (2000). Biomonitoring of environmental tobacco smoke (ETS)-related exposure to 4-(methylnitrosamino)-1-(3-pyridyl)-1-butanone (NNK). *Biomarkers,* 5, 33–45.

Melchior, W. B. Jr, Marques, M. M., and Beland, F. A. (1994). Mutations induced by aromatic amine DNA adducts in pBR322. *Carcinogenesis*, 15, 889–99.

Melikian, A. A., Amin, S., Huie, K., Hecht, S. S., and Harvey, R. G. (1988). Reactivity with DNA bases and mutagenicity toward *Salmonella typhimurium* of methylchrysene diol epoxide enantiomers. *Cancer Research*, 48, 1781–7.

Melikian, A. A., Fudem Goldin, B., Prahalad, A. K., and Hecht, S.S. (1990). Modulation of benzo[a]pyrene-DNA adducts in hamster cheek pouch by chronic ethanol consumption. *Chemical Research in Toxicology*, 3, 139–43.

Merlo, F., Andreassen, A., Weston, A., Pan, C. F., Haugen, A., Valerio, F., et al. (1998). Urinary excretion of 1-hydroxypyrene as a marker for exposure to urban air levels of polycyclic aromatic hydrocarbons. *Cancer Epidemiology, Biomarkers and Prevention*, 7, 147–55.

Milunsky, A., Carmella, S. G., Ye, M., and Hecht, S. S. (2000). A tobacco-specific carcinogen in the fetus. *Prenatal Diagnosis*, 20, 307–10.

Misra, R. R., Page, J. E., Smith, G. T., Waalkes, M. P., and Dipple, A. (1998). Effect of cadmium exposure on background and *anti*-5-methylchrysene-1,2-dihydrodiol 3,4-epoxide-induced mutagenesis in the *supF* gene of pS189 in human Ad293 cells. *Chemical Research in Toxicology*, 11, 211–16.

Moriya, M. (1993). Single-stranded shuttle phagemid for mutagenesis studies in mammalian cells: 8-oxoguanine in DNA induces targeted G·C→T·A transversions in simian kidney cells. *Proceedings of the National Academy of Sciences of the United States of America*, 90, 1122–6.

Mumford, J. L., Li, X., Hu, F., Lu, X. B., and Chuang, J. C. (1995). Human exposure and dosimetry of polycyclic aromatic hydrocarbons in urine from Xuan Wei, China with high lung cancer mortality associated with exposure to unvented coal smoke. *Carcinogenesis*, 16, 3031–6.

Murphy, S. E., Carmella, S. G., Idris, A. M., and Hoffmann, D. (1994). Uptake and metabolism of carcinogenic levels of tobacco-specific nitrosamines by Sudanese snuff dippers. *Cancer Epidemiology, Biomarkers and Prevention*, 3, 423–8.

Nair, J., Barbin, A., Velic, I., and Bartsch, H. (1999). Etheno DNA-base adducts from endogenous reactive species. *Mutation Research*, 424, 59–69.

Nan, H. M., Kim, H., Lim, H. S., Choi, J. K., Kawamoto, T., Kang, J. W., et al. (2001). Effects of occupation, lifestyle and genetic polymorphisms of CYP1A1, CYP2E1, GSTM1 and GSTT1 on urinary 1-hydroxypyrene and 2-naphthol concentrations. *Carcinogenesis*, 22, 787–93.

National Cancer Institute (1999). *Health effects of exposure to environmental tobacco smoke: The report of the California Environmental Protection Agency*. Smoking and Tobacco Control Monograph, No. 10. US Dept of Health and Human Services, National Institutes of Health, National Cancer Institute, Bethesda, MD, NIH Pub. No. 99–4645.

National Cancer Institute (2001). *Risks associated with smoking cigarettes with low machine-measured yields of tar and nicotine*. Smoking and Tobacco Control Monograph, No. 13. US Dept of Health and Human Services, National Institutes of Health, National Cancer Institute, Bethesda, MD, NIH Pub. No. 99–4645.

National Toxicology Program (1986). *Toxicology and carcinogenesis studies of benzene (CAS No. 71–43–2) in F344/N rats and B6C3F$_1$ mice (gavage studies)*. NTP Technical Report, No. 289. National Toxicology Program.

National Toxicology Program (1993). *Toxicology and carcinogenesis studies of 1,3-butadiene*. NTP Technical Report, No. 434. National Toxicology Program.

Nerurkar, P. V., Okinaka, L., Aoki, C., Seifried, A., Lum-Jones, A., Wilkens, L. R., et al. (2000). CYP1A1, GSTM1, and GSTP1 genetic polymorphisms and urinary 1-hydroxypyrene excretion in non-occupationally exposed individuals. *Cancer Epidemiology, Biomarkers and Prevention*, 9, 1119–22.

Nesnow, S., Ross, J. A., Stoner, G. D., and Mass, M. J. (1995). Mechanistic linkage between DNA adducts, mutations in oncogenes and tumorigenesis of carcinogenic environmental polycyclic aromatic hydrocarbons in strain A/J mice. *Toxicology*, **103**, 403–13.

Noori, P. and Hou, S. M. (2001). Mutational spectrum induced by acetaldehyde in the HPRT gene of human T lymphocytes resembles that in the *p53* gene of esophageal cancers. *Carcinogenesis*, **22**, 1825–30.

Owen, P. E., Glaister, J. R., Gaunt, I. F., and Pullinger, D. H. (1987). Inhalation toxicity studies with 1,3-butadiene. 3. Two year toxicity/carcinogenicity study in rats. *American Industrial Hygiene Association Journal*, **48**, 407–13.

Parsons, W. D., Carmella, S. G., Akerkar, S., Bonilla, L. E., and Hecht, S. S. (1998). A metabolite of the tobacco-specific lung carcinogen 4-(methylnitrosamino)-1-(3-pyridyl)-1-butanone (NNK) in the urine of hospital workers exposed to environmental tobacco smoke. *Cancer Epidemiology, Biomarkers and Prevention*, **7**, 257–60.

Pastorelli, R., Guanci, M., Restano, J., Berri, A., Micoli, G., Minoia, C., *et al.* (1999). Seasonal effect on airborne pyrene, urinary 1-hydroxypyrene, and benzo(a)pyrene diol epoxide-hemoglobin adducts in the general population. *Cancer Epidemiology, Biomarkers and Prevention*, **8**, 561–5.

Pauly, G. T., Peterson, L. A. and Moschel, R. C. (2002). Mutagenesis by O^6-[4-oxo-4-(3-pyridyl)-butylguanine] in *Escherichia coli* and human cells. *Chemical Research in Toxicology*, **15**, 165–9.

Penning, T. M., Burczynski, M. E., Hung, C. F., McCoull, K. D., Palackal, N. T., and Tsuruda, L. S. (1999). Dihydrodiol dehydrogenases and polycyclic aromatic hydrocarbon activation: Generation of reactive and redox active o-quinones. *Chemical Research in Toxicology*, **12**, 1–18.

Peto, R., Lopez, A. D., Boreham, J., Thun, M., Heath, C. Jr, and Doll, R. (1996). Mortality from smoking worldwide. *British Medical Bulletin*, **52**, 12–21.

Pfeifer, G. P., Denissenko, M. F., Olivier, M., Tretyakova, N., Hecht, S. S., and Hainaut, P. (2002). Tobacco smoke carcinogens, DNA damage and p53 mutations in smoking-associated cancers. *Oncogene* (submitted).

Phillips, D. H. (1996). DNA adducts in human tissues: biomarkers of exposure to carcinogens in tobacco smoke. *Environmental Health Perspectives*, **104** (Suppl. 5), 453–8.

Poirier, M. C. and Weston, A. (1996). Human DNA adduct measurements: state of the art. *Environmental Health Perspectives*, **104** (Suppl. 5), 883–93.

Preussmann, R. and Stewart, B. W. (1984). N-Nitroso carcinogens. In: *Chemical carcinogens* (2nd edn) (ed. C. E. Searle), ACS Monograph 182, Vol. 2, pp. 643–828. American Chemical Society, Washington, DC.

Pryor, W. A. (1997). Cigarette smoke radicals and the role of free radicals in chemical carcinogenicity. *Environmental Health Perspectives* **105**, 875–82.

Recio, L., Saranko, C. J., and Steen, A. M. (2000). 1,3-Butadiene: cancer, mutations, and adducts. Part II: Roles of two metabolites of 1,3-butadiene in mediating its in vivo genotoxicity. *Research Report/Health Effects Institute*, **2000**, 49–87.

Reznik-Shuller, H. M. (1983). Cancer induced in the respiratory tract of rodents by *N*-nitroso compounds. In: *Comparative respiratory tract carcinogens* (ed. H. M. Reznik-Shuller), pp. 109–59. CRC Press, Boca Raton, FL.

Richie, J. P., Carmella, S. G., Muscat, J. E., Scott, D. G., Akerkar, S. A., and Hecht, S. S. (1997). Differences in the urinary metabolites of the tobacco-specific lung carcinogen 4-(methylnitrosamino)-1-(3-pyridyl)-1-butanone in black and white smokers. *Cancer Epidemiology, Biomarkers and Prevention*, **6**, 783–90.

Rivenso, A., Hoffmann, D., Prokopczyk, B., Amin, S., and Hecht, S. S. (1988). Induction of lung and exocrine pancreas tumors in F344 rats by tobacco-specific and *Areca*-derived N-nitrosamines. *Cancer Research* **48**, 6912–17.

Roggi, C., Minoia, C., Sciarra, G. F., Apostoli, P., Maccarini, L., Magnaghi, S., *et al.* (1997). Urinary 1-hydroxypyrene as a marker of exposure to pyrene: an epidemiological survey on a general population group. *Science of the Total Environment*, **199**, 247–54.

Rojas, M., Alexandrov, K., Cascarbi, I., Brockmoller, J., Likhachev, A., Pozharisski, K., *et al.* (1998). High benzo[*a*]pyrene diol-epoxide DNA adduct levels in lung and blood cells from individuals with combined CYP1A1 MspI/MspI-GSTM1*0/*0 genotypes. *Pharmacogenetics*, **8**, 109–18.

Ronai, Z., Gradia, S., Peterson, L. A., and Hecht, S. S. (1993). G to A transitions and G to T transversions in codon 12 of the Ki-*ras* oncogene isolated from mouse lung tumors induced by 4-(methylnitrosamino)-1-(3-pyridyl)-1-butanone (NNK) and related DNA methylating and pyridyloxobutylating agents. *Carcinogenesis*, **14**, 2419–22.

Ross, J. A. and Nesnow, S. (1999). Polycyclic aromatic hydrocarbons: correlations between DNA adducts and ras oncogene mutations. *Mutation Research*, **424**, 155–66.

Santella, R. (1999). Immunological methods for detection of carcinogen-DNA damage in humans. *Cancer Epidemiology, Biomarkers and Prevention*, **8**, 733–9.

Scherer, G. and Richter, E. (1997). Biomonitoring exposure to environmental tobacco smoke (ETS): a critical reappraisal. *Human Experimental Toxicology*, **16**, 449–59.

Scherer, G., Conze, C., Tricker, A. R., and Adlkofer, F. (1992). Uptake of tobacco smoke constituents on exposure to environmental tobacco smoke (ETS). *Clinical Investigation*, **70**, 352–67.

Scherer, G., Frank, S., Riedel, K., Merger-Kossien, I., and Renner, T. (2000). Biomonitoring of exposure to polycyclic aromatic hydrocarbons of nonoccupationally exposed persons. *Cancer Epidemiology, Biomarkers and Prevention*, **9**, 373–80.

Schüller, H. M., Jorquera, R., Reichert, A., and Castonguay, A. (1993). Transplacental induction of pancreas tumors in hamsters by ethanol and the tobacco-specific nitrosamine 4-(methylnitrosamino)-1-butanone. *Cancer Research*, **53**, 2498–501.

Sellakumar, A. and Shubik, P. (1974). Carcinogenicity of different polycyclic hydrocarbons in the respiratory tract of hamsters. *Journal of the National Cancer Institute*, **53**, 1713–19.

Seo, K. Y., Jelinsky, S. A., and Loechler, E. L. (2000). Factors that influence the mutagenic patterns of DNA adducts from chemical carcinogens. *Mutation Research*, **463**, 215–46.

Simon, P., Lafontaine, M., Delsaut, P., Morele, Y., and Nicot, T. (2000). Trace determination of urinary 3-hydroxybenzo[a]pyrene by automated column-switching high-performance liquid chromatography. *Journal of Chromatography. B, Biomedical Sciences Applications*, **748**, 337–48.

Simpson, C. D., Wu, M. T., Christiani, D. C., Santella, R. M., Carmella, S. G., and Hecht, S. S. (2000). Determination of r-7,t-8,9,c-10-tetrahydroxy-7,8,9,10-tetrahydrobenzo[*a*]pyrene in human urine by gas chromatography-negative ion chemical ionization-mass spectrometry. *Chemical Research Toxicology*, **13**, 271–80.

Singer, B. and Grunberger, D. (1983). *Molecular biology of mutagens and carcinogens*, pp. 45–94. Plenum Press, New York.

Sithisarankul, P., Vineis, P., Kang, D., Rothman, N., Caporaso, N., and Strickland, P. (1997). The association of 1-hydroxypyrene-glucuronide in human urine with cigarette smoking and broiled or roasted meat consumption. *Biomarkers*, **2**, 217–21.

Siwinska, E., Mielzynska, D., Bubak, A., and Smolik, E. (1999). The effect of coal stoves and environmental tobacco smoke on the level of urinary 1-hydroxypyrene. *Mutation Research—Genetics Toxicology and Environmental Mutagens*, **445**, 147–53.

Skipper, P. L. and Tannenbaum, S. R. (1990). Protein adducts in the molecular dosimetry of chemical carcinogens. *Carcinogenesis*, 11, 507–18.

Sodum, R. S. and Fiala, E. S. (1998). N2-amination of guanine to 2-hydrazinohypoxanthine, a novel in vivo nucleic acid modification produced by the hepatocarcinogen 2-nitropropane. *Chemical Research in Toxicology*, 11, 1453–9.

Solt, D. B., Polverini, P. J., and Claderon, L. (1987). Carinogenic response of hamster buccal pouch epithelium to 4 polycyclic aromatic hydrocarbons. *Journal of Oral Pathology*, 16, 294–302.

Spiegelhalder, B. and Bartsch, H. (1996). Tobacco-specific nitrosamines. *European Journal of Cancer Prevention*, 5, 33–8.

Swenberg, J. A., Kerns, W. D., Mitchell, R. I., Gralla, J., and Pavkov, K. L. (1980). Induction of squamous cell carcinomas of rat nasal cavity by inhalation exposure to formaldehyde vapor. *Cancer Research*, 40, 3398–402.

Swenberg, J. A., Bogdanffy, M. S., Ham, A., Holt, S., Kim, A., Morinello, E. J., *et al.* (1999). Formation and repair of DNA adducts in vinyl chloride- and vinyl fluoride-induced carcinogenesis. *IARC Scientific Publications*, 29–43.

Szaniszlo, J. and Ungvary, G. (2001). Polycyclic aromatic hydrocarbon exposure and burden of outdoor workers in Budapest. *Journal of Toxicology and Environmental Health A*, 62, 297–306.

Szeliga, J. and Dipple, A. (1998). DNA adduct formation by polycyclic aromatic hydrocarbon dihydrodiol epoxides. *Chemical Research in Toxicology*, 11, 1–11.

Taioli, E., Garbers, S., Bradlow, H. L., Carmella, S. G., Akerkar, S., and Hecht, S. S. (1997). Effects of indole-3-carbinol on the metabolism of 4-(methylnitrosamino)-1-(3-pyridyl)-1-butanone (NNK) in smokers. *Cancer Epidemiology, Biomarkers and Prevention*, 6, 517–22.

Thornton-Manning, J. R., Dahl, A. R., Bechtold, W. E., Griffith, W. C. Jr, and Henderson, R. F. (1995). Disposition of butadiene monoepoxide and butadiene diepoxide in various tissues of rats and mice following a low-level inhalation exposure to 1,3-butadiene. *Carcinogenesis*, 16, 1723–31.

Tretyakova, N., Lin, Y., Sangaiah, R., Upton, P. B., and Swenberg, J. A. (1997). Identification and quantitation of DNA adducts from calf thymus DNA exposed to 3,4-epoxy-1-butene. *Carcinogenesis*, 18, 137–47.

Upadhyaya, P., Kenney, P. M. J., Hochalter, J. B., Wang, M., and Hecht, S. S. (1999). Tumorigenicity and metabolism of 4-(methylnitrosamino)-1-(3-pyridyl)-1-butanol (NNAL) enantiomers and metabolites in the A/J mouse. *Carcinogenesis*, 20, 1577–82.

Upadhyaya, P., McIntee, E. J., and Hecht, S. S. (2001). Preparation of pyridine-*N*-glucuronides of tobacco-specific nitrosamines. *Chemical Research in Toxicology*, 14, 555–61.

van Delft, J. H., Steenwinkel, M. S., van Asten, J. G., de Vogel, N., Bruijntjes-Rozier, T. C., Schouten, T., *et al.* (2001). Biological monitoring the exposure to polycyclic aromatic hydrocarbons of coke oven workers in relation to smoking and genetic polymorphisms for GSTM1 and GSTT1. *Annals of Occupational Hygiene*, 45, 395–408.

Van Rooij, J. G., Veeger, M. M., Bodelier-Bade, M. M., Scheepers, P. T., and Jongeneelen, F. J. (1994). Smoking and dietary intake of polycyclic aromatic hydrocarbons as sources of interindividual variability in the baseline excretion of 1-hydroxypyrene in urine. *International Archives of Occupational and Environmental Health*, 66, 55–65.

Venier, P., Clonfero, E., Cottica, D., Gava, C., Zordan, M., Pozzoli, L., *et al.* (1985). Mutagenic activity and polycyclic aromatic hydrocarbon levels in urine of workers exposed to coal tar pitch volatiles in an anode plant. *Carcinogenesis*, 6, 749–52.

Vineis, P., Marinelli, D., Autrup, H., Brockmoller, J., Cascorbi, I., Daly, A. K., *et al.* (2001). Current smoking, occupation, N-acetyltransferase-2 and bladder cancer: a pooled analysis of genotype-based studies. *Cancer Epidemiology, Biomarkers and Prevention*, 10, 1249–52.

Wang, M., McIntee, E. J., Cheng, G., Shi, X., Villalta, P. W., and Hecht, S. S. (2000a). Identification of DNA adducts of acetaldehyde. *Chemical Research and Toxicology*, **13**, 1149–57.

Wang, M., McIntee, E. J., Cheng, G., Shi, Y., Villalta, P. W., and Hecht, S. S. (2000b) Identification of paraldol-deoxyguanosine adducts in DNA reacted with crotonaldehyde. *Chemical Research and Toxicology*, **13**, 1065–74.

Wang, M., McIntee, E. J., Cheng, G., Shi, Y., Villalta, P. W., Hecht, S. S. (2001a). A Schiff base is a major DNA adduct of crotonaldehyde. *Chemical Research and Toxicology*, **14**, 423–30.

Wang, M., McIntee, E. J., Shi, Y., Cheng, G., Upadhyaya, P., Villalta, P. W., *et al.* (2001b). Reactions of α-acetoxy-N-nitrosopyrrolidine with deoxyguanosine and DNA. *Chemical Research and Toxicology*, **14**, 1435–45.

Weston, A., Bowman, E. D., Carr, P., Rothman, N., and Strickland, P. T. (1993). Detection of metabolites of polycyclic aromatic hydrocarbons in human urine. *Carcinogenesis*, **14**, 1053–5.

Wilson, V. L., Weston, A., Manchester, D. K., Trivers, G. E., Roberts, D. W., Kadlubar, F. F., *et al.* (1989). Alkyl and aryl carcinogen adducts detected in human peripheral lung. *Carcinogenesis*, **10**, 2149–53.

World Health Organization (1997). *Tobacco or health: A global status report*, pp. 10–48. WHO, Geneva.

Zhao, C., Tyndyk, M., Eide, I., and Hemminki, K. (1999). Endogenous and background DNA adducts by methylating and 2-hydroxyethylating agents. *Mutation Research*, **424**, 117–25.

Zhao, C., Vodicka, P., Sram, R. J., and Hemminki, K. (2000). Human DNA adducts of 1,3-butadiene, an important environmental carcinogen. *Carcinogenesis*, **21**, 107–11.

Part 3

Nicotine and addiction

Chapter 6

Pharmacology of nicotine addiction

Jack E. Henningfield and Neal L. Benowitz

Since the 1980s, it has become recognized by clinicians, researchers, and public health experts that tobacco products are among the most addictive and deadly of all dependence producing substances (Royal College of Physicians 2000; WHO 2001). Nicotine meets all of the standard criteria for a dependence-producing drug and all types of tobacco products are capable of delivering dependence-producing levels of nicotine (US DHHS 1988; Royal Society of Canada 1989; Royal College of Physicians 2000). These conclusions are consistent with the neuropharmacology of nicotine (Henningfield *et al.* 1996), with clinical studies of nicotine dependence and withdrawal (e.g. Hughes *et al.* 1990; Henningfield *et al.* 1995*a*), and with the epidemiology of tobacco use and dependence (Giovino *et al.* 1995). In fact, if evaluated against the criteria used to determine the level of psychoactive scheduling set by the U.S. Controlled Substance Act or the World Health Organization's Convention on Psychotropic Substances (described by McClain and Sapienza 1989; Vocci 1989), nicotine could be appropriately categorized as a controlled substance (Food and Drug Administration 1995, 1996).

However, nicotine is not categorized as a controlled substance and there are several reasons for the relatively recent widespread recognition of its dependence-producing effects (e.g. as compared to the role of morphine in opium use). For example, although the effects of nicotine on the nervous system have been investigated since the nineteenth century (e.g. Langley 1905), and the role of nicotine in tobacco since early in the twentieth century (e.g. Johnston 1942; Finnegan *et al.* 1945), it was not until the 1980s that an overwhelming body of research established that nicotine itself met all criteria for a dependence-producing drug (National Institute on Drug Abuse 1984; US DHHS 1988).

Tobacco dependence and withdrawal were listed in the Diagnostic and Statistical Manual (DSM) of the American Psychiatric Association (APA) in its third edition in 1980. The International Classification of Diseases (ICD) of the World Health Organization (WHO) listed tobacco dependence and withdrawal in its tenth edition, in 1992. Although the APA identified the disorders of tobacco dependence and tobacco withdrawal in 1980, it did not list nicotine dependence and nicotine withdrawal until it revised the DSM III in 1987 (APA 1980, 1987). In 1980, the APA had concluded that there was not sufficient evidence to confirm that nicotine, independent of tobacco, could produce dependence and withdrawal. By 1987, the APA concluded that the role of nicotine was sufficiently well established to merit the classification of nicotine dependence and nicotine withdrawal disorders. In contrast, WHO (1992) continues to refer to the substance 'tobacco' as opposed to its drug, 'nicotine' just as it refers to the substance 'cannabinoids' as opposed to their drug, tetrahydrocannabinol. This is based on the reasoning that even though nicotine is the critical drug that defines the disorders, in practice, withdrawal signs from pure nicotine systems (e.g. nicotine gum and patches) are generally weak and the establishment of dependence on pure nicotine preparations is not a known public health problem.

Both the APA and WHO approaches have merit and scientific rationale. The WHO approach to emphasize the importance of the tobacco vehicle is highly relevant to recent advances in the understanding of tobacco use that have begun to unravel the contributions of tobacco product ingredients and designs, which may be determinants of the risk, severity, and prevalence of nicotine addiction. These issues will be addressed in the present analysis. Despite the many research questions that need to be explored to fully understand the mechanisms underlying dependence on tobacco and nicotine, there is a strong science foundation upon which to guide policy aimed at reducing the prevalence of tobacco use and eradicating tobacco-caused diseases.

Pharmacology of nicotine

Nicotine is an alkaloid that is present in concentrations of about 1–3% in tobacco cultivated for commercial tobacco products (Browne 1990). The concept that the pharmacologic effects of tobacco primarily reflect the actions of nicotine has been widely accepted, at least since Lewin's analysis from the 1920s (translated into English in 1931 and reprinted in 1964) in which he concluded. 'The decisive factor in the effect of tobacco, desired or undesired, is nicotine...' For example, prominent effects of tobacco on muscle tone, heart rate, and blood pressure, as well as behavioral and mood altering effects, can be mimicked by administration of nicotine (Benowitz 1990; Henningfield et al. 1996; Taylor 1996).

Nicotine is a potent and powerful agonist of several subpopulations of nicotinic receptors of the cholinergic nervous system (Henningfield et al. 1996; Vidal 1996; Paterson and Nordberg 2000). Acute doses of 1 mg per 70 kg accelerate heart rate and alter mood, although daily users are substantially less sensitive to such effects than non-users (US DHHS 1988; Soria et al. 1996; Taylor 1996; Foulds et al. 1997). The half-life of nicotine averages approximately 2 h but is longer in persons in the presence of a genetic polymorphism of the liver enzyme CYP2A6, which is the primary metabolic pathway of nicotine (Tyndale and Sellers 2001; Benowitz et al. 2002). The prevalence of CYP2A6 alleles that are associated with reduced enzymatic activity is higher in Asians than in Caucasians or African Americans, and this difference may contribute to lower daily cigarette consumption and a lower risk of lung cancer in Asians compared to Caucasians and African Americans. (Ahijevych 1999; Tyndale and Sellers 2001; Benowitz *et al.* 2002). A primary nicotine metabolite, cotinine, has an 18–20 h half-life and distribution in blood, urine, and saliva that makes it useful for studies of nicotine intake in the laboratory and at the population level (Benowitz 1996, 1999).

The peripheral nervous system actions of nicotine on ganglionic cholinergic receptors have been studied since the nineteenth century. Studies of nicotinic agonists and antagonists contributed to advances in methods, which formed the foundation for modern neuroscience research, including the use of selective agonists and antagonists to explore the mechanism of action of neurons and the concept of the 'receptive substance' as a mediator of effects (e.g. Langley 1905). The peripheral actions of nicotine include relaxation or stimulation of muscles, depending upon the dose and the muscle group, as well as a high dose 'paralysis,' which can lead to respiratory depression and death; the latter is a mechanism exploited in the use of nicotine as a pesticide (Taylor 1996).

Central nervous system actions of nicotine are diverse. The importance of variation in the structural and functional properties of nicotinic cholinergic receptors throughout the brain is an especially active area of neuropharmacological research. Identifying selective nicotinic agonists and antagonists could yield clinically important advances in medications for aiding smoking cessation as well as for treating disorders that appear to involve the various nicotinic receptor subpopulations, e.g. Parkinson's disease, Alzheimer's disease, attention deficit hyperactivity disorder, Tourette's Syndrome, and various affective disorders (Newhouse and Hughes 1991; Balfour and Fagerstrom 1996 Levin *et al.* 1996; Vidal 1996; Newhouse *et al.* 1997; Paterson and Nordberg 2000; Santos *et al.* 2002).

Abuse liability and physical dependence potential

All commercially successful tobacco products contain and deliver behaviorally active amounts of nicotine to their users (FDA 1995, 1996). Tobacco products without nicotine are not well accepted by chronic tobacco users (e.g. Finnegan *et al.* 1945) and are not well accepted in the market place (FDA 1995, 1996). The abuse liability and physical dependence potential of nicotine have been well characterized and further exploration of the mechanism of these effects is an active area of research. In brief, nicotine produces dose-related psychoactive effects in humans that are identified as stimulant-like, and it elevates scores on standardized tests for liking and euphoria that are relied upon by WHO for assessing abuse potential (US DHHS 1988; Henningfield *et al.* 1995; Jones *et al.* 1999; Royal College of Physicians 2000). The subjective effects of nicotine are reduced by the centrally acting nicotinic cholinergic receptor blocker, mecamylamine (Rose *et al.* 1989; Lundahl *et al.* 2000), but not by the peripherally acting blocker, pentolinium (Stolerman *et al.* 1973). Drug discrimination testing in animals has similarly revealed that nicotine is discriminated in a dose-related fashion and that these effects are blocked by centrally but not peripherally acting nicotinic cholinergic receptor blockers (US DHHS 1988; Henningfield *et al.* 1996).

Nicotine can serve as a potent and powerful reinforcer for both humans and animals as demonstrated by intravenous self-administration studies (Goldberg *et al.* 1983; Goldberg and Henningfield 1988; Corrigall 1999), patterns of self-administration are more similar to those of stimulants than of other drug classes (Griffiths *et al.* 1980). However, the range of conditions under which it functions as a reinforcer is smaller than that under which cocaine serves as a reinforcer.

Intravenous nicotine self-administration is reduced by centrally acting nicotinic cholinergic receptor blockers, but not by peripherally acting blockers (Corrigall 1999). Patterns of tobacco product self-administration are influenced by nicotine dose with manipulations of delivery resulting in changes in behavior that tend to sustain similar levels of nicotine intake (Gritz 1980; Henningfield 1984; US DHHS 1988). Nicotine exposure results in a high degree of tolerance, which is mediated by several mechanisms, and which includes acute and long-term components (Swedberg *et al.* 1990; Perkins *et al.* 1993; Perkins 2002).

Tolerance. Tolerance to some effects may be related to the up-regulation of central nervous system nicotine receptors, but genetic factors also modulate nicotine effects including development of tolerance (Collins and Marks 1989). A practical consequence is that whereas first time tobacco users often become profoundly sick and intoxicated, these effects generally dissipate within a few hours and are rarely experienced again due to a combination of learning to avoid overdosing, and tolerance (US DHHS 1988; Royal College of Physicians 2000). Laboratory studies of intravenous nicotine (Soria *et al.* 1996) and nicotine gum administration (Heishman and Henningfield 2000) have demonstrated greater sensitivity to the mood altering and behavioral effects of nicotine in subjects who do not use tobacco compared to tobacco users. The development of snuff products that are marketed as starter products in which the products delivered lower doses of nicotine more slowly than do the maintenance products takes advantage of the tolerance phenomenon and minimizes the likelihood that the initial users experience will be unpleasant (Connolly 1995; FDA 1995, 1996). With respect to cigarettes, because the nicotine dosing is puff by puff, with the physiologic response occurring quite quickly after each puff, this problem is less of a barrier to the acquisition of smoking than it is for the acquisition of snuff use (in which the dose is determined by the amount of snuff put in the mouth) (Connolly 1995; Slade 1995).

Physical dependence and withdrawal. Tobacco withdrawal signs and symptoms, including changes in brain electrical activity, cognitive performance, anxiety, and response to stressful stimuli can be altered by administration of pure nicotine in a variety of forms (e.g. gum, patch, nasal delivery) (Hughes *et al.* 1990; Heishman *et al.* 1994;

Pickworth *et al.* 1995; Shiffman *et al.* 1998). Humans report generally similar subjective effects from intravenous nicotine as from smoked tobacco (Henningfield *et al.* 1985; Jones *et al.* 1999). Tobacco craving is only partially relieved by pharmaceutical forms of nicotine, reflecting the facts that (1) cravings can be elicited by factors that are not mitigated by nicotine (e.g. the smell of smoke, the sight of other people smoking, and tobacco advertisements), and (2) tobacco smoke constituents other than nicotine (e.g. 'tar' and other smoke constituents) can reduce craving independently of nicotine (Butchsky *et al.* 1995) and may have synergistic effects with nicotine in cigarettes to provide more effective nicotine relief than cigarette smoke-delivered nicotine (Rose *et al.* 1993).

Rodent models of nicotine withdrawal have been developed and serve in the evaluation of medications for treating withdrawal (e.g. Malin *et al.* 1992, 1998*a*, *b*). The most useful is one in which the frequency of signs are observed and coded from a checklist which includes writhes and gasps, wet shakes and tremors, ptosis, bouts of teeth chattering and chewing, and miscellaneous less frequent signs such as foot licks, scratches, and yawns (Malin *et al.* 1992). Episodes of locomotor immobility lasting longer than a minute are also recorded. Another rodent model that might be of particular relevance to disruption of behavioral performance in humans is one in which acute nicotine abstinence disrupted food-maintained learned behaviors (Carroll *et al.* 1989).

Dose-related effects

As with many drugs, understanding the mechanisms of the effects of nicotine is complicated by the fact total dose, rate of delivery, and amount of prior exposure are important determinants (Ernst *et al.* 2001). For example, 1 mg nicotine delivered by smoke inhalation may produce cardiac acceleration and mood alteration, whereas the approximately 1 mg nicotine delivered per hour by transdermal nicotine patch produces no reliable change in mood or cardiovascular measure (Benowitz 1990; Pickworth *et al.* 1994). Furthermore, observed effects involve a diverse array of mechanisms, which operate differentially at different dosages. For example, stimulation of nicotinic cholinergic receptors in the spinal cord may directly alter muscle tone, whereas heart rate acceleration and mood alteration appear to be primarily mediated by catecholamines release that is modulated by nicotine (e.g. release of norepinephrine and increased brain dopamine, respectively) (Benowitz 1990; Balfour and Fagerstrom 1996; Henningfield *et al.* 1996).

Nicotine is rapidly and efficiently absorbed when inhaled into the lung (Benowitz 1990). It is also well absorbed through the skin, nasal passages, and the oral mucosa, although the speed of its absorption through the mucosa is directly related to the fraction of nicotine that is in a 'free-base' or unionized state, as opposed to that which is in the 'bound' or in the ionized state. The alkaloid nature of nicotine implies that the percentage of unionized nicotine molecules in tobacco material can be influenced by the pH of the product or its aqueous medium, with the concentration of free base nicotine increasing logarithmically as a function of increasing pH (Henningfield *et al.* 1995*b*). The pKa of nicotine is 8, and thus 50% of the nicotine is unionized and free to be rapidly absorbed at an aqueous pH of 8. The alkaline smoke typical of cigars (typically 7.0–8.5) enables efficient absorption of nicotine through the mouth without inhalation (Henningfield *et al.* 1999; Baker *et al.* 2000). The mildly acidic smoke of cigarettes (pH 5.5–6.5) produces less throat irritation and is easier to inhale than higher pH cigar smoke, but no nicotine is absorbed in the mouth and smoke must be inhaled to absorb nicotine (Hoffman and Hoffman 1997). Since addictive drug effects are intensified by faster delivery (O'Brien 1996), the dual consequence of a potentially more addictive form of nicotine delivery and the well-documented greater lung toxicity due to the repetitive exposure of the lung to the smoke results (Hoffman and Hoffman 1997). Therefore, even though a cigar potentially delivers more nicotine and toxins, the risk of lung disease is less than that associated with cigarette smoking (National Cancer Institute 1998; Baker *et al.* 2000).

Smokeless tobacco products such as snuff, include 'starter' products (tobacco industry term) that are generally at pH levels of approximately 7.0, whereas products that experienced users tend to 'graduate' to (tobacco industry term) generally show an aqueous pH of 7.5–8.5) (Henningfield *et al.* 1995*b*). Snuff products with higher pH levels than products with similar nicotine content produce more rapidly rising and higher plasma nicotine levels as well as higher heart rates and stronger subjective effects (Fant *et al.* 1999).

An additional consequence of smoke inhalation is the generation of arterial plasma nicotine spikes that can be up to ten times greater than simultaneously measured venous levels within the first minute following the smoking of a cigarette (Henningfield *et al.* 1993). Similar effects occur with smoked cocaine and appear to contribute to its powerful reinforcing effects (Evans *et al.* 1996). Consistent with these observations, tobacco products that deliver nicotine more rapidly are demonstrated to be of higher abuse liability in standard testing than pharmaceutical products, which deliver nicotine more slowly (Henningfield and Keenan 1993; Stitzer and De Witt 1998). These observations are consistent with product design and ingredients: Whereas, tobacco products are designed to maximize addictive potential, pharmaceutical products are designed and labeled to minimize the risk of addiction and abuse (Henningfield and Slade 1998; Slade and Henningfield 1998).

Cross population variation in nicotine metabolism. There is much individual variability in the CYP2A6 activity of human liver samples, and much variability in the rate of nicotine metabolism among individuals and populations. Studies of racial/ethnic differences have shown slower metabolism of nicotine and cotinine in Chinese Americans, and slower metabolism of cotinine African Americans compared to

American Caucasians and Hispanics (Perez-Stable *et al.* 1998; Benowitz *et al.* 2002). As mentioned previously the slower metabolism of nicotine and cotinine by Asians can be explained by the high frequency of CYP2A6 gene alleles that are associated with diminished or absent enzyme activity (Oscarson 2001). Slower metabolism of nicotine among Asians may explain, at least in part, lower cigarette consumption among Asians compared to Caucasians (Benowitz *et al.* 2002). African Americans also metabolize nicotine and cotinine via the glucuronidation pathway more slowly than do Caucasians (Benowitz *et al.* 1999). The genetic basis and biological consequences of slower glucuronidation among African Americans have not yet been determined. Pregnancy is associated with a marked acceleration of nicotine and cotinine metabolism (Dempsey *et al.* 2002). Thus the pregnant woman may require higher dose of nicotine medication to aid smoking cessation compared to the non-pregnant woman. Ageing has been reported to be associated with slower metabolism of nicotine, as has the presence of kidney disease (Molander *et al.* 2000, 2001). The importance of individual differences in nicotine metabolism in determining cigarette consumption and/or addiction risk is a subject of ongoing investigation.

Tobacco-delivered nicotine

Tobacco products are a means of storing nicotine and serve as vehicles for its delivery. Tobacco companies use a variety of techniques to control the nicotine dosing characteristics of cigarettes. The modern cigarette is elaborately designed, involving numerous patents for wrappers, manufacturing, filter systems, and processes for making 'tobacco' filler out of tobacco materials and other substances (Browne 1990; FDA 1995, 1996). The function of the cigarette has been described eloquently by senior Philip Morris researcher William Dunn, as reprinted in Hurt and Robertson (1998):

> The cigarette should be conceived not as a product but as a package. The product is nicotine. Think of the cigarette pack as a storage container for a day's supply of nicotine... Think of the cigarette as dispenser for dose unit of nicotine... Think of a puff of smoke as the vehicle of nicotine. Smoke is beyond question the most optimized vehicle of nicotine and the cigarette the most optimized dispenser of smoke.

Although both the tobacco industry and non-industry scientists and agencies have described cigarettes as nicotine delivery systems, not all of their effects are explained by nicotine delivery (e.g. FDA 1995, 1996; Slade *et al.* 1995; Hurt and Robertson 1998; WHO 2001). Most of the toxicity of the products is due to substances other than nicotine. Substances in tobacco smoke, in addition to nicotine, may also contribute to the development and maintenance of tobacco use (FDA 1995, 1996; Slade *et al.* 1995; Hurt and Robertson 1998; WHO 2001).

Because the speed and nature of the absorption process is a strong determinant of the effects of nicotine, it is not surprising that the tobacco industry has focused much attention on tobacco product development and the control of nicotine dosing characteristics by means such as pH manipulation of tobacco and tobacco smoke (FDA 1995, 1996; Slade *et al.* 1995; Kessler *et al.* 1996; Hurt and Robertson 1998). For example, buffering compounds in smokeless tobacco products (FDA 1995, 1996; Tomar and Henningfield 1997) can alter the speed and amount of nicotine delivery of the products. Similarly, menthol, and perhaps compounds such as levulinic acid (Bates *et al.* 1999), may alter the effects of nicotine delivered by smoke by enabling smokers to inhale larger quantities of smoke by making the smoke feel less harsh and by reducing concerns about the smoke toxicity because of the perceived smoothness (Henningfield *et al.* 2002). Product design and ingredients can also be employed to control the mean particle size to optimize the efficient inhalation of nicotine deep into the lungs where absorption is rapid and virtually complete (Royal College of Physicians 2000). Characteristics that contribute to larger amounts of smoke being more deeply absorbed into the lung could also contribute to more rapid absorption of nicotine as well as increasing the probability of diseases such as deep lung adenocarcinomas (Hoffman and Hoffman 1997; Thun and Burns 2001).

The idea that cigarette smoke is a chemical cocktail that produces effects beyond those produced by nicotine and/or which may modulate nicotine's effects has received increasing support since the 1990s. This has led to the conclusion that tobacco-delivered nicotine is not only more toxic, but more addictive than pure nicotine forms (Henningfield *et al.* 2000; Royal College of Physicians 2000). Additionally, it appears that non-nicotine components of cigarette smoke inhibit monoamine oxidase which could contribute to an antidepressant effect of smoking (Volkow *et al.* 1999). Acetaldehyde, a metabolite of alcohol, which contributes to its subjective effects, is present in cigarette smoke and can act synergistically with nicotine to produce stronger reinforcing effects than either nicotine or acetaldehyde alone (FDA 1995, 1996; Bates *et al.* 1999). Research on this topic was conducted by the tobacco industry and modern cigarettes can be engineered to increase their delivery of acetaldehyde either by adding the substance or by including certain sugars, which yield acetaldehyde upon pyrolysis (FDA 1995, 1996; Bates *et al.* 1999).

Nicotine toxicology

Although nicotine can be a lethal poison at very high dosages, relative to those typically delivered by use of tobacco or nicotine replacement medications, its toxicological effects in tobacco use are modest compared to the many carcinogens and other toxins present in tobacco products and the many more produced when tobacco products are burned (Hoffman and Hoffman 1997; Benowitz 1998). Nonetheless, nicotine delivered by tobacco products and medications is not entirely benign. Nicotine can produce a variety of potential adverse effects depending upon the dose and pattern of administration. 'For example, nicotine is a fetal neuroteratogen in rats and there is concern that nicotine from cigarette smoking during pregnancy might contribute to developmental and behavioral problems in children of mothers who smoke.'

(US DHHS 2001). At doses delivered by nicotine replacement medications, the risk of adverse effects from nicotine during pregnancy appears substantially lower than by smoking. But because the possibility of risks cannot be ruled out, it is generally recommended that a doctor be consulted concerning use of the medications during pregnancy (Windsor *et al.* 2000). Similarly, nicotine is a possible contributor to coronary artery disease leading to labeling on nicotine medications advising persons with histories of heart disease to consult with a doctor before using the products.

Comparison across addictive drugs

As indicated by the foregoing discussion, nicotine delivered by tobacco meets the criteria as a dependence-producing drug. Moreover, there is sufficient epidemiological and clinical evidence for a systematic comparison of cigarettes to other addictive drugs. One such comparison was provided in a table (pp. 299–303) in the 1988 Surgeon Generals Report (US DHHS 1988), and another by Henningfield *et al.* (1995*a*), which was adapted for presentation in the report of the Royal College of Physicians (2000) (Table 6.1). The following comparison of drugs is based upon these prior analyses. Key findings were that the apparent severity of addictive effects of the various drugs depends upon the measure under consideration; no addictive drug exceeds all others on all points; nicotine delivered by tobacco is a highly addictive drug. Nonetheless, differences in specific features of addictive drugs and differences in consequences of their use have implications for regulatory approaches appropriate to each drug and for

Table 6.1 Ranking of nicotine in relation to other drugs in terms of addiction factors of concern (Royal College of Physicians 2000)

Dependence among users	nicotine > heroin > cocaine > alcohol > caffeine
Difficulty achieving abstinence	(alcohol = cocaine = heroin = nicotine) > caffeine
Tolerance	(alcohol = heroin = nicotine) > cocaine > caffeine
Physical withdrawal severity	alcohol > heroin > nicotine > cocaine > caffeine
Societal impact	serious effects due to secondary deaths (nicotine), accidents (alcohol) or crime (heroin, cocaine); no substantial impact for caffeine
Deaths	nicotine > alcohol > (cocaine = heroin) > caffeine
Importance in user's daily life	(alcohol = cocaine = heroin = nicotine) > caffeine
Intoxication	alcohol > (cocaine = heroin) > caffeine > nicotine
Animal self-administration	cocaine > heroin > (alcohol = nicotine) > caffeine
Liking by non-drug abusers	cocaine > (alcohol = caffeine = heroin = nicotine)
Prevalence	caffeine > nicotine > alcohol > (cocaine = heroin)

clinical approaches to treating individuals which are determined by the particular drug under consideration (Goldstein 1994).

Incidence, prevalence, and risk of progression. Following initial use, development of dependence to nicotine is far more common than that to cocaine, heroin, or alcohol, and the rate of graduation from occasional use to addictive levels of intake is highest for nicotine (Anthony *et al.* 1994; Giovino *et al.* 1995). Depending upon the definition used for occasional use, between 33% and 50% escalate to become daily smokers in the US (US DHHS 1994). In contrast, even when highly addictive dosage forms of cocaine (i.e. smokable 'crack' cocaine) are readily available in the US, the risk of progression from any use to regular use is the exception and not the rule.

Remission and relapse. An evaluation of several data sets indicates that rates and patterns of relapse are similar for nicotine, heroin, and alcohol (e.g. Hunt and Matarazzo 1973; Maddux and Desmond 1986), and probably for cocaine (e.g. Wallace 1989). A closer analysis of relapse to cigarette smoking showed that in the context of a minimal treatment intervention approach, approximately 25% of persons relapsed within 2 days of their last cigarette and approximately 50% within 1 week (Kotke *et al.* 1989), and that among people quitting on their own, two-thirds were smoking within 3 days of their scheduled quit date (Hughes *et al.* 1992).

Reports of addictiveness by drug abusers. Two studies evaluated ratings across addictions by polydrug abusers. The first study found that when rating the degree of 'liking', tobacco, cocaine, and heroin were rated similarly and all were rated more highly than alcohol, and that tobacco was among the most highly rated drugs on a 'need' scale (Blumberg *et al.* 1974). Another study found that compared to other substances, tobacco was associated with equal or greater levels of difficulty in quitting and urge to use, but its use was not as pleasurable (Kozlowski *et al.* 1989).

Psychoactivity and euphoria. One correlate of addiction liability is that a drug produces pleasurable or euphoriant effects in standard tests of drug liking and morphine-benzedrine group scale (MBG) scores of the Addiction Research Center Inventory (Jasinski 1979; Fischman and Mello 1989). Intravenous nicotine mimics mood-altering effects of tobacco and, when rapidly administered by intravenous injections in a similar manner as cocaine is often abused, nicotine produces qualitatively similar effects as cocaine in poly drug abusers (Henningfield *et al.* 1995*a*; Jones *et al.* 1999).

Reinforcing effects. As discussed earlier, nicotine serves as a reinforcer for a variety of species. Its reinforcing effects are related to the dose and are increased when sensory stimuli are associated with injections and by food deprivation (US DHHS 1988; Corrigall 1999).

Physical dependence. Among addictive drugs, the most severe withdrawal syndromes are those that occur following acute deprivation of extended administration of alcohol or short-acting barbiturates; morphine-like opioids can also produce an overtly recognizable syndrome (O'Brien 1996). Deprivation after extended administration of cocaine and cannabis can also produce a diagnosable withdrawal syndrome; however, it is only since the mid 1980s that addiction experts have come to generally concur that these drugs can produce syndromes of withdrawal that can be distinguished from the lack of the effects of the drugs themselves; the role of the withdrawal syndromes in sustaining cocaine and cannabis use remains unclear (Gawin and Kleber 1986; O'Brien 1996). Acute deprivation from extended tobacco use produces a syndrome of withdrawal signs and symptoms that is intermediate between that of the opioids and cocaine in that it has been recognized for several decades, and is generally understood to serve as a barrier to even short-term efforts to achieve tobacco abstinence. Tobacco withdrawal can be occupationally and socially debilitating, but other than standing as a barrier to extended cessation, is not life-threatening in its own right (American Psychiatric Association 1996).

Tolerance. A high degree of tolerance develops to the acute effects of nicotine, and some degree of tolerance is gained during each day of smoking and lost during the approximately 8 hours of tobacco deprivation during sleeping hours (Swedberg *et al.* 1990). Tolerance to nicotine has been systematically explored for more than a century (e.g. Langley 1905). Its mechanisms are diverse and the time course of gain and loss of tolerance varies across responses under evaluation (Collins and Marks 1989; Balfour and Fagerstrom 1996; Royal College of Physicians 2000; Perkins 2002). Comparing drugs of abuse on measures of tolerance is complicated by the varying potential range of measures that can be considered, however, the general degree of tolerance that is produced by repeated nicotine exposure is comparable to that produced by other addictive drugs that produce high levels of tolerance such as the opioids.

Implications for treatment of tobacco dependence

Although many people are able to quit smoking without formal intervention, this generally occurs only after many cessation attempts and after sufficient harm has been done to substantially increase the risks of premature mortality (Royal College of Physicians 2000; US DHHS 2000). For others, perhaps as a consequence of the pathological changes in brain structure and function produced by long-term nicotine exposure, achieving remission from dependence without treatment may be no more readily achievable than achieving remission from coronary artery disease or oral cancer without treatment. In fact, following surgery for coronary artery disease and lung cancer caused by smoking, many smokers resume smoking in face of the extraordinarily high risks (US DHHS 1988) (Fig. 6.1). The U.S. Clinical Practice Guideline: Treating Tobacco Use and Dependence (Fiore *et al.* 2000) and reports from the U.S. Surgeon General (US DHHS 2000) and Royal College of Physicians (2000) describe behavioral and pharmacological treatment interventions that approximately double

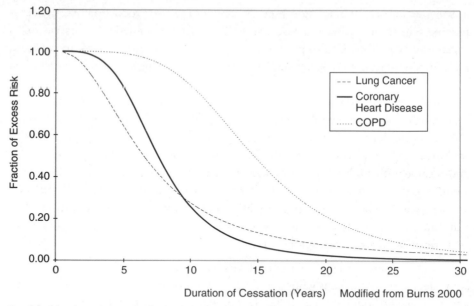

Fig. 6.1 Fraction of excess risk remaining with increasing duration of cessation.

the chances of achieving cessation. These include intensive group behavioral counseling, other individualized behavior therapies and several types of pharmacotherapy. Pharmacotherapies include different nicotine replacement medications (gum, patch, lozenge, oral inhaler, and nasal spray) and bupropion, as well as medications that have been demonstrated to be effective but have not been explicitly approved or marketed for smoking cessation (nortriptyline and clonidine). Many other substances have been used but show little evidence of efficacy (Henningfield *et al.* 1998; Fiore *et al.* 2000; US DHHS 2000).

Acknowledgements

Preparation of this paper was supported, in part, by a Robert Wood Johnson Foundation Innovators Combating Substance Abuse Award to Dr. Henningfield. Dr. Henningfield provides consulting services regarding treatments for tobacco dependence to GlaxoSmithKline Consumer Health Care through Pinney Associates, and also has a financial interest in a nicotine replacement product under development, and serves as an expert witness in litigation against the tobacco industry by the U.S. Department of Justice and other plaintiffs. Dr. Benowitz work was supported, in part, by U.S. Public Health Service Grants DA02277 and DA 12393. We greatly appreciate the editorial assistance of Christine A. Rose, whose efforts were supported by the Innovators award to JEH.

References

Ahijevych, K. (1999). Nicotine metabolism variability and nicotine addiction. *Nicotine & Tobacco Research*, **1** (Suppl.), S59–S62.

American Psychiatric Association (1980). *Diagnostic and statistical manual of mental disorders.* (3rd edn). American Psychiatric Association, Washington, DC.

American Psychiatric Association (1987). *Diagnostic and statistical manual of mental disorders.* American Psychiatric Association, Washington, DC.

American Psychiatric Association (1996). *Practice guideline for the treatment of patients with nicotine dependence.* American Psychiatric Association, Washington, DC.

Anthony, J. C., Warner, L. A., and Kessler, R. C. (1994). Comparative epidemiology of dependence on tobacco, alcohol, controlled substance, and inhalants: Basic findings from the National Comorbidity Survey. *Experimental and Clinical Psychopharmacology*, **2**, 244–68.

Baker, F., Ainsworth, S. R., Dye, J. T., Crammer, C., Thun, M. J., Hoffmann, D., *et al.* (2000). Health risks associated with cigar smoking. *Journal of the American Medical Association*, **284** (6), 735–40.

Balfour, D. J., and Fagerstrom, K. O. (1996). Pharmacology of nicotine and its therapeutic use in smoking cessation and neurodegenerative disorders. *Pharmacology and Therapeutics*, **72** (1), 51–81.

Bates, C., Connolly, G. N., and Jarvis, M. (1999). *Tobacco additives: cigarette engineering and nicotine addiction.* Action on Smoking and Health, London, U.K.

Benowitz, N. L. (1990). Pharmacokinetic considerations in understanding nicotine dependence. In: *The biology of nicotine dependence* (ed. G. Bock and J. Marsh), pp. 186–209. John Wiley and Sons Ltd, London, U.K.

Benowitz, N. L. (1996). Biomarkers of cigarette smoking. In: *The FTC cigarette test method for determining tar, nicotine, and carbon monoxide yields of U.S. cigarettes: report of the NCI Expert Committee.* pp. 93–111. National Institutes of Health, and National Cancer Institute, Bethesda, MD.

Benowitz, N. L. (ed.) (1998). *Nicotine safety and toxicity.* Oxford University Press, Oxford.

Benowitz, N. L. (1999). Biomarkers of environmental tobacco smoke exposure. *Environmental Health Perspectives*, **107** (2), 349–55.

Benowitz, N. L., Perez-Stable, E. J., Herrera, B., and Jacob, P., III. (2002). Slower metabolism and reduced intake of nicotine from cigarette smoking in Chinese-Americans. *Journal of the National Cancer Institute*, **94** (2), 108–15.

Blumberg, H. H., Cohen, S. D., Dronfield, B. E., Mordecal, E. A., Roberts, J. C., and Hawks, D. (1974). British opiate users I. People approaching London drug treatment centers. *International Journal of Addiction*, **9**, 1–23.

Browne, C. L. (1990). *The design of cigarettes* (3rd edn). Filter Products Division Hoechst Celanese Corporation, Charlotte, North Carolina.

Butschky, M. F., Bailey, D., Henningfield, J. E., and Pickworth, W. B. (1995). Smoking without nicotine delivery decreases withdrawal in 12-hour abstinent smokers. *Pharmacology Biochemistry and Behavior*, **50** (1), 91–6.

Carroll, M. E., Lac, S. T., Asencio, M., and Keenan, R. M. (1989). Nicotine dependence in rats. *Life Sciences*, **45**, 1381–8.

Collins, A. C., and Marks, M. J. (1989). Chronic nicotine exposure and brain nicotinic receptors – influence of genetic factors. In: *Progress in brain research* (ed. A. Nordberg, K. Fuxe, B. Holmstedt, and A. Sundwall), Vol. 79.

Connolly, G. N. (1995). The marketing of nicotine addiction by one oral snuff manufacturer. *Tobacco Control*, **4** (1), 73–9.

Corrigall, W. A. (1999). Nicotine self-administration in animals as a dependence model. *Nicotine and Tobacco Research*, **1**, 11–20.

Ernst, M., Matochik, J. A., Heishman, S. J., Van Horn, J. D., Jons, P. H., Henningfield, J. E., and London, E. D. (2001). Effect of nicotine on brain activation during performance of a working memory task. *Proceedings of the National Academy of Sciences of the United States of America*, **98** (8), 1728 33.

Evans, S. M., Cone, E. J., and Henningfield, J. E. (1996). Arterial and venous cocaine plasma concentrations in humans: relationships to route of administration, cardiovascular effects and subjective effects. *Journal of Pharmacology and Experimental Therapeutics*, **279**, (3), 1345–56.

Fant, R. V., Henningfield, J. E., Nelson, R., and Pickworth, W. B. (1999). Pharmacokinetics and pharmacodynamics of moist snuff in humans. *Tobacco Control*, **8**, 387–92.

Finnegan, J. K., Larson, P. S., and Haag, H. B. (1945). The role of nicotine in the cigarette habit. *Science*, **102**, 94–6.

Fiore, M. C., Bailey, W. C., Cohen, S. J., et al. (2000). *Treating tobacco use and dependence. Clinical practice guideline.* U.S. Department of Health and Human Services. Public Health Service, Rockville, MD.

Fischman, M. W., and Mello, N. K. (ed.) (1989). *Testing for abuse liability of drugs in humans.* NIDA Research Monograph, No. 92. Washington, DC, U.S. Government. Printing Office, 73-100.

Food and Drug Administration (1995). 21 CFR Part 801, *et al.* Regulations restricting the sale and distribution of cigarettes and smokeless tobacco products to protect children and adolescents; proposed rule analysis regarding FDA's jurisdiction over nicotine-containing cigarettes and smokeless tobacco products; notice. *Federal Register*, **60** (155), 41314–792.

Food and Drug Administration (1996). 21 CFR Part 801, *et al.* Regulations restricting the sale and distribution of cigarettes and smokeless tobacco to protect children and adolescents; final rule. *Federal Register*, **61** (168), 44396–5318.

Foulds, J., Stapleton, J., Bell, N., Swettenham, J., Jarvis, M. J., and Russell, M. A. H. (1997). Mood and physiological effects of subcutaneous nicotine in smokers and never-smokers. *Drug and Alcohol Dependence*, **44**, 105–15.

Gawin, F. H., and Kleber, H. D. (1986). *Abstinence symptomatology and psychiatric diagnosis in cocaine abusers, archives of general psychiatry*, Vol. 43, pp. 107–13.

Giovino, G. A., Henningfield, J. E., Tomar, S. L., Escobedo, L. G., and Slade, J. (1995). Epidemiology of tobacco use and dependence. *Epidemiologic Reviews*, **17** (1), 48–65.

Goldberg, S. R., Spealman, R. D., Risner, M. E., and Henningfield, J. E. (1983). Control of behavior by intravenous nicotine injections in laboratory animals. *Pharmacology Biochemistry and Behavior*, **19**, 1011–20.

Goldberg, S. R., and Henningfield, J. E. (1988). Reinforcing effects of nicotine in humans and experimental animals responding under intermittent schedules of IV drug injection. *Pharmacology Biochemistry and Behavior*, **30**, 227–34.

Goldstein, A. (1994). *Addiction: from biology to drug policy.* W.H. Freeman and Company, New York.

Griffiths, R. R., Bigelow, G. E., and Henningfield, J. E. (1980). Similarities in animal and human drug-taking behavior. In: *Advances in substance abuse* (ed. N. K. Mello), pp. 1–90. JAI Press, Inc., Greenwich, Connecticut.

Gritz, E. R. (1980). Smoking behavior and tobacco use. *Advances in Substance Abuse*, **1**, 91–158.

Heishman, S. J., Taylor, R. C., and Henningfield, J. E. (1994). Nicotine and smoking: a review of effects on human performance. *Experimental and Clinical Psychopharmacology*, **2** (4), 345–95.

Heishman, S. J., and Henningfield, J. E. (2000). Tolerance to repeated nicotine administration on performance, subjective, and physiological responses in nonsmokers. *Psychopharmacology*, **152**, 321–33.

Henningfield, J. E. (1984). Behavioral pharmacology of cigarette smoking. In: *Advances in behavioral pharmacology*, Vol. 4 (ed. T. Thompson, P.B. Dews, and J. Barrett), pp. 131–210. Academic Press, New York.

Henningfield, J. E., Miyasato, K., and Jasinski, D. R. (1985). Abuse liability and pharmacodynamic characteristics of intravenous and inhaled nicotine. *Journal of Pharmacology and Experimental Therapeutics*, **234** (1), 1–12.

Henningfield, J. E., and Keenan, R. M. (1993). Nicotine delivery kinetics and abuse liability. *Journal of Consulting and Clinical Psychology*, **61** (5), 1–8.

Henningfield, J. E., Schuh, L. M., and Jarvik, M. E. (1995*a*). Pathophysiology of Tobacco Dependence. In: *Psychopharmacology: The Fourth Generation of Progress* (ed. F. E. Bloom and D. J. Kupfer), pp. 1715–29. Raven Press, Ldt., New York.

Henningfield, J. E., Stapleton, J. M., Benowitz, N. L., Grayson, R. G., and London, E. D. (1993). Higher levels of nicotine in arterial than in venous blood after cigarette smoking. *Drug and Alcohol Dependence*, **33**, 23–9.

Henningfield, J. E., Radzius, A., and Cone, E. J. (1995*b*). Estimation of available nicotine content of six smokeless tobacco products. *Tobacco Control*, **4** (1), 57–61.

Henningfield, J. E., Keenan, R. M., and Clarke, P. B. S. (1996). Nicotine. In: *Pharmacological Aspects of Drug Dependence* (ed. C. R. Schuster and M. Kuhar), pp. 272–314. Springer-Verlag, Berlin.

Henningfield, J. E., Fant, R. V., and Gopalan, L. (1998). Non-nicotine medications for smoking cessation. *The Journal of Respiratory Diseases*, **19**(8), S33–S42.

Henningfield, J. E., and Slade, J. (1998). Tobacco-dependence medications: public health and regulatory issues. *Food and Drug Law Journal*, **53** (Suppl.), 75–114.

Henningfield, J. E., Fant, R. V., Radzius, A., and Frost, S. (1999). Nicotine concentration, smoke pH and whole tobacco aqueous pH of some cigar brands and types popular in the United States. *Nicotine and Tobacco Research*, **1**, 163–8.

Henningfield, J. E., Fant, R. V., Shiffman, S., and Gitchell, J. (2000). Tobacco dependence: scientific and public health basis of treatment. *The Economics of Neuroscience*, **2** (1), 42–6.

Henningfield, J. E., Benowitz, N. L., Ahijevych, B., Garrett, G., Connolly, G., and Ferris Wayne, G. (2002). Developing leadership in reducing substance abuse. *Nicotine and Tobacco Research* (in press).

Hoffmann, D., and Hoffmann, I. (1997). The changing cigarette, 1950–1995. *Journal of Toxicology and Environmental Health*, **50**, 307–64.

Hughes, J. R., Higgins, S. T., and Hatsukami, D. (1990). Effects of abstinence from tobacco—a critical review. In: *Research advances in alcohol and drug problems* (ed. L. T. Kozlowski, H. M. Annis, H. D. Cappell, Fr. B. Glaser, M. S. Goodstadt, Y. Israel, H. Kalant, E. M. Sellers, and E. R. Vingilis), pp. 317–98. Plenum Publishing Corporation.

Hughes, J. R., Gulliver, S. B., Fenwick, J. W., Valliere, W. A., Cruser, K., Pepper, S., Shea, P., Solomon, L. J., and Flynn, B. S. (1992). Smoking cessation among self-quitters, *Health Psychology*, **11**, 331–4.

Hunt, W. A., and Matarazzo, J. D. (1973). Three years later: recent developments in the experimental modification of smoking behavior. *Journal of Abnormal Psychology*, **31** (2), 107–114.

Hurt, R. D., and Robertson, C. R. (1998). Prying open the door to the tobacco industry's secrets about nicotine: the Minnesota Tobacco Trial. *Journal of the American Medical Association*, **280** (13), 1173–81.

Institutes of Medicine (1997). *Dispelling the myths about addiction: strategies to increase understanding and strengthen research.* National Academy Press, Washington, DC.

Jasinski, D. R. (1979). Assessment of the abuse potentiality of morphine-like drugs (methods used in man). *British Medical Journal,* 7, (Suppl.), 287S–290S.

Johnston, L. M. (1942). Tobacco smoking and nicotine. *Lancet,* 2, 742.

Jones, H. E., Garrett, B. E., and Griffiths, R. R. (1999). Subjective and physiological effects of intravenous nicotine and cocaine in cigarette smoking and cocaine abusers. *Journal of Pharmacology and Experimental Therapeutics,* 288 (1), 188–97.

Kessler, D. A., Witt, A. M., Barnett, P. S., Zeller, M. R., Natanblut, S. L., Wilkenfeld, J. P., *et al.* (1996). The Food and Drug Administration's regulation of tobacco products. *New England Journal of Medicine,* 335 (13), 988–94.

Kotke, T. E., Breeke, M. L., Solberg, L. I., and Hughes, J. R. (1989). A randomized trail to increase smoking intervention by physicians, doctors helping smokers. Round 1. *Journal of American Medical Association,* 261, 2101–6.

Kozlowski, L. T., Wilkinson, D. A., Skinner, W., Kent, C., Franklin, T., and Pope, M. (1989). Measuring the heaviness of smoking: using self-reported time to the first cigarette of the day and number of cigarettes smoked per day. *British Journal of Addiction,* 84(7), 791–9.

Langley, J. N. (1905). On the reaction of cells and of nerve-endings to certain poisons, chiefly as regards the reaction of striated muscle to nicotine and to curari. *Journal of Physiology (London),* 33, 374–413.

Levin, E. D., Wilson, W., Rose, J., and McEvoy. (1996). Nicotine-haloperidol interactions and cognitive performance in schizophrenics. *Neuropsychopharmacology,* 15 (5), 429–36.

Lewin, L. (1964). *Phantastica: Narcotic and stimulating drugs, their use and abuse.* E.P. Dutton and Company, New York.

Lundahl, L. H., Henningfield, J. E., and Lukas, S. E. (2000). Mecamylamine blockade of both positive and negative effects of IV nicotine in human volunteers. *Pharmacology Biochemistry and Behavior,* 66 (3), 637–43.

Maddux, J. F., and Desmond, D. P. (1986). Relapse and recovery in substance abuse careers. In: *Relapse and recovery in drug abuse, NIDA research monograph* (ed. F.M. Tims and C.G. Leukefeld), 72. (pp. 49–71). Bethesda, MD: US Department of Health and Human Services, Public Health Service, Alcohol, Drug Abuse, and Mental Health Administration, National Institute of Drug Abuse. DHHS Publication No. (ADM) 88–1473.

Malin, D. H., Lake, J. R., Newlin-Maultsby, P., Roberts, L. K., Lanier, J. G., Carter, V. A., *et al.* (1992). Rodent model of nicotine abstinence syndrome. *Pharmacology, Biochemistry and Behavior,* 43, 779–84.

Malin, D. H., Lake, J. R., Shenoi, M., Upchurch, T. P., Johnson, S. C., Schweinle, W. E., and Cadle, C. D. (1998*a*). The nitric oxide synthesis inhibitor nitro-L-arginine (L-NNA) attenuates nicotine abstinence syndrome in the rat. *Psychopharmacology,* 140, 371–7.

Malin, D. H., Lake, J. R., Upchurch, T. P., Shenoi, M., Rajan, N., and Schweinle, W. E. (1998*b*). Nicotine abstinence syndrome precipitated by the competitive nicotinic antagonist dihydro-beta-erythroidine. *Pharmacology Biochemistry and Behavior,* 60, 609–13.

McClain, H. and Sapienza, F. (1989). The role of abuse liability testing in drug procedures. In: *Testing for abuse liability of drugs in humans. NIDA research monograph no. 92* (ed. M.W. Fischman, and N.K. Mello), pp. 21–42. DHHS publication number (ADM) 89–1613. U.S. Department of Health and Human Services, Rockville, MD.

Molander, L., Hansson, A., and Lunell, E. (2001). Pharmacokinetics of nicotine in health of elderly people. *Clinical Pharmacology and Therapeutics,* 69, 57–65.

Molander, L., Hansson, A., Lunell, E., Alainentalo, L., Hoffmann, M., and Larsson, R. (2001). Pharmacokinetics of nicotine in kidney failure. *Clinical Pharmacology and Therapeutics*, **68**, 250–60

National Institute on Drug Abuse (1984). *Drug abuse and drug abuse research, first triennial report to congress.* National Institute on Drug Abuse, Rockville, MD.

National Cancer Institute (1998). *Cigars: health effects and trends. Smoking and tobacco control monograph No. 9.* U.S. Department of Health and Human Services, Public Health Service, National Institutes of Health National Cancer Institute.

Newhouse, P. A., and Hughes, J. R. (1991). The role of nicotine and nicotinic mechanisms in neuropsychiatric disease. *British Journal of Addiction*, **86** (5), 521–6.

Newhouse, P. A., Potter, A., and Levin, E. D. (1997). Nicotinic system involvement in Alzheimer's and Parkinson's-diseases—implications for therapeutics. *Nicotine and Neurodegenerative Diseases*, **11** (3), 206–28.

O'Brien, C. P. (1996). Drug addiction and drug abuse. In: *Goodman and Gilman's The Pharmacological Basis of Therapeutics* (ed. J. G. Hardman, A. G. Gilman, and L. E. Limbird), pp. 557–77. McGraw-Hill, New York.

Oscarson, M. (2001). Genetic polymorphism in the cytochrome P450 2A6 gene: Implications for interindividual differences in nicotine metabolism. *Drug Metab. Disp.*, **29**, 91–5.

Paterson, D., and Nordberg, A. (2000). Neuronal nicotinic receptors in the human brain. *Progress in Neurobiology*, **61** (1), 75–111

Perkins, K. (2002). Chronic tolerance to nicotine in humans and its relationship to tobacco dependence. *Nicotine and Tobacco Research*, **4**, 405–22.

Perez-Stable, E. J., Herrera, B., Jacob, P., III, and Benowitz, N. L. (1998). Nicotine metabolism and intake in black and white smokers. *Journal of the American Medical Association*, **280**, 152–6.

Perkins, K. A., Grobe, J. E., Epstein, L. H., Caggiula, A. R., Stiller, R. L., and Jacob, R. G. (1993). Chronic and acute tolerance to subjective effects of nicotine. *Pharmacology Biochemistry and Behavior*, **45**, 375–81.

Pickworth, W. B., Bunker, E. B., and Henningfield, J. E. (1994). Transdermal nicotine: reduction of smoking with minimal abuse liability. *Psychopharmacology*, **115**, 9–14.

Pickworth, W. B., Heishman, S. J., and Henningfield, J. E. (1995). Relationships between EEG and performance during nicotine withdrawal and administration. In: *Brain Imaging of Nicotine and Tobacco Smoking* (ed. E. F. Domino), NPP Books, Ann Arbor, pp. 275–87.

Rose, J. E., Sampson, A., Levin, E. D., and Henningfield, J. E. (1989). Mecamylamine increases nicotine preference and attenuates nicotine discrimination. *Pharmacology Biochemistry and Behavior*, **32**, 933–8.

Rose, J. E., Behm, F. M., and Levin, E. D. (1993). Role of nicotine dose and sensory cues in the regulation of smoke intake. *Pharmacology Biochemistry and Behavior*, **44**, 891–900.

Royal College of Physicians of London (2000). *Nicotine addiction in Britain: a report of the Tobacco Advisory Group of the Royal College of Physicians.* Royal College of Physicians, London, U.K.

Royal Society of Canada (1989). *Tobacco nicotine and addiction: a committee report prepared at the request of the Royal Society of Canada.* Royal Society of Canada, Ottawa, Canada.

Santos, M. D., Alkondon, M., Pereira, E. F., Aracava, Y., Eisenberg, H. M., Maelicke, A., and Albuquerque, E. X. (2002). The nicotinic allosteric potentiating ligand galantamine facilitates synaptic transmission in the mammalian central nervous system. *Molecular Pharmacology*, **61** (5), 1222–34.

Shiffman, S., Mason, K. M., and Henningfield, J. E. (1998). Tobacco dependence treatments: review and prospectus. *Annual Review of Public Health*, **19**, 335–58.

Slade, J. (1995). Are tobacco product drugs? Evidence from U.S. tobacco. *Tobacco Control*, 4(1), 1–2.

Slade, J., Bero, L. A., Hanauer, P., Barnes, D. E., and Glantz, S. A. (1995). Nicotine and addiction. The Brown and Williamson documents. *Journal of the American Medical Association*, 274 (3), 225–33.

Slade, J., and Henningfield, J. E. (1998). Tobacco product regulation: context and issues. *Food and Drug Law Journal*, 53 (Suppl), 43–74.

Soria, R., Stapleton, J. M., Gilson, S. F., Sampson-Cone, A., Henningfield, J. E., and London, E. D. (1996). Subjective and cardiovascular effects of intravenous nicotine in smokers and non-smokers. *Psychopharmacology (Berl)*, 128 (3), 221–6.

Stitzer, M. L., and De Wit, H. (1998). Abuse liability of nicotine. In: *Nicotine safety and toxicity* (ed. N.L. Benowitz), pp. 119–31. Oxford University Press, NY.

Stolerman, I. P., Goldfarb, T., Fink, R., and Jarvik, M. E. (1973). Influencing cigarette smoking with nicotine antagonists. *Psychopharmacologia*, 28, 217–59.

Swedberg, M. D. B., Henningfield, J. E., and Goldberg, S. R. (1990). Nicotine dependency: animal studies. In: *Nicotine psychopharmacology: molecular, cellular, and behavioural aspects* (ed. S. Wonnacott, M. A. H. Russell, and I. P. Stolerman), pp. 38–76. Oxford University Press.

Taylor, P. (1996). Agents acting at the neuromuscular junction and autonomic ganglia. In: *Goodman and Gilman's The Pharmacological basis of therapeutics* (ed. J.G. Hardman, L.E. Limbrid, P.B. Molinoff, R.W. Ruddon, and A.G. Gilman, T.), pp. 177–97. McGraw-Hill, NY.

Tomar, S. L., and Henningfield, J. E. (1997). Review of the evidence that pH is a determinant of nicotine dosage from oral use of smokeless tobacco. *Tobacco Control*, 6, 219–25.

Thun, M. J., and Burns, D. M. (2001). Health impact of 'reduced yield' cigarettes: a critical assessment of the epidemiological evidence. *Tobacco Control*, 10 (Suppl 1), i4–i11.

Tyndale, R. F., and Sellers, E. M. (2001). Variable CYP2A6-mediated nicotine metabolism alters smoking behavior and risk. *Drug Metabolism and Disposition*, 29(4 Pt 2), 548–52.

U.S. Department of Health and Human Services (1988). *The health consequences of smoking: nicotine addiction, a report of the Surgeon General*. U.S. Government Printing Office, Washington, DC.

U.S. Department of Health and Human Services (1994). *Preventing tobacco use among young people. A report of the Surgeon General*. U.S. Government Printing Office, Washington, DC.

U.S. Department of Health and Human Services (2000). *Reducing tobacco use. A report of the Surgeon General*. U.S. Government Printing Office, Washington, DC.

U.S. Department of Health and Human Services (2001). *Women and Smoking: a report of the Surgeon General*. U.S. Department of Health and Human Services, Public Health Service, Office of the Surgeon General, Rockville, MD.

Vidal, C. (1996). Nicotinic receptors in the brain. Molecular biology, function, and therapeutics. *Molecular Chemistry and Neuropathology*, 28 (1–3), 3–11

Vocci, F. J. (1989). The necessity and utility of abuse liability evaluations in human subjects: the FDA perspective. In M.W. Fischman, and N.K. Mello (ed.), *Testing for abuse liability of drugs in humans. NIDA research monograph no. 92* (pp. 7–20). DHHS publication number (ADM) 89–1613. U.S. Department of Health and Human Services, Rockville, MD.

Volkow, N. D., Fowler, J. S., Ding, Y. S., Wang, G. J., and Gatley, S. J. (1999). Imaging the neurochemistry of nicotine actions: studies with positron emission tomography. *Nicotine and Tobacco Research*, 1 (Suppl 2), S127–S132

Wallace, B. C. (1989). Psychological and environmental determinants of relapse in crack cocaine smokers. *Journal of Substance Abuse Treatment*, 6, 95–106.

Windsor, R., Oncken, C., Henningfield, J. E., Hartmann, K., and Edwards, N. (2000). Behavioral and pharmacological treatment methods for pregnant smokers: issues for clinical practice. *Journal of the American Medical Women's Association*, **55** (5), 304–10.

World Health Organization (1992). *The ICD-10 classification of mental and behavioural disorders: clinical description and diagnostic guidelines.* World Health Organization, Geneva, Switzerland.

World Health Organization (2001). *Advancing knowledge on regulating tobacco products.* World Health Organization, Geneva, Switzerland.

Chapter 7

Behavioral pharmacology of nicotine reinforcement

Bridgette E. Garrett, Linda Dwoskin,
Michael Bardo, and Jack E. Henningfield

Introduction

A key feature of drug addiction is compulsive and highly controlled drug seeking and self-administration, which often occur, despite the users' awareness of harmful effects (O'Brien 1996; American Psychiatric Association 1994; World Health Organization 1992). Addictive drugs, in turn, are defined in part by their ability to act as reinforcers as a result of their actions in the brain; these actions are often associated with desirable alterations of mood and feeling state (O'Brien 1996; US DHHS 1988).

The 1998 U.S. Surgeon General's conclusion that nicotine met all criteria for an addictive drug was based in part on findings that nicotine could produce (1) highly controlled or compulsive use, (2) psychoactive or mood-altering effects, and (3) that the drug functioned as a reinforcer (US DHHS 1988). The fact that tobacco use could be compulsive and that nicotine could alter mood and produce psychoactive effects had been known for centuries before the Surgeon General's report, but the determination that it met the most stringent criteria for a reinforcer was one of the pivotal findings supporting the conclusion of the 1988 report.

Understanding the nature and determinants of the reinforcing effects of nicotine and how these can be modulated by tobacco delivery systems is a key factor in understanding tobacco addiction and for developing more effective means to prevention and treatment. The field of science that addresses such issues is termed 'behavioral pharmacology' (Thompson and Schuster 1968) and a behavioral pharmacological analysis of nicotine reinforcement will be the focus of this chapter.

Drug reinforcement. A drug is said to be reinforcing, or capable of producing reinforcement, when its administration can be used to strengthen behavior leading to its presentation (Thompson and Schuster 1968). This is a key behavioral pharmacological mechanism, by which highly controlled or compulsive drug use can be established namely, through the strengthening of behavior produced by the presentation of the drug. The strength of the resultant behavior is related to factors such as the chemistry of the drug itself, which can lead to controlled behavior. The reinforcing effects are generally related to the dose of the drug such that doses that are very low might produce no behavioral effect whereas very large doses might produce noxious effects that are avoided and not sought.

The reinforcing effects can also be enhanced or reduced by the administration of other chemicals, producing 'chemical cocktails', which can be of increased or decreased addictiveness but are frequently of increased toxicity (O'Brien 1996). As will be discussed, nicotine itself can serve as a reinforcer and other substances in tobacco and tobacco smoke can result in a chemical cocktail that may be a stronger reinforcer than nicotine alone. This finding was crucial in the analysis of the U.S. Food and Drug Administration's determination that cigarettes and smokeless tobacco products were highly engineered drug delivery systems designed to maximize the potential addictive effects of nicotine (Kessler 2000).

Interestingly, even more persistent behavior can be established when the presentation of the drug is paired with environmental stimuli such that the environmental stimuli themselves come to be able to establish and sustain behavior as has been demonstrated with cocaine and nicotine in animals and human models of drug taking ('self-administration') (Goldberg *et al.* 1983; Goldberg and Henningfield 1988; Katz 1990). This is termed 'conditioned reinforcement' because the effectiveness of the stimulus (e.g. visual, auditory, olfactory, or taste) is derived from the association of the drug with the stimulus.

When such drug-associated stimuli acquire the ability to control behavior in their own right, they can sustain robust patterns of conditioned behavior even when the drug is not actually administered, although if the drug is consistently absent, the behavior eventually will weaken or 'extinguish' (Thompson and Schuster 1968; US DHHS 1988). Nicotine reinforcement can be measured using both human and animal models, which will be discussed in the following sections.

Human models of nicotine reinforcement

Self-administration

The potential of a drug to serve as a reinforcer can be directly assessed in laboratory models of drug self-administration. In self-administration studies, a specific response (e.g. lever press, squeeze on nasal spray bottle, inhalation of cigarette smoke) is required before the drug is administered, and the degree to which a drug is self-administered more than an inactive substance (e.g. placebo) is typically used to quantify its reinforcing value (Perkins 1999a). Nicotine, like cocaine and heroin, is self-administered by both animals and humans, demonstrating addictive potential and strength as a reinforcer.

In animal models of self-administration, nicotine is generally self-administered intravenously (as discussed below), whereas cigarette smoking is typically used in human laboratory studies, as humans primarily self-administer nicotine in this way.

However, even though cigarette smoking is the most common way for smokers to self-administer nicotine in the laboratory setting, the intravenous route of nicotine administration has also been used to demonstrate nicotine reinforcement in humans (Henningfield *et al.* 1983), confirming the importance of nicotine in tobacco reinforcement and addiction. This study showed that smokers will lever-press to self-administer intravenous nicotine in place of cigarettes. In this procedure, subjects were allowed to choose between nicotine and placebo and they preferentially chose nicotine, clearly demonstrating its positive reinforcing effects. Two important conclusions from the Henningfield *et al.* study are (1) intravenous nicotine self-administration in humans produced euphoric effects similar to those produced by morphine and cocaine, two typically abused drugs with powerful reinforcing effects, and (2) intravenous nicotine self-administration in humans is a viable method for measuring nicotine reinforcement, as patterns resembled those of humans smoking cigarettes and animals self-injecting psychomotor stimulants under similar experimental conditions.

There are several factors that can influence nicotine self-administration including the availability of nicotine, concurrent drug use, and environmental and social factors, but the primary factor that influences nicotine self-administration is the speed of nicotine delivery. When tobacco smoke is inhaled, nicotine is rapidly absorbed into the lungs, enters the arterial circulation and is rapidly distributed to body tissues (Benowitz 1996; Henningfield *et al.* 1993). Following tobacco smoke inhalation, nicotine reaches the brain within a matter of seconds, thus contributing to the powerful reinforcing effects of the cigarette. The importance of speed in nicotine reinforcement is further evidenced by the fact that therapeutic forms of nicotine, such as the gum and patch, are generally not addictive because of the slow speed with which they deliver nicotine to the brain, typically taking many minutes or even hours (Henningfield and Keenan 1993).

Nicotine is also self-administered to avoid unpleasant withdrawal effects (i.e. negative reinforcement) which (frequently?) occur after abrupt cessation or reduction of nicotine in the individual who has become physically dependent on it. Physical dependence results when chronic administration of the drug alters the physiology and behavior in such a way that physical and behavioral functioning are disrupted when drug intake is abruptly reduced (O'Brien 1996; US DHHS 1988). The nicotine withdrawal syndrome is characterized by: dysphoric or depressed mood; insomnia; irritability, frustration, or anger; anxiety; difficulty concentrating; restlessness; decreased heart rate; increased appetite or weight gain (American Psychiatric Association 1994). Although tobacco users acquire preferences for particular types of tobacco products, and even for particular brands within types of products, the withdrawal syndrome can be at least partially relieved by a wide range of nicotine delivery forms including, for example, the substitution of chewing tobacco for cigarettes, or the administration of nicotine in the form of gum, patches, or intravenous injections (US DHHS 1988; O'Brien 1996).

Thus, tobacco use can be powerfully driven both to avoid the aversive effects of withdrawal as well as to produce the directly reinforcing and mood altering effects sought by so many smokers (Henningfield 1984). When it is understood that nicotine can also produce effects that are considered useful in their own right such as reduced body weight and the small but potentially useful improvements in attention, the biological base for the strength of the addiction becomes more evident (US DHHS 1988).

Subjective effects

Smoking is a complex behavior that involves not only nicotine delivery but also an array of interoceptive stimulus effects that are important in the acquisition and maintenance of smoking behavior. Tests of subjective effects are generally used to measure the interoceptive effects of nicotine in humans. Although not easily definable, the subjective effects of nicotine are a combination of actual and perceived effects that an individual experiences as a result of tobacco use. It is thought that the interoceptive stimulus effects of a drug are critical in determining its reinforcing efficacy (Jasinski and Henningfield 1989), thus, a key to understanding nicotine reinforcement in humans may be its relatively subtle but important subjective effects (Henningfield *et al.* 1985; US DHHS 1988; Perkins *et al.* 1993).

Subjective effects of nicotine and other drugs have typically been assessed with various standardized or study-specific self-report measures such as paper and pencil questionnaires and computerized test batteries. Some of the more widely used tests include the Profile of Mood States (POMS), the Addiction Research Center Inventory (ARCI), and the Visual Analog Scale (VAS). For the POMS and ARCI, scores are added across items within a subscale to obtain a score for a particular subjective effect (e.g. POMS 'tension', ARCI 'euphoria' scale; Perkins and Stitzer 1998). The VAS questionnaire is a series of items usually on a scale from 0 to 100 on which the subject rates the degree of the subjective state described by the particular item (e.g. 'lightheaded', 'dizzy', 'head rush', 'jittery', 'tired'; Perkins and Stitzer 1998).

Subjective measures of nicotine's interoceptive effects have shown that nicotine produces euphoric effects similar to those produced by cocaine. In a study by Henningfield *et al.* (1985), nicotine elevated scores on the MBG (Morphine Benzedrine Group) scale of the ARCI, indicative of euphoria. This and other similar studies have shown that nicotine is identified as a stimulant (like cocaine or amphetamine), and produces similar effects to cocaine on a number of subjective ratings including increases in 'drug effect', 'rush', 'good effects', and 'high' (Henningfield *et al.* 1983, 1985; Jones *et al.* 1999; Garrett and Griffiths 2001).

Discriminative stimulus effects

Although tests of subjective effects are used to measure the interoceptive effects of nicotine, these tests are limited in their ability, as subjects are required to use experimenter-defined descriptors, which may vary in familiarity and meaning across subjects

(Fischman and Foltin 1991). Another method for assessing the interoceptive effects of nicotine is the drug discrimination procedure, in which the perceived stimulus effects can be directly observed (Preston and Bigelow 1991).

Nicotine, like other dependence-producing drugs, displays drug discrimination, inducing changes in the central nervous system that are distinct and identifiable. These changes can be blocked by a central (mecamylamine), but not a peripheral (trimethaphan) nicotine antagonist, demonstrating that the discriminative stimulus effects of nicotine are centrally mediated (Perkins *et al.* 1999*b*). The discriminative stimulus effects of nicotine are thought to be critical in understanding both nicotine reinforcement and addiction as these effects of nicotine may cue further drug-seeking behavior, supplementing the primary reinforcing effects of nicotine (Jasinski and Henningfield 1989; Stolerman and Jarvis 1995).

A drug's discriminative stimulus effect is thought to be closely related to its subjective effects (Preston and Bigelow 1991). However, unlike subjective effects, the discrimination procedure uses observable behavioral responses to determine whether a drug's stimulus effects have been perceived by the subject (Preston and Bigelow 1991). Discriminative stimulus effects of nicotine are demonstrated by training subjects to explicitly associate the drug effect to a specific response that leads to reinforcement (Di Chiara 2000). In a drug discrimination procedure, subjects learn, through repeated exposure to the drug, to recognize its interoceptive characteristics and employ these characteristics to discriminate different drugs or different doses of the same drug (Duka *et al.* 2002).

Most human drug discrimination studies use a similar testing method (Perkins *et al.* 1997). Initially, subjects learn to discriminate nicotine from placebo (Discrimination Training). During discrimination training, subjects are presented with training doses of nicotine and placebo that are labeled 'A' and 'B'. During the first presentation of each, subjects are told which one they received. There are then subsequent presentations, in random order, in which subjects must guess if they received 'A' or 'B' (Discrimination Testing). The criterion for reliable discrimination is at least 80% correct identification of the letter code with ten or fewer sessions. After reliably discriminating the training dose of nicotine from placebo, subjects are administered a range of doses for generalization testing to determine how similar these doses are to the training doses ('A' and 'B'). Using this method, studies have consistently found that smokers can reliably discriminate nicotine from placebo.

Animal models of nicotine reinforcement

Nicotine locomotor stimulant effects

Consistent with its effects in humans, nicotine produces psychostimulant effects in laboratory animals. Acute nicotine administration produces a dose-dependent, transient decrease in locomotor activity, followed by a dose-dependent, more prolonged locomotor activity increase in rats (Morrison and Lee 1967; Clarke and Kumar 1983; Clarke 1990; Ksir 1994). Repeated nicotine administration (0.1–0.4 mg/kg, once daily) results in tolerance to the initial depressant effect of nicotine and behavioral sensitization or enhancement of its stimulant effects (Stolerman *et al.* 1973; Clarke and Kumar 1983; Benwell and Balfour 1992; Ksir 1994). Mecamylamine and dihydro β erythroi dine, classical centrally acting, noncompetitive and competitive antagonists, respectively, inhibit the effects of both acute and chronic nicotine treatment on the locomotor activity in rodents (Clarke and Kumar 1983; Balfour and Benwell 1993; Martin *et al.* 1990; Stolerman *et al.* 1997), thereby indicating that the effects of nicotine on locomotor activity are the result of activation of neuronal nicotinic receptors.

Repeated nicotine administration results in neuroadaptive responses and dynamic changes in neuronal function, which can be expressed as behavioral sensitization in animals and addiction in smokers. Behavioral sensitization following repeated drug administration has been hypothesized to model the changes that occur with recurrent use and addiction in humans(?) (Wise and Bozarth 1987; Koob 1992; Robinson and Berridge 1993). Behavioral sensitization has been characterized as consisting of two distinct processes, initiation (events leading to sensitization) and expression (enduring behavioral changes) (Pierce and Kalivas 1997). Mecamylamine has been shown to inhibit the initiation of locomotor sensitization to nicotine in rats following 15 consecutive daily injections (Ericson *et al.* 2000), as well as the expression of sensitization following 5 consecutive daily injections of nicotine (Clarke and Kumar 1983). Thus, the latter results suggest that both initiation and expression of sensitization to nicotine following repeated, daily nicotine administration for days to weeks results from stimulation of nicotinic receptors.

Behavioral sensitization to nicotine has also been demonstrated following infrequent nicotine administration, i.e. once-weekly injections (Miller *et al.* 2001). In this study, long-lasting acute tolerance to the hypoactive effect of nicotine was observed 1 week following a single nicotine injection. After the fourth weekly injection, sensitization to the hyperactive effect of nicotine was clearly evident. Sensitization persisted across a 21-day period during which nicotine was not administered. The enduring behavioral adaptation to this infrequent nicotine administration was the result of nicotinic receptor activation, since pretreatment with mecamylamine attenuated both the initiation and expression of sensitization. Thus, even infrequent nicotine administration initiates neuroadaptive processes associated with nicotine addiction. In this regard, neuroplasticity evident in the mesolimbic dopamine system has been reported following a single nicotine injection into the ventral tegmental area (e.g. long-term increases in basal dopamine levels in the nucleus accumbens, increases in tyrosine hydroxylase mRNA and GluR1 mRNA levels ventral tegmental area) (Ferrari *et al.* 2002). As such, the development of behavioral sensitization is significant, since such neural adaptation likely precedes nicotine addiction, and the persistence of sensitization represents heightened drug sensitivity. The enduring adaptive changes observed in animal models following repeated, infrequent and even acute nicotine administration are consistent with its high addiction liability in smokers and suggest that even a seemingly trivial and/or limited exposure to nicotine can lead to relapse long after cessation of regular tobacco use.

Nicotine drug discrimination

The interoceptive properties of nicotine are thought to be important for their rewarding effects, dependence and abuse liability. As such, the ability of nicotine to serve as a discriminative stimulus is likely necessary for nicotine self-administration. To assess the interoceptive properties of nicotine, rats and more recently mice, are trained typically to press a lever under a fixed ratio schedule for food reinforcement, although other more complex operant schedules, such as tandem fixed ratio variable interval schedules have also been utilized. Once responding stabilizes, nicotine discrimination training is instituted using a two-lever procedure. On alternating days, nicotine is administered at a particular training dose; during these experimental sessions, pressing of one of the two levers results in food pellet reinforcement, whereas pressing the second lever has no programmed consequence. On alternate days, saline is administered prior to the session and the lever that delivers food is reversed from the previous day. Thus, the animal learns to use the presence or absence of the nicotine cue to signal which lever leads to food reinforcement. Sessions are typically terminated after a predetermined number of reinforcements are earned or after a predetermined time has elapsed. Drug discrimination is established when animals reliably make drug- and saline-appropriate responses under a brief test condition when food reinforcement is omitted. During subsequent test sessions, dose response for nicotine generalization may be determined to ascertain if nicotine is discriminated accurately from the vehicle. Other drugs may be substituted for nicotine to ascertain their ability to generalize to the discriminative stimulus effects of nicotine (stimulus generalization or substitution tests). Alternatively, drugs may be administered prior to or concurrently with nicotine to determine their ability to block the discriminative stimulus of nicotine (stimulus antagonism tests). In experiments employing humans as the subjects, examples of subjective effects assessed concurrently with behavioral discrimination reveal that nicotine discrimination is guided by interoceptive cues such as 'stimulated', 'alert', and 'jittery' (Perkins *et al.* 1994; Perkins and Stitzer 1998).

Mecamylamine and dihydro-β-erythroidine have been shown to inhibit completely the discriminative stimulus effects of nicotine in drug discrimination studies (Stolerman *et al.* 1984, 1997; Brioni *et al.* 1994; Shoaib *et al.* 2000); and thus, the discriminative stimulus effects of nicotine are mediated by neuronal nicotinic receptors. Interestingly, the discriminative stimulus effects of nicotine were not attenuated by methyllycaconitine (Brioni *et al.* 1996; Gommans *et al.* 2000), indicating that homomeric α7 nicotinic receptors are not likely involved. However, more than one subtype of nicotinic receptor may contribute to the discriminative stimulus produced by nicotine, which is one interpretation of results from generalization studies with cytisine, a potent, partial agonist at α4β2 receptors (Chandler and Stolerman 1997). In the latter study, the discriminative stimulus effects of nicotine and cytisine were similar, but subtle differences, such as asymmetrical cross-generalization and differences in susceptibility to antagonism by mecamylamine, were evident. The development of subtype-selective nicotinic receptor antagonists will aide in the elucidation of the specific nicotinic receptor subtype(s) responsible for the discriminative stimulus effects of nicotine (Dwoskin and Crooks 2001).

Nicotinic receptors containing β2 subunits play a major role in nicotine discrimination, as indicated by the demonstration that mutant mice lacking this subunit fail to acquire nicotine discrimination at doses which clearly engender discrimination in wild-type mice (Shoaib *et al.* 2002). Furthermore, dopaminergic neurotransmission has also been suggested to play a major role in the discriminative stimulus effects of nicotine. α-Methyl-p-tyrosine and 6-hydroxydopamine (both of which lead to dopamine depletion) and clozapine (the D4 dopamine receptor antagonist) have been shown to attenuate the discriminative stimulus effects of nicotine (Schechter and Rosecrans 1972; Roscrans *et al.* 1976; Brioni *et al.* 1994).

Interestingly, antagonists at D1 and/or D2 dopamine receptors (cis-flupentixol, haloperidol, spiperone, and SCH23390) did not block the discriminative stimulus effects of nicotine (Brioni *et al.* 1994; Corrigall and Coen 1994), perhaps suggesting a dissociation of the mechanisms mediating nicotine discrimination and reinforcement. Interestingly, local administration of nicotine into the medial prefrontal cortex has been shown to substitute for peripheral nicotine administration, and local administration into the nucleus accumbens and ventral tegmental area also produced partial substitution (Miyata *et al.* 2002). Thus, the latter work implicates the mesolimbic dopamine system is an important neuroanatomical substrate mediating the discriminative stimulus properties of nicotine.

Nonetheless, it is likely that the effects of nicotine are not exclusively mediated by the dopaminergic system (Meltzer and Rosecrans 1981; Shoaib and Stolerman 1996). This is consistent with the clinical finding that a variety of types of medications, including antidepressants which work by both dopaminergic and nondopaminergic mechanisms are potentially useful in relieving nicotine cravings when smoking cessation is attempted (Royal College of Physicians 2000). The apparent involvement of multiple brain pathways also supports the possibility that a variety of types of medications might eventually prove useful for the treatment of tobacco dependence.

Nicotine Conditioned Place Preference (CPP)

In a typical CPP experiment, rats are exposed to an apparatus that consists of two distinct contexts that differ in several stimulus dimensions (e.g. visual, tactile, olfactory cues). Conditioning involves pairing a drug with one context and pairing vehicle with the other compartment. Following repeated drug-context pairings, the rat is allowed to choose between the two compartments while in a drug-free state. An increase in time spent in the drug-paired context relative to a vehicle-paired context is taken as evidence that the drug is rewarding. Most drugs of abuse have been shown to produce CPP in rats.

While stimulant drugs such as amphetamine and cocaine have consistently been shown to produce CPP (Bardo and Bevins 2000), evidence for nicotine CPP is mixed. An initial report indicated that nicotine produces dose-dependent CPP in rats (Fudala *et al.* 1985). However, subsequent reports have not always found nicotine CPP, but instead have found either a place aversion (Jorenby *et al.* 1990) or no effect (Parker 1992). One likely explanation for the discrepancy among studies is that the positive findings of nicotine CPP have been obtained generally using a 'biased' design, in which rats are conditioned with nicotine in the nonpreferred compartment. In contrast, the negative findings have been obtained using a 'nonbiased' design, in which rats are conditioned with nicotine to either compartment in a counterbalanced manner. The nicotine CPP obtained with the biased design is problematic, because it does not rule out the possibility that nicotine is simply reducing aversion to the nonpreferred compartment, rather than producing a true preference. In addition, other work has shown that nicotine CPP is dependent of the rat strain tested (Horan *et al.* 1997). Thus, until the parameters required to establish reliable nicotine CPP are elucidated, this paradigm may provide only limited information about the rewarding effect of nicotine.

Nicotine self-administration

In contrast to nicotine CPP, evidence for the rewarding effects of nicotine in laboratory animals appears more consistent using the intravenous drug self-administration paradigm. Since laboratory animals do not inhale tobacco smoke voluntarily, use of the intravenous route of administration is advantageous because it tends to mimic the rapid absorption of nicotine that occurs in human cigarette smokers. Although response rates for intravenous nicotine tend to be lower compared with response rates for other stimulants such as amphetamine or cocaine, reliable rates of nicotine self-administration have been observed under fixed ratio (FR) schedules of reinforcement in a variety of species, including monkeys (Goldberg *et al.* 1981), dogs (Risner and Goldberg 1983), rats (Corrigall and Coen 1989), and mice (Rasmussen and Swedberg 1998).

In the widely used method of Corrigall and Coen (1989), food-restricted rats are first given brief training to press a lever for food and then they are trained to self-administer nicotine through an indwelling intravenous catheter using a two-lever operant conditioning procedure. One lever delivers a rapid (~1 sec) infusion of nicotine that is signaled by a cue light, whereas the second lever has no programmed consequence. Responding is first reinforced on a fixed ratio (FR) 1 schedule, and then the schedule is incremented gradually to an FR5 until responding stabilizes. The reinforcing effect of nicotine is demonstrated as a significant increase in responding on the active lever leading to the nicotine infusion compared with responding on the inactive lever.

Many factors are known to alter nicotine self-administration in laboratory animals and the extensive list is beyond the scope of the current chapter. However, in the method of Corrigall and Coen (1989), one important factor known to alter response rates is the restricted food regimen. This regimen facilitates lever pressing for nicotine and, without it, response rates for nicotine are quite low (Shoaib et al. 1997). In addition, the sex of the subject is known to alter nicotine self-administration, with females acquiring more rapidly than males (Donny et al. 2000). These results from laboratory animals may have important clinical implications for human female smokers who report using cigarettes to control their body weight.

Nicotine self-administration in rats is described by an inverted U-shaped dose effect curve, with maximal responding occurring at a training dose of about 0.03 mg/kg per infusion (Corrigall and Coen 1989). The ascending limb of the dose–response curve presumably reflects an increase in reinforcing efficacy that is not readily satiated, whereas the descending limb presumably reflects satiation, as well as potentially aversive or response-suppressant properties of high unit doses of nicotine. However, relative to other stimulant drugs such as cocaine, the dose–response curve for nicotine self-administration tends to be relatively flat. Rose and Corrigall (1997) have argued that the nicotine dose–response curve is relatively flat because the regulation of nicotine levels in the body is crude and that this finding in rats is consistent with available data on regulation of nicotine levels in human tobacco smokers. In support of this notion, Lynch and Carroll (1999) found that the regulation of intravenous nicotine intake in rats is not as precise as with cocaine.

While FR schedules typically yield an inverted U-shaped dose–response curve with drugs of abuse, progressive ratio (PR) schedules tend to yield monophasic increases in responding up to a plateau. In a PR schedule, the response requirement following presentation of each drug infusion within the session is increased (e.g. FR 1, 2, 5, 9, etc.) until the animal stops responding for a prolonged (e.g. 60 min) interval. The total number of infusions earned within the session is defined as the breakpoint, which presumably reflects the reinforcing efficacy of a given unit dose. Donny et al. (1999) examined nicotine self-administration across varied unit doses using a PR schedule in 4-h daily sessions. Rats displayed an increase in the breakpoint on the PR schedule, with the breakpoint being higher for nicotine than for heroin. Thus, when combined with the data for human tobacco smokers, it would appear that nicotine is a positive reinforcer capable of controlling behavior.

The nicotine self-administration procedure has also been useful for investigating the role of various factors in triggering a relapse among tobacco smokers who are attempting to quit. The paradigm that most frequently has been used for addressing this important clinical issue is the reinstatement test. With the reinstatement test, rats are first trained to self-administer a drug until stable rates of responding are acquired. Saline is then substituted for the drug and, when responding extinguishes to a low rate, a priming injection of drug is administered prior to the session. Although rats still only respond for saline (not drug), the typical finding is that the drug prime increases or reinstates the extinguished response. Shaham *et al.* (1997) showed that a priming injection of nicotine can dose-dependently reinstate nicotine-seeking behavior in rats. In addition, they also found that nicotine seeking was reinstated when rats were simply rested in their home cage for a 21-day period. Thus, the mere passage of time was a sufficient condition to produce spontaneous recovery of the extinguished response. These preclinical results attest to the frequently reported craving and relapse that occurs in abstinent human smokers even following a long period of abstinence. The reinstatement model has also been used to examine the effect of potential smoking cessation treatments (e.g. immunization conjugates) to reduce relapse in nicotine dependence (Lindblom *et al.* 2002).

It is important to understand that the fact that pure nicotine can serve as reinforcer does not mean that the reinforcing effects of cigarette smoke are fully accounted for by nicotine. As discussed earlier sensory effects can acquire conditioned reinforcing properties. In addition, other chemicals present in smoke can interact with nicotine to produce stronger reinforcing effects. For example, Philip Morris researchers found that acetaldehyde (which is present in cigarette smoke) can serve as a reinforcer in its own right for animals (DeNobel and Mele as reported by the U.S. Food and Drug Administration 1996 and Royal College of Physicians, 2000). These investigators found that when nicotine and acetaldehyde were simultaneously administered, the reinforcing effects were stronger than those produced by either drug alone. Other substances have also been investigated such as the tobacco alkaloid and active nicotine metabolite nornicotine which is self-administered in rats (Bardo *et al.* 1999), and which also produces psychomotor stimulant and discriminative stimulus effects (Bardo *et al.* 1997; Dwoskin *et al.* 1999). Such work has important implications for understanding the powerfully addicting effects of tobacco-delivered nicotine as discussed in the Royal College of Physicians (2000).

Neurochemical mechanisms

The subunit composition of nicotinic receptor subtypes mediating the behavioral effects of nicotine have not been elucidated conclusively. Distinguishing between native nicotinic receptors subtypes involved in nicotine-induced alterations of behavior has been difficult considering the current lack of availability of subtype-selective pharmacological tools (Dwoskin and Crooks 2001). Furthermore, defining the subunit composition of nicotinic receptors mediating the effects of nicotine on dopaminergic systems has also been a major challenge (Klink *et al.* 2001; Champtiaux *et al.* 2002; Picciotto and Corrigall 2002). Evidence indicates that nicotinic receptors containing the β2 subunit are clearly involved in the locomotor activating, subjective and rewarding effects of nicotine (Corrigall *et al.* 1994; Picciotto *et al.* 1998). Designation of the subunits which when combined with β2 constitute the nicotinic receptor subtype mediating nicotine's behavioral effects has been controversial. Putatively, a role for subtypes containing pairs of subunits (e.g. α3β2 and α6β2), as well as highly heterogeneous compositions (e.g. $\alpha 4\alpha 6\alpha 5(\beta 2)_2$) have been suggested. Although a potential role for nicotinic receptors containing α7 subunits has also been suggested (Panagis *et al.* 2000), α7 subtype mediation of these effects is not supported by others (Grottick *et al.* 2000; Kempsill and Pratt 2000). Continuing developments in nicotinic receptor pharmacophores, neural circuitry and molecular genetics will certainly enhance our understanding of the specific mechanisms underlying nicotine effects on behavior, nicotine reinforcement and abuse.

Implications for tobacco control

Understanding tobacco use as a form of nicotine self-administration in which the behavior is modulated by diverse pharmacological and behavioral mechanisms helps to explain the persistence of the behavior. In essence, the behavior is controlled and guided by the direct reinforcing effects of nicotine itself, by the ability of self-administered nicotine to relieve cravings and other withdrawal symptoms, by the subjective and discriminative effects of nicotine, by the sensory stimuli that come to be associated with the effects of nicotine, and by a variety of potentially useful effects of nicotine. The neurochemical mechanisms underlying these actions are increasingly well understood making it clear that there is a strong biological basis for tobacco dependence. When it is then understood that the tobacco products are not only 'dirty' from a toxicological perspective but also insofar as they provide chemical cocktails that are potentially more reinforcing than pure nicotine alone, we begin to understand their powerful addictive grip. In addition, and compounding the risk that people will be exposed to tobacco and able to readily obtain addictive doses of nicotine are tobacco product marketing factors, social variables, and a regulatory framework that does little to discourage efforts by tobacco companies to establish addiction in nonusers and to sustain it in those who have already begun to use as discussed elsewhere in this volume (see also, Kessler 2000)

Since the development of models for nicotine self-administration in the 1980s, scientific progress has been quite rapid, and has moved on from the relatively simple determination of whether or not nicotine met criteria as a psychoactive and reinforcing drug to the evaluation of the potential behavioral pharmacological factors which influence its strength as a reinforcer. This work has implications for the development of potential new medications for treating tobacco dependence because it suggests a variety of potential targets for therapeutics. It also has implications for regulating tobacco products because it suggests that just as the toxicity of the products is related to tobacco product ingredients and emissions, so to should the reinforcing effects of tobacco products be influenced by the ingredients and emissions of tobacco products. Just as it should be possible to reduce cigarette toxicity even short of eliminating toxicity, it may be possible to reduce tobacco addictiveness even without eliminating the nicotine or eliminating addiction potential (Henningfield and Zeller 2003; World Health Organization 2003). Behavioral pharmacological analyses may then prove to be as important as toxicology studies in guiding the regulation of tobacco product ingredients and emissions.

Acknowledgments

Preparation of this paper was supported, in part, by a Robert Wood Johnson Foundation Emerging Leadership Program Award to B.E. Garrett, and a Robert Wood Johnson Foundation Innovators Combating Substance Abuse Award to J.E. Henningfield. J.E. Henningfield provides consulting services regarding treatments for tobacco dependence to GlaxoSmithKline Consumer Health Care through Pinney Associates. J.E. Henningfield also has a financial interest in a nicotine replacement product under development, and serves as an expert witness in litigation against the tobacco industry by the U.S. Department of Justice and other plaintiffs. We greatly appreciate the editorial assistance of Christine A. Rose, whose efforts were supported by the Innovators award to JEH.

References

American Psychiatric Association (APA) (1994). Diagnostic and Statistical Manual of Mental Disorders, 4th ed. Washington (DC): American Psychiatric Association.

Balfour, D. J. K. and Benwell, M. E. M. (1993). The role of brain dopamine systems in the psychopharmacological responses to nicotine. *Asia Pac J Pharmacol*, **8**, 153–67.

Bardo, M. T., Bevins, R. A., Klebaur, J. E., Crooks, P. A., and Dwoskin, L. P. (1997). Nornicotine partially substitutes for (+)-amphetamine in a drug discrimination paradigm in rats. *Pharmacol Biochem Behav*, **58**, 1083–7.

Bardo, M. T., Green, T. A., Crooks, P. A., and Dwoskin, L. P. (1999). Nornicotine is self-administered intravenously by rats. *Psychopharmacol*, **146**, 290–6.

Bardo, M. T. and Bevins, R. A. (2000). Conditioned place preference: what does it add to our preclinical understanding of drug reward? *Psychopharmacol*, **153**, 31–43.

Benowitz, N. L. (1996). Pharmacology of nicotine: addiction and therapeutics. *Annu Rev Pharmacol Toxicol*, **36**, 597–613.

Benwell, M. E. and Balfour, D. J. K. (1992). The effects of acute and repeated nicotine treatment on nucleus accumbens dopamine and locomotor activity. *Br J Pharmacol*, **105**, 849–56.

Brioni, J. D., Kim, D. J., and O'Neill, A. B. (1996). Nicotine cue: lack of effect of the α7 nicotinic receptor antagonist methyllycaconitine. *Eur J Pharmacol*, **301**, 1–5.

Champtiaux, N., Han, Z. Y., Bessis, A., Rossi, F. M., Zoli, M., Marubio, L., *et al.* (2002). Distribution and pharmacology of α6-containing nicotinic acetylcholine receptors analyzed with mutant mice. *J Neurosci*, **22**, 1208–17.

Chandler, C. J. and Stolerman, I. P. (1997). Discriminative stimulus properties of the nicotinic agonist cytisine. *Psychopharmacol*, **129**, 257–64.

Clarke, P. B. S. (1990). Dopaminergic mechanisms in the locomotor stimulant effects of nicotine. *Biochem Pharmacol*, **40**, 1427–32.

Clarke, P. B. S. and Kumar, R. (1983). The effect of nicotine on locomotor activity in non-tolerant and tolerant rats. *Br J Pharmacol*, **78**, 329–37.

Corrigall, W. A. and Coen, K. M. (1989). Nicotine maintains robust self-administration in rats on a limited-access schedule. *Psychopharmacol*, **99**, 473–8.

Corrigall, W. A. and Coen, K. M. (1994). Dopamine mechanisms play at best a small role in the nicotine discriminative stimulus. *Pharmacol Biochem Behav*, **48**, 817–20.

Corrigall, W. A., Coen, K. M., and Adamson, K. L. (1994). Self-administered nicotine activates the mesolimbic dopamine system through the ventral tegmental area. *Brain Res*, **653**, 278–84.

DiChiara, G. (2000). Role of dopamine in the behavioral actions of nicotine related to addiction. *Eur J Pharmacol*, **393**, 295–314.

Donny, E. C., Caggiula, A. R., Mielke, M. M., Booth, S., Gharib, M. A., Hoffman, A., *et al.* (1999). Nicotine self-administration in rats on a progressive ratio schedule of reinforcement. *Psychopharmacol*, **147**, 135–42.

Donny, E. C., Caggiula, A. R., Rowell, P. P., Gharib, M. A., Maldovan, V., Booth, S., *et al.* (2000). Nicotine self-administration in rats: estrous cycle effects, sex differences and nicotinic receptor binding. *Psychopharmacol*, **151**, 392–405.

Duka, T., Seiss, E., and Tasker, R. (2002). The effects of extrinsic context on nicotine discrimination. *Behav Pharmacol*, **13**, 39–47.

Dwoskin, L. P., Crooks, P. A., Teng, L., Green, T. A., and Bardo, M. T. (1999). Acute and chronic effects of nornicotine on locomotor activity in rats: altered response to nicotine. *Psychopharmacol*, **145**, 442–51.

Dwoskin, L. P. and Crooks, P. A. (2001). Competitive neuronal nicotinic receptor antagonists: a new direction for drug discovery. *J Pharmacol Exp Ther*, **298**, 345–402.

Ericson, M., Olausson, P., Engel, J. A., and Soderpalm, B. (2000). Nicotine induces disinhibitory behavior in the rat after subchronic peripheral nicotine acetylcholine receptor blockade. *Eur J Pharmacol*, **397**, 103–11.

Ferrari, R., Le Novere, N., Picciotto, M. R., Changeux, J. P., and Zoli, M. (2002). Acute and long-term changes in the mesolimbic dopamine pathway after systemic or local single nicotine injections. *Eur J Neurosci*, **15**, 1810–18.

Fischman, M. W. and Foltin, R. W. (1991). Utility of subjective effects measurements in assessing abuse liability of drug in humans. *Br J Addict*, **86**, 1563–70.

Fudala, P. J., Teoh, K. W., and Iwamoto, E. T. (1985). Pharmacologic characterization of nicotine-induced conditioned place preference. *Pharmacol Biochem Behav*, **22**, 237–41.

Garrett, B. E. and Griffiths, R. R. (2001). Intravenous nicotine and caffeine: subjective and physiological effects in cocaine abusers. *J Pharmacol Exp Ther*, **296**, 486–94.

Goldberg, S. R. and Henningfield, J. E. (1998). Reinforcing effects of nicotine in humans and experimental animals responding under intermittent schedules of i.v. drug injection. *Pharmacol Biochem Behav*, **30**, 227–34.

Goldberg, S. R., Spealman, R. D., and Goldberg, D. M. (1981). Persistent behavior at high rates maintained by intravenous self-administration of nicotine. *Science*, **214**, 573–5.

Goldberg, S. R., Spealman, R. D., Risner, M. E., and Henningfield, J. E. (1983). Control of behavior by intravenous nicotine injections in laboratory animals. *Pharmacol Biochem Behav*, **19**, 1011–20.

Gommans, J., Stolerman, I. P., and Shoaib, M. (2000). Antagonism of the discriminative and aversive stimulus properties of nicotine in C57BL/6J mice. *Neuropharmacol*, **39**, 2840–7.

Grottick, A. J., Trube, J., Corrigall, W. A., Huwyler, J., Malherbe, P., Wyler, R., *et al.* (2000). Evidence that nicotinic α7 receptors are not involved in the hyperlocomotor and rewarding effects of nicotine. *J Pharmacol Exp Ther*, **294**, 1112–19.

Henningfield, J. E., Miyasato, K., and Jasinski, D. (1983). Cigarette smokers self-administer intravenous nicotine. *Pharmacol Biochem Behav*, **19**, 887–90.

Henningfield, J. E. (1984). Behavioral Pharmacology of Cigarette Smoking. In: Thompson T, Dews PB and Barrett JE editors. *Advances in Behavioral Pharmacology*, Vol. IV. New York: Academic Press, pp. 131–210.

Henningfield, J. E., Miyasato, K., Jasinski, D. R. (1985). Abuse liability and pharmacodynamic characteristics of intravenous and inhaled nicotine. *J Pharmacol Exp Ther*, **234**, 1–12.

Henningfield, J. E. and Keenan, R. (1993). Nicotine delivery kinetics and abuse liability. *Journal of Consulting Clin Psychol*, **61**, 743–50.

Henningfield, J. E., Stapleton, J. M., Benowitz, N. L., and London, E. D. (1993). Higher levels of nicotine in arterial than in venous blood after cigarette smoking. *Drug Alcohol Depend*, **33**, 23–9.

Henningfield, J. E. and Zeller, M. (2003). Could science-based regulation make tobacco products less addictive. *Yale Journal of Health Policy*, Law and Ethics, in press.

Horan, B., Smith, M., Gardner, E. L., Lepore, M., and Ashby, C.R. (1997). Nicotine produces conditioned place preference in Lewis, but not Fischer 344 rats. *Synapse*, **26**, 93–4.

Jasinski, D. R. and Henningfield, J. E. (1989). Human abuse liability assessment by measurement of subjective and physiological effects. In: Fischman MW, Mello NK, ed. Testing for abuse liability of drugs in humans. NIDA Research Monograph 92. Washington (DC): US Government Printing Office, pp. 73–100.

Jones, H. E., Garrett, B. E., and Griffiths, R. R. (1999). Subjective and physiological effects of intravenous nicotine and cocaine in cigarette smoking cocaine abusers. *J Pharmacol Exp Ther*, **288**, 18–197.

Jorenby, D. E., Steinpreis, R. E., Sherman, J. E., and Baker, T. B. (1990). Aversion instead of preference learning indicated by nicotine place conditioning in rats. *Psychopharmacol*, **101**, 533–8.

Katz, J. L. (1990). Models of relative reinforcing efficacy of drug and their predictive utility. *Behav Pharmacol*, **1**, 283–301.

Kempsill, F. E. J. and Pratt, J. A. (2000). Mecamylamine but not the α7 receptor antagonist α-bungarotoxin blocks sensitization to the locomotor stimulant effects of nicotine. *Br J Pharmacol*, **131**, 997–1003.

Kessler, D. (2000). A Question of Intent: A Great American Battle with a Deadly Industry. New York: Public Affairs.

Koob, G. F. (1992). Neural mechanisms of drug reinforcement. *Ann NY Acad Sci*, **564**, 171–91.

Klink, R., de Kerchove d'Exaerde, A., Zoli, M., and Changeux, J. P. (2001). Molecular and physiological diversity of nicotinic acetylcholine receptors in the midbrain dopaminergic nuclei. *J Neurosci*, **21**, 1452–63.

Ksir, C. (1994). Acute and chronic nicotine effects on measures of activity in rats: a multivariate analysis. *Psychopharmacol*, **15**, 105–9.

Lanca, A. J., Sanelli, T. R., and Corrigall, W. A. (2000). Nicotine-induced fos expression in the pedunculopontine mesencephalic tegmentum in the rat. *Neuropharmacol*, **39**, 2808–17.

Lindblom, N., De Villiers, S. H., Kalayanov, G., Gordon, S., Johansson, A. M., and Svensson, T. H. (2002). Active immunization against nicotine prevents reinstatement of nicotine seeking behavior in rats. *Respiration*, **69**, 254–60.

Lynch, W. J. and Carroll, M. E. (1999). Regulation of intravenously self-administered nicotine in rats. *Exp Clin Psychopharmacol*, **7**, 198–207.

Martin, T. J., Suchocki, J., May, E. L., and Martin, B. R. (1990). Pharmacological evaluation of the antagonism of nicotine's central effects by mecamylamine and pempidine. *J Pharmacol Exp Ther*, **254**, 45–51.

Meltzer, L. T. and Rosecrans, J. A. (1981). Investigations on the CNS sites of action of the discriminative stimulus effects of arecoline and nicotine. *Pharmacol, Biochem and Behav*, **15**, 21–6.

Miller, D. K., Wilkins, L. H., Bardo, M. T., Crooks, P. A., and Dwoskin, L. P. (2001). Once weekly administration of nicotine produces long-lasting locomotor sensitization in rats via a nicotinic receptor-mediated mechanism. *Psychopharmacol*, **156**, 469–76.

Miyata, H., Ando, K., and Yanagita, T. (2002). Brain regions mediating the discriminative stimulus effects of nicotine in rats. *Ann NY Acad Sci*, **965**, 354–63.

Morrison, C. F. and Lee, P. N. (1967). A comparison of the effects of nicotine and physostigmine on a measure of activity in the rat. *Psychopharmacologia*, **13**, 210–21

O'Brien, C. P. (1996). Drug addiction and drug abuse. In: JG Hardman, AG Gilman, and LE Limbird, ed. Goodman and Gilmans's *The Pharmacologic Basis of Therapeutics*, New York: McGraw Hill, pp. 557–77.

Panagis, G., Kastellakis, A., Spyraki, C., and Nomikos, G. (2000). Effects of methyllycaconitine (MLA), an α7 nicotinic receptor antagonist, on nicotine- and cocaine-induced potentiation of brain stimulation reward. *Psychopharmacol*, **149**, 388–96.

Parker, L. A. (1992). Place conditioning in a three- or four-choice apparatus: role of stimulus novelty in drug-induced place conditioning. *Behav Neurosci*, **106**, 294–306.

Perkins, K. A., Grobe, J. E., Epstein, L. H., Caggiula, A. C., Stiller, R. L., and Jacob, R. G. (1993). Chronic and acute tolerance to subjective effects of nicotine. *Pharmacol Biochem Behav*, **45**, 375–81.

Perkins, K. A., DiMarco, A., Grobe, J. E., and Fonte, C. (1994). Nicotine discrimination in male and female smokers. *Psychopharmacol*, **116**, 407–13.

Perkins, K. A., Sanders, M., D'Amico, D., and Wilson, A. (1997). Nicotine discrimination and self-administration in humans as a function of smoking status. *Psychopharmacol*, **131**, 361–70.

Perkins, K. A. and Stitzer, M. (1998). Behavioral pharmacology of nicotine. In: Tarter R, Ammerman PT, Ott P, ed. Handbook of substance abuse: *Neurobehavioral Pharmacology*. New York: Plenum Press, pp. 299–317.

Perkins KA. (1999*a*). Nicotine self-administration. *Nicotine Tob Res*, **1**, S133–S137.

Perkins, K. A., Sanders, M., Fonte, C., Wilson, A. S., White, W., Stiller, R., *et al.* (1999*b*). Effects of central and peripheral nicotine blockade on human nicotine discrimination. *Psychopharmacol*, **142**, 158–64.

Picciotto, M. R. and Corrigall, W. A. (2002). Neuronal systems underlying behaviors related to nicotine addiction: Neural circuits and molecular genetics. *J Neurosci*, **22**, 3338–41.

Picciotto, M. R., Zoli, M., Rimondini, R., Lena, C., Marubio, L. M., Pich, E. M., *et al.* (1998). Acetylcholine receptors containing the beta2 subunit are involved in the reinforcing properties of nicotine. *Nature*, **391**, 173–7.

Pierce, R. C. and Kalivas, P. W. (1997). A circuitry model for the expression of behavioral sensitization to amphetamine-like psychostimulants. *Brain Res Rev*, **25**, 192–216.

Preston, K. L. and Bigelow, G. E. (1992). Subjective and discriminative effects of drugs. *Behav Pharmacol*, **2**, 293–313.

Rasmussen, T. and Swedberg, M. D. B. (1998). Reinforcing effects of nicotinic compounds: intravenous self-administration in drug-naive mice. *Pharmacol Biochem Beh*, **60**, 567–73.

Risner, M. E. and Goldberg, S. R. (1983). A comparison of nicotine and cocaine self-administration in the dog: fixed-ratio and progressive-ratio schedules of intravenous drug infusion. *J Pharmacol Exp Ther*, **224**, 319–26.

Robinson, T. E. and Berridge, K. C. (1993). The neural basis of drug craving: an incentive-sensitization theory of addiction. *Brain Res Rev*, **18**, 247–91.

Rose, J. E. and Corrigall, W. A. (1997). Nicotine self-administration in animals and humans: similarities and differences. *Psychopharmacol*, **130**, 28–40.

Rosecrans, J. A., Chance, W. T., and Schechter, M. D. (1976). The discriminative stimulus properties of nicotine, d-amphetamine and morphine in dopamine depleted rats. *Psychopharmacol Communications*, **2**, 349–56.

Royal College of Physicians of London (2000). Nicotine addiction in Britain: a report of the Tobacco Advisory Group of the Royal College of Physicians. London: Royal College of Physicians.

Schechter, M. D. and Rosecrans, J. A. (1972). Nicotine as a discriminative stimulus in rats depleted of norepinephrine or 5-hydroxytryptamine. *Psychopharmacologia*, **24**, 417–29.

Shoaib, M. and Stolerman, I. P. (1996). Brain sites mediating the discriminative stimulus effects of nicotine in rats. *Behav Brain Res*, **78**, 183–8.

Shaham, Y., Adamson, L. K., Grocki, S., and Corrigall, W. A. (1997). Reinstatement and spontaneous recovery of nicotine seeking in rats. *Psychopharmacol*, **130**, 396–403.

Shoaib, M., Schindler, C. W., and Goldberg, S. R. (1997). Nicotine self-administration in rats: strain and nicotine pre-exposure effects on acquisition. *Psychopharmacol*, **129**, 35–43.

Shoaib, M., Zubaran, C., and Stolerman, I. P. (2000). Antagonism of stimulus properties of nicotine by dihydro-beta-erythroidine (DHbetaE) in rats. *Psychopharmacol*, **149**, 140–6.

Shoaib, M., Gommans, J., Morley, A., Stolerman, I. P., Grailhe, R., and Changeux, J. P. (2002). The role of the nicotinic receptor beta-2 subunits in nicotine discrimination and conditioned taste aversion. *Neuropharmacol*, **42**, 530–9.

Stolerman, I. P., Fink, R., and Jarvic, M. E. (1973). Acute and chronic tolerance to nicotine measured by activity in rats. *Psychopharmacol*, **30**, 329–42.

Stolerman, I. P., Garcha, H. S., Pratt, J. A., and Kumar, R. (1984). Role of training dose in discrimination of nicotine and related compounds by rats. *Psychopharmacol*, **84**, 413–9.

Stolerman, I. P. and Jarvis, M. J. (1995). The scientific case that nicotine is addictive. *Psychopharmacol*, **117**, 2–10.

Stolerman, I. P., Chandler, C. J., Garcha, H. S., and Newton, J. S. (1997). Selective antagonism of the behavioral effects of nicotine by dihydro-β-erythroidine in rats. *Psychopharmacol*, **129**, 390–7.

Thompson, T. and Schuster, C. R. (1968). Behavioral Pharmacology, Englewood Cliffs (NJ) Prentice-Hall.

US Department of Health and Human Services (1998). The health consequences of smoking: nicotine addiction. A report of the Surgeon General. Washington (DC): US Government Printing Office.

US Food and Drug Administration (1996). 21 CFR Part 801, *et al.* Regulations restricting the sale and distribution of cigarettes and smokeless tobacco to protect children and adolescents; final rule, Federal Register, 61(168) Washington (DC): Government Printing Office, pp. 44396–5318.

Wise, R. A. and Bozarth, M. A. (1987). A psychomotor stimulant theory of addiction. *Psychological Rev*, **94**, 469–92.

World Health Organization (1992). The ICD-10 classification of mental and behavioural disorders: clinical description and diagnostic guidelines. Geneva, Switzerland: World Health Organization.

World Health Organization, Scientific Advisory Committee on Tobacco Product Regulation (2003). Recommendation on Tobacco Product Ingredients and Emissions.

Chapter 8

Cigarette science: Addiction by design

Jeff Fowles and Dennis Shusterman

Introduction

The addictive property of cigarettes is widely attributed to the presence of the naturally occurring nicotine alkaloid in tobacco (U.S. Surgeon General 1988; U.S. National Institute on Drug Abuse 2000). Signs of addiction to nicotine can be seen in a matter of days following initiation of smoking (Charlton *et al.* 2000), and addiction is firmly established by one year of smoking (RCP 2000). However, although the physiological and biochemical impacts of nicotine on the central and peripheral nervous systems have been extensively studied and reviewed (U.S. Surgeon General 1988), the process of addiction to tobacco is still not entirely understood.

Complicating our understanding of how cigarettes are addictive are the long lists of additives and ingredients used by tobacco companies (UK Department of Health 1998; NZ Ministry of Health 2000). Some of these compounds or extracts are clearly added to impart a 'flavour' to the smoke, or to alter the 'character' of the smoke. These substances are added to increase a cigarette's marketability, either through manufacturing considerations or direct appeal to consumers. It is likely that the appeal of cigarettes to smokers would include added substances that influence taste and odour, compounds that reduce feelings of membrane irritation, and compounds that directly or indirectly enhance tobacco's addictiveness. Research on the influence of these additives on initiation or quitting smoking is not available because the information on brand-specific additives has been kept from disclosure under the argument of proprietary secret.

Cigarette pharmacology

Nicotine addiction

The U.S. Surgeon General report (1988) defines addiction as: "the compulsory use of a drug that has psychoactivity and that may be associated with tolerance and physical dependence (i.e. may be associated with withdrawal symptoms after the cessation of drug use)". Most smokers are probably addicted to nicotine according to this criterion. Fewer than 7 per cent of those smokers in the U.S. who try to quit smoking unaided by various therapies are successful for one year or longer (National Institute on Drug Addiction 2000).

Nicotinic pyridine alkaloids in cigarettes

Tobacco contains at least 20 different, pyridine alkaloids, 16 of which are shown in Fig. 8.1. Of these, the dominant alkaloid is nicotine, making up nearly 88% of the total alkaloid content of some tobaccos, and it has been reported that the average nicotine content of tobacco is 1.5% by weight (Benowitz *et al.* 1983). Cigarettes can essentially be described as nicotine delivery devices. For example, it can be seen from chromatograms of cigarette smoke tar, that nicotine is among the few compounds that is delivered in milligram quantities. Most of the remaining compounds in cigarette smoke are delivered in microgram or nanogram quantities.

The relative pharmacological potency of nicotine is 1.2–2.5 times that of nornicotine and anabasine, depending on the test system and animal model used (U.S. Surgeon General 1988). The alkaloid profile appears to vary substantially with

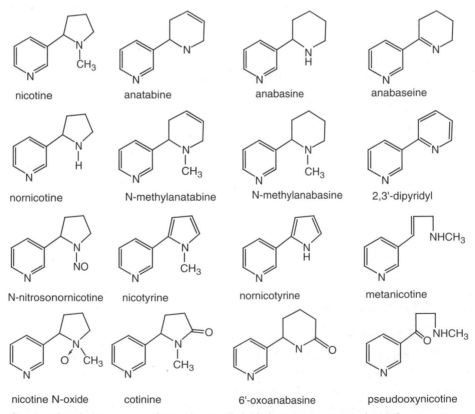

Fig. 8.1 Chemical structures of 16 tobacco alkaloids (US Surgeon General 1988).

different tobacco strains, but these additional alkaloids are not routinely quantified and their contribution to the pharmacological effect of smoking is not precisely known.

Tobacco cultivars vary widely in their yield of nicotine and other chemicals by strain and growing condition. Cigarettes are therefore made from blended tobaccos to arrive at a target yield of nicotine delivery. (U.S. Surgeon General 1988).

Pharmacological effects of nicotine

Nicotine has potent pharmacological and toxicological effects that result in dependence (US Surgeon General 1988; RCP 2000). While nicotine may be the dominant pharmacological agent in cigarette smoke, it is of interest to note that the effects of nicotine do not account for all the pharmacological or behavioural influences seen with smoking (Cherek *et al.* 1989; Pickworth *et al.* 1999). It has been demonstrated that nicotine replacement therapies do not completely mimic the neuropharmacological changes seen with smoking, even when the blood nicotine levels are essentially identical (Cherek *et al.* 1989). This may, in part, be due to the rapid absorption of nicotine through the inhalation route, which elicits discernible central effects in just seven seconds (Kobayashi *et al.* 1999).

Epidemiology studies have revealed the unexpected finding that smoking prevalence is inversely related to the incidence of Parkinson's disease in which brain nicotine receptor numbers are significantly lowered at autopsy compared with people without Parkinson's disease (Kelton *et al.* 2000; Mihailescu and Drucker-Colin 2000). There is also indication that nicotine may help alleviate symptoms of Alzheimers disease (Kelton *et al.* 2000). Given the extensive neuropharmacological activity of nicotine in the brain, it is possible that certain individuals smoke in order to treat their own neurological disorders. It has become known, for example, that smoking prevalence is very high among people who have been diagnosed as having attention deficit/hyperactivity disorder (ADHD) (Lambert and Hartsough 1998; Riggs *et al.* 1999).

Nicotine stimulates epinephrine release and increases general metabolism, and is known to reduce body weight. Smokers are, on average, seven pounds lighter than non-smokers, and people who quit smoking often gain weight (Benowitz *et al.* 1994). This may add to a psychological dependence on smoking in the case of people trying to lose weight.

The nicotine receptor

Neuronal nicotinic acetylcholine receptors (nAChRs) represent a large family of ligand-gated cation channels with diverse structures and properties. The physiological functions of neuronal nAChRs are not well defined to date. Behavioral studies indicate that brain nAChRs participate in complex functions such as attention, memory, and cognition, whereas clinical data suggest their involvement in the pathogenesis of certain neuropsychiatric disorders, including Alzheimer's and Parkinson's diseases,

Tourette's syndrome, schizophrenia, and depression (Belluardo *et al.* 2000). For some of these disorders, the use of nAChRs' agonists may represent either a preventative or a symptomatic treatment (Mihailescu and Drucker-Colin 2000).

Nicotine binding to receptors in the brain, augments the release of numerous neurotransmitters, including dopamine, serotonin, norepinephrine, acetylcholine, gamma-aminobutyric acid, and glutamate (Quattrocki *et al.* 2000). The binding of nicotine to the receptor increases the production of acetylcholine receptors in neurons and affects neural tissue through this stimulus in the presence of acetylcholine.

The result of chronic receptor-mediated stimulation of these tissues is an alteration of nearly all components of the neuroendocrine system including the corticosteroids, adrenal hormones, serotonin, and pituitary hormones (US Surgeon General 1988).

It is important to note that the nicotine receptor is able to bind a wide range of compounds as agonists (e.g. acetylcholine, epibatidine, imperialine, pyridine) and receptor antagonists (e.g. succinylcholine). This raises the possibility that some of the compounds in the complex mixture of cigarette smoke have nicotinic (or anti-nicotinic) activity that is not factored into the standard nicotine yield measurements.

While chronic agonist stimulation of most neuroreceptors results in a down-regulation of receptor numbers in tissues, the nicotine receptor is apparently up-regulated in the hippocampus and thalamus regions of the brain under such conditions (Kobayashi *et al.* 1999). The up-regulation of these receptors precedes the development of tolerance to nicotine (Kobayashi *et al.* 1999). The degree of nicotine receptor binding correlates with the number of cigarettes smoked per day (Benhammou *et al.* 2000). The role of non-nicotine factors in this up-regulation is not clear, and there have been suggestions that other compounds in tobacco smoke (e.g. anabasine) influence this regulation (Yates *et al.* 1995). It has been shown that ethanol treatment *in vitro* results in a reduced level of receptor up-regulation (Gorbounova *et al.* 1998).

Nicotine receptors on human neurological cells *in vitro* can serve as biomarkers for nicotinic activity in cigarette total particulate matter. Such *in vitro* assay systems have the potential to help determine the biological nicotinic activity of cigarette smoke. If 'denicotinized' cigarettes were to become marketed, biological measures such as this would be needed to ensure that the removal of nicotine is accompanied by a removal of nicotinic activity in the smoke.

Factors that influence the absorption or delivery of nicotine

The standard measured nicotine yield of a cigarette is determined by:

- The nicotine content of the tobacco
- The static burn rate or amount of tobacco consumed during puffing
- The pressure drop of the tobacco column
- Porosity of the wrapper and or ventilation at the filter

- ◆ The pressure drop of the filter
- ◆ The filter material including its surface area, and
- ◆ The affinity of the filter material for nicotine particularly as a function of smoke pH.

Nicotine content and yield

Through the combination of the above variables, plant genetics, and commercial processes to remove nicotine from tobacco, it is possible to manipulate the machine-measured yield of nicotine from about 0.1 mg to 4 mg per cigarette (Benowitz 1989; Baldinger *et al.* 1995). However, in practice, the so called 'ultra-low' nicotine cigarettes do not deliver the low levels of nicotine to smokers that are implied by the yield rating (Benowitz *et al.* 1983). Similarly, smoking fewer cigarettes per day does not necessarily translate into a lower tar or nicotine exposure for a smoker. This is because smokers compensate for the reduced nicotine in a conventional puff, and smoke much more intensively to achieve the desired nicotine blood level (Benowitz 1986). Some cigarettes appear to be designed to provide low yields by conventional machine testing, while still delivering roughly equivalent nicotine and tar levels. This can be seen especially in the case of light and mild brands when tested under 'intense' or 'realistic' smoking conditions (Smoke Constituents 2000; MACTC 2001).

According to Benowitz and Henningfield (1994) the proportion of nicotine in cigarettes that is physically available for absorption is up to about 40%. If cigarettes were to be re-designed physically and/or chemically it is possible that this limit could change and the degree of bioavailability would need to be reassessed.

Altering the cigarette burn rate

Cigarette manufacturers apparently design certain features into cigarette tobacco during blending that can affect nicotine delivery (Robertson 2000). For example, cigarette filling power (bulk), pressure drop or resistance to draw, and static burn rate are all decreased with ascending stalk position on the tobacco plant. A decrease in the burn rate increases the puff count, and thereby results in the delivery of more nicotine to the smoker because less tobacco is burned between puffs (US Federal Register 1995).

Chemicals that affect pH changes in cigarette smoke

A number of chemicals are added to cigarettes with the effect of increasing or buffering the pH of the inhaled smoke (NZ Ministry of Health 2000; Robertson 2000). Ammonia compounds, for example, are added in significant quantities to cigarettes; some industry reports showing up to 1.5% by weight (NZ Ministry of Health 2000; UK Department of Health 1998). Ammonia, with a pKa of 9.25, increases pH of the tobacco smoke. Nicotine is a weak base with a pKa of 8.0 (U.S. Surgeon General 1988). As the pH of cigarette smoke increases, the relative amount of unionized nicotine (and other alkaloids) will increase. This is important because 'free base' compounds, including unionized nicotine, are more volatile than their ionized counterparts. As chemicals become more volatile and separate from the particulate (tar droplet) phase to the vapour phase, they diffuse more rapidly and are better distributed throughout the lung more quickly, gaining access to lung membranes (Pankow 1999). In addition, the free base nicotine content in the tobacco rod has a lower boiling point, which means that more nicotine can be transferred from the tobacco to the aerosol. In addition, unionized compounds traverse biological membranes with greater ease than the equivalent chemicals when ionized (Rozman Klaassen 1994).

Other compounds in cigarette smoke that may influence addiction

It has been observed in experiments that de-nicotinized cigarettes, while not exerting the same pharmacological effects as conventional cigarettes, do retain the ability to lessen some of the cravings of smokers in abstinence (Pickworth *et al.* 1999). Rose *et al.* (2001) found that platelet monoamine oxidase was inhibited by non-nicotine factors in de-nicotinized cigarettes. Therefore, while nicotine appears to dominate the pharmacological effects of smoking, the pharmacology of and possibly the addiction to cigarette smoking may extend beyond nicotine alone.

Acetaldehyde

A number of reports show that acetaldehyde exerts biological effects that may contribute to addiction (Wrona *et al.* 1997). Acetaldehyde is a metabolite of ethanol. It has been shown that nicotine is more reinforcing in patients with a prior history of alcoholism (Hughes *et al.* 2000). Acetaldehyde is suspected to act as a synergist with nicotine, though the precise mechanism has not been identified (Gray 2000).

It has been observed that ethanol and acetaldehyde exposures in animals lead to a build up of cellular amines that are closely related to opioid compounds such as morphine (Smith 1975). Cellular amino acid derivatives react with acetaldehyde *in vitro* to form alkaloids such as isoquinoline and carboline. These compounds have pharmacological activity in the nervous system that may help explain the withdrawal symptoms from alcohol. In the brain, acetaldehyde has been found to react with endogenous 5-hydroxytryptamine (5-HT) to form 1-methyl-6-hydroxy-1,2,3,4-tetrahydro-beta-carboline, and oxygen radical derivatives of this alkaloid (Wrona *et al.* 1997). Research is ongoing on the mechanisms of acetaldehyde neurotoxicity and the effects the ensuing biochemical changes in the brain may have in terms of addiction, as this chemical is derived from both smoking and alcohol consumption (Han and Dryhurst 1996).

Acetaldehyde is formed from combustion of organic material, and is formed in particularly high concentrations upon combustion of sugars. It is present in high concentrations in cigarette smoke, with a mean yield of about 700 micrograms per cigarette (NZ Ministry of Health 2000).

Nitrosamines

Nitrosamines are biologically reactive compounds formed by a reaction between amine groups and nitrate. Nitrates are found in tobacco naturally, particularly as a result of plant uptake from fertilisers (Fischer *et al.* 1990). The rate of the nitrosamine reaction is enhanced under heat and combustion. Many of the important nitrosamines in cigarette smoke are nitrosated derivatives of the nicotine alkaloids (*N*-Nitrosonornicotine or NNN, and 4-*N*-nitrosomethylamino)-1-(3-pyridyl)-1-butanone or NNK are the nitrosamine derivatives of nornicotine and nicotine, respectively). A high-affinity binding of NNK to nicotinic acetylcholine receptors in neuroendocrine tissues has been described (Plummer *et al.* 2000), but the relative contribution of this binding to overall nicotinic activity has not been reported.

Cigarette smoke particles

There is occupational evidence that particles between 0.5 and 5.0 microns in size are more 'breathable' and persist in the bronchial apparatus up to 120 days (Orto *et al.* 1996). Cigarette smoke particles range from 0.1 to 1.0 micron, or near the low end of the range for optimal persistence (Li and Hopke 1993). For the R.J. Reynolds Premier® product, the particle size of its prototypes were in the range of approximately 1–2 microns (R.J. Reynolds 1988). It has been reported that 47% of cigarette smoke particles fall in the range of 0.2–0.4 microns (Polydorova 1961). A geometric mean diameter for particle size of mainstream cigarette smoke was determined to be 0.18 microns (Okada *et al.* 1977), while the standard deviation of the particle size distribution was 0.4 microns. Therefore a considerable fraction of the smoke particles would be expected to occur in the optimal persistence range. Overall, the smoke particle retention in the lungs is about 80% (range 63–89% for average and moderate smokers). Therefore, these particles, by virtue of their size and content, make a very effective drug delivery system.

Increasing palatability of cigarette smoke

In many countries, tobacco products are sweetened and flavoured, although most industry returns do not contain information on any given product, making it impossible to use the returns to assess the contribution of these constituents on initiating and maintaining smoking. This does not hold true, however, for Canada, where "additives" are not permitted in cigarettes (Dr Murray Kaiserman 2002).

In some additive lists in industry reports, up to 12.7% of a cigarette by weight may be added sugars and sweeteners (NZ Ministry of Health 2000). Undoubtedly the high sugar content affects the palatability and flavour of cigarettes to smokers. Since children are well known to seek out sweet tasting foods (Watt *et al.* 2000) it is not unreasonable to assume that any added sweetness in tobacco smoke would be received favourably by a child. De Graaf and Zandstra (1999) found that the optimal sucrose concentrations in taste tests increase in adolescents and even more so in children compared with adults.

Licorice is also reportedly added in quantities of up to 1.3% by weight according to industry reports (NZ Ministry of Health 2000). This is potentially significant since licorice has a long history of use in the food industry as a sweetening enhancer. The constituent of licorice, glycyrrhizin, is 50 times sweeter than sugar (http://www.go-symmetry.com/licorice.htm).

Although a considerable percentage of cigarette weight could be cocoa and chocolate extracts (up to 3.2%), it is not known and could not be found to what degree this influences flavour of the mainstream or sidestream smoke, or more specifically how this might influence smoking initiation among youth. Similarly, the influence of coffee extract on inhaled smoke flavour is unknown.

The flavouring additives vanillin and ethyl-vanillin are added in substantial quantities to tobacco (NZ Ministry of Health 2000). Vanilla, when compared with a range of spices was judged to be the most similar to sugar (Blank and Mattes 1990).

Sensory irritation and the deadening of peripheral nerves

Cigarette smoke, like any other combustion product, is inherently irritating to the mucous membranes of the nasal and airway passages, as well as to the eyes. This irritation is a natural warning sign by the body of an ongoing harmful exposure. Principal identified irritants in cigarette smoke include aldehydes (formaldehyde, acetaldehyde, acrolein) and organic acids (formic, acetic, propionic), although more complex compounds found in cigarette smoke (e.g. nicotine) also have irritant properties (Ayer and Yeager 1982). To counter this effect, cigarette manufacturers add a number of agents to temporarily lessen this sensation of irritation, essentially removing a natural barrier for avoidance of cigarette smoke. This would affect the attractiveness of cigarettes.

The pathophysiology of mucous membrane irritation from smoking

True allergy to tobacco smoke constituents is rare (Stankus *et al.* 1988). Irritation, on the other hand, is a dose-dependent phenomenon. 'Sensory' [eye, nose, and throat] irritation involves stimulation of both specific and non-specific receptors on airway (and ocular) nociceptive nerves. These nerves belong to the C- and Aδ-classes, and, depending upon the specific location within the upper respiratory tract, originate in the trigeminal (5th cranial), glossopharyngeal (9th cranial), or vagus (10th cranial) nerves (Widdicombe 1986). One specific receptor involved in cigarette smoke-mediated irritation is the so-called 'neuronal nicotine receptor' (see below). Two other receptors—the capsaicin (or VR1) receptor, and the acid-sensitive ion channel (ASIC) respond to acidic and/or thermal stimuli (Caterina *et al.* 1997; Waldmann *et al.* 1997). A secondary mechanism of neuronal activation for reactive aldehydes and organic acids may be sensory nerve stimulation by endogenous mediators (e.g. purines, prostaglandins) released secondary to actual tissue damage (Barnes 2001).

Airway irritation may trigger a variety of reflexes, including alterations in respiratory behavior (coughing, sneezing, breath-holding), hypersecretion, and changes in airway caliber (mediated principally by vascular dilatation in the upper airway, and by smooth muscle contraction in the lower airway) (Widdicombe 1986). The threshold for CO_2- (irritant-) induced 'transient reflex apnea' (reflexive arrest of inspiration in the presence of an irritant) is higher in smokers than in nonsmokers, suggesting that long-term exposure to irritants in cigarette smoke either produces neuronal adaptation or alters the barrier qualities of nasal mucous in smokers (Cometto-Muniz and Cain 1982).

Compounds in smoke that mask mucous membrane irritation

Eugenol is an organic compound found in clove oil, and is known to have local anaesthetic properties and was used for this purpose in surgeries (Wicker 1994). Although the reported level of clove 'extract' is only 0.0001% in some industry documents, the amount of eugenol and its contribution to the numbing effect of the peripheral nerves in the upper airways is unknown.

Menthol has local anaesthetic properties on nerves linked with taste and irritation of the mouth and throat (Green and McAuliffe 2000). Some tobacco industry documents list menthol as up to 0.71% by weight of the cigarette (NZ Ministry of Health 2000). The reported limit in cigarettes is approximately equal to the amount of menthol that can be found in a typical cough drop, and probably serves to add flavour while simultaneously deadening local nerve endings to reduce the feeling of irritation from inhalation of the various combustion products.

Humectants assist with aerosol formation, dissolving more nicotine into tar droplets, and making the smoke less irritating to the smoker's throat and easier to inhale. Glycerol and methylglycerol are added to cigarettes as humectants, to decrease the sensory irritation of the inhaled smoke. Although not toxic by itself, when burnt, glycerol forms acrolein. Acrolein is a small reactive aldehyde that causes localized inflammation and membrane irritation when inhaled, or to the eyes (HSDB 2000). Acrolein was found to be the leading contributor from tobacco smoke to respiratory and eye irritation in a previous risk assessment (ESR 2000).

Masking the irritation and odour from sidestream smoke

It has been reported that the tobacco industry has for many years and is currently researching ways to mask the unpleasantness of sidestream smoke for smokers and non-smokers (Connolly et al. 2000). Efforts to produce socially acceptable cigarettes include 'Premier' by RJ Reynolds, 'Vantage Excel', and 'Chelsea' (reintroduced in 1990 as 'Horizon'). Though these brands did not succeed in the marketplace, research is apparently ongoing in this area and is likely to continue as regulations affecting sidestream smoke become more strict internationally.

Additives to the cigarette paper, including potassium citrate and aluminium and other metal hydroxides, have been patented by the tobacco industry as paper wrapper additives aimed to reduce particulate visibility by making droplet sizes smaller, though not affecting total emissions (Connolly *et al.* 2000).

A number of additives apparently have the purpose of reducing sidestream smoke unpleasant odour. These include acetylpyrazine, anethole, and limonene — compounds with low odour thresholds and few components that would affect the trigeminal nerve endings in the upper airways. Polyanethol, and cinnamic aldehyde pinanediol acetal produced a fresher 'less cigarette-like' aroma than controls (Connolly *et al.* 2000). A summary table of additives that have been reported to reduce sidestream smoke irritation or alter sidestream smoke odour to lessen complaints is found in Connolly *et al.* (2000).

The effect of nicotine on upper airway mucosa

In addition to its neuropsychological properties as a stimulant, nicotine is also a mucous membrane irritant, producing, at high concentrations, a sensation of 'burning' or 'stinging'. In point of fact, nicotine is the single cigarette smoke constituent for which a specific receptor has been identified in the nasal mucosa (Blank *et al.* 1997). Evidence of the operation of a specific nicotine receptor in the upper airway comes from both psychophysical and electrophysiologic studies. Investigators have shown distinct psychophysical stimulus potencies *and* sensory qualities for R- and S-nicotine, implying the operation of a specific receptor (Thuerauf *et al.* 1999). Electrophysiologically, researchers have shown selective blocking of nicotine- but not cyclohexanone-induced trigeminal activity in rats after administration of a nicotinic blocker (Alimohammadi and Silver 2000). Notwithstanding its potential as an aversive stimulus, it is unclear to what degree low-level irritation of the upper respiratory tract due to nicotine may actually constitute a reinforcing aspect of cigarette smoking (Thuerauf *et al.* 2000).

Conclusions

Cigarettes are highly engineered to optimize the delivery of nicotine to the smoker. A host of chemical additives and ingredients may serve to further this goal, directly or indirectly. The effects of these compounds include: improving flavour and/or increasing sweetness of the smoke, reduction of feelings of sensory irritation (though not decreasing irritation itself), altering pH of the smoke, and potentially causing pharmacological effects in addition to those caused by nicotine.

Many of the flavours used are fruit extracts and sweeteners, which conceivably increase the attractiveness of tobacco products to children. Similarly, compounds that mask membrane irritation would effectively lessen any avoidance of cigarettes for first time smokers, while compounds that reduce odour and irritation from secondhand smoke are an attempt to lessen the rejection of smoking behaviour by non-smokers.

Physical design features of cigarettes that work to optimize nicotine delivery include paper permeability and ventilation hole placement, which can lead to underestimates of actual delivery using ISO smoking machine tests. The particle size distributions of cigarette smoke ensure that these particles will penetrate deep into the lung and be retained.

The possibility that some of the compounds, among the thousands in cigarette smoke, have 'nicotinic' activity has not been adequately addressed. Some of the combustion products of these chemicals, such as acetaldehyde, may have pharmacological effects that are relevant to addiction. There has been no systematic evaluation of the public health impacts of additives or their combustion products. The development of bioassays to characterize the activity of cigarette smoke has some potential to help address some of these questions.

In most countries, the structure of the tobacco industry reports does not permit an examination of the chemical content of any particular brand or its smoke. Therefore, it is not currently possible to conduct a risk assessment on the products that are being sold, or to follow changes in these products which may be leading to increases in smoking or nicotine addiction. Regulatory agencies should be able to require disclosure of additives and ingredients, as well as constituents of cigarette smoke in order to enable such efforts.

References

Alimohammadi, H., Silver, W. L. (2000). Evidence for nicotinic acetylcholine receptors on nasal trigeminal nerve endings of the rat. *Chemistry of the Senses*, **25**, 61–6.

Ayer, H. E. and Yeager, D. W. (1982). Irritants in cigarette smoke plumes. *American Journal of Public Health*, **72**, 1283–5.

Baldinger, B., Hasenfratz, M., and Battig, K. (1995). Switching to ultralow nicotine cigarettes: Effects of different tar yields and blocking of olfactory cues. *Pharmacology, Biochemistry and Behaviour*, **50**(2), 233–9.

Barnes, P. J. (2001). Neurogenic inflammation in the airways. *Respiratory Physiology*, **125**, 145–154.

Belluardo, N., Mudo, G., Blum, M., and Fuxe, K. (2000). Central nicotinic receptors, neurotrophic factors and neuroprotection. *Behaviour and Brain Research*, **113**(1–2), 21–34

Benhammou, K., Lee, M., Strook, M., Sullivan, B., Logel, J., Raschen, K., Gotti, C., and Leonard, S. (2000). [3H]Nicotine binding in peripheral blood cells of smokers is correlated with the number of cigarettes smoked per day. *Neuropharmacology*, **39**, 2818–29.

Benowitz, N. (1986). Dosimetric studies of compensatory cigarette smoking. In: Wald, N. and P. Froggatt (ed.) *Nicotine, Smoking and the Low Tar Programme*. New York: Oxford University Press. pp. 133–50.

Benowitz, N. (1989). Health and public policy implications of the 'low yield' cigarette. *New England Journal of Medicine*, **320**(24), 1619–21.

Benowitz, N., Hall, S. M., Herning, R. I., Jacob, P., Jones, R. T., and Osman, A. L. (1983). Smokers of low yield cigarettes do not consume less nicotine. *New England Journal of Medicine*, **309**(3), 139–42.

Benowitz, N., and Henningfield, J. (1994). Establishing a nicotine threshold for addiction. *New England Journal of Medicine*, **331**(2), 123.

Blank, D. M. and Mattes, R. D. (1990). Sugar and spice: similarities and sensory attributes. *Nursing Research*, **39**(5), 290–3.

Blank, U., Ruches, C., Clauss, W., and Weber, W-M. (1997). Effects of nicotine on human nasal epithelium: Evidence for nicotinic receptors in non-excitable cells. *European Journal of Physiology*, **434**, 581–6.

Caterina, M. J., Schumacher, M. A., Tominaga, M., Rosen, T. A., Levine, J. D., and Julius, D. (1997). The capsaicia receptor: a heat-activated ion channel in the pain pathway. *Nature*, **389**(6653), 816–824.

Charlton, A., Moyer, C., Gupta, P., and Hill, D. (2000). Youth and cigarette smoking. International Union Against Cancer website. (http://factsheets.globalink.org/en/youth.shtml). Website accessed January 2001.

Cherek, D. R., Bennett, R. H., Kelly, T. H., Steinberg, J. L., and Benowitz, N. L. (1989). Effects of nicotine gum and tobacco smoking on human avoidance responding. *Pharmacology and Biochemistry of Behaviour*, **32**(3), 677–81.

Cometto-Muniz, J. E. and Cain, W. S. (1982). Perception of nasal pungency in smokers and nonsmokers. *Physiology of Behaviour*, **29**(4), 727–31.

Connolly, G. N., Wayne, G. D., Lymperis, D., and Doherty, M. C. (2000). How cigarette additives are used to mask environmental tobacco smoke. *Tobacco Control*, **9**, 283–91.

De Graaf, C. and Zandstra, E. H. (1999). Sweetness intensity and pleasantness in children, adolescents, and adults. *Physiology of Behaviour*, **67**(4), 513–20.

NZ Ministry of Health (2000). The chemical constituents of cigarettes and cigarette smoke: Priorities for harm reduction. A report by the Institute of Environmental Science and Research (ESR) for the New Zealand Ministry of Health (New Zealand National Drug Policy website: www.ndp.govt.nz).

Fischer, S., Spiegelhalder, B., Eisenbarth, J., and Preussman, R. (1990). Investigations on the origin of tobacco-specific nitrosamines in mainstream smoke of cigarettes. *Carcinogenesis*, **11**(5) 723–30.

Gorbounova, O., Svensson, A., Jonsson, P., Mousavi, M., Miao, H., Hellstrom-Lindahl, E., and Nordberg, A. (1998). Chronic ethanol treatment decreases [3H] epibatidine and 3[H] nicotine binding and differentially regulates mRNA levels of nicotinic acetylcholine receptor subunits expressed in M10 and SH-SY5Y neuroblastoma cells. *Journal of Neurochemistry*, **70**, 1134–42.

Gray, N. (2000). Reflections on the saga of tar content: Why did we measure the wrong thing? *Tobacco Control*, **9**, 90–4.

Green, B. G. and McAuliffe, B. L. (2000). Menthol desensitization of capsaicin irritation. Evidence of a short-term anti-nociceptive effect. *Physiology of Behaviour*, **68**(5), 631–9

Han, Q. P. and Dryhurst, G. (1996). Influence of glutathione on the oxidation of 1-methyl-6-hydroxy-1,2,3,4-tetrahydro-beta-carboline: Chemistry of potential relevance to the addictive and neurogenerative consequences of ethanol use. *Journal Medicine and Chemistry*, **39**(7), 1494–1508.

Hazardous Substances Data Base (HSDB). (2000). TOMES Microdmedex, Inc. Englewood, Colorado, USA.

Hughes, J. R., Rose, G. L., and Callas, P. W. (2000). Nicotine is more reinforcing in smokers with a past history of alcoholism than in smokers without this history. *Alcohol Clinical Experimental Research*, **24**(11), 1633–8.

Dr Murray Kaiserman (December 2002). Health Canada. Personal communication.

Kelton, M. C., Kahn, H. J., Conrath, C. L., and Newhouse, P. A. (2000). The effects of nicotine on Parkinson's disease. *Brain Cognition*, **43**(1–3), 274–82

Kobayashi, H., Suzuki, T., Kamata, R., Saito, S., Sato, I., Tsuda, S., and Matsusaka, N. (1999). Recent progress in the neurotoxicology of natural drugs associated with dependence or addiction, their endogenous agonists and receptors. *J Toxicol Sci*, **24**(1), 1–16.

Lambert, N. M. and Hartsough, C. S. (1998). Prospective study of tobacco smoking and substance dependencies among samples of ADHD and non-ADHD participants. *Journal of Learning Disability*, **31**(6), 533–44.

Li, W., and Hopke, D. K. (1993). Initial Size Distributions and Hygroscopicity of Indoor Combustion Aerosol Particles. *Aerosol Science and Technology*, **19**(3), 305–16.

Mihailescu, S., and Drucker-Colin, R. (2000). Nicotine, brain nicotinic receptors, and neuropsychiatric disorders. *Archives Medical Research*, **31**(2), 131–44.

Ministerial Advisory Council on Tobacco Control (MACTC) (2001). Putting an end to deception. A report to the Canadian Minister of Health. September 2001.

National Institute on Drug Addiction website. 2000. (http://www.NIDA.NIH.Gov/researchreports/nicotine/nicotine2html#addictive). Website accessed December 2000.

Okada, T., Ishizu, Y., and Matsunuma, K. (1977). Determination of particle-size distribution and concentration of cigarette smoke by a light-scattering method. *Beitr. Tabakforsch*, **9**(3), 153–60.

Orto, D., Valfre, F., Svoini, G., and Enne, G. (1996). Animal feed and good agricultural practice. Residues of veterinary drugs and mycotoxins in animal products: new methods for risk assessment and quality control. Proceedings of the Teleconference held on Internet (Listserver Meatqual) from April 15–August 31, 1994. pp. 101–109.

Pankow, J. F. (1999). Behavior of nicotine and N-nitrosamines in tobacco smoke. Crisp Data Base National Institutes of Health. Bethesda MD, USA.

Pickworth, W. B., Fant, R. V., Nelson, R. A., Rohrer, M. S., and Henningfield, J. E. (1999). Pharmacodynamic effects of new de-nicotinised cigarettes. *Nicotine and Tobacco Resarch*, **1**(4), 357–64.

Plummer, H. K., Sheppard, B. J., and Schuller, H. M. (2000). Interaction of tobacco-specific toxicants with nicotinic cholinergic regulation of fetal pulmonary neuroendocrine cells: implications for pediatric lung disease. *Experimental Lung Research*, **26**(2), 121–35.

Polydorova, M. (1961). An attempt to determine the retention of tobacco smoke by means of membrane filters. In Davies CN (ed.) *Inhaled Particles and Vapours*. Proceedings of the International Symposium organized by the British Occupational Hygiene Society.

Quattrocki, E., Baird, A., and Yurgelun-Todd, D. (2000). Biological aspects of the link between smoking and depression. *Harvard Reviews in Psychiatry*, **8**(3), 99–110

Riggs, P. D., Mikulich, S. K., Whitmore, E. A., and Crowley, T. J. (1999). Relationship of ADHD, depression, and non-tobacco substance use disorders to nicotine dependence in substance-dependent delinquents. *Drug Alcohol Dependence*, **54**(3), 195–205

Reynolds, R. J.(1988). *Chemical and Biological Studies on New Cigarette Prototypes that Heat Instead of Burn Tobacco*; Published by R.J. Reynolds Tobacco Company, Winston-Salem, North Carolina, 1988.

Robertson, C. (2000). The design and engineering of a cigarette. WHO Conference: Advancing Knowledge on Regulating Tobacco Products. Oslo, Norway. Feb 2000.

Rose, J. E., Behm, F. M., Ramsay, C., and Ritchie, J. C. Jr. (2001). Platelet monoamine oxidase, smoking cessation, and tobacco withdrawal sypmtoms. *Nicotine and Tobacco Research*, **3**, 383–90.

Royal College of Physicians (2000). *Nicotine Addiction in Britain*. A report of the Tobacco Advisory Group of the Royal College of Physicians. London.

Rozman, K. K. and Klaassen, C. D. (1994). Absorption, distribution, and excretion of toxicants. In: Klaassen CD (ed.) *Cassarett and Doull's Toxicology*. McGraw-Hill, New York.

Smith, A. A. (1975). Interaction of biogenic amines with ethanol. *Advances in Experimental Medicine and Biology*, **56**, 265–75.

Smoke constituents (2000). Available (2002) from Government of British Columbia, Ministry of Health Services web site: http://www.hlth.gov.bc.ca/ttdr/pdf/sc.html

Stankus, R. P., Sastre, J., Salvaggio, J. E. (1988). Asthma induced by exposure to low molecular weight compounds and cigarette smoke. In: Simmons DH. (ed.) *Current Pulmonology—Volume 9*. Chicago: Year Book Medical Publishers. pp. 369–94.

Thuerauf, N., Kaegler, M., Dietz, R., Barocka, A., Kobal, G. (1999). Dose-dependent stereoselective activation of the trigeminal sensory system by nicotine in man. *Psychopharmacology*, 142, 236–43.

Thuerauf, N., Kaegler, M., Renner, B., Barocka, A., and Kobal, G. (2000). Specific sensory detection, discrimination, and hedonic estimation of nicotine enantiomers in smokers and nonsmokers: Are there limitations in replacing the sensory components of nicotine? *Journal of Clinical Psychopharmacology*, 20, 472–8.

U.K. Department of Health (1998). Permitted additives to tobacco products in the United Kingdom. London. September 1998.

U.S. Federal Register: August 11, 1995 (Volume 60, Number 155). Industry manipulation and control of nicotine delivery in marketed tobacco products.

U.S. National Institute on Drug Addiction website. 2000. Is nicotine addictive? *(http://www.nida. nih.gov/researchreports/nicotine/nicotine2.html#addictive)*. Website accessed December 2000.

U.S. Surgeon General Report. 1988. *The Health Consequences of Smoking: Nicotine Addiction.* Department of Health and Human Services, Centers for Disease Control. Atlanta GA.

Waldmann, R., Champigny, G., Bassilana, F., Heurteaux, C., and Lazdunski, M. (1997). A proton-gated cation channel involved in acid-sensing. *Nature*, 386(6621), 173–7.

Watt, R. G., Dykes, J., and Sheiham, A. (2000). Preschool children's consumption of drinks: implications for dental health. *Community Dent Health*, 17(1), 8–13.

Wicker, P. (1994). Local anaesthesia in the operating theatre. *Nurs. Times*, 90(46), 34–5.

Widdicombe, J. G. (1986). Reflexes from the upper respiratory tract. In: Cherniack NS, Widdicombe JG (ed.) *Handbook of Physiology*. Bethesda, MD, American Physiological Society, pp. 363–94.

Wrona, M. Z., Wakiewicz, J., Han, Q. P., Han, J., Li, H., and Dryhurst, G. (1997). Putative oxidative metabolites of 1-methyl-6-hydroxy-1,2,3,4-tetrahydro-beta-carboline of potential relevance to the addictive and neurogenerative consequences of ethanol abuse. *Alcohol*, 14(3), 213–23.

Yates, S. L., Bencherif, M., Fluhler, E. N., and Lippiello, P. M. (1995). Up-regulation of nicotnic acetylcholine receptors following chronic exposure of rats to mainstream cigarette smoke or a4b2 receptors to nicotine. *Biochemical Pharmacology*, 50(12), 2001–8.

Chapter 9

Nicotine dosing characteristics across tobacco products

Mirjana V. Djordjevic

Introduction

Nicotiana tabacum L., the most commonly cultivated tobacco worldwide, is a hybrid between two species, *N. sylvestris* and *N. tomentosiforemis* or *octophora* (Tso 1990). *Nicotiana rustica*, another *N.* species used in tobacco products, is primarily grown in Russia, the Ukraine, and other Eastern European countries, including Georgia, Moldavia, and Poland. It is also grown in South America and, to a limited extent, in India. In the US, there is a collection of 1500 tobacco germplasms. They represent a wide range of variations of chemical constituents, including nicotine, and smoke deliveries despite plants being grown at the same location under similar treatment. Tobacco usage is primarily due to the stimulant effect of nicotine. Through tobacco smoke inhalation, it takes 10–19 seconds for nicotine to pass from the cigarette to the brain (Benowitz 1999).

Nicotine, a 3-pyridyl derivative, is a principal alkaloid in commercial tobaccos (in 34 out of 65 species of *N. tabacum*) followed by nornicotine (the main alkaloid in 19 species), anabasine, anatabine, oxynicotine, myosmine, cotinine, 2,3'-dipyridyl, 3-acetylpyridine, nicotine amide, nicotinic acid, and others (Tso 1990). Indole alkaloids, such as harmane and norharmane were also reported but in minute quantity. Tobacco types, plant parts, cultural practices, degree of leaf ripening and fertilizer treatment, and climate condition, are among some prominent factors which determine the levels of alkaloids in *N. tabacum* plants. In fact, every step in tobacco growing that affects plant metabolism will influence the level of alkaloid content to a certain degree. The Maryland and sun-cured (a.k.a. oriental, Turkish) tobaccos are generally low in nicotine; the flue-cured (a.k.a. bright, blond, or Virginia) tobacco, air-cured (a.k.a. burley) tobacco, Cuban and Connecticut cigar wrapper contain medium levels of nicotine; and the Pennsylvania, dark fire-cured tobacco, and especially *N. rustica*, are high in nicotine content. Tobacco leaves have the highest content of nicotine, roots have less, and stalks have the least. Within a plant, the levels of nicotine vary by stalk position (bottom leaves containing the lowest amount of nicotine and top leaves the highest). Within a leaf, the tip and outer area usually have higher alkaloid content than the base and inner area (Burton *et al.* 1992). Alkaloid levels increases as a plant matures, especially during the period after topping. Marked increase of nicotine is generally associated with the increased rate of nitrogen fertilization. Under favorable conditions, *N. rustica* produces double the quantity of nicotine measured in ordinary tobacco (Tso 1990). The curing and processing technologies (Peele *et al.* 1995; Wiernik *et al.* 1995), as well as the storage conditions (Burton *et al.* 1989), also have a profound influence on the alkaloid content in tobacco.

The wide variation of nicotine content in commercial tobaccos (from 0.17 to 4.93%; Tso 1990) enables manufacturers to achieve, easily, desired nicotine delivery in a specific product by tobacco blending. In the past, flue-cured tobaccos were used exclusively for cigarettes in the United Kingdom, Finland, Canada, Japan, China, and Australia. Air-cured tobaccos were the preferred choice for cigarettes in France, southern Italy, some parts of Switzerland and Germany, and South America. Cigarettes made from sun-cured tobacco are smoked predominantly in Greece and Turkey. In the US, cigarettes are made by blending flue-, air-, and sun-cured tobaccos as well as reconstituted tobacco sheets. Currently, the American-blend cigarette is gaining market share worldwide (Hoffmann and Hoffmann 2001).

Apart from its well-documented effects on the central nervous and cardiovascular system (Benowitz 1998*a*, *b*), nicotine plays an important role in tobacco-associated carcinogenesis. Nicotine is the major source of the three carcinogenic tobacco-specific *N*-nitrosamines (TSNA): 4-(methylnitrosamino)-1-(3-pyridyl)-1-butanone (NNK), 4-methylnitrosamino)-1-(3-pyridyl)-1-butanol (NNAL), and *N'*-nitrosonornicotine (NNN) (Hoffmann *et al.* 1994). The minor secondary amine tobacco alkaloids such as nornicotine, anatabine, and anabasine also give rise to corresponding *N*-nitrosamines: NNN, *N'*-nitrosoanatabine and *N'*-nitrosoanabasine, respectively. NNK and NNAL are very potent procarcinogens, which, upon metabolic activation induce lung cancer in all laboratory animals tested, regardless of dose and the route of administration (Hecht 1998, 1999). NNN, in addition to inducing lung cancer in mice, is predominantly responsible for esophageal and nasal tumors in rats. The data emerging from testing the potential impact of nicotine itself on pulmonary carcinogenesis suggest that chronic non-neoplastic lung diseases such as bronchitis, bronchiolitis, chronic obstructive pulmonary disease, emphysema, and asthma, are highly associated with both active and involuntary smoking and may pose an additional risk factor for lung cancer (Schuller 1998). Most recently, nicotine has been reported to be a possible promoter of cancer progression in human lung cells grown in the laboratory (West *et al.* 2003).

Nicotine content in tobacco products

The most commonly used tobacco products worldwide are cigarettes, both manufactured and hand made (a.k.a. roll-your-own). However, there are many countries in the world, especially in South Asia, where smokeless tobacco use is a significant part of the overall world tobacco burden (World Health Organization 1997). In the US, 4.2 pounds of tobacco were consumed per person in 1999: 83% in cigarettes, 6% in cigars, 5% as snuff, 5% as chewing tobacco, and 1% as smoking tobacco (Giovino 2002).

Commercial cigarettes

Tobacco

Unlike systematic monitoring and reporting of emissions of nicotine, tar, and carbon monoxide in the mainstream smoke (MS) of cigarettes (e.g. U.S. Federal Trade Commission 2000), there is no official requirement, in any country in the world, for the reporting on nicotine content in the tobacco blend of commercial products. The latter is especially puzzling since the chemical composition of cigarette smoke (both qualitative and quantitative), as well as addictive and carcinogenic properties of any given product, depend directly on the profile of preformed tobacco constituents.

The data in Table 9.1 show an international comparison of the levels of nicotine, nitrate, and the two carcinogenic, nicotine-derived, N-nitrosamines in commercial cigarette tobacco. The assays of a large number of brands from the US, Canada, the United Kingdom (UK), Japan, and other countries have demonstrated that there is a wide variation in concentrations of nicotine in the tobacco filler (from 7.2 to 23.5 mg/g tobacco), as well as concentrations of nitrate (from 0.3 to 20.6 mg/cigarette), NNN (from 45-58 000 ng/g tobacco), and NNK (from not detected to 10 745 ng/cigarette; detection limit <10–50 ng/cigarette) (Djordjevic et al. 1989, 1990, 1991, 2000b, c; Fisher et al. 1989a, 1990a, b; Nair et al. 1989; Tricker et al. 1991; Kozlowski et al.1998). The country of origin plays a profound role in the chemical composition of the product; cigarettes from India and Italy contained extremely high levels of TSNA, up to 58 000 ng/g NNN and 10 745 ng/cigarette NNK. The cigarettes manufactured in the former USSR contained the lowest amounts of nicotine and TSNA (Djordjevic et al. 1991).

The chemical composition of tobacco from different types of blended cigarettes (oriental, Virginia, American blend, dark tobacco) is shown in Table 9.2, as well as the composition of tobacco from different types of cigarettes as it relates to nicotine and tar yields in the mainstream smoke. [*The terms 'ultra low-, low-, medium-, and high-yield' used in Table 9.2 are not official government designates but a part of trademarked names of products that inform on the smoke yields obtained by machine-smoking using standardized protocols (Pillsbury et al. 1969; CORESTA 1991). In general, ultra low-yield products deliver less than 5 mg tar per cigarette, low-yield between 5 and 10 mg of tar, regular 'full-flavored' cigarettes deliver between 10 and 20 mg of tar, and very high-yield products deliver over 20 mg of tar per cigarette (IARC 1986) although different research groups make their own classifications; Stratton et al. 2001*]. The data in Table 9.2 indicate no difference in the content of tobacco nicotine, within a blend category, among cigarettes that deliver different smoke yields as measured using standard machine-smoking methods. For example, Virginia blend cigarettes sold in

Table 9.1 The ranges of concentrations of nicotine, nitrate, and preformed TSNA in tobacco from commercial cigarettes. International comparison

	NO$_3^-$ (mg/cigt.)	Nicotine (mg/g)	NNN (ng/cigt.)	NNK (ng/cigt.)	Reference
Austria	4.2–8.0	n.a.[a]	306–1122	92–310	Fisher et al. 1990b
Belgium	1.8–10.8	n.a.	504–1939	219–594	Fisher et al. 1990b
Canada	0.3–3.3	8.0–18.3	288–982	447–884	Fisher et al. 1990a, Kozlowski et al. 1998
Germany	0.6–20.6	n.a.	45–5340	n.d.[b]–1120	Fisher et al. 1990b, 1989a; Tricker 1991
France	1.5–19.4	10.7	120–6019	57–990	Djordjevic et al. 1989; Fisher et al. 1990b
India	n.a.	n.a.	1300–58 000 ng/g	40–4800 ng/g	Nair et al.1989
Italy	6.2–13.3	n.a.	632–12 454	153–10 745	Fisher et al. 1990b
Japan	3.7–13.1 mg/g	11.4–23.5 mg/g	360–1110 ng/g	190–330 ng/g	Djordjevic et al. 2000c; Fukumoto et al. 1997
Netherlands	1.5–8.8	n.a.	58–1647	105–587	Fisher et al. 1990b
Poland	4.4–12.8	n.a.	870–2760	140–450	Fisher et al. 1990b
			670–4870 ng/g	70–660 ng/g	Djordjevic et al. 2000b
Sweden	2.4–5.4	n.a.	544–1511	192–569	Fisher et al. 1990b
Switzerland	6.4–7.8	n.a.	1280–2208	450–554	Fisher et al. 1990b
UK	1.4–8.0	9.0–17.5	140–1218	92–433	Fisher et al. 1990b; Kozlowski et al. 1998
USA	6.2–13.5	7.2–13.4	993–1947	433–733	Fisher et al. 1990b; Kozlowski et al. 1998
	7.8–15.9 mg/g	16.9–17.9	1290–3050 ng/g	420–920 ng/g	Djordjevic et al. 1990, 2000c
USSR	1.7–9.1	n.a.	60–850	n.d.–150	Fisher et al. 1990b
	4.2–17.2 mg/g	7.6–9.4	360–850 ng/g	n.d.[c]–70 ng/g	Djordjevic et al. 1991

[a]n.a., not available.

[b]n.d., not detected (NNK detection limit <50 ng/g, Fisher et al. 1989a, b).

[c]n.d., not detected (NNK detection limit <10 ng/g, Djordjevic et al. 1991).

Canada contain 8.0–18.3 mg nicotine per gram of tobacco whereas US American blend cigarettes contain 16.9–17.9 mg nicotine (Fisher et al. 1990a; Djordjevic et al. 1990; 2000c; Kozlowski et al. 1998). Cigarettes manufactured in Japan contain a somewhat wider range of nicotine, from 11.4 to 23.5 mg per gram of tobacco, although there is no difference between medium- and high-yield brands (Fukumoto et al. 1997).

Table 9.2 The ranges of nicotine, nitrate, and preformed TSNA concentrations in tobacco from commercial cigarettes with a wide range of FTC nicotine and 'tar' yields. International comparison

Country	Cigarette type	F/NF[a]	NO$_3^-$ (mg/cigt.)	Nicotine (mg/g)	NNN (ng/cigt.)	NNK (ng/cigt.)	Reference
Germany	Blend	F	2.2–7.8	n.a.[b]	400–1390	100–410	Tricker et al. 1991
(n = 20)	Blend	NF	5.4–12.3	n.a.	660–2670	270–500	
	Dark	NF	14.2–20.6	n.a.	4500–5340	800–960	
Germany	Oriental		0.6–2.7	n.a.	45–432	n.d.–177	Fisher et al. 1989a
(n = 55)	Virginia		0.7–3.3	n.a.	133–330	170–580	
	American blend		1.8–5.4	n.a.	500–2534	160–696	
	Dark		10.9–14.4	n.a.	3660–5316	370–1120	
Canada	Ultra-low yield (V)		0.3–3.2	11.2–14.4§	288–982	447–785	Fisher et al. 1990a
(n = 25)	Low yield (V)		0.4–0.6	12.4–16.7§	292–527	510–884	Kozlowski et al. 1998§
	Moderate yield (V)		0.4–0.8	11.9–15.6§	337–407	585–705	
	High yield (V)		0.3–1.0	8.0–18.3§	259–381	495–663	
U.S.	Ultra-low yield (AB)		13.6–14.0	17.6–17.9	1750–1980	500–580	Djordjevic et al. 1990
(n = 13)	Low yield (AB)		9.0–12.3	17.9	1900–3050	490–800	Djorcjevic et al. 2000c
	Moderate yield (AB)		7.8–15.9	16.9	1780–2890	420–920	
	High Yield (AB)		11.7	17.9	1290	770	
Japan	Low yield		5.7–13.1	11.4–18.6	810–1110	190–330	Djordjevic et al. 2000c
(n = 6)	Medium yield		3.7–7.5	16.1–24.3	360–1040	200–320	Fukumoto et al. 1997
(n = 17/nic)	High Yield		n.a.	17.7–23.5	n.a.	n.a.	

[a]Abbreviations: F, filtered cigarettes; NF, non-filtered cigarettes; V, Virginia type cigarettes; AB, American blend cigarettes.

[b]n.a.: not available.

Canadian and Japanese brands contained the lowest amounts of preformed NNN in tobacco (from 259 to 1110 ppb), while the US brands contained the highest (from 1750 to 3050 ppb). Cigarettes made with dark tobaccos contain the highest amounts of NNN (up to 5534 ppb). NNK content was of the same order of magnitude in both Canadian and US brands (up to 920 ppb), whereas Japanese cigarettes contained the lowest concentrations of preformed NNK in tobacco (up to 330 ppb).

The significance of nicotine content in tobacco: An international comparison of cigarettes with a wide range of the FTC nicotine and tar MS yields (0.1–1.3 mg nicotine and 1–17 mg tar per cigarette) showed very similar levels of nicotine in tobacco (Kozlowski *et al.* 1998). One gram of tobacco from American-blended cigarettes (*n*=32) contained on average 10.2 mg nicotine (7.2–13.4 mg range); the tobacco from Canadian Virginia blend cigarettes (*n*=23) contained on average 13.5 mg nicotine (8.0–18.3 mg range); tobacco from British Virginia blend cigarettes (*n*=37), 12.5 mg nicotine (9.0–17.5 mg range). The similar potential of cigarettes, regardless of their labeling and marketing claims (filtered vs non-filtered; low- vs high-yield), to deliver any amount of nicotine and carcinogens in the MS can partially explain an ever-increasing trend in lung cancer incidence and mortality rates, especially among women (Jemal *et al.* 2002), despite the fact that a significant reduction of smoke yields has occurred during the past five decades (Hoffmann and Hoffmann 1997). Smokers responded to changing cigarettes by changing their behavior to obtain a desired amount of nicotine (Burns and Benowitz 2001). They switched to lower-yield products, smoked greater number of cigarettes per day, and increased the intensity of smoking (e.g. drawing larger puffs more frequently and blocking the ventilation holes on filter tips) to obtain the desired dose of nicotine. As a consequence, more intense smoking not only increased the dose of nicotine in smoke, but also the dose of carcinogens. The most recent evaluation of risks associated with smoking cigarettes with low machine-measured yields of tar and nicotine revealed that switching to low-yield cigarettes had no, or very little, effect on reducing cancer risk (Burns *et al.* 2001). In summary, the presence of a large pool of nicotine in tobacco enables the smoker, driven by a physiological need, to titrate his or her own dose by engaging in compensatory (more intense) smoking behaviors (Henningfield *et al.* 1994; Kozlowski *et al.* 1998; Djordjevic *et al.* 2000*a*). Hence, both the qualitative and quantitative composition of tobacco blend need to be taken into consideration when evaluating the addicting and carcinogenic potential of cigarettes.

Mainstream smoke

Mainstream smoke yields as measured with standard machine-smoking methods

The MS yields of cigarettes are influenced primarily by filtration, ventilation, and the choice of tobacco processing and blending. As with any agricultural product, there is a natural variation of tobacco composition from year to year. In the interest of manufacturing a consistent product, tobacco blends are usually made using the crops from previous years. The burning rate of cigarettes also influences smoke yields (a faster burn rate results in a lower tar yield).

In 1998, there were 1294 brands of cigarettes on the US market for which the emissions of tar, nicotine, and carbon monoxide (CO) had been established (U.S. FTC 2000). These emissions have been systematically reported by the U.S. Federal Trade Commission (FTC) since 1969. The reported values were based on a standardized machine-smoking procedure first described by Bradford *et al.* in 1936 and later adopted, with some modifications, by the U.S. FTC (Pillsbury *et al.* 1969). According to this method, the smoking machine is set up to draw 35-mL puffs of 2 seconds duration once per minute until the predetermined butt length has been reached (23 mm for non-filtered cigarettes, or the length of filter over wrapping paper plus 3 mm for filtered cigarettes). Ventilation holes (when applicable) are not blocked during machine-smoking. The FTC method which is used in the US is very similar to the methods of the International Standard Organization (ISO) and Cooperation Center for Scientific Research Relative to Tobacco (CORESTA) which are used throughout the rest of the world (Eberhardt and Scherer 1995; Baker 2002).

The MS yields of contemporary brands in the US range from < 0.05 to 2 mg nicotine, < 0.5 to 27 mg tar, and < 0.5 to 18 mg CO per cigarette. The sales-weighted average nicotine and tar smoke yields are now 0.9 and 12 mg per cigarette, compared to 1.4 and 21.6 mg, respectively, in 1968: a decrease of 40% (U.S. FTC 2000). The tar and nicotine reduction has been achieved by several methods, including reducing tobacco weight, increasing filtration, implementing air dilution through ventilation holes on the filter tips or using porous wrapping paper, reconstituted and expanded tobacco, chemical additives (to control the combustion rate), and performing specific agronomic practices.

In the United Kingdom, sales-weighted average machine-measured tar yields have declined steadily: in 1999 were 9.2 mg per cigarette, less than half their 1972 level (Jarvis 2001). Over the same period, nicotine yields have come down from 1.33 to 0.8 mg per cigarette. Carbon monoxide yields have shown smaller declines. At the same time as absolute yields have declined, there have also been changes in tar to nicotine ratios. In 1999, smokers in the UK were exposed to 22% less tar per unit of nicotine than in 1973. During 1983–1990, a number of studies investigated the yields and range of additional smoke constituents (e.g. hydrogen cyanide, aldehydes, acrolein, nitric oxide, low-molecular weight phenols and polynuclear aromatic hydrocarbons [PAH]) and their inter-relationship with the routinely monitored agents (Philips and Waller 1991). The authors concluded that the routinely monitored tar, nicotine, and CO provide an adequate guide to the deliveries of other analytes of interest in MS of British cigarettes except of nitric oxide, which is strongly dependent on tobacco type, and some phenols, and PAH.

The data presented in Table 9.3 show a wide range of emissions of nicotine (0.1–2.7 mg per cigarette), tar (1–44 mg per cigarette), and TSNA in the mainstream smoke of

Table 9.3 The ranges of mainstream smoke yields of select constituents in commercial cigarettes (FTC/CORESTA/ISO machine smoking method). International comparison

	Tar (mg/cigt.)	Nicotine (mg/cigt.)	CO (mg/cigt.)	BaP (ng/cigt.)	NNN (nn/cigt.)	NNK (ng/cigt.)	Reference
Austria	9–15	0.7–0.9	n.a.[b]	n.a.	42–172	12–100	Fisher et al. 1990b
Belgium	13–16	1.0–1.3	n.a.	n.a.	38–203	29–150	Fisher et al. 1990b
Canada	0.7–19	0.1–1.4	1–21	3.4–28.4	4–37	6–97	Rickert et al. 1985; Fisher et al. 1990a; Kaisermar and Rickert 1992a, b; Kozlowski et al. 1998
Germany	1–28	0.1–2.0	n.a.	n.a.	5–625	n.d.[a]–470	Fisher et al. 1989a, 1990b; Tricker 1991
France	6–44	0.3–2.7	n.a.	n.a.	11–1000	20–498	Djordjevic et al. 1989; Fisher et al. 1990b
India	18–28[c]	0.9–1.8	n.a.	n.a.	6–401	n.d.–34.4	Nair et al. 1989; Pakhale et al. 1989
Italy	n.a.	n.a.	n.a.	n.a.	21–1353	8–1749	Fisher et al. 1990b
Japan	7–16	0.1–2.4	6–19	5.1–13.3	36–129	37–58	Djordjevic et al. 1996; Fukumoto et al. 1997
Netherlands	1–18	0.2–1.5	n.a.	n.a.	9–163	5–102	Fisher et al. 1990b

Poland	19	1.4	n.a.	n.a.	68–347	36–105	Fisher et al. 1990b; Djordjevic et al. 2000b
Sweden	9–23	0.8–1.8	n.a.	n.a.	44–141	27–84	Fisher et al. 1990b
Switzerland	12–15	0.9–1.2	n.a.	n.a.	121–127	69–124	Fisher et al. 1990b
Thailand	5–28	0.2–2.4	n.a.	n.a.	28–730	16–369	Brunnemann et al. 1996; Mitacek et al. 1991
(US brands)	9–26	0.6–1.5	n.a.	n.a.	209–278	156	
UK	1–13	0.2–1.2	1–17	n.a.	17–123	18–103	Fisher et al. 1990b; Kozlowski et al. 1998
USA	1–24	0.1–2.0	1–20	2.2–26.2	14–1007	6–425	Adams et al. 1987; Fisher et al. 1990b; Djordjevic et al. 1990, 1996; Brunnemann et al. 1994; Kozlowski et al. 1998
USSR	22–29	0.9–1.4	n.a.	16.1–27.3	23–389	4–145	Fisher et al. 1990b; Djordjevic et al. 1991

[a] n.d., not detected limit: <4 ng/cigt.

[b] n.a., not available.

[c] Dry TPM (total particulate matter).

cigarettes sold globally. The highest concentrations of TSNA were measured in non-filtered cigarettes sold in France and Italy (up to 1353 ng NNN and up to 1740 ng NNK per cigarette). These are the same brands that contained the highest amounts of preformed TSNA (Fisher *et al.* 1990*b*). The lowest emissions were found in blended cigarettes from Canada, the UK, Netherlands, Sweden, and Japan, with upper values as low as 58 ng NNK. Surprisingly, the NNK levels in MS of two cigarette brands from India were extremely low, from not detected to 34.4 ng per cigarette, given the extremely high levels of preformed NNK in tobacco (Nair *et al.* 1989).

The comparative assessment of the MS composition of three popular US brands of filtered cigarettes purchased on the open markets in 29 countries worldwide showed a dramatic variation in the levels of tar, nicotine, NNN, and NNK within each brand (Table 9.4; Gray *et al.* 2000). While the variation in tar levels in MS ranged from 25% to 50%, the yields of NNK varied from 3- to 9-fold. NNK and NNN yields were highly correlated ($r = 0.88$). These data created great concern among the public health officials, who called for setting upper limits for carcinogen levels by establishing the marker median as an initial upper limit (Gray *et al.* 2000; Gray and Boyle 2002).

Mainstream smoke yields as measured using more intense, human-like, smoking conditions

The fact that the rates of death from lung cancer, which is 81.6% attributable to cigarette smoking (U.S. CDC 2002), did not parallel the reduction of toxic emissions (Burns *et al.* 2001) indicated that smokers responded to low-yield cigarettes by spontaneously changing their smoking behaviors so that they could obtain desired amount of nicotine, the major pharmacoactive agent in tobacco and tobacco smoke that induces tobacco dependence. More intense smoking, to overcome draw resistance due to filtration and air dilution, resulted in higher exposure to both nicotine and carcinogens (Djordjevic *et al.* 2000*a*). Kozlowski *et al.* (1998) showed that nicotine concentrations in MS are highly correlated with that of tar which harbor non-volatile carcinogens ($r = 0.97$ [0.93–0.99]).

To obtain more realistic estimates of smokers' exposure to toxic and carcinogenic agents from cigarette smoke, the puffing characteristics of 133 adult smokers of cigarettes rated by the FTC at 1.2 mg of nicotine or less (56 smokers of low-yield

Table 9.4 The chemical composition of the three global brands sold in 29 countries worldwide (Gray *et al.* 2000)

	Tar (mg/cigt.)	Nicotine (mg/cigt.)	NNK (ng/cigt.)
Brand I	10.6–15.7	0.85–1.3	50–100
Brand II	11.8–20.4	0.85–1.3	50–225
Brand III	8.4–15.9	0.68–1.25	50–325

cigarettes [≤0.8 mg nicotine/cigarette] and 77 smokers of medium-yield cigarettes [0.9–1.2 mg nicotine per cigarette]) were assessed by a pressure transducer system (Djordjevic *et al.* 2000*a*). The smoking profiles for a randomly chosen subset of 72 individuals were then programmed into a piston-type machine to generate smoke from each smoker's usual brand of cigarettes for assays of nicotine, tar, and lung cancer-causing agents such as benzo(*a*)pyrene (BaP) and NNK. The FTC protocol was also used to assess levels of targeted compounds in the 11 brands most frequently smoked by study subjects. Compared with the FTC protocol values, smokers of low- and medium-yield brands took statistically significantly larger puffs (48.6- and 44.1-mL puffs, respectively) at statistically shorter intervals (21.3 and 18.5 seconds, respectively) and drew larger total smoke volumes than specified in the FTC parameters (the total volume drawn through the cigarette is the main factor responsible for the nicotine and TSNA delivery in MS; Rickert *et al.* 1986; Fisher *et al.* 1989*b*; Melikian *et al.* 2002). Subsequently, smokers received 2.5 and 2.2 times more nicotine and 2.6 and 1.9 times more tar, respectively, than FTC-derived amounts and approximately double the levels of BaP and NNK. Smokers of medium-yield cigarettes received higher doses of all components when compared with smokers of low-yield cigarettes. The major conclusion of this study was that the FTC protocol underestimates nicotine and carcinogen doses to smokers and overestimates the proportional benefit of low-yield cigarettes (Burns and Benowitz 2001).

The most comprehensive data on the chemical composition of the MS of contemporary cigarettes generated by machine under more intense conditions were compiled in 'The 1999 Massachusetts Benchmark Study. Final Report' (Borgerding *et al.* 2000). Eighteen leading US brands (26 brand styles), delivering from 1 to 26 mg FTC 'tar' per cigarette, were screened. All the brands (0.05–9% market share by brand style) were American blend cigarettes made by mixing different tobacco types and grades, including reconstituted tobacco sheets, expanded tobacco, and additives. Cigarette smoke was generated for the assays of 44 constituents both in a vapor and particulate phase by machine-smoking using both the FTC method and the Massachusetts machine-smoking method: 45-ml puffs of 2 seconds duration drawn twice a minute until the predetermined butt length of 23 mm for non-filter cigarettes; or the length of filter over wrapping paper plus 3 mm for filter cigarettes. The ventilation holes on filter tips, when applicable, are 50% blocked during machine-smoking (U.S. FTC 1997). The 'more intense' Massachusetts machine-smoking protocol was developed in response to the debate on the validity of the FTC method for the assessment of smokers exposure (Hoffmann *et al.* 1996). The nicotine levels of the 26 tested brands ranged from 0.56 to 3.32 mg/cigarette. The yields of other toxic and carcinogenic MS constituents obtained by machine-smoking of 26 brands of cigarettes using the Massachusetts method were published by Gray and Boyle (2002).

The Tobacco Sales Act 2002 of British Columbia, Canada (http://www.qp.gov.bc.ca/statreg/reg/T/TobaccoSales/282_98.htm#schedulea), mandates the machine-smoking method for cigarette testing that utilizes even more stringent settings than the Massachusetts method prescribes: puff volume—55 mL, puff interval—30 seconds, puff duration—2 seconds, and 100% of the ventilation holes must be blocked during smoking. The British Columbia Ministry of Health (http://www.healthservices.gov.bc.ca/ttdr/index.html) provides information on MS deliveries of 11 constituents in commercial leading Canadian cigarettes (top 22 brands in British Columbia are accounting for 70–80% of the market) under both standard FTC and more intense (human-like) smoking conditions (HSC). When machine smoked using more intense parameters, the leading Canadian, Japanese, and the UK brands sold in British Columbia deliver on average, 3.3 mg, 2.4 mg, and 2.9 mg nicotine per cigarette, respectively, and 36 mg, 28 mg, and 34 mg tar per cigarette, respectively.

The drawback of both the Massachusetts and Health Canada methods is that they do not take into account that cigarettes with different FTC tar and nicotine yields are designed to guide smokers to smoke them differently (Burns *et al.* 2001). Therefore, one single set of even more intense machine-smoking parameters will not adequately reflect individual puffing characteristics and delivered dosages of nicotine and carcinogens to smokers. Moreover, the very large inter- and intra-individual variations in smoking topography among smokers of the same brand (Djordjevic *et al.* 2000*a*) needs to be considered during the exposure assessment. To demonstrate this, the Massachusetts smoke yields for the leading US full flavor regular and mentholated brands were compared with the values obtained by mimicking the puffing patterns of two individuals who smoked those two brands (Table 9.5). The smoker of the mentholated brand drew in 5.6 mg nicotine per cigarette and the smoker of non-mentholated cigarette drew 4.1 mg nicotine, double the amounts than those estimated by the Massachusetts method. Moreover, the smoker of non-mentholated brand took in four times more of the carcinogens NNN and NNK (Djordjevic *et al.* 2000), than determined by the 'intense' Massachusetts method and approximately eight times more than determined by the FTC method. When the Thai cigarette was machine-smoked at a rate of two puffs per minute, the emission of nicotine in the MS was 5.6 mg per cigarette (Mitacek 1990).

Roll-your-own cigarettes

Roll-your-own (RYO) cigarettes are a cheaper substitute for commercially manufactured brands and are gaining in popularity worldwide. Smokers of RYO tend to be concentrated in the lower socio-economic levels. In Europe, the major markets for RYO are the Netherlands and Germany (Dymond 1996). In Canada, sales of RYO accounted for approximately 14% of the Canadian cigarette market by the end of 1989 (Kaiserman and Rickert 1992*a*). In the United Kingdom, in 1994, more than 20% of male smokers used RYO products as compared to 4% of female smokers (Darrall *et al.* 1998). In the US, 3.4 billion RYO cigarettes were smoked in 1994 (2000 Maxwell Tobacco Fact Book).

Table 9.5 The chemical composition of the mainstream smoke of the two US leading full flavor filter cigarettes smoked by two randomly chosen individuals

	Non-mentholated cigarette			Mentholated cigarette		
	Mass[a]	HSC[b]	HSC/Mass	Mass	HSC	HSC/Mass
Nicotine (mg/cigt.)	2.1	4.1	2.0	2.6	5.6	2.2
BaP (ng/cigt.)	27.8	34.6	1.2	31.2	34.3	1.1
NNN (ng/cigt.)	202.0	794.0	3.9	243.1	537.0	2.2
NNK (ng/cigt.)	184.0	714.0	3.9	198.4	239.0	1.2

Abbreviations: FTC, Federal Trade Commission; HSC, human smoking conditions.
[a]Borgerding et al. 2000.
[b]Djordjevic et al. 2000a.

In the study by Darrall and co-workers, 57% of RYO cigarettes produced higher levels of tar than the 15 mg/cigarette, which is the current maximum allowed in manufactured cigarettes in the UK. Seventy-seven percent of RYO smokers made cigarettes with smoke nicotine yields greater than the current UK maximum of 1.1 mg/cigarette. Dutch consumers make RYO cigarettes that deliver, on average, 13.2 mg tar and 1.2 mg nicotine per cigarette (Dymond 1996). The smoke yields for 31 brands of RYO tobaccos tested in Canada were: 15.5 mg tar and 1.1 mg nicotine per cigarette (Kaiserman and Rickert 1992b). In the latter study it was emphasized that it is the tube and filter combination that controls the delivery of toxic constituents to smokers.

Three varieties of hand-rolled cigarettes from Thailand yielded 28.5–40.8 mg tar and 1.1–5.5 mg nicotine per cigarette in MS (Mitacek et al. 1991). No data are presently available on the levels of nicotine-derived TSNA in the smoke of RYO cigarettes, or on smoking topography and true deliveries of smoke constituents of these cigarettes as the result of individual smoking behaviors.

Cigars

A cigar is any roll of tobacco wrapped in leaf tobacco or any other substance containing tobacco. There are four main types of cigars: little cigars, small cigars ('cigarillos'), regular cigars, and premium cigars (Stratton et al. 2001). Little cigars contain air-cured and fermented tobacco and are wrapped either in reconstituted tobacco or in cigarette paper that contains tobacco and/or tobacco extract. Some little cigars have cellulose acetate filter tips and are shaped like cigarettes. Cigarillos are small, narrow cigars with no cigarette paper or acetate filter. Regular and premium cigars are available in various shapes and sizes and are rolled to a tip at one end. The dimensions of cigars are from 110 to 150 mm in length and up to 17 mm in diameter. Regular cigars weigh between 5 and 17 grams. Premium cigars (exclusively handmade from natural, long-cut filler tobacco) vary in size, ranging from 12 to 23 mm in diameter and

127 to 214 mm in length. Although the use of cigarettes declined throughout the 1990s (18% decrease from 1990 to 1999; 2000 Maxwell Tobacco Fact Book), large cigar and cigarillo consumption increased by 58% during the same period (from 2.34 billion to 3.72 billion pieces).

In 1997, the leading US brands of little, large, and premium cigars (ranging in length from 8.65 to 17.6 cm and in weight from 1.24 to 8.1 g) were analysed for levels of nicotine and select carcinogens in the MS (Table 9.6; Djordjevic *et al.* 1997). The results were obtained by machine-smoking of cigars under standard smoking conditions as defined by the International Committee for Cigar Smoke Study (20-mL puffs of 1.5 seconds duration drawn once per minute to the predetermined butt length of 23 mm; ICCSS 1974). The delivered dosages of nicotine, tar, and carbon monoxide increased exponentially from cigarettes to premium cigars. When compared to cigarettes, the levels of nicotine, BaP and NNK were 3 times, 7 times, and 17 times, respectively, higher in the MS of premium cigars.

When little cigars were machine-smoked simulating the puffing characteristics of smokers, the emissions of the total tobacco-specific *N*-nitrosamines were two times higher than those determined using the standard ICCSS method (Djordjevic *et al.* 1997), the similar trend as described for cigarettes (Djordjevic *et al.* 2000a). A similar 2.2-fold difference in all smoke constituents due to more 'intense smoking' was reported by Rickert and Kaiserman (1999). In the latter study, under standard conditions, MS constituent yields generated from cigarettes and cigars were substantially different (ammonia: 12.7 *vs* 327 µg/unit; NNN: 41.5 *vs* 932 ng/unit; nitrogen oxides: 1.6 *vs* 35.9 µg/unit). In an earlier study, Rickert and his co-workers (1985) reported that small cigars delivered, on average, 38 mg tar and 2.1 mg nicotine into the

Table 9.6 Smoke yields of the leading US cigarettes and little, large, and premium cigars

	Medium-yield cigarettes (0.9–1.2 mg FTC nicotine)[a,c]	Cigars[b,d]		
		Little	Regular	Premium
Nicotine (mg/unit)	1.11	1.5	1.4	3.4
Tar (mg/unit)	15.4	24	37	44
Carbon monoxide (mg/unit)	14.6	38	98	133
BaP (ng/unit)	14.0	26.2	96	97.4
NNK (ng/unit)	146.2	290	805	2490

[a]Djordjevic *et al.* 2000a.

[b]Djordjevic *et al.* 1997.

[c]The cigarettes were smoked under FTC conditions: 1 puff/min, 35 mL volume, 2-second puff duration, butt length: the length of filter overwrap plus 3 mm (Pillsbury *et al.* 1969).

[d]The cigars were smoked under the ICCSS (International Committee for Cigar Smoke Study 1974) conditions: 1 puff/40 seconds, 20 mL, 1.5-second puff duration, butt length 33 mm.

MS whereas a large cigar delivered 17.5 mg tar and 1.37 mg nicotine. To control for varying volumes of smoke emitted from cigarettes and cigars, standardized comparisons in milligrams of toxic substance per liter of smoke were created. Using this method, the mean deliveries of tar, nicotine, and CO per liter of smoke were found to be the highest for small cigars, followed by hand-rolled and manufactured cigarettes while large cigars had the lowest mean deliveries.

The analysis of 17 cigar brands (weight range: 0.53–21.5 g per piece) revealed a considerable variation in the total tobacco nicotine content (5.7–336.2 mg per cigar) and the acidity of aqueous solution of cigar tobacco (pH range: 5.7–7.8) (Henningfield *et al.* 1999). The MS pH values of the smallest cigars were generally acidic, changed little across the puffs, and more closely resembled the profiles previously reported for typical cigarettes. Curiously, the smoke pH of smaller cigars and cigarillos only became acidic after the first third of the rod and then remained acidic thereafter. Larger cigars were acidic during the first third of the rod and became quite alkaline during the last third . The acidity/basicity of cigar smoke is of significance since it has an impact on the bio-availability of nicotine.

Thai products delivered 7.95–11.4 mg nicotine, 91–201 mg tar, and 111–819 mg CO per cigar in the MS (Mitacek *et al.* 1991). The tobacco from an Indian cigar contained 25 000 ng preformed NNN and 8900 ng NNK per gram of tobacco (Nair *et al.* 1989).

Bidis

Bidis are hand-rolled cigarettes which are predominantly used in India and rural areas of several Southeast Asian countries. Bidis are made by rolling a dried tobacco leaf into a conical shape around approximately 0.2 g of sun-dried, flaked tobacco and securing the roll with a thread. Bidi smoking is a well-established risk factor for cancers of the upper aerodigestive tract (IARC 2002) as well as cardiovascular and respiratory diseases. The mainstream smoke yields of the total dry particulate matter and nicotine in bidis smoked in India, as measured with a standard machine-smoking method, ranged from 26 to 41 mg and 1.9 to 2.8 mg per piece, respectively (Pakhale *et al.* 1989). These emissions were much higher than those measured in the MS of cigarettes in the same study (Table 9.3).

In recent years, bidis have become increasingly popular among US teenagers because they are perceived by some as a safer, more natural alternative to conventional ciga-rettes. American versions of bidis were shown to have higher percentage of tobacco by weight (94% *vs* 42.5%, respectively) than Indian bidis (Malson *et al.* 2001). The nicotine concentration in tobacco of American bidis (21.2 mg/g) is higher than in tobacco of commercial filter cigarettes (mean: 16.mg/g—Malson *et al.* 2001; mean: 17.5 mg/g—Djordjevic *et al.* 1990; Mean: 10.2 mg/g—Kozlowski *et al.* 1998) and non-filtered cigarettes (13.5 mg/g; Malson *et al.* 2001). In 'an open-label, within the subject design' study, it was determined that time required to smoke a bidi cigarette and number of puffs per bidi were significantly higher than for a conventional cigarette (Malson and Pickworth 2002; Malson *et al.* 2002). In smokers who switched to Irie bidi cigarettes, plasma nicotine levels increased above the levels observed when they smoked their regular cigarettes (26 ng/mL *vs* 18.5 ng/mL). Based on the higher content of nicotine in the tobacco and similar or higher nicotine and CO deliveries in the MS, it is unlikely that bidis can be considered as a safer alternative to smoking regular cigarettes. The levels of preformed NNN and NNK in bidi tobacco are from 6200 ng to 12 000 ng/g and from 400 ng to 1400 ng/g tobacco, respectively (Nair *et al.* 1989). In the MS of bidis, the NNN levels ranged from 11.6 ng to 250 ng per cigarette and the NNK levels ranged from not detected to 40 ng per cigarette. These concentrations were comparable to those determined in the MS of Indian cigarettes (Table 9.3).

Chutta

Chutta is a smoking product exclusively used in India. Reverse smoking of chutta (burning end inside the mouth), which is prevalent among women in the rural communities of Andhra Pradesh, has been associated with cancer of the upper palate. Chutta is also smoked as a normal cigar. The tobacco levels of preformed NNN and NNK in chutta were reported to be extremely high (from 21 100 ng to 295 000 ng and from 12 600 ng to 210 300 ng/g, respectively) (Nair *et al.* 1989). The reverse smoker inhales both the mainstream and sidestream smoke. The NNN and NNK levels in the MS of Chutta ranged from 288 ng to 1260 ng per cigarette and from 150 ng to 2650 ng, respectively.

Kreteks

Kreteks are a type of small cigar containing tobacco (approximately 60%), ground clove buds (40%), and cocoa, which gives a characteristic flavor and 'honey' taste to the smoke (Stratton *et al.* 2001). Kreteks are indigenous to Indonesia, but are also available in the US. The chemical composition of kreteks that was used to compare their acute toxicity with that of American blended cigarettes in male and female rats was as follows: total particulate matter, 52.3 mg/kretek cigarette *vs* 19 mg/per conventional cigarette; nicotine, 2.4 mg vs 1.0 mg; CO, 23.7 vs 15 mg (Clark 1989).

Novel potentially reduced-exposure products

During the past five decades there has been a continuous trend in developing and marketing 'safer' (reduced-exposure, reduced-toxicity) tobacco products in order to reduce adverse health effects. The latest review of the field (Burns *et al.* 2001) revealed that the changes in cigarette design made since the 1950s have resulted in about a 60% reduction in machine-smoking measured yields of tar (smoke condensate that harbors numerous carcinogenic constituents), but have had little or no effect on reducing cancer risk. The minor decrease in risk occurred only among the exclusive users of low-yield cigarettes, not among the switchers from high- to low-yield products.

In recent years, there has been a proliferation of new potential reduced-exposure products (PREPs) from which specific agents, particularly cancer-causing compounds, have been selectively removed or substantially reduced using advanced technologies (Stratton *et al.* 2001). To date, the tobacco industry's toxicological research claims have not been validated by any independent institution. These new products have been targeted at smokers who cannot or do not want to quit, smokers who want to exercise the option of choosing a product that contains lower amount of cancer-causing agents, and smokers who want an alternative to cigarettes when they are in smoke-free environment they confront on a daily basis (such as workplace, home, during travel, and other environment) (Henningfield and Fagerström 2001).

Currently, there are several categories of tobacco products on world markets that purport to reduce harm: (i) cigarettes made with modified tobacco containing reduced levels of cancer-causing agents, such as NNK (the most potent lung adenocarcinoma-causing agent) and PAH (especially BaP, lung squamous cell carcinoma-causing agent); (ii) cigarettes made with a genetically modified nicotine-free tobacco; (iii) cigarette-like delivery devices engineered to reduce tobacco toxin exposure using advance technologies; and (iv) smokeless tobacco products, especially moist snuff, made with tobacco from which cancer-causing agents, such as NNK, were either completely eliminated or significantly reduced.

The chemical composition of the MS of one cigarette brand that is being test-marketed as a reduced-nitrosamine product (http://www.starscientific.com/066745321909/advancesmoke.html) is shown in Table 9.7. The yields of select smoke components for this cigarette were compared with the average yields for three commercial brands with the same FTC ranking and the reduction of emissions were calculated. It is notable that nicotine concentration in MS of the new cigarette did not change. Although the NNN and NNK levels were significantly lower than in commercial cigarettes (up to 85%), the reduction of other constituents was not as pronounced. The tar yield, in which many carcinogens including PAH reside, was reduced by only 8.4% (20.8 mg per cigarette under more intense machine-smoking conditions). The levels of carcinogenic 1,3-butadiene increased slightly and formaldehyde levels went up by 47% compared with commercial cigarettes. Another cigarette brand which claims reduced-lung carcinogens delivers comparable tar, nicotine, BaP yields as commercial brands and much higher yields of nitric oxide and formaldehyde (http://www.omnicigs.com/frameset_test.asp?home.asp). In summary, similar levels of nicotine between the modified and non-modified cigarettes indicate that the addictive properties of new products were not reduced, nor was the possibility of endogenous formation of TSNA. The biological relevance of selective reduction/removal of specific carcinogens has yet to be investigated.

Another example of novel reduced-exposure products is a cigarette-like device that employs unconventional technology to deliver nicotine to the smoker (deBethizy *et al.* 1990; Borgerding *et al.* 1997). The intended purpose of this cigarette which heats rather

Table 9.7 The yields of select toxic and carcinogenic agents in the MS of a novel nitrosamine-free cigarette test-marketed in the US (http://www.starscientific.com/066745321909/advancesmoke.html)

Compound	FTC method	Massachusetts method	% Reduction (compared to 2 commercial brands (Mass method)
Nicotine (mg/cigt.)	0.8	1.7	(−) 0
Tar (mg/cigt.)	10.8	20.8	(−) 8.4
CO (mg/cigt.)	8.7	18.7	(−) 17.2
BaP (ng/cigt.)	8.1	18.4	(−) 8.0
4-ABP (ng/cigt.)	2.1	3.5	(−) 18.6
Formaldehyde (µg/cigt.)	36.0	81.2	(+) **46.8**
NOx (µg/cigt.)	101.5	215.3	(−) 56.7
Ammonia (µg/cigt.)	12.8	28.0	(−) 33.0
Acrolein (µg/cigt.)	39.7	102.0	(−) 10.5
1,3-Butadiene (µg/cigt.)	46.9	94.3	(+) **1.1**
Benzene (µg/cigt.)	29.6	66.9	(−) 14.9
NNN (ng/cigt.)	39.8	73.0	(−) 75.4
NNK (ng/cigt.)	15.6	30.2	(−) 84.4

than burns tobacco is to simplify the chemical composition and reduce the biological activity of the mainstream and sidestream smoke, and to achieve a significant reduction of environmental tobacco smoke. While this cigarette burns some tobacco, it does not use tobacco as the fuel to sustain combustion and to provide heat to the cigarette. Rather, this new cigarette primarily heats tobacco, thereby reducing products of smoke formation mechanisms such as tobacco combustion, tobacco pyrolysis, and pyrosynthesis. The MS composition from a cigarette based on the new design has been characterized in comparative chemical testing with two Kentucky reference cigarettes using the FTC machine-smoking method. The data shown in Table 9.8 indicate that the mainstream concentrations of most targeted compounds are significantly lower in this unconventional cigarette than in KY 1R4F reference low-yield cigarette. Although the new product delivered a lower amount of nicotine, the absorption of nicotine from this cigarette was not found to be significantly different from nicotine delivered by tobacco-burning cigarettes (Benowitz *et al.* 1997). Carboxyhemoglobin (COHb) and expired breath CO levels were elevated by 24.4 and 30.6%, respectively, in smokers after switching to new product that heats tobacco (Smith *et al.* 1998). In contrast, the urine mutagenicity of smokers of the new cigarette was significantly lower

Table 9.8 The yields of select toxic and carcinogenic agents in the MS of a novel cigarette that heats rather than burns tobacco (Borgerding *et al.* 1997)

Compound	Eclipse	Reference KY 1R4F cigarette	% Reduction
Nicotine (mg/cigt.)	0.2	0.8	(–) 76.5
Tar (mg/cigt.)	2.9	8.8	(–) 67.0
CO (mg/cigt.)	7.5	11.1	(–) 32.4
BaP (ng/cigt.)	0.6	5.0	(–) 88.0
4-ABP (ng/cigt.)	n.d.	3.3	(–) 100
Formaldehyde (μg/cigt.)	1.2	11.8	(–) 89.8
NOx (μg/cigt.)	35.0	279.0	(–) 87.4
Ammonia (μg/cigt.)	5.5	19.8	(–) 72.2
Acrolein (μg/cigt.)	20.0	72.0	(–) 72.0
1,3-Butadiene (μg/cigt.)	1.6	35.0	(–) 95.5
Benzene (μg/cigt.)	6.2	38.0	(–) 84.0
NNN (ng/cigt.)	11.0	68.0	(–) 84.0
NNK (ng/cigt.)	14.0	67.0	(–) 79.0

($p < 0.05$) than that of smokers of conventional cigarettes and it was not significantly different ($p > 0.10$) from that of non-smokers (deBethizy *et al.* 1990).

Another new technology, an electrically heated cigarette was introduced to the US market in 1998. The prototype, containing a tobacco filler wrapped in a tobacco mat, is kept in constant contact with eight electrical heater blades in a microprocessor-controlled lighter. This cigarette contains about half the amount of tobacco of a conventional cigarette. Under the FTC-standardized smoking conditions, the cigarette delivers 1 mg nicotine while all other analysed smoke constituents were significantly lower than those measured in the MS of conventional low-yield reference cigarette. The carcinogenic PAH were below the detection level (Hoffmann *et al.* 2001). However, formaldehyde yields were significantly higher.

None of the new products that claim reduced harm have been widely used in larger populations and their toxicology is generally unknown, as is their potential impact on both individual and public health. The outcome of a small, short-term, clinical study (10 male and 10 female smokers) suggested that neither of two products that employ unconventional nicotine delivery technologies is likely to be an effective reduced-exposure product for smokers (Breland *et al.* 2002a). In another study by the same group of researchers, 12 smokers who switched to a reduced-nitrosamine cigarette, received lower exposure to the lung carcinogen NNK than when using regular cigarettes, but more NNK exposure than when not smoking (Breland *et al.* 2003). Relative to smokers' own brands, low-nitrosamine cigarettes produced similar withdrawal suppression and heart rate increase and higher plasma nicotine concentrations (Breland *et al.* 2002*b*). These three studies represent the limited state of the non-tobacco industry funded published literature in that they are far too small to develop conclusions regarding the products tested.

References

Adams, J. D., O'Mara-Adams, K. J., and Hoffmann, D. (1987). Toxic and carcinogenic agents in undiluted mainstream smoke and sidestream smoke of different types of cigarettes. *Carcinogenesis*, **8**, 729–31.

Baker, R. R. (2002). The development and significance of standards for smoking-machine methodology. *Beitr. Tabakforsch., Intl.*, **20**, 23–41.

Benowitz, N. L. (1998*a*). Nicotine pharmacology and addiction. In: *Nicotine safety and toxicology* (ed. N. L. Benowitz), pp. 3–16. Oxford University Press.

Benowitz, N. L. (1998*b*). Cardiovascular toxicity of nicotine: pharmacokinetic and pharmacodynamic considerations. In: *Nicotine safety and toxicology* (ed. N. L. Benowitz), pp. 19–28. Oxford University Press.

Benowitz, N. L., Jacob, P. J., III, and Slade, J. (1997). Nicotine content of the Eclipse nicotine delivery device. *Am. J. Publ. Health*, **87**, 1865–6.

Benowitz, N. (1999). Nicotine addiction. *Primary Care*, **26**, 611–31.

Borgerding, M. F., Bodnar, J. A., Chung, H. L., Mangan, P. P., Morrison, C. C., Risner, C. H., *et al.* (1997). Chemical and biological studies of a new cigarette that primarily heats tobacco. Part I. Chemical composition of mainstream smoke. *Fd. Chem. Toxicol.*, **36**, 169–82.

Borgerding, M. F., Bodnar, J. A., and Wingate, D. E. (2000). The 1999 Massachusetts Benchmark Study—Final Report (2000). A research study conducted after consultation with the Massachusetts Department of Health.

Bradford, J. A., Harlan, W. R., and Hanmer, H. R. (1936). Nature of cigarette smoke. Technic of experimental smoking. *Ind. Engi. Chem.*, **28**, 836–9.

Breland, A. B., Buchhalter, A. R., Evans, S. E., and Eissenberg, T. (2002*a*). Evaluating acute effects of potential reduced-exposure products for smokers: Clinical laboratory methodology. *Nicotine & Tobacco Research*, S131–S140

Breland, A. B., Evans, S. E., Buchhalter, A. R., and Eissenberg, T. (2002*b*). Accute effects of Advance™: A potential reduced exposure product for smokers. *Tob Contr.* **11**, 376–8.

Breland, A. B., Acosta, M. C., and Eissenberg, T. (2003). Tobacco-specific nitrosamines and potential reduced exposure products for smokers: Preliminary evaluation of Advance™ (Submitted for publication).

Brunnemann, K. D., Hoffmann, D., Garioala, C. G., and Lee, B. C. (1994). Low ignition propensity cigarettes: Smoke analysis for carcinogens and testing for mutagenic activity of the smoke particulate matter. *Fd. Chem. Toxicol.*, **32**, 917–22.

Brunnemann, K. D., Mitacek, E. J., Liu, Y., Limsila, T., and Suttaajit, M. (1996). Assessment of major carcinogenic tobacco-specific nitrosamines in Thai cigarettes. *Cancer Detection & Prevention*, **20**, 114–21.

Burns, D. M. and Benowitz, N. L. (2001). Public health implication of changes in cigarette design and marketing. In: *Smoking and tobacco control monograph no. 13: Risks associated with smoking cigarettes with low machine-measured yields of tar and nicotine*. U.S. Department of Health and Human Services. Public Health Service. National Institutes of Health, National Cancer Institute, pp. 1–12.

Burns, D. M., Major, J. M., Shanks, T. G., Thun, M. J., and Samet, J. (2001). Smoking lower yield cigarettes and disease. In: *Smoking and tobacco control monograph no. 13: Risk associated with smoking cigarettes with low-machine measured yields of tar and nicotine.* U.S. Department of Health and Human Services. Public Health Service. National Institutes of Health, pp. 65–158.

Burton, H. R., Djordjevic, M. V., and Bush, L. P. (1989). Influence of temperature and humidity on the accumulation of tobacco-specific nitrosamines in stored burley tobacco. *J. Agric. Food Chem.,* **37,** 1372–7.

Burton, H. R., Dye, N. K., and Bush, L. P. (1992). Distribution of tobacco constituents in tobacco leaf tissue 1. Tobacco-specific nitrosamines, nitrate, nitrite, and alkaloids. *J. Agric. Fd. Chem.,* **40,** 1050–5.

Clark, G. C. (1989). Comparison of the inhalation toxicity of kretek (clove cigarette) smoke with that of American cigarette smoke. I. One day exposure. *Arch. Toxicol.,* **63,** 1–6.

CORESTA Standard Method No. 23 (1991). Determination of total and nicotine-free dry particulate matter using a routine analytical cigarette smoking machine. Determination of total particulate matter and preparation for water and nicotine measurements. *CORESTA Inform. Bull.,* **Special Vol. 1991–3,** 141–57.

Darrall, K. G., Figgins, J. A., Brown, R. D., and Phillips, G. F. (1998). Determination of benzene and associated volatile compounds in mainstream cigarette smoke. *Analyst,* **123,** 1095–101.

deBethizy, J. D., Borgerding, M. F., Doolitle, D. J., Robinson, J. H., McManus, K. Y. T., Rahn, C. A., *et al.* (1990). Chemical and biological studies of a cigarette that heats rather than burns tobacco. *J. Clin. Pharmacol.,* **30,** 755–63.

Djordjevic, M. V., Brunnemann, K. D., and Hoffmann, D. (1989). Identification and analysis of a nicotine-derived N-nitrosamino acid and other nitrosamino acids in tobacco. *Carcinogenesis,* **10,** 1725–31.

Djordjevic, M. V., Sigountos, C. W., Brunnemann, K. D., and Hoffmann, D. (1990). Tobacco-specific nitrosamine delivery in the mainstream smoke of high- and low-yield cigarettes smoked with varying puff volume (1990). In: *CORESTA Symposium Proceedings, Smoke Study Group,* pp. 54–62. Kallithea, Greece.

Djordjevic, M. V., Sigountos, C. W., Hoffmann, D., Brunnemann, K. D., Kagan, M., Bush, L. P., *et al.* (1991). Assessment of major carcinogens and alkaloids in the tobacco and mainstream smoke of USSR cigarettes. *Int. J. Cancer,* **47,** 348–51.

Djordjevic, M. V. D., Eixarch, L., Bush, L. P., and Hoffmann, D. (1996). A comparison of the yields of selected components in the mainstream smoke of the leading U.S. and Japanese Cigarettes. In: *CORESTA Congress Proceedings, Joint Smoke and Technology Groups.* Yokohama, Japan, pp. 200–17.

Djordjevic, M. V. D., Eixarch, L., and Hoffmann, D. (1997). Self-administered and effective dose of cigar smoke constituents. *51st Tobacco Chemist's Research Conference.* Winsnton-Salem, NC, September 14–17, 1997.

Djordjevic, M. V., Stellman, S. D., and Zang, E. (2000a). Dosages of nicotine and lung carcinogens delivered to cigarette smokers. *J. Natl. Cancer Inst.,* **92,** 106–11.

Djordjevic, M. V., Prokopczyk, B., and Zatonski, W. (2000b). Tobacco-specific *N*-nitrosamines (TSNA) in tobacco and mainstream smoke of the leading Polish cigarettes: a comparison with the U.S. and Japanese brands. *CORESTA Congress, Smoke Study Group.* ST1, Lisbon, Portugal, Oct. 15–19, 2000.

Djordjevic, M. V., Stellman, S. D., Takezaki, T., and Tajima, K. (2000c). Cigarette composition as a possible explanation of US-Japan differences in lung cancer rates. *91st Annual Meeting of the American Association for Research on Cancer.* Vol. 41, Abstr. # 1561, San Francisco, CA, April 1–5, 2000.

Dymond, H. F. (1996). Making habits of roll-your-own smokers in the Netherlands and tar and nicotine yields from the resultant products. *Tob. Sci.*, **40**, 87–91.

Eberhardt, H. J. And Scherer, G. (1995). Human smoking behavior in comparison with machine smoking methods. *Beitr. Tabakforsch., Intl.*, **16**, 131–40.

Fisher, S., Spiegelhalder, B., and Preussmann, R. (1989*a*). Preformed tobacco-specific nitrosamines in tobacco—role of nitrate and influence of tobacco type. *Carcinogenesis*, **1**, 1511–7.

Fisher, S., Spiegelhalder, B., and Preussmann, R. (1989*b*). Influence of smoking parameters on the delivery of tobacco-specific nitrosamines in cigarette smoke—a contribution to relative risk evaluation. *Carcinogenesis*, **10**, 1059–66.

Fisher, S., Castonguay, A., Kaiserman, M., Spiegelhalder, B., and Preussmann, R. (1990*a*). Tobacco-specific nitrosamines in Canadian cigarettes. *Cancer Res. Clin. Oncology*, **116**, 563–8.

Fisher, S., Spiegelhalder, B., and Preussmann, R. (1990*b*). Tobacco-specific nitrosamines in European and USA cigarettes. *Archiv Geschwulstforshung*, **60**, 169–77.

Fukumoto, M., Kubo, H., and Ogamo, A. (1997). Determination of nicotine content of popular cigarettes. *Veterinary and Human Toxicology*, **39**, 225–7.

Giovino, G. A. (2002). Epidemiology of tobacco use in the United States. *Oncogene*, **21**, 7326–40.

Gray, N., Zaridze, D., Robertson, C., Krivosheva, L., Sigaccieva, N., Boyle, P., and The International Cigarette Variation Group (2000). Variation within global cigarette brands in tar, nicotine and certain nitrosamines: Analytic study. Letters to the Editor. *Tob. Control*, **9**, 351.

Gray, N. and Boyle, P. (2002). Regulation of cigarette emissions. Editorial. *Annales Oncology*, **13**, 19–21.

Hecht, S. S. (1998). Biochemistry, biology, and carcinogenicity of tobacco-specific *N*-nitrosamines. *Chem. Res. Toxicol.*, **11**, 559–603.

Hecht, S. S. (1999). Tobacco smoke carcinogens and lung cancer. *J. Natl. Cancer Inst.*, **91**, 1194–210.

Henningfield, J. E., Kozlowski, L. T., and Benowitz, N. L. (1994). A proposal to develop meaningful labeling for cigarettes. *J. Am. Med. Assoc.*, **272**, 312–14.

Henningfield, J. E., Radzius, A., and Cone, E. J. (1995). Estimation of available nicotine content of six smokeless tobacco products. *Tob. Control*, **4**, 62–6.

Henningfield, J. E., Fant, R. V., Eadzius, A., and Frost, S. (1999). Nicotine concentration, smoke pH and whole tobacco aqueous pH of some cigar brands and tobacco types popular in the United Sates. *Nicotine and Tob. Res.*, **1**, 163–8.

Henningfield, J. E. and Fagerström, K. (2001). Swedish Match Company, Swedish snus and public health: A harm reduction experiment in progress? *Tobacco Control*, **10**, 253–7.

Hoffmann, D., Brunnemann, K. D., Prokopczyk, B., and Djordjevic, M. V. (1994). Tobacco-specific *N*-nitrosamines and areca-derived N-nitrosamines: Chemistry, biochemistry, carcinogenicity, and relevance to humans. *Journal of Toxicology and Environmental Health*, **41**, 1–52.

Hoffmann, D., Djordjevic, M. V., and Brunnemann, K. D. (1996). Changes in cigarette design and composition over time and how they influence the yields of smoking constituents. In: *Smoking and tobacco control monograph no. 7: The FTC cigarette test method for determining tar, nicotine, and carbon monoxide yields of US. cigarettes.* pp. 15–37. U.S. Department of Health and Human Services, Public Health Service, National Institutes of Health, National Cancer Institute.

Hoffmann, D. and Hoffmann, I. (1997). Changing cigarettes. 1950–1995. *J. Toxicol. Environ. Health*, **50**, 307–64.

Hoffmann, D. and Hoffmann, I. (2001). The changing cigarette: Chemical studies and bioassays. In: *Smoking and tobacco control monograph no. 13: Risks associated with smoking cigarettes with low machine-measured yields of tar and nicotine.* U.S. Department of Health and Human Services. Public Health Service. National Institutes of Health, National Cancer Institute, pp. 159–91.

International Agency for Research on Cancer (1986). Tobacco Smoking. *IARC monographs on the evaluation of the carcinogenic risks to humans*, Vol. 38, p. 61. International Agency for Research on Cancer, Lyon, France.

International Agency for Research on Cancer (2002). Tobacco Smoke and Voluntary Smoking. *IARC monographs on the evaluation of the carcinogenic risks to humans*. Vol. 83. International Agency for Research on Cancer, Lyon, France. http://monographs.iarc.fr/htdocs/indexes/vol83index.html

International Committee for Cigar Smoke Study (1974). Machine smoking of cigars. *CORESTA Inform. Bull.*, **1**, 31–4.

Jarvis, M. J. (2001). Trend in sales weighted tar, nicotine, and carbon monoxide yields of UK cigarettes. *Thorax*, **56**, 960–3.

Jemal, A., Thomas, A., Murray, T., and Thun, M. (2002). Cancer statistics, 2002. *CA Cancer J. Clin.*, **52**, 23–47.

Kaiserman, M. J. and Rickert, W. S. (1992*a*). Carcinogens in tobacco smoke: Benzo(*a*)pyrene from Canadian cigarettes and cigarette tobacco. *Am. J. Publ. Health*, **82**, 1023–6.

Kaiserman, M. J. and Rickert, W. S. (1992*b*). Hand made cigarettes. It's the tube that counts. *Am. J. Publ. Health*, **87**, 107–9.

Kozlowski, L. T., Mehta, N. Y., Sweeney, C. T., Schwartz, S. S., Vogler, Jarvis, M. J., and West, R. J. (1998). Filter ventilation and nicotine content of tobacco of cigarettes from Canada, the United Kingdom, the United States. *Tob. Control*, **7**, 369–75.

2000 Maxwell Tobacco Fact Book (Table 15, RYO; Table 3, cigarettes; Table 9, cigars). 2000SpecComm International, Inc. (USA).

Malson, J. L., Sims, K., Murty, R., and Pickworth, W. B. (2001). Comparison of the nicotine content of tobacco used in bidis and conventional cigarettes. *Tob. Control*, **10**, 181–3.

Malson, J. L. and Pickworth, W. B. (2002). Bidis-hand-rolled, Indian cigarettes: Effects on physiological, biochemical and subjective measures. *Pharmacology, Biochemistry and Behavior*, **72**, 443–7.

Malson, J. L., Lee, E. M., Moolchan, E. T., and Pickworth, W. B. (2002). Nicotine delivery from smoking bidis and an additive-free cigarettes. *Nic. Tob. Res.*, **4**, 485–90.

Melikian, A. A., Djordjevic, M. V., Chen, S., Hosey, J., Zhang, J., Muscat, Hoffmann, D., and Stellman, S. D. (2002). The relationships of smoking behavior and mainstream cigarette smoke yields of toxic chemicals: Comparison between men and women. *56th Tobacco Science Research Conference*, Poster # 14, Lexington, KY, Sept. 29–Oct. 02, 2002.

Mitacek, E., Brunnemann, K. D., and Poledanak, A. P. (1990). 'Tar', nicotine, and carbon monoxide content in Thai cigarettes, and implications for cancer prevention in Thailand. *Cancer Detect. Prev.*, **14**, 515–20.

Mitacek, E., Brunnemann, K. D., Poledanak, A. P., Hoffmann, D., and Suttajit, M. (1991). Composition of popular tobacco products in Thailand and its relevance to disease prevention. *Prev. Med.*, **20**, 764–73.

Nair, J., Pakhale, S. S., and Bhide, S. V. (1989). Carcinogenic tobacco-specific nitrosamines in Indian tobacco products. *Fd. Chem. Toxic.*, **27**, 751–3.

Pakhale, S. S., Jayant, K., and Bhide, S. V. (1989). Total Particulate matter and nicotine in Indian bidis and cigarettes: A comparative study of standard machine estimates and exposure levels in smokers in Bombay. *Indian J. Cancer*, **26**, 227–32.

Peele, D. M., Danehower, D. A., and Goins, G. D. (1995). Chemical and biochemical changes during flue curing. *Rec. Adv. Tob. Sci.*, **21**, 81–133.

Philips, G. F. and Waller, R. E. (1991). Yields of tar and other smoke components from UK cigarettes. *Fd. Chem. Toxic.*, **29**, 469–74.

Pillsbury, H. C., Bright, C. C., O'Connor, K. J., and Irish, F. W. (1969). Tar and nicotine in cigarette smoke. *J. Assoc. Offic. Anal. Chem.*, **52**, 458–62.

Rickert, W. S., Robinson, J. C., Bray, D. F., Rogers, B., and Collishaw, N. (1985). Characterization of tobacco products: Comparative study of the tar, nicotine, and carbon monoxide yields of cigars, manufactured cigarettes, and cigarettes made from fine-cut tobacco. *Prev. Med.*, **14**, 226–33.

Rickert, W. S., Collishaw, N. E., Bray, D. F., and Robinson, J. C. (1986). Estimates of maximum or average cigarette tar, nicotine, and carbon monoxide yields can be obtained from yields under standard conditions. *Prev. Med.*, **15**, 82–91.

Rickert, W. S. and Kaiserman, M. J. (1999). Application of proposed Canadian test methods to the analysis of cigarette filler, fine cut tobacco, and tobacco smoke. Abstr. # 16, *53rd Tobacco Science Research Conference*, Montreal, Canada, Sept. 12–15, 1999.

Schuller, H. (1998). Nicotine and lung cancer. In: *Nicotine safety and toxicology* (ed. N. L. Benowitz), pp. 77–88. Oxford University Press.

Smith, C. J., Guy, T. D., Stiles, M. F., Morton, M. J., Collie, B. B., Ingebrethsen, B. J., and Robinson, J. H. (1998). A repeatable method for determination of carboxyhemoglobin levels in smokers. *Human and Experimental Toxicol.*, **17**, 29–34.

Stratton, K. S., Shetty, P., Wallace, R., and Bondurant S. (ed.) (2001). Products for tobacco exposure reduction. *Clearing the smoke: Assessing the science base for tobacco harm reduction*, pp. 4-1 to 4-10. National Academy Press, Washington, DC.

Tricker, A. R., Ditrich, C., and Preussmann (1991). N-nitroso compounds in cigarette tobacco and their occurrence in mainstream tobacco smoke. *Carcinogenesis*, **12**, 257–61.

Tso, T. C. (1990). Organic metabolism—alkaloids. In: *Production, physiology and biochemistry of tobacco plant*, pp. 427–86. IDEALS, Inc. Institute of International Development & Education in Agriculture and Life sciences. Beltsville, MD.

U.S. Federal Trade Commission. Part III. (1997). Cigarette Testing: Request for Public Comment; Notice. *Federal Register*, September 12, 1997.

U.S. Federal Trade Commission (2000). 'Tar', nicotine, and carbon monoxide of the smoke of 1294 varieties of domestic cigarettes for the year 1998. FTC, Washington, DC.

U.S. Centers for Disease Control (CDC) (2002). Annual smoking-attributable mortality, years of potential life lost, and economic costs—United States, 1995–1999. *Morbidity and Mortality Weakly Reports (MMWR)*, **51**, 300–3.

West, K. A., Brognard, Clark, A. S., Linnoila, I. R., Yang, X., Swain, S. M., Harris, C., Belinski, S., and Dennis, P. A. (2003). Rapid Akt activation by nicotine and a tobacco carcinogen modulates the phenotype of normal human airway epithelial cells. *J. Clin. Invest.*, **111**, 81–90.

Wiernik, A., Christakopolous, A., and Johansson, L. (1995). Effect of air curing on the chemical composition of tobacco. *Rec. Adv. Tob. Sci.*, **21**, 39–80.

World Health Organization (1997). *Tobacco or health, a global status report*. WHO, Geneva.

Part 4

Tobacco use: Prevalence, trends, influences

Chapter 10

Tobacco in Great Britain

Patti White

The British love affair with tobacco began in the sixteenth century with the pipe smoking Elizabethan pirates who sailed with Hawkins and Drake. While many mid-sixteenth century Europeans were exploring the supposed curative properties of tobacco, the English seized upon this new import from the Americas as a substance to be enjoyed. By the end of Elizabeth I's reign, smoking was observed in all classes of society (Corti 1931).

Elizabeth's successor, James I, is renown for fulminating against smoking in his *A Counterblaste to Tobacco* (1604) but, not for the last time, the commercial value of tobacco ultimately overcame all objections. The sale of tobacco grown in the Jamestown colony became the saviour of the whole English colonial enterprise in America (Borio 1998). By the late 1620s about 500 000 lbs of Virginia tobacco were being imported into London every year; the tobacco trade was a major business by the second half of the century (RCP 2000).

Snuff taking, a French habit that became fashionable with the restoration of the monarchy in the latter seventeenth century, gave way to the rise of the cigar in the nineteenth century. A popular culture of smoking emerged accompanied by the publication of pamphlets, books, and periodical articles preaching the 'art of smoking' to the expanding middle class.

The cigarette, initially seen as rather effeminate, had been brought to England by soldiers returning from the Crimean War (1853–56). In 1854, Philip Morris, a Bond Street tobacconist, began to manufacture his own brand of handmade cigarettes and in 1880, Richard Benson and William Hedges opened a shop nearby (Borio 2001). But it was in the twentieth century, with the mechanization of cigarette manufacture, that smoking became a mass habit.

A twentieth century epidemic

Tobacco consumption changed dramatically in Great Britain during the twentieth century, doubling in the first half of the century from 4.1 g per adult per day in 1905 to 8.8 g in 1945/46 (RCP 2000). Very few women smoked before the 1920s but the tobacco industry began marketing cigarettes to women using images of emancipation and power and smoking prevalence began to rise in the 1930s and 1940s. The highest recorded level of smoking prevalence among men was 82 per cent in 1948 (Wald and Nicolaides-Bouman 1991).

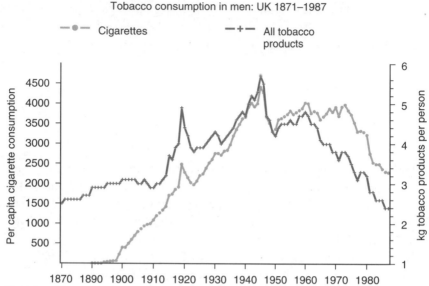

Fig.10.1 The different ways tobacco was used from the late nineteenth to late twentieth century among UK males, with the rise of the cigarette around the turn of the century and the decline of other forms of tobacco use. (The scale on the left is per capita cigarette consumption, and on the right, kilogrammes of tobacco.) (Source: M. Jarvis from Wald and Nicolaides-Bouman 1991.)

Like many other love affairs, Britain's dalliance with tobacco began to sour. The groundbreaking work of Richard Doll and Sir Austin Bradford Hill in 1950 proving the link between smoking and lung cancer attracted professional attention but went largely unreported in the British press. The government of the day not only failed to act to reduce smoking, but even went out of its way to downplay the weight of evidence. Finally, frustrated by its failure to address the problem through traditional channels, the Royal College of Physicians of London made its first intervention in a public health debate since 1725 when it had opposed cheap gin (RCP/ASH 2002). The publication of *Smoking and Health* (1962) was a landmark event in public health in the United Kingdom. Nine years later the RCP founded Action on Smoking and Health (ASH) and tobacco control advocacy moved into the public arena.

Tobacco control had a big job on its hands. By the end of the twentieth century, smoking annually caused more than 120 000 deaths in the United Kingdom of people aged 35 and older; one in five deaths at all ages. Cigarette smoking caused 46 000 deaths from cancer, 40 000 from circulatory disease and 34 000 from respiratory disease. Nine in ten lung cancer deaths in men and three in four in women were caused by smoking. Smoking caused 30 per cent of all deaths from cancer. More than two in five deaths under 65 from ischaemic heart disease and two in five from stroke were caused by smoking. Some 14 people—nine men and five women—died every hour because of their smoking (Callum 1998).

Adult smoking

Since 1972, smoking prevalence in Great Britain has been measured regularly in a nationally representative population sample as part of the General Household Survey. These surveys show that the prevalence of cigarette smoking fell substantially in the 1970s and early 1980s. Since then the decline has slowed and there has been little change in adult prevalence since 1992 (Fig. 10.2).

In December 1998, the UK government for the first time set out a comprehensive strategy to tackle smoking in its White Paper, *Smoking Kills*, and set a target for to decrease smoking prevalence in adults, school children (11–15 years), and among pregnant women in England (DH 1998). It has subsequently set targets to narrow the gap in smoking between manual and non-manual social classes (DH 2000).

Gender

Prior to the mid-1980s, men in Great Britain were much more likely to be cigarette smokers than were women, but since then the difference in prevalence has been decreasing. However, Fig 10.2 does not account for pipe or cigar smoking and British women rarely use these forms of tobacco. Taking cigar and pipe smoking into consideration, about 32 per cent of men smoke any tobacco product compared to 26 per cent of women (Walker *et al.* 2001).

Adult age groups

In 2000, cigarette smoking prevalence was highest among those aged 20–34. Prior to the 1990s, prevalence was similar in all age groups except the youngest (16–19) and the oldest (60 and over) (Walker *et al.* 2001).

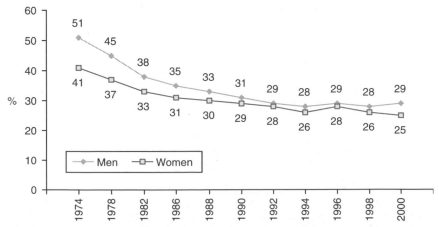

Fig. 10.2 Prevalence of cigarette smoking by age and sex: 1974–2000 Great Britain, Persons 16 years and over. (Source: Walker *et al.* 2001.)

Minority ethnic communities

Levels of smoking prevalence vary considerably between ethnic groups. In England in 1999, Black Caribbean, Bangladeshi, and Irish men and women all had prevalence rates above that of the general population while both Chinese men and women were much less likely to smoke (Erens *et al.* 2001). There are also large variations in smoking by sex. In South Asian communities few women smoke, but some do use oral tobacco. This is most pronounced among Bangladeshi women, only about 1 per cent of whom report smoking cigarettes, compared to over a quarter who say they chew tobacco (Erens *et al.* 2001).

Region

Cigarette smoking prevalence has tended to be higher in Scotland than in England and Wales, at least since regular national surveys of smoking prevalence began in the 1970s. In 2000, about 30 per cent of men in Scotland smoked compared with 29 per cent in England and 25 per cent in Wales. For women, the figures were 30, 25, and 24 per cent, respectively (Walker *et al.* 2001).

Young people

Regular surveys of smoking among schoolchildren aged 11–15 have been carried out in Great Britain since 1982. In nearly 20 years, regular smoking—defined as usually smoking one cigarette a week—has fluctuated, but has been fairly stable (Fig. 10.3).

One notable feature has been that since the mid-1980s, girls have been more likely than boys to be regular smokers, although boys smoke more. In the 2000 survey,

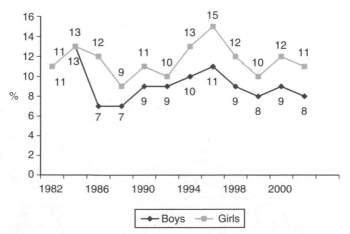

Fig. 10.3 Cigarette smoking by sex, secondary school children in England 1982–2001. (Source: Department of Health 2002.)

boys who were regular smokers reported smoking 50 cigarettes in the past week compared with girls' 44. The number of cigarettes smoked by regular smokers has been stable since 1982 (DH 2001).

Smoking prevalence increases sharply with age: in 2001, about 1 per cent of 11 year olds smoked regularly compared with 22 per cent of 15 year olds (DH 2002). Gender differences in regular smoking appear about age 13 and are maintained at 14 and 15.

Laws prohibiting the sale of tobacco to young people have existed since 1908, and currently under the Children and Young Persons (Protection from Tobacco) Act 1991, it is an offence to sell any tobacco product to anyone under the age of 16. In 2000, 80 per cent of regular underage smokers said they usually bought cigarettes from shops. This proportion is lower than the period 1982–98, but greater proportions of pupils mentioning other sources of cigarettes, such as purchasing from vending machines or friends, has broadly increased over that period (DH 2001).

Socio-economic group

A clear social class gradient in smoking prevalence has existed in Great Britain for more than 20 years. The general decline in smoking in the last quarter century has been less pronounced among those in manual occupational groups and as a result smoking has become increasingly concentrated in these groups. In 2000, in social class I (professional), around 15 per cent of men and 13 per cent of women smoke cigarettes; in social class V (unskilled manual), prevalence among men is 39 per cent and 34 per cent among women (Walker *et al.* 2001). These figures, however, disguise very high prevalence rates among the most deprived groups—such as lone mothers living on state benefit—among whom prevalence reaches over 70 per cent (Marsh and Mackay 1994).

Smoking and deprivation

The government has identified smoking as the greatest single factor contributing to the gap in healthy life expectancy between the best and the worst off (DH 1998). Among men, smoking accounts for over half of the difference in risk of premature death between the social classes. Premature deaths from lung cancer are five times higher among men in unskilled manual compared with those in professional work (Jarvis and Wardel 1999).

The success of better-off smokers is not due to motivation. Surveys have shown consistently that about seven in ten smokers in England say they want to stop smoking and those in lower socio-economic groups are just as motivated to quit as those in professional groups. There is evidence to suggest both from survey data and from quantitative measures that nicotine dependence increases with deprivation (Jarvis and Wardel 1999). As part of its comprehensive tobacco programme, the government has made pharmaceutical aids to quit smoking available on National Health Service prescription. It has also funded, through the NHS since 2000, a national network of smoking cessation services that are free of charge.

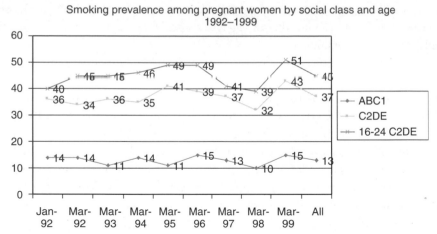

Fig. 10.4 Prevalence of cigarette smoking among pregnant women by social class and age: 1992–1999. (Source: Owen and Penn 1999.)

Smoking in pregnancy

From 1992 to 2000, the Health Education Authority (HEA) conducted annual surveys among pregnant women in England. The proportion of pregnant smokers fluctuated over that time (Owen and Penn 1999). In 1999 nearly a third of women (31.5%) smoked during pregnancy compared to 27 per cent in 1992. Smoking was especially prevalent among women who were single, separated, or divorced, in social groups DE, living in rented social housing or who had left full-time education at 15 and 16 years old. In this period, smoking remained consistently high among young women from manual social groups (Fig. 10.4).

Looking at current smoking by trimester of pregnancy shows that the proportion of women who stop smoking during pregnancy is small; stopping tends to happen in the first trimester. On average across the nine surveys, 32 per cent of women were smoking in the first trimester, compared with 27 per cent in the second trimester and 25 per cent in the third (Owen and Penn 1999).

Conclusion

Britain has had a long association with tobacco, both through trade and domestic use. After the declines in cigarette smoking prevalence of the last quarter century, it would be tempting to think that the affair was drawing to an end, but it is far from over. Over a quarter of the adult population still smokes cigarettes and there has been little change in prevalence over a decade. Smoking is stubbornly high among pregnant women, secondary schoolchildren and the most disadvantaged members of society. The UK government has set its sights on cutting deaths from coronary heart disease and cancer, and bringing about better equality in health among all members of society. While it has put in place a number of new initiatives to help achieve this, health professionals and advocates in the UK will have to apply themselves with urgency and vigour to bring a four centuries-old affair to an end.

References

Borio, G. (1998). *A brief history of Jamestown, Virginia.*
    http://www.tobacco.org/resources/history/Jamestown.html.

Borio, G. (2001). *Tobacco timeline.* http://www.tobacco.org/resources/history.

Callum, C. (1998). *The UK smoking epidemic: deaths in 1995.* HEA, London.

Department of Health (1998). *Smoking kills: a White Paper on tobacco.* The Stationery Office, London.

Department of Health (2000). *The cancer plan.* The Stationery Office, London.

Department of Health (2001). *Smoking, drinking and drug use among young people in England in 2000.* The Stationery Office.

Department of Health (2002). *Drug use, smoking and drinking among young people in England in 2001: preliminary results.* Statistical Press Notice 15/3/02.

Erens, B., Primatesta, P., and Prior, G. (2001). *Health Survey for England: the health of minority ethnic groups 1999.* The Stationery Office, London.

Jarvis, M. and Wardel, J. (1999). Social patterning of individual health behaviours: the case of cigarette smoking. In: *Social determinants of health* (ed. M. Marmot and R. Wilkinson). Oxford University Press, Oxford.

Marsh, A. and McKay, S. (1994). *Poor smokers.* Policy Studies Institute, London.

Owen, L. and McNeill, A. (2001). Saliva cotinine as indicator of cigarette smoking in pregnant women. *Addiction* **96**, 1001–6.

Owen, L. and Penn, G. (1999). *Smoking and pregnancy: a survey of knowledge, attitudes and behaviour 1992–1999.* Health Education Authority, London.

Royal College of Physicians (2000). *Nicotine addiction in Britain.* Royal College of Physicians of London, London.

Royal College of Physicians and ASH (2002). *Forty fatal years.* Royal College of Physicians of London, London.

Walker, A., Maher, J., Coulthard, M., Goddard, E., and Thomas, M. (2001). *Living in Britain: results from the 2000 general household survey.* National statistics. The Stationery Office, London.

Chapter 11

The epidemic of tobacco use in China

Yang Honghuan

Introduction

Tobacco use was first introduced into China during the sixteenth and seventeenth century from the west, via the Philippines and Vietnam, to the south of China, and via Korea to the Northeast of China (Wu and Zhang).

During 1889, the American Tobacco Company, and 1890 the British American Company came into the Chinese market after which the domestic tobacco company started to set up. The growing of tobacco started in Taiwan province then extended to the central and southeast areas of China. During 1931–35, the area growing tobacco reached 290 000 hectare in 23 provinces, annual product of tobacco was 330 000 metric tons. Many famous film stars worked in Tobacco advertisements, smoking was accepted by Chinese society and was a fashionable activity (Chart 1).

Since 1949, all tobacco companies have become state-ownership enterprises. The Chinese government published a 'Draft of regulation on monopoly on cigarette' in 1951. China started a monopoly business of cigarette manufacture controlled by the State. In 1950 the tobacco produced was 154 000 metric ton; then it increased to 2 238 000 metric ton by 1990, when it was 33 per cent of the world's tobacco product (Food and Agricultural Organization) (WCOO). Cigarette production was 17 040 000 cartons (1 carton equal 50 000 cigarettes) in 1980, then quickly increased to 34 800 000 cartons in 1995, then decreased a little to 33 349 000 cartons in 2000. The cigarettes were mainly sold in the domestic market, sales volume was 33 336 000, the tax revenue achieved 105 billion RBM (Newletter of Smoking and Health in China 2001), which was 9 per cent of total tax revenue (Fig. 11.1).

China, home of 1.2 billion people and the world's fastest growing economy, is the most sought-after target of the transnational companies. Multinational companies are moving quickly to establish themselves in China after half a century during which they withdrew from the Chinese market. In Asia, they have had the support of US trade negotiators in forcing open tobacco markets previously closed to foreign companies. Since the mid-1980s, Japan, South Korea, Thailand, and Taiwan have all given in to pressure from Washington and allowed the sale of foreign cigarettes. In Japan, foreign cigarettes now make up nearly 20 percent of the country's cigarette market. RJ Reynolds has manufactured Camel and Winston cigarettes in Chinese factories

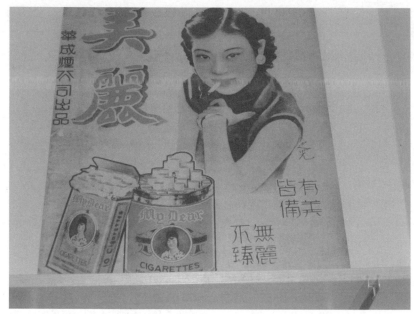

Chart 1 (From the brand of Beauty made by Hua-Chen Tobacco Company in 1925. The chart from website: Shanghai.online.sh.cn/business/shzz/shzz-03.htm)

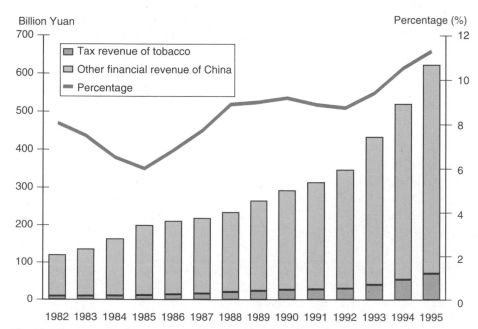

Fig. 11.1 Revenue of tobacco compared with national total revenue, 1982–95.

since the late 1980s. In 2001, Philip Morris reached an agreement with the Chinese government-run tobacco company to manufacture Marlboro and other PM brands in China (Shenon 1984).

In the background, the prevalence of tobacco use was quickly increasing, and the hazards of tobacco use were starting to appear.

Prevalence of tobacco use

General picture

There was no national picture on tobacco-use behavior before the 1984' national survey. The World Health Organization estimated annual per capita consumption of cigarettes per Chinese adult 15 years of age and above to be 730 in 1970–72, 1290 in 1980–82, and 1900 in 1990–92 (WHO).

In 1984 the first national survey on the prevalence of tobacco use was carried out by the National Patriotic Health Campaign Committee, which covered all 29 provinces, autonomous regions and municipalities. 519 600 persons (258 422 males and 261 178 females) aged 15 years and above surveyed by stratified random sampling. The average smoking rate among Chinese was 34.45 per cent, with 61.01 per cent for males and 7.04 per cent for females (Weng 1987). The average number of cigarettes was 13 per day for males and 11 per day for females. The 1996 national prevalence survey on smoking behavior was conducted in all urban and rural areas of the Mainland China. The total sample size was 130 657 by three-stage probability sample. Of the originally sampled population of 128 766, a total of 120 783 (93.8%) persons provided complete data and were included in the final analysis. There were 63 793 male and 56 020 female participants (with 485 not identifying gender), of whom two-thirds came from rural and one-third from urban areas. The indicators for smoking rates were based on the WHO classification of smoking definitions: *ever smokers* included persons who had ever smoked for at least 6 months during their lives; *current smokers* were smoking tobacco products at the time of the survey; *regular smokers* were persons smoking at least one cigarette daily; and *heavy smokers* at the time of the survey smoked at least 20 cigarettes daily (World Health Organization 1983). *Passive smoke exposure* was defined as being exposed to another person while he or she is smoking for at least 15 minutes daily for more than 1 day per week. Overall smoking rates were calculated using a pre-weighting method and with age-standardization to the 1990 national census (Chinese Academy of Preventive Medicine 1996).

In the 1996 survey, overall prevalence rates for smokers were 66.9% for males and 4.2% for females, with an overall prevalence of 37.6% among China's population older than 15 years of age. Most smokers started smoking at the age of 20, three years younger than what was found in the 1984 national survey. Daily per capita consumption in 1996 was 15 cigarettes, two cigarettes more per day than in 1984. The age of starting to smoke increased with age in both men and women. Compared to 1984,

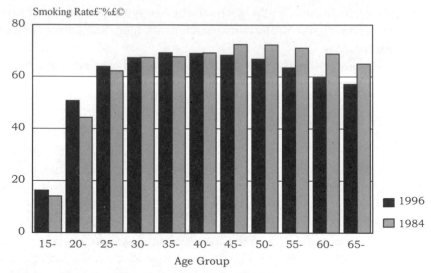

Fig. 11.2 Prevalence of smoking in males, 1996 vs. 1984.

the regular smoking rate of 35.1% for 1996 was higher by 3.4%. The prevalence of smoking increased in males less than 30 years old, and decreased in those older than 45 years compared with the data from 1984 (Fig. 11.2). Between the two surveys, the ages at which males and females reported starting to smoke dropped by about three years. For men, the average age of starting to smoke in the 1996 data was about 19 years compared to about 22 years in 1984. For women, the age of starting to smoke dropped from 28 years to 25 years (Yang *et al.* 1999). Similar results have been obtained from other epidemiological surveys, such as 1991 national survey on prevalence of hypertension, which reported the current smoking rate (Wu *et al.* 1995). Based on the results of the 1996 survey, more than 300 million men and 20 million women smokers were estimated, making China the world's largest actual and potential national market for cigarettes. In 1994 about 1.7 trillion cigarettes were produced in China and about 900 million were imported (WHO 1997). In detail smoking behavior from the 1996 survey is as follows:

♦ Smoking rates increased rapidly from 18% among those 15–19 years old, to 55% in the next 5-year age category, while for women, the smoking prevalence increased slowly to about 5% at 45 years of age and then more rapidly to over 14% for those 65 years of age and older. In older males, the current smoking rate declined as the percentage of ex-smokers increased.

♦ The average number of cigarettes smoked per day by men rose from about 2 per day at 15–19 years of age to 12 cigarettes a day at 20–25 years, and then up to an average of 15 cigarettes per day by age 30 years. Women smoked slightly more than 10 cigarettes per day at all ages above 20 years of age.

◆ Among males, smoking rates were lowest among those with at least a college education (54.2%) and highest among those with no more than primary schooling (72.4%). Smoking rates among males also varied by occupational group. Over 70% of farmers, factory workers, service people, private company employees, those self-employed, and the floating or itinerant population with no fixed residence were smokers. Smoking rates for male health professionals (60%) and male teachers (56%)—two key groups of male role models for prevention—were also high. Among women, smoking rates by occupation were distinctly different, with the highest rates among retired persons (11%), and those working at home (8%).

◆ The smoking rate for rural males (68.4%) was slightly higher than for urban males (64%) at all ages. Older women living in urban areas smoked more than women in rural areas, with a peak prevalence rate of 16% at age 65 years. Regional distributions show that among males, smoking rates were high throughout China, but especially so in the southwest. For females, there was significant variation in smoking rates by region, with the highest rates in the northeast and north of China (10.2%) and the lowest (2.5%) in the south.

◆ Most smokers used filtered cigarettes, which dominated the market, especially among the young. Only about 20% of the men and women smoked unfiltered brands. Smoking practices varied across the country, reflecting different cultural practices by ethnic groups. The Chinese pipe was commonly smoked in particular areas, primarily the south and southeast, and hand-rolled cigarettes were used in the northeast, where for example, 20% of older men and middle-aged women smoked pipe tobacco.

Smoking in women

The prevalence of tobacco use in Chinese women was lower than in men, which was related to the social and cultural background of China. However, the prevalence of tobacco use was not same for different generations of women. There were several stages: the prevalence among women born in 1921–40 was higher, almost 10–15 per cent, which was consistent with the tobacco industry's marketing strategy during 1930–40. Meanwhile the prevalence of tobacco use was higher among the Northeast women than in other areas and was similar to tobacco use from Korea to the Northeast. The reason for this is worth studying.

Smoking in adolescence

In recent years there have been over ten studies on smoking prevalence and smoking-related knowledge, attitudes and behaviors among adolescents in China, including the Global Youth Tobacco Survey (GYTS) (Wang *et al.* 1994; Li *et al.* 1999; Warren *et al.* 2000) and a 1998 survey which covered 12 urban areas and 12 rural areas located in 16 provinces. The GYTS included over 10 000 students aged 13–15 years, from four cities. The 1998 survey primarily focused on middle school students, but also included non-students of middle school age in the 12 rural areas. The survey outlined the transition from non-smoker to smoker among adolescent.

• Overall, the reported prevalence rates of experimenting were 47.8% for boys and 12.8% for girls aged 12–18; the corresponding figures for ever-smoking were 9.4% for boys and 0.6% for girls (Yang *et al.* in press). The China GYTS also indicated that 32.5% of the male students and 13% of the female students aged 12–15 had tried smoking and the average age of smoking initiation was 10.7 years of age (Warren *et al.* 2000). There was a slight increase of prevalence among middle school students in a later survey compared with earlier surveys; the smoking rate among male students was still significantly higher than that of the female students, but the smoking rate among female students in the big cities of China is increasing.

• The prevalence of experimenting increased sharply with age for boys and the majority of 15–16-year-olds had experimented. While the prevalence of experimenting also increased with age for girls, less than 20% of 15–16-year-olds had experimented.

• By region, the prevalence rates of experimenting for boys were similar in the urban and rural locations (48.1% vs. 47.4% respectively) (Table 11.1). For girls, the prevalence rates for experimenting were twice as high in the urban areas (15.6%) compared with the rural areas (7.6%).

• With regard to the age of initiation, about 6% of boys and 2% of girls took their first puffs by age 10 years, and 3% of boys and 0.3% of girls were smoking by age 15 years.

• The source of the first cigarette smoked was most commonly peers (44.0%); another 18.5% obtained the cigarette themselves and only 4.6% obtained the cigarette from a family member.

• The major of reasons for initiation of smoking were (1) out of curiosity, (2) due to peer pressure, and (3) because of the need of social interaction.

• The China GYTS indicated that 92% of the students surveyed believed that smoking is harmful to people's health and 81% believed that passive smoking is harmful. About 85% of the students said that their parents had advised them not to smoke (Warren *et al.* 2000). But there was not an association between knowledge and behavior for tobacco-use.

• From 1988 to 2000 several studies also focused on the factors related to the beginning of smoking among adolescents. A variety of risk factors may push young people to begin smoking, while other factors may steer them away from smoking. Weak performance in school was a relevant personal factor associated with experimenting. Peer smoking and school performance were even stronger determinants for becoming a smoker than for experimenting (Zhu *et al.* 1988; Crowe *et al.* 1994; Osaki *et al.* 1999). Outside environmental factors, such as cigarette advertising were related to attitudes on smoking in adolescence (Lam *et al.* 1998). And social-economical,

Table 11.1 Smoking among adolescents in China

	Male (n = 11 378)						Female (n = 9932)					
	Puff		Ever		Current		Puff		Ever		Current	
	No.	%	No.	%	No.	%	No.	%	No.	%	No.	%
Total	5441	47.8	1074	9.4	984	8.6	1267	12.8	55	0.6	43	0.4
Urban	3222	28.3	696	6.1	637	5.6	998	10.0	49	0.5	40	0.4
Rural	2219	19.5	378	3.3	347	3.0	269	2.7	6	0.06	3	0.03
Nun student	228	2.0	106	0.9	102	0.9	13	0.1	0	0	0	0

Source: Yang GH, Ma JM, Jon Samet, et al. Smoking in adolescent in China, *J. British Medicine* (in press).

cultural, and other environmental factors, such as the social norms on smoking also related to smoking behavior among adolescents (Sun *et al.* 1997).

Smoking cessation

Cessation can prevent some deaths related to tobacco use, but there are many barriers to it. The picture of cessation among Chinese smokers was different from western countries. Systematic large-scale research on cessation was not very plentiful, but the 1996 survey drew an outline of the cessation process among Chinese smokers (Yang *et al.* 2001).

+ Only 16.76 per cent current smokers wanted to quit the habit, but without any plan;

+ The proportion of quitting and relapse were almost equal. 9.5 per cent of ever smokers were quitting, another 10.6 per cent quit once but were smoking at the survey.

+ Only 3.5 per cent among ever-smokers have currently quit successfully for at least 2 years.

+ The numbers of those willing to quit, trying to quit, and successfully quitting increased with age. There are very obvious differences between groups with different educational levels and occupations.

+ The most common reason for quitting was illness, which explained why the rate of quitting was higher in older people.

+ Among the students who smoke, 72% said that they wanted to quit, but only 58% of them had tried to quit. Their reasons for trying to quit were (1) because of the harmfulness of tobacco use to their health (66%), (2) due to the opposition to smoke from parents and friends (16%), and (3) to save money (Warren *et al.* 2000).

In summary, the percentage of former smokers and smokers contemplating quitting was low in China.

Environmental tobacco smoke exposure

Various methods were used in describing prevalence of environmental tobacco smoke exposure in China. They range from simple questionnaire reports to measurements of tobacco combustion products in air of indoor environments and of biomarkers of tobacco smoke in human fluids and tissues. Studies comparing questionnaire indexes of ETS exposure to levels of biomarkers have shown that these different indicators are correlated, although their results are not perfectly concordant. The term passive smoking was used to describe ETS exposure as measured by the questionnaire.

In China there were large-scale epidemiological surveys on ETS exposure with questionnaires, such as 1996 national survey, and small-scale epidemiological survey with biomarkers.

In the 1996 national survey in China, of all current non-smokers, 53.58% reported exposure to ETS, defined as being in the presence of passive smoke at least 15 minutes per day on more than one day a week. The prevalence rate of ETS exposure in females

(57%) was higher than in males (45%). The highest prevalence of exposure to ETS was in women in the reproductive age range, up to 60%, with higher exposure in younger groups than in older age groups. The majority of passive smokers were exposed to ETS every day, with 71.2% reporting exposure at home, 25.0% reporting ETS exposure in their work environments, and 32.5% in public places (multiple choices offered) (Chinese Academy of Preventive Medicine 1996). The level was higher compared with that in other countries, such as the United States (37% in men and women over 18 years in 1993, and 31% in 1997) (Yang et al. 1999).

ETS exposure in children is strongly associated with a number of adverse effects, particularly involving the respiratory tract. The vast majority of children exposed to tobacco smoke do not choose to be exposed. Children's exposure is involuntary, arising from smoking, mainly by adults, in places where children live, work, and play. Unfortunately there were a few reports on ETS exposure in Chinese children. A survey on distribution, frequency, and intensity of asthma was carried out among 71 867 subjects in six areas of Guangdong province. The overall prevalence rate was 0.94%. The group with high prevalence of asthma focused on children less than 7 years old. Among patients with asthma frequent exposure to side-stream smoke was reported by 54.7% (Tang et al. 2000). A cross-sectional survey on 1449 never-smoking pregnant women who made their first prenatal visit to the Women and Children's Hospital of Guangzhou, China during 1996–97, found that 60.2% (95% Confidence Interval 57.7–62.7%) of the never-smoking pregnant women had a husband who currently smoked. Women with smoking husbands ($n=872$) were more exposed to ETS than those with non-smoking husbands ($n=577$) at home (71% vs. 33%), in public places (77% vs. 66%), and at work (60% vs. 50% of working women), and they took less action against passive smoking in public places (Loke et al. 2000). In general passive smoking is an important public health problem in China, especially in women and children.

Summary

The present situation of tobacco use in China is alarming from a public health perspective. On the one hand, tobacco use is on the increase in China while it is decreasing steadily in most of the developed countries. On the other hand, smoking rates among women may be relatively low at present, but it is most likely to go up when big international tobacco companies swarm into China when China enters the World Trade Organization. The big international tobacco companies will undoubtedly target Chinese women and adolescents. This situation requires strategic efforts to reduce tobacco use among men and control the possible increase among women and youth.

The hazards of tobacco use

The most useful epidemiological studies for assessing the health risks of tobacco were cohort studies initiated in the 1950s, 1960s, and 1970s, with follow-up mortality analyses pertaining to this period as well (Peto et al. 1994). In the USA, UK, and Canada, where men had been smoking in large numbers for decades before these studies were carried out, smoking was typically associated with a 70–80% excess mortality from all causes.

In China a report from long-term disease surveillance pointed out that the diseases related to tobacco use, such as lung cancer, stroke, and COPD had been increasing. Mortality rate of lung cancer was on average increasing 4.5 per cent each year since 1990 (Chinese Academy of Preventive Medicine).

In China there were a series of epidemiological studies on tobacco and mortality, first in Shanghai (Gao *et al.* 1987; Zhong *et al.* 1999), then the world's largest retrospective and prospective studies were carried out by researchers from two leading Chinese scientific institutions (Chinese Academy of Preventive Medicine and Chinese Academy of Medical Sciences) in collaboration with researchers from Oxford University, England and Cornell University, USA. This retrospective study of novel design interviewed the families of one million dead people to find out whether the dead person had smoked. In addition an ongoing nationally representative prospective study, in which a quarter of a million adults were interviewed about their own smoking habits, have been followed for several years to see what they die from. The objective was to assess the hazards at an early phase of the growing epidemic of deaths from tobacco in China and, by continuing the prospective study for another few decades, to monitor the future growth of the epidemic. The retrospective study compared the smoking habits of 0.7 million adults who had died of cancer, respiratory or vascular causes with those of a 'reference group' of 0.2 million adults who had died of other causes (calculating, for example, the excess risk of lung cancer among smokers from the excess of smokers among those who had died from lung cancer). The fieldwork involved over 500 interviewers in 24 major cities and 74 rural counties that are reasonably nationally representative of China.

The prospective study sought out a quarter of a million men aged over 40 from nationally representative disease surveillance points and weighed, measured, interviewed, and carried out medical tests on 225 000 persons. Mortality and causes of death have been monitored by annual visits. This prospective study will continue for decades, tracing the growth of the epidemic.

Its preliminary results confirm the more detailed findings of the retrospective study. The key findings from the retrospective study are the following:

There was 51 per cent excess of cancer deaths, 31 per cent excess of respiratory deaths, and 15 per cent excess of vascular deaths among male smokers aged 35–69. There was 39 per cent excess of cancer deaths, 54 per cent excess of respiratory deaths, and 6 per cent excess of vascular deaths among male smokers aged 70 and over. Fewer females smoked, but those who did had smoking-attributed risks of lung cancer and respiratory disease about as great as for males (Liu *et al.* 1998). The main way that smoking kills people in China is by making diseases that are already common, even more common. For example, among men in urban China those smoking more than

20 cigarettes a day had double the non-smoker TB death rates. So, in 1990, tobacco caused 0.6 million Chinese deaths, 0.3 million deaths at ages 35–69, increasing to 0.8 million in the year 2000 of which 0.4 million at ages 35–69. The tobacco deaths were 12 per cent of total deaths for male, and 3 per cent for female.

When the young smokers of today reach old age, tobacco will be causing about 3 million deaths a year, 33 per cent of male deaths and 1 per cent of female deaths.

The main findings from the prospective study were that the overall mortality was greatest among those who started smoking in early adult life; the excess mortality among smokers chiefly involved cancer, respiratory and vascular disease; and these associations are largely causal, so tobacco currently causes 12% of all male deaths in China. The overall risk ratio for smokers starting before the age of 20 is already 1.34, implying that even at current death rates about 1 in 4 smokers will be killed by tobacco. But, this risk ratio has already grown much bigger in the cities and will do likewise in rural areas, as the generations that did not smoke cigarettes regularly are succeeded by the generations that have done so. In urban areas, where a greater proportion of tobacco use involves cigarettes, the risk ratio for those who began before age 20 is already approaching 2, suggesting that half of all smokers will be killed by tobacco (Niu *et al.* 1998).

In general, the prospective study and the retrospective study both indicate that in the early 1990s smoking was already responsible for about 12% of all adult male deaths, which currently corresponds to 0.7 million male deaths, plus about 3% (0.1 million) of all adult female deaths. The current health effects, however, chiefly reflect past smoking patterns. On present smoking patterns, the death rates of smokers will become double those of nonsmokers of the same age, suggesting that about half of today's young smokers will eventually be killed by tobacco.

References

Chinese Academy of Preventive Medicine, Ministry of Health, *et al.* (1996). National survey on prevalence of smoking in China. China Science and Technology Press, August 1997.

Chinese Academy of Preventive Medicine, Ministry of Health, A serious of surveillance report from National System of Disease Surveillance Points, Yang GH, editor in chief, Beijing Medical University and Chinese Union Medical University Press, Nov., in 1990–2001.

Crowe, J. W., Torabi, M. R., and Nakornkhet, N. (1994). Cross-cultural study of samples of adolescents' attitudes, knowledge, and behaviors related to smoking. *Psychol Rep*, Dec, **75**(3 Pt 1), 1155–61.

Food and Agriculture Organization. Statistical database.

Gao, Y. T., Blot, W. J., Zheng, W., Ershow, A. G., Hsu, C. W., Levin, L. I., *et al.* (1987). Lung cancer among Chinese women. *Int J Cancer*, **40**, 604–9.

Lam, T. H., Chung, S. F., Betson, C. L., *et al.* (1998). Tobacco advertisements: one of the strongest risk factors for smoking in Hong Kong students. *Am J Prev Med*, Apr **14**(3), 217–23.

Liu, B. Q., Peto, R., Chen, Z. M., Boreham, J., Wu, Y. P., Li, J. Y., *et al.* (1998). Emerging tobacco hazards in China: 1. Retrospective proportional mortality study of one million deaths. *BMJ*, **317**(7170), 1411–22.

Li, X., Fang, X., and Stanton, B. (1999). Cigarette smoking among schoolboys in Beijing, China. *Journal of Adolescence*, Oct, **22**(5), 621–5.

Loke, A. Y., Lam, T. H., Pan, S. C., Li, S. Y., Gao, X. J., and Song, Y. Y. (2000). Exposure to and actions against passive smoking in non-smoking pregnant women in Guangzhou, China. *Acta Obstet Gynecol Scand*, Nov, **79**(11), 947–52 Related Articles, Books, LinkOut PMID: 11207006 [PubMed—indexed for MEDLINE].

Newsletter of Smoking and Health in China, No 40, February 2001.

Niu, S. R., Yang, G. H., Chen, Z. M., Wang, J. L., He, X. Z., Schoepff, H., *et al.* (1998). Emerging tobacco hazards in China: 2. early mortality results from a prospective study. *BMJ*, **317**, 1423–4.

Osaki, Y., Minowa, M., and Mei, J. (1999). A comparison of correlates of cigarette smoking behavior between Jiangxi province, China and Japanese high school students. *J Epidemiol*, Aug, **9**(4), 254–60.

Peto, R., Lopez, A. D., Boreham, J., Thun, M., and Heath, C. (1994). *Mortality from smoking in developed countries, 1950–2000*. Oxford University Press, Oxford.

Philip Shenon, 'Asia's Having One Huge Nicotine Fit,' New York Times, May 15, 1994, sec. 4, p. 1. (sdb5/16/94) 'Mr. Butts Promotes Gender Equality'.

Sun, W. Y. and Ling, T. (1997). Smoking behavior among adolescents in the city, suburbs, and rural areas of Shanghai. *Am J Health Promot*, May-Jun, **11**(5), 331–6.

Tang, T., Ding, Y., and Zhen (2000). Epidemiological survey and analysis on bronchial asthma in Guangdong Province. *J Zhonghua Jie He He Hu Xi Za Zhi*, Dec, **23**(12), 730–3 Related Articles, Books, LinkOut.

Wang, S. Q., Yu, J. J., Zhu, B. P., Liu, M., and He, G. Q. (1994). Cigarette smoking and its risk factors among senior high school students in Beijing, China, 1988. *Tobacco Control*, **3**(2), 107–14.

Warren, C. W., Riley, L., Asma, S., Erikson, M. P., Green, L., Blanton, C., *et al.* (2000). Tobacco use by youth: A surveillance report from the global youth tobacco survey project. *Bulletin of the World Health Organization*, **78**(7), 868–76.

Weng Xinzhi Hong Zhaoguang Cheng Danyang (1987). Smoking prevalence in Chinese aged and above. *Chinese Medical Journal*, **100**(11), 886–92.

WHO (1997). The World Health Organization Report 1997. Conquering suffering; enriching humanity. Geneva.

WHO, Tobacco or Health: a global status report, P25 ISBN 92 4 156184X.

World Health Organization (1983). *Guidelines for the conduct of tobacco smoking surveys for the general population*. Report Number Technical Document No. WHO/SMO/83.4, WHO, Geneva.

Wu, X. G., Duan, X. F., Hao, D. S. H., *et al.* (1995). Prevalence of hypertension and trend in China, *Chinese Journal of Hypertension*, Apr. **3**(Suppl.), pp. 7–13.

Wu, Y., Zhang, Z. H. P. The history of tobacco in China.

Yang, G. H., Fan, L. X., Samet, J., *et al.* (1999). Smoking in China: findings of the 1996 National Prevalence Survey. *JAMA*, Oct 6, **282**(13), 1247–53.

Yang, G. H., Ma, J. M., Jon Samet, *et al.* Smoking in adolescent in China, *J British Medicine* (in press).

Yang, G. H., Ma, J. M., Samet, M. J. (2001). Smoking cessation in China: finding from the 1996 national prevalence survey, *Tobacco Control*, **10**, 170–4.

Zhong, L., Goldberg, M. S., Gao, Y. T., Jin, F. (1999). A case-control study of lung cancer and environmental tobacco smoke among nonsmoking women living in Shanghai, China. *Cancer Causes and Control*, **10**(6), 607–16.

Zhu, B. P., Liu, M., Wang, S. Q. *et al.* (1992). Cigarette smoking among junior high school students in Beijing, China, 1988. *Int J Epidemiol*, Oct, **21**(5), 854–61.

Chapter 12

Patterns of smoking in Russia

David Zaridze

Russia is the fourth largest cigarette market in the world, and one of the fastest-growing. Russians consume about 300 billion cigarettes a year. According to official statistics in 1985 Russians consumed 240 billion cigarettes.

The smoking rate in Russia was already quite high in mid-1980s, 46–48% among men and 3–12% among women (The principal investigators. The MONICA Project 1989). Since then smoking rates in men increased by about 10–15% and the rates in women have at least doubled. In the survey carried out in Karelia in 1992 (Puska *et al.* 1993), highest smoking rates were recorded among people aged 25–34 years, 77% and 20% in men and women, respectively. Proportion of smokers among men aged 35–44 and 45–54 was 61% and 68% respectively. In women, in these age groups smoking rates were lower, 13% and 3%, respectively. Lowest rates were observed in those aged 55–64 years, 57% in men and 3% in women (Table 12.1).

The results of the survey undertaken by the Russian Centre for Public Opinion Research in 1996, which covered 69 urban and rural areas and included 1599 interviews have shown that smoking is common in all areas of Russia (McKee *et al.* 1998). Among men aged 18–24 years, 65% smoked, rising to 73% in those aged 25–34 and falling steadily to reach 41% in those aged 65 years and older. Among women, smoking was much more common among young (27% in those aged 18–34) than among middle aged and elderly (5% in those aged 55+) (Table 12.1). Smoking was much more common among living in urban areas than in rural areas. Differences in smoking rates were more pronounced for women: 30%, 15–18%, 13%, and 9% among women living in Moscow, in other cities, in small towns, and rural areas, respectively.

Highest rates of smoking in women were recorded in Moscow (Levshin *et al.* 1998). According to this study 31% and 28% of women in the age 20–30 and 30–39 smoked. Among men of the same age groups 66 and 69% were smokers (Table 12.1). Kamardina *et al.* (2002) have recently reported very high rates of smoking among women in Moscow: 29% of women in the age 25–64 years are smokers. In the survey of Oganov and Tkachenko (2001) 63% of men and 10% of women in Moscow smoke. However smoking rates are much higher in men (74%) and women (25%) aged 30–35 years.

Table **12.1** Smoking prevalence (%) in Russia

Age group	Puska et al. (1993)	RLMS VI[1]	McKee et al. 1998	Levshin et al. (1998)	Zaridze et al. (in press)		
					Barnaul	Tomsk	Tyumen
Men							
15–24	NA	52	65 (18–24)	NA	NA	NA	NA
25–34	77	71	73	66 (20–29)	71	71	71
35–44	61	66	71	69 (30–39)	72	71	69
45–54	68	60	64	59 (40–49)	68	65	61
55–64	57	50	49	48 (50–59)	54	51	50
65+	NA	34	42	32 (60–69)	34	33	32
Women							
15–24	NA	17	27 (18–24)	NA	NA	NA	NA
25–34	20	17	28	31 (20–29)	18	23	22
35–44	13	11	14	28 (30–39)	13	18	16
45–54	6	7	12	20 (40–49)	9	13	10
55–64	3	2	5	11 (50–59)	3	4	3
65+	NA	1	5	2 (60–69)	2	2	1

RMLS – Russian Longitudinal Monitoring survey. (Quoted from McKee et al. 1998.)

Ignatova *et al.* (1993) reported the results of a small household survey from Chelyabinsk, based on the personal interviews of 859 men and 1222 women, among which 62% men and 5% women smoked. Alexeeva and Alexeev (2002) reported from Novosibirsk that smoking rates in men since 1985 have not changed and remained at about 60%, while smoking in women increased from 3% in 1985 to 12% in 1997.

According to the most recent survey the proportion of current, former, and never smokers in Moscow, in men aged 18–75 years is 58%, 20%, and 22% respectively. The proportion of current, former, and never smokers in women of the same age is 27%, 12%, and 62%, respectively (Levshin and Fedichkina 2001). In the study reported by McKee *et al.* (1998) the proportion of ex-smokers increased from 13% in the age groups 18–24, 25–34, and 35–44 to 34% in men aged 55–64. High proportions of ex-smokers were recorded in young women aged 18–24 and 25–34 (12% and 13%, respectively) and low proportions in women aged 45 years and older (7%).

Smoking prevalence is higher in less-educated people. Probability of smoking is higher in men who graduated secondary and primary schools, than in men with university background, relative risk for smoking being 2.6 (95%CI 1.9–3.7) among men with secondary education and 6.2 (95% CI 3.2–12.4) with primary education, in comparison with those who graduated from university (Levshin and Fedichkina 2001). McKee *et al.* (1998) did not find any association between education and smoking, however, they report higher smoking rates in economically deprived individuals. Probability of smoking was statistically significantly higher among the most deprived. Relative risk in men was 1.7 (95% CI 1.1–2.7) and 2.0 (95% CI 1.0–3.9) in women.

Smoking prevalence is very high among young clerks: 75% and 38% in men and women of 20–29 years, 79% and 38% in men and women of 30–39 years old (Levshin *et al.* 1998). Smoking rate is also quite high among physicians: 59% among men and 10% among women (Oderova 2001). Levshin *et al.* (1998) reported that proportion of smokers among male and female physicians in Moscow is 41% and 13%, respectively. Smoking rate was also very high in medical students aged 20–25 years, 44% and 29% among men and women, respectively. It is important to note that students start smoking during their tenure as medical faculty. Smoking frequency is lower among medical students in their first year in university: 24% and 6% among men and women, respectively. According to the same authors 11%. Female nurses are smokers.

Smoking habit is influenced by marital status. Probability of smoking is significantly higher among divorced, than among married men (RR 2.3, 95% CI 1.00–5.3) (Levshin and Fedichkina 2001). The smoking habit of an individual is also influenced by smoking in the family and among friends (Levshin and Fedichkina 2001). Probability of smoking is statistically significantly increased if parents, spouse, and/or friends are/were smokers.

In 1998–99 we have carried out a large household survey in Barnaul, Tomsk, and Tyumen, towns situated in western Siberia. Populations of these towns are 500 000, 350 000, and 300 000, respectively. Personal interviews on lifestyle habits including smoking and alcohol consumption were conducted with 53 097 men (20 092 in

Barnaul, 16 076 in Tomsk, 16 929 in Tyumen) and 76 968 women (29 694 in Barnaul, 22 939 in Tomsk, 24 335 in Tyumen) in the age 25 years and older. Highest proportion of smokers among men was observed in the age group 35–44 years (71% in all three towns) and in the age group 45–54 years (72% in Barnaul, 71% in Tomsk, and 69% in Tyumen). With increase in age, percentage of smokers among those interviewed declined. However, smoking rates were still quite high among elderly men: 32–34% in men 65 years and older. Proportion of ex-smokers increased with age from 5–7% among men 25–34 years of age up to 31–34% in men aged 65 years and older (Table 12.2). It should be noted that proportion and age distribution of smokers among men in these three cities were very similar (Zaridze *et al.* in press).

Smoking rates were significantly higher among young women, 18%, 23%, and 22% in Barnaul, Tomsk, and Tyumen, respectively. Proportion of current smokers was also quite high among women 35–44 years old—13%, 18%, and 16% in Barnaul, Tomsk, and

Table 12.2 Smoking prevalence in men (%) in Russia

Age	Barnaul	Tomsk	Tyumen
25–34			
Never	24.3	23.8	22.2
Ex	5.1	5.5	6.5
Current	70.6	70.7	71.3
35–44			
Never	21.5	22.3	23.0
Ex	7.0	6.9	8.0
Current	71.5	70.8	68.9
45–54			
Never	21.9	24.3	26.6
Ex	10.1	10.9	12.0
Current	67.9	64.8	61.4
55–64			
Never	26.6	29.4	28.6
Ex	18.9	20.1	21.4
Current	54.4	50.5	50.0
65+			
Never	32.7	35.8	32.3
Ex	34.7	31.0	35.8
Current	34.0	32.8	32.3
Total	20 092	16 076	16 929

Tyumen, respectively. With increasing age, the proportion of smokers declined to
1–2% among women 65 years and older. The proportion of ex-smokers was very low
in all age groups (Table 12.3).

Smoking in Russia has become a 'paediatric epidemic'. The proportion of smokers
among teenagers in Russia is very high and continues to increase, suggesting that eventually there will be a big increase in tobacco-related premature death in Russia. A survey of school children in Nalchik reported that 38% of boys and 12% of girls smoked
at least one cigarette per week (Skvortsova 2002). Surveys conducted by our group in
mid-1990s have shown that proportion of smokers among teenagers attending
secondary schools were 13%, 26%, and 49% in boys 12–13, 14–16, and 17–18 years
old, respectively. In girls, proportion of smokers is 7, 24, and 30% in age-groups 12–13,
14–16, and 17–18 years, respectively. Seventy five per cent of boys and 31% girls aged
17–18 years attending professional-technical schools were smokers (Levshin *et al.* 1998).

Table 12.3 Smoking prevalence in women (%) in Russia

Age	Barnaul	Tomsk	Tyumen
25–34			
Never	79.4	72.4	75.2
Ex	2.5	4.0	2.6
Current	18.1	23.1	22.2
35–44			
Never	84.8	78.4	82.4
Ex	1.8	3.8	2.0
Current	13.4	17.8	15.6
45–54			
Never	89.9	84.4	88.3
Ex	1.3	2.8	1.5
Current	8.9	12.8	10.1
55–64			
Never	96.7	95.0	95.7
Ex	0.5	1.3	0.9
Current	2.8	3.7	3.4
65+			
Never	95.4	96.1	97.8
Ex	1.3	1.8	1.1
Current	1.7	2.2	1.2
Total	29 694	22 939	24 335

Smoking was frequently associated with alcohol consumption and drug abuse. Among boys who smoked 40% took alcoholic beverages at least once per month, while only 19% of non-smoking boys took alcohol. Thirty seven per cent of boys who smoked used drugs once or more times, while only 6% of non-smoking boys used drugs once or more times.

Vyshinsky (2002) reports that 46% boys and 38% girls in the age of 15–16 years living in Moscow smoke. It is estimated that in Russia about 40% boys and 28% girls in the age 15–17 years are current smokers (Skvortsova 2002).

In summary, nationwide smoking prevalence in Russia increased from approximately 50% in 1985 to 65–70% in men and from about 5% to 15–20% in women. Peto *et al.* (1994) estimated that in 1990 smoking accounted for 30% of male and 4% of female deaths in Russia. Proportion of death attributed to smoking was higher for the age group 35–69 years: 42% and 6% for men and women, respectively. The observed increase in smoking rates in Russia will contribute to further increase, especially in women, of tobacco-related death.

Increases in smoking in Russia particularly in young people and women could be largely attributed to the aggressive promotion practices employed by multinational tobacco companies, including 'seductive' promotion primarily targeting women and teenagers. Russia has relatively strict laws limiting tobacco advertising. Although cigarette ads have been banned on TV, and printed advertisements must carry health warnings, tobacco products are among the most heavily advertized in this country. The multinational companies have devised a myriad of marketing tricks to win over Russian consumers. Tobacco companies sponsor different cultural events such as, for example, art exhibitions, competitions and tournaments in music and sport. In Russia you still can see free distribution of cigarettes in the streets, at different sport and rock events, which attract mostly young people and teens. But what is most outrageous is that cigarettes were imported to Russia as a humanitarian aid tax free and were given away to the army, and also sold in black markets.

Multinational tobacco companies are in the lead in investing in Russia and other countries of former Soviet Union. The declared size of investment in local tobacco industry amounts to US$ 1.6 billion. In Russia and Ukraine multinationals already control more than 90% of local tobacco production.

In 2001 Russian Duma (the Lower House of Russian Parliament) passed the law on smoking control, which includes bans on sale of cigarettes to minors (individuals 18 years or less), prohibition of smoking in all public places and workplace in the broadest sense, prohibition of smoking in TV shows, prohibition of billboards within 300 meters of schools and medical institutions etc. However, there is little enforcement of this law.

Smoking is a major health hazard in Russia. While, much of tobacco-related death that Russia faces is avoidable, vigorous public health actions are needed to reduce the magnitude of the tobacco problem in this country.

References

Alexeeva, N. and Alexeev, O. (2002). Current tobacco control situation in Novosibirsk, Russia. 3rd European Conference on Tobacco or Health, 20–22 June, Warsaw, Poland, Abstracts, C.7, p. 62.

Ignatova, G., Volkova, E., and Ionin, A. (1993). Epidemiologic situation in Chelyabinsk. Conference on priorities in prevention of non-communicable diseases. Moscow, Abstracts, vol. 2, p. 308 (in Russian).

Kamardina, T., Glasunov, L., Lukitcheva, L., and Sokolova, L. (2002). Smoking epidemic among females in Russia. 3rd European Conference on Tobacco or Health, 20–22 June, Warsaw, Poland. Abstracts, A.3, p. 4.

Levshin, V., Drojachich, V., and Fedichkina, T. (1998). Epidemiology of tobacco smoking. *Nyjegorodskyi med. J.*, **1**, 10–11 (in Russian).

Levshin, V. and Fedichkina, T. (2001). Prevalence of smoking in Moscow. *Vratch*, **7**, 26–28 (in Russian).

Mc Kee, M., Bobak, M., Rosre, R., Shkolnikov, V., Chenet, L., and Leon, D. (1998). Patterns of smoking in Russia. *Tob Control*, **7**, 22–6.

Oganov, R. and Tkachenko, G. (2001). Priorities in prevention of tobacco smoking. Conference on smoking pattern in Russia, Moscow, Abstracts, pp. 21–2 (in Russian).

Oderova, I. (2001). Smoking control as a part of prevention programs. Conference on smoking patterns in Russia, Moscow, Abstracts, pp. 63–4 (in Russian).

Peto, R., Lopez, A. D., and Borenham, J., *et al.* (1994). Mortality from smoking in developed countries 1950–2000, Oxford University Press, Oxford.

Puska, P., Matilainen, T., and Jousilahti, P. (1993). Cardiovaskular risk factors in the Republick of Karelia, Russia, and North Karelia, Finland. *Int. J. Epidemiol.*, **22**, 1048–55.

Skvortsova, E. S. (2002). The tendencies of consumption of tobacco among teenagers in Russia. 3rd European Conference on Tobacco or Health, 20–22 June, Warsaw, Poland, Abstracts, B.5, p. 43.

The principal investigator (1989). The MONICA Project: a worldwide monitoring system for cardiovascular disease. WHO: world health statistics annual. World Health Organization, Geneva, 27–149.

Vyshinsky, K. (2002). Cigarette smoking in Moscow. 3rd European Conference on Tobacco or Health, 20–22 June, Warsaw, Poland. Abstracts, B.7, p. 43.

Zaridze, D., Borenham, J., Igitov, V., Karpov, R., Konobeevskaya, I., Lazarev, V., *et al.* Smoking patterns in Russia (in press).

Chapter 13

Tobacco smoking in central European countries: Poland

Witold Zatoński

Two simultaneous health phenomena developed in eastern and central Europe after World War II. On the one hand, the incidence of infectious diseases and perinatal/ neonatal mortality fell abruptly. However, at the same time the incidence of and mortality from man-made diseases began to rise rapidly. In the 1970s and 1980s, the incidence of lung cancer, liver cirrhosis (especially in south-eastern Europe), cardiovascular diseases and injury-related mortality (especially in the then Soviet Union) in young and middle-aged adults (particularly among men) reached levels never previously recorded in the world (Feachem 1994; Zatoński and Jha 2000). As a result of the above, at the end of the 1980s the levels of mortality due to infectious diseases and mortality among infants or children and youth before age 20 were comparable to Western standards (World Bank 1996; Zatoński and Jha 2000). At the same time, adult health represented a public health catastrophe. Premature mortality, especially among young and middle-aged adult men had reached the highest level in the developed world. The WHO report from 1990 showed that fewer 15-year-old boys from Poland and other CEE countries would reach the age of 60 than their peers not only in western Europe but also in Latin America, China or even India (Murray and Lopez 1994). Very high premature mortality in Poland and other eastern European countries is mainly due to man-made diseases: nearly 50% of this burden is attributable to cigarette smoking (Peto *et al.* 1994). The incidence of lung cancer (a disease that almost exclusively effects cigarette smokers) in Poland (and other central European countries) had reached a level not seen anywhere else in Europe (Zatoński *et al.* 1996). The heath, economic, and social costs of smoking became a major challenge facing Poland and eastern Europe (Zatoński and Boyle 1996).

Introduction

The adult health catastrophe, unusual in peacetime, cannot be understood without first tracing the history of exposure to tobacco smoke in EE populations.

Before WWII tobacco consumption in EE countries was lower than in most western European countries (Forey *et al.* 2002). There was some diversification and tobacco was mostly consumed as hand-made cigarettes, most smokers being males.

After World War II the manufacturing of tobacco products was standardized across the entire Soviet bloc. National tobacco monopolies were ruled and the tobacco market consisted nearly exclusively of factory-made cigarettes. The state promoted cigarettes as important basic goods, representing equality and socialist welfare and democratization.

But good quality information about frequency of smoking in EE countries is fragmentary, with data on sales (consumption of tobacco/cigarettes) being the only source (Forey *et al.* 2002). However, trends in smoking seem to be similar throughout the region. The political and economic homogeny of all Soviet bloc countries also embraced the smoking of cigarettes.

In the militarized societies of EE countries, cigarette production became a state priority. In the army, everyone, including non-smokers, received a quota of cigarettes, and non-smoking soldiers were looked at suspiciously and harassed. The prices of cigarettes were low, and the product itself was widely available. Smoking was allowed everywhere and at any time, except where it interfered with occupational safety (fire hazard). This situation practically did not change until the end of the 1980s.

The closed societies of the Soviet empire were deprived of information on the harmful effects of smoking. Reports from scientific studies of the relation of smoking to cancer and other diseases, undertaken since the 1950s chiefly in the UK and the USA (Doll, in this book), did not reach EE countries or, perhaps, were censored. Awareness of the harm to health due to smoking was very low until the 1980s (Zatoński and Przewoźniak 1992). There were more smokers among better educated and better-off people, especially among women (this observation is corroborated, among others, by data about the incidence of lung cancer in the over-65 age group, which is higher among women with university education than among those who only attended elementary school) (Zatoński and Przewoźniak 1992).

This attitude towards tobacco, which could be observed in EE countries almost until the end of the 1980s, put these countries on top of the list of world tobacco consumption from the early 1960s until the end of the twentieth century (WHO 1996).

A rapid rise in tobacco consumption in eastern Europe after WWII naturally resulted in a similarly fast increase in the incidence of diseases caused by the inhalation of tobacco smoke (Peto *et al.* 1994).

From the early 1980s onward, the incidence of lung cancer (almost exclusively afflicting smokers) in men (especially in Poland, Hungary, former Czechoslovakia, or some areas in Russia) remained at the highest level ever recorded in the world (particularly in young and middle-aged adults) (Zatoński 1995; Zatoński *et al.* 1996). Lung cancer rates in EE women also well reflect the rise in exposure: the incidence of lung cancer in Hungarian under-65 women at the end of the twentieth century was higher than the corresponding rates in men under 65 years old from most western European countries (Fig. 13.3 and 13.4) (Zatoński *et al.* 1996).

Naturally, tobacco consumption is determined not only by public attitude to this product but also by the market situation (the availability of cigarettes and their prices).

The development of the tobacco market ran an identical course in all Soviet bloc countries until the beginning of the 1980s decade. The economic and political crisis which affected the entire economy in the 1980s disturbed the tobacco market in EE countries. The closed socialist economy was not able to produce a sufficient number of cigarettes. This insufficiency had its most drastic consequences first in Poland in the early 1980s (cigarettes were rationed in the martial law period) and then in the Soviet Union towards the end of the decade (lack of cigarettes under Gorbachev's rule provoked social unrest, with smokers staging demonstrations). Eventually, a considerable proportion of Soviet federal gold reserves was exchanged for cigarettes supplied by transnational tobacco companies (Zatoński, Case study of Poland's experience … [in print*a*]).

The systemic and economic transformation in the 1990s quickly restored a normal cigarette market. The tobacco industry was the first to undergo privatization and cigarette manufacturers were almost completely taken over by transnational companies. A structured market was soon established. Constant availability was ensured while prices were kept at a very low level. In the early 1990s in Poland, the price of a pack of cigarettes was on average lower than the price of a loaf of bread (Zatoński and Przewoźniak 1996). It is still the same now, at the turn of the twenty-first century, in some countries in south-eastern Europe. Cigarettes also became the most heavily advertised product. For example, in the late 1990s, the industry was spending one hundred million USD in Poland (Krajowe. NTIA 1998) (about 40 million inhabitants, a little less than 10 million smokers) a year. (Since 2001 tobacco advertising has been completely banned in Poland.) (Dz. U. Nr 96, 1999.)

Rather unexpectedly for the tobacco industry, a new factor began to affect tobacco consumption—activity of health advocates. Having identified smoking as an important factor determining health and the potential for development, including macroeconomic development (Zatoński, Case study of Poland's experience … [in print*a*]), they began to make efforts aiming at reduction of tobacco consumption.

With the return to democracy after 1990, the health advocacy movement began their struggle to avert the tobacco-related health catastrophe in these countries. In Poland, for example, with the advent of a democratic system and freedom of speech, a significant health advocacy movement started to exploit the opportunities afforded by the new political paradigm. In collaboration with MPs (among whom, in those early days of democracy, were many medical professionals), they prepared comprehensive legislation for reducing the harmful health consequences of tobacco smoking, during a five-year confrontation with international tobacco companies, which took over nearly all domestic cigarette manufacturers after 1990 (Zatoński, Case study of Poland's experience … [in print*a*]).

It was only the return of parliamentary democracy and free mass-media in the early 1990s that made effective tobacco control action possible in Poland as the pioneer country in EE. Following five years of animated public debate, the health advocates (mostly medical professionals) in 1995 finally succeeded in having a parliamentary act adopted in Poland, with bipartisan support (Dz. U. Nr 10, 1996). It was not possible to ban all tobacco advertising in 1995, but in October 1999 Parliament voted to extend tobacco control, passing a total ban on advertising and promotion (billboards from 2000, newspapers from 2001) again by a vast majority of votes. A sum equivalent to 0.5% of tobacco excise is now dedicated to tobacco control. The ban on sponsorship of political parties by tobacco companies is the first such regulation worldwide (Dz. U. Nr 96, 1999). Other provisions include:

- smoking bans in health care establishments, schools, and other educational facilities;
- smoking bans in workplaces;
- a ban on selling tobacco products to minors under 18, by vending machines in small packs or individual units;
- health warnings on cigarette packs (30% of pack, front and back);
- a ban on selling tobacco products in vending machines;
- a ban on selling tobacco products in health care establishments, schools and other educational facilities, and in sports facilities;
- gradual reduction of tar and nicotine levels;
- the free provision of treatment for smoking dependence;

The law included all the tasks outlined in WHOs gold standard for tobacco control. The Polish legislation effectively provided for the protection of non-smokers and introduced the world's largest health warnings on cigarette packs. The law also obligated the government to prepare annual action programmes for controlling the health consequences of cigarette smoking. Implementation reports have since been presented to Parliament every year (Roemer, in this book).

The law promotes better health by reducing exposure to tobacco smoke. Workplace smoking regulations are being successfully enforced, especially in private enterprises. The first compensation claim regarding forced passive smoking in the workplace has been won recently. Local health-oriented tobacco control initiatives are growing. A national 'Quit and win' campaign has a major public health intervention since 1991, with over 2.5 million people reported to have quit smoking, thanks to it (Akcja. The Great Polish Smoke-out 1999; Jaworski *et al.* 2000).

Educational campaigns, the media, and legislation became an important factor influencing tobacco consumption.

After 1990, tobacco consumption in Poland began to decrease for the first time (Michaels 1999).

The developments in Poland are comparable with what happened in the 1990s in some other countries in central Europe (Slovenia, Czech Republic, Slovakia), but at the same time quite different from the situation in most countries of the region, especially post-Soviet countries, where the 1990s were a period of stagnation (no significant changes) in tobacco consumption (WHO report 2002).

History of tobacco exposure in central Europe: The case of Poland

Material and methods

My analysis of the development of exposure to tobacco smoke in eastern European countries will be based on data regarding Poland, the country I know best and one where the relevant data are of quite good quality (Zatoński and Przewoźniak 1992, 1996).

Analysis of the developments in epidemiology of exposure to tobacco smoke in Poland will be based on four sources of information:

1. Country's sale statistics. Data on the sales of cigarettes in Poland in 1923–1999 were derived from state statistical sources (yearbooks of the Central Statistical Office). These were quite accurate in the postwar period until 1989 owing to centralized trade (including import) of cigarettes and reliable information on the sales. Since 1990 the data have been much less credible, being disclosed rather reluctantly by privatized tobacco companies for taxation-related reasons.

2. Surveys. Surveys regarding smoking were initiated in 1974 and since 1980 they have been carried out annually (sometimes twice a year). The studies are invariably based on a representative sample of the adult Polish population (16 and more years old). The three-degree, proportionally stratified, randomized sampling design has not changed since the first study. In 1974–1991 sample size was 1000 individuals. Since 1991 this number has been 1500. The response rate has always been higher than 70% (80–90% on average). The questionnaire has almost not changed, either. Smoking categories are defined according to WHO recommendations (Lewith 1983). Every year the study has been prepared and conducted by the same research team from the Department of Cancer Epidemiology and Prevention at the Center of Oncology in Warsaw (Zatoński and Przewoźniak 1992, 1996) and carried out by the same public opinion research center (OBOP) almost every year.

3. The Household Survey from 1996. In April 1996, the Polish Central Statistical Office (GUS) together with its Dutch counterpart carried out a household survey regarding health of Polish population. One of the questions was concerned with smoking (it followed the standards used in the annual smoking surveys in Poland). The study was based on a randomized and representative sample of households in Poland. The sample comprised 19 203 households, with a total of 47 924 occupants. The response rate was 88% (GUS [Central Statistical Office] 1997).

4. Lung cancer mortality data from 1963 onward from Central Statistical Office (Statistical Yearbooks of Poland; Zatoński and Becker 1988; Zatoński et al. 1996).

Indicators of tobacco exposure

Sale

The consumption of tobacco was relatively low after World War I and did not rise significantly until World War II (Fig. 13.1) (Forey et al. 2002). After World War II the sales of cigarettes (cigarettes were almost the only tobacco product sold in Poland, and also in the other EE countries, after 1950) rose exponentially until the early 1980s. In the 1980s, sales were frozen due to an economic crisis brought about by political developments (Zatoński and Przewoźniak 1996). In the 1990s tobacco consumption fell by as much as 10% for the first time in the twentieth century (Michaels 1999).

Surveys

The first survey carried out in 1974 showed that cigarettes accounted for more than 99% of all tobacco used. 59.3% of men more than 16 years old and 17.8% of women more than 16 years old were smokers (Zatoński and Przewoźniak 1992). In the male population, there was not much difference in smoking frequency by age group, place of residence or level of education. In women, the popularity of smoking was strongly age-dependent (birth generation, place of residence) and education (Oleś 1983; Zatoński and Przewoźniak 1992). A study from the early 1980s revealed that the frequency of smoking in men had somewhat increased. In women, the frequency of smoking had risen between 1974 and 1982 from 18% to 30% (Zatoński and Przewoźnaik 1992). An additional factor that affected the distribution of cigarette smoking was the introduction (due to a political and economic crisis that resulted in a lack of cigarettes on the market) of rationing of cigarettes so that everyone, smokers and non-smokers, received a quota. As a result there was a steep rise in the number of both everyday and occasional smokers by more than one million. In 1982 the incidence of smoking among men (62–65%) and women (30%) was the highest in history (Zatoński and Przewoźniak 1992).

In the 1980s, market shortages led to the freezing of consumption levels, also regarding cigarettes (Fig. 13.1). The proportion of young male never-smokers rose slightly (due to the market shortages) while rates of smoking among women kept increasing (Zatoński and Przewoźniak 1996). In the 1990s, for the first time in history, smoking rates fell both among men and among women (Fig. 13.2). In the male population, the decrease can be observed in all age groups, being most marked among the elderly. It is seen across all defined categories of education, but is much more pronounced among those better educated, better-off and more religious (Zatoński and Przewoźniak 1996).

In women, smoking rates have fallen only in the younger age groups. Generally, the reduction has been most marked in the youngest (20–29) age group; over the last decade, smoking rates among women have fallen by half (Fig. 2). The greatest reduction has occurred among young, well-educated women (Zatoński and Przewoźniak 1996).

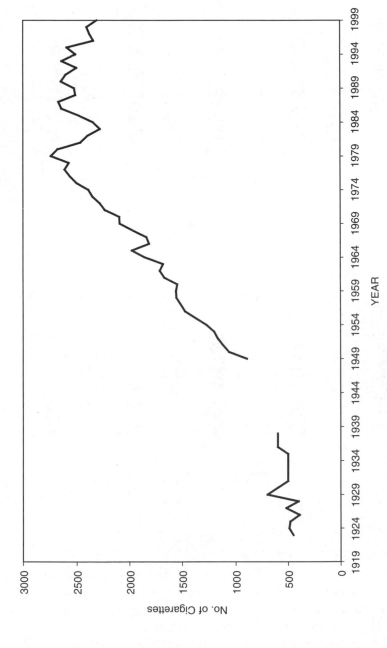

Fig. 13.1 Cigarette consumption (per capita) in Poland, 1923–1999.

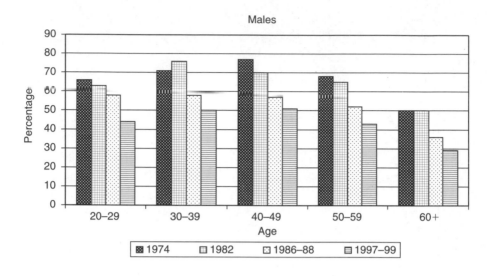

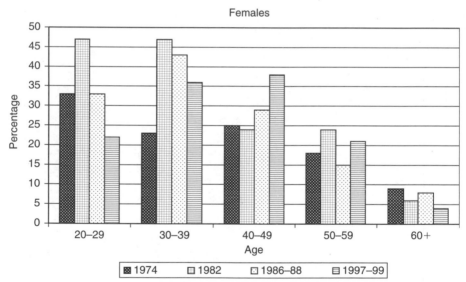

Fig.13.2 Smoking frequency by age groups in Poland in 1975a, 1982, 1986–88, 1997–99.

The Household Survey from 1996

In 1996, a large survey was carried out by the Central Statistical Office which, despite being a one-off project, confirmed earlier survey data. Additionally, the large sample made possible precise analyses of smoking rates by age group and birth cohort with additional data breakdown based on education or place of residence (GUS [Central Statistical Office] 1997). The analysis shows that in 1990s it was the level of education rather than gender that made one a potential smoker. While smoking rates among young men and women are becoming similar, the habit is rare among the best educated (and financially best-off) but continues to be popular among those less well educated and economically handicapped (Zatoński *et al.* in preparation).

Time trends in lung cancer by age groups

Lung cancer incidence and mortality rates seem to be a good indicator of population exposure to tobacco smoke. Trends in lung cancer mortality may also indicate changing exposure (efficacy of tobacco control).

Lung cancer in Europe occurs nearly exclusively in cigarette smokers. Attributed risk in eastern Europe (but also in other countries in Europe and North America) is especially high. In a group of 21,242 cases of lung cancer in Poland only 1107 (5.2%) had been diagnosed in never-smokers (database of Tuberculosis and Pulmonary Diseases Institute in Warsaw). Moreover, epidemiological assessments indicate that a half of lung cancer in never-smoking population may be due to forced exposure to passive smoking (ETS) (Doll 1998). At the beginning of the twenty-first century, lung cancer is still rare among never-smokers (Peto *et al.* 1994; Thun and Henley in this book).

Thus, the monitoring of trends in lung cancer supplies interesting and important (as validated by epidemiological studies) indicators of exposure to tobacco smoke. Additionally, by analysing trends in lung cancer, starting from young adults (20–44 years) and middle-aged persons (45–64 years), changes can be documented relatively quickly (Fig. 13.3 and 13.4).

In Poland, analyses of trends in mortality from lung cancer in men have made it possible to detect falling mortality within several years after a reduction in exposure (with a concomitant increase in the proportion of never-smokers in the younger age groups), first in the 20–44 age group, and then, about 10 years later, in older men, 45–64 years old. It must be added that in the over-65 age group, mortality still has been rising (Fig. 13.3).

Trends in lung cancer mortality among Polish women, which is still on the increase (perhaps with the exception of the last 5 years in the youngest age group, i.e. 20–44 years), also correspond with trends in smoking (Fig. 13.4).

Polish data are in excellent agreement with cancer mortality trends in the same age groups observed in the UK and the USA (Fig. 13.3 and 13.4). Additionally, Hungary appears to be a good reference country, supporting the usability of observations of time trends in lung cancer mortality in selected age groups. Hungary is also the country where lung cancer mortality in young (20–44 years) adult women reached, in 1990s, levels higher than in USA and UK among men (Peto *et al.* 2000).

The product

Since the 1950s, in Poland and other eastern European countries, tobacco has been smoked nearly exclusively in the form of cigarettes. The kind of tobacco previously used for making cigarettes was usually domestic black shag. Cigarettes were usually

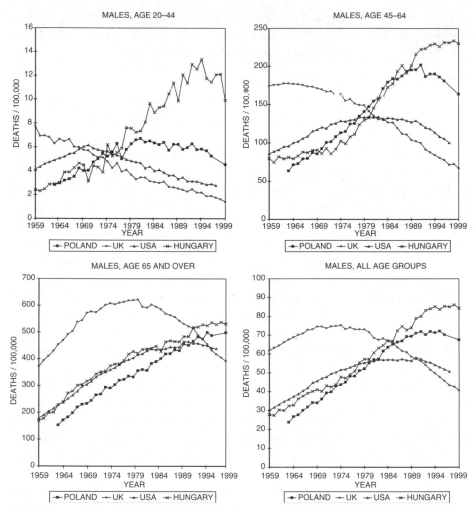

Fig. 13.3 Mortality trends from lung cancer, selected countries 1959–1999.

made without additives. They had a relatively high content of nicotine (about 2 mg/piece in the 1980s) and tar (about 20 mg/piece in the 1980s) (Przewoźniak *et al.* 1987; Zatoński and Przewoźniak 1987, 1988). Cigarettes seldom had filters. In 1982, 28% of men and 74% of women smoked filter cigarettes; in 1988, 48% of cigarettes sold had filters (Zatoński and Przewoźniak 1992; Forey *et al.* 2002). After 1990 international tobacco companies successively took over almost the entire tobacco industry in Poland (and in other EE countries). Now cigarettes are manufactured according to international formulas and standards. Their toxic properties, 'power' additives and taste enhancers are similar to those used in the western world (Djordjevic *et al.* 2002).

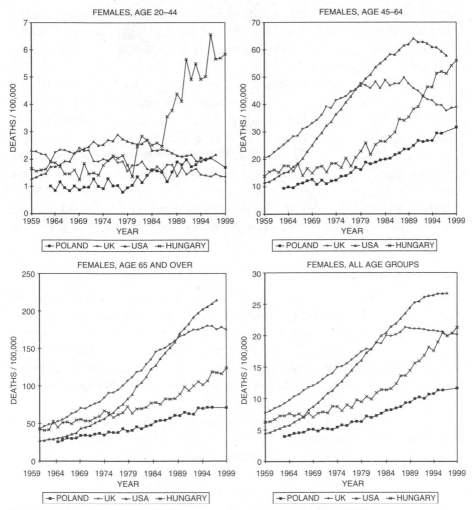

Fig.13.4 Mortality trends from lung cancer, selected countries 1959–1999.

Smoking among children and youth

In paternalistic and conservative societies of eastern Europe, cigarette smoking was strongly forbidden among children, particularly girls. Estimates based on the fragmentary data available indicate that in the early 1980s about 25% of 15-year-old boys and less than 10% of girls smoked cigarettes at least once a week, which was much less than in western Europe (Zatoński and Przewoźniak 1992).

However, there was also another social norm. Entering adulthood on the eighteenth birthday meant acquiring the right to smoke officially, also at school. Consequently, smoking rates rose abruptly among 18-year-olds and later. With every recruit given cigarettes for free, army service was a good school in smoking. For this reason, smoking rates among young (20–29 years old) men were 70–80% (depending on the level of education) in the early 1980s. Smoking was also quite widespread among young women, of whom nearly a half were smokers (Fig. 13.2).

The transformation of the late 1980s/early 1990s brought about changes in norms and behaviour. Access of children to cigarettes increased (Westernization?!). International studies of 13–15-year-old children carried out in the 1990s showed the rates of smokers (at least 1 cigarette a week) in boys at an unchanged level of 30% and a rapid rise in girls—from 16% (in 1990) to 28% in 1999 (Mazur *et al.* 2000). Still, these rates, especially among girls, are again lower than in western European countries (Mazur *et al.* 2000).

At the same time, the steep rise in smoking rates in early adulthood has been stopped, at least in Poland (1999 data for 20–29-year-old men and women: 49% and 22% respectively) (Fig. 13.2).

Smoking among women

Historically, smoking was rare among women in eastern Europe. Women from rural areas did not smoke at all before World War II. The smoking habit was spreading among better educated women living in towns and cities. This is confirmed by epidemiological data on lung cancer (Zatoński *et al.* 1996). After World War II, the popularity of smoking among women rose rapidly, with 18% of adult women smoking in 1974, and 30% in 1982. The 1974 survey revealed considerable differences in successive birth cohorts (Fig. 13.2).

The smoking habit begins to increase more rapidly among less well-educated women, but is still grossly limited to the urban female population. There are still much fewer smokers among women from rural areas, also at the end of the twentieth century (not only in Poland but in most EE countries). These observations are confirmed by data on the distribution of lung cancer, which is invariably rare among women from rural areas (Zatoński *et al.* 1996).

Data from the 1980s and 1990s reveal a picture of a rapid diversification of smoking rates among Polish women by level of education. For example, in the early 1990s about 40% of pregnant women with elementary education and about 10% of those with university education smoked cigarettes (Szamotulska *et al.* 2000). A change in attitude towards smoking led to a rapid decline in smoking rates among the youngest women, especially those better educated (Fig. 13.2). Between 1980s and 1999, the rate of women smokers in the 20–29 age group fell nearly by half (from 36% to 22%). There is still a large population of never-smoking adult Polish women (66% in 1999) (Zatoński 2002*b*).

Now, at the turn of the century, smoking is much more popular among less well-educated women, unlike the pattern that was prevalent as late as the mid-1970s. This is again well illustrated by epidemiological data on the incidence of lung cancer.

According to data collected at the end of the 1990s decade, in the 20–44 age group, lung cancer mortality among women with primary education was five times higher than among those with university education, while in women above 65 years of age lung cancer is more prevalent among better educated women (Zatoński 2002b).

Never-smokers

Smoking was a norm in the male populations of eastern European countries, while non-smoking was an exception. A 1974 survey in Poland revealed that in certain male birth cohorts, the proportion of never-smokers was less than 10% (Oleś 1983; Zatoński and Przewoźniak 1992).

The increasing number of never-smokers in the 1980s and 1990s has been a major achievement in creating an anti-smoking climate in Poland (Fagerström et al. 2001). Since 1985 this proportion has risen from 28% (1985) to 47% (1999) among 20–29-year-old men and from 50% (1985) to 70% (1999) among women in this age group (Zatoński 2002b).

The proportion of never-smoking women in EE countries remains high. Among Polish adult women, this figure has never been lower than 60% (70% in 1974, 63% in 1982, 66% in 1999) (Zatoński and Przewoźniak 1996; Zatoński 2002b).

Smoking cessation

It was only in the 1980s that the attitude towards smoking in Poland began to change. The number of people quitting smoking has also been growing since that time. It is estimated that more than 2.5 million smokers quit smoking in the 1990s (the Great Polish Smoke Out, organized in November and December every year, plays an important role, mobilizing people to quit and helping them to achieve this goal) (Jaworski et al. 2000).

The introduction of large (30% of both larger surfaces of a pack) clear health warnings (smoking causes cancer, smoking causes heart disease) on cigarette packs provided a stimulus to quit for many smokers, especially those less well educated (Dz. U. Nr 96, 1999; Zatoński, Health warnings... [in printb]).

In recent years, Poland has introduced a total ban on tobacco advertising (tobacco billboards disappeared in December 2000, and newspaper ads for cigarettes have been banned since December 2001) (Dz. U. Nr 96, 1999), which considerably improved the antismoking climate (Fagerström et al. 2001) and will significantly encourage quitting. At the end of the 1990s, over 70% of Polish smokers wanted to quit (Fagerström et al. 2001). In 1996, the number of quit attempts in the smoking population was assessed— more than half of all smokers had made 1–3 quit attempts and more than 25% had made 4–10 quit attempts (Boyle et al. 2000; Zatoński 2002b).

An increasing number of heavy smokers (assessed by Fagerström's Test for Nicotine Dependence, FTND) can be seen in Poland—the FTND from a random sample of Polish smokers in 1993 was 3.59 compared with 3.91 six years later (Zatoński, Gaining... [in printc]). This figure can be compared with a FTND of 4.30 for US smokers when assessed in 1994 (Fagerström *et al.* 1996). Among Polish ex-smokers, merely 2% had been aided in their efforts by health professionals. Tobacco control campaigns continuing over a number of years result in the accumulation of heavily dependent smokers, who stand little chance of quitting solely 'on strong will'.

Smoking among medical doctors

At the end of the 1990s, smoking rates among medical doctors in certain countries of south-eastern Europe and ex-Soviet countries were higher than in the general population. In Poland, the earliest study from 1983 found that 45% of male physicians and 36% of female physicians were smokers (compared to 62% of men and 30% of women in the general population in 1982) (Kaczmarczyk-Chałtas *et al.* 1984). In the last 20 years, smoking rates have fallen to about 30% among male physicians and 11% among female physicians (Przewoźniak and Zatoński 2000). The decline has been particularly marked among women and in younger medical doctors. It should be mentioned that in such countries as the USA or Finland, the proportion of smokers in the medical profession is very low, 2–5% (Adriaanse and Van Reek 1989).

Exposure to enforced passive smoking

In eastern Europe, just like in many western European countries, smoking in the presence of non-smokers (including little children) is still an accepted social norm. A 1986 study found cotinine in urine in 92% of a sample of non-smoking Polish women. Cotinine is a metabolite of nicotine and a marker of exposure to tobacco smoke (through enforced smoking) (Becher *et al.* 1992). The proportion of smokers among pregnant women was about 30% in the early 1990s (Szamotulska *et al.* 2000). More than a half of all smokers admit that they smoke in the presence of children and 25% will sometimes smoke in the presence of a pregnant woman (Zatoński 2002b). Sixty-five per cent of children aged 13–15 are exposed to enforced passive smoking (Mazur *et al.* 2000). Over the last decade, following the introduction of tobacco control legislation, exposure to tobacco smoke in the workplace and in public places has been greatly reduced. In the early 1990s, 84% of non-smoking women and 86% of non-smoking men stated that they were passive smokers; the respective percentages for 2001 were 49% and 59% (Zatoński and Przewoźniak 1996). The frequency of smoking among pregnant women fell from 30% to 20% in the period 1990–1999 (Brzeziński *et al.* 1998; Zatoński 2002b).

Summary

The development of the tobacco smoking situation in Poland, presented in the last part of this paper, seems to parallel that in some CE countries (Slovenia, the Czech Republic, Slovakia, and recently Hungary and the Baltic countries as well). In other countries (Bulgaria, Romania, former Yugoslavia countries) the situation does not appear to be changing (the levels of tobacco consumption remain high and steady) (WHO report 2002).

Unfortunately, available data on the development of tobacco smoking in CE countries apart from Poland are fragmentary and not based on representative population studies using the same standardized research techniques over a number of years (WHO report 2002). Thus it is not possible to reliably compare these countries and Poland with respect to long time trend in tobacco smoking. Still, for instance, studies carried out under the MONICA program in the Czech Republic involve representative samples of the Czech population and always use the same research procedures. These studies likewise show a decrease in smoking frequency among 25–64-year-old men (49% in 1985, 27% in 1998) and stabilization in women (27% in 1988, 25% in 1998) (Bruthans 2000). Similarly, trends regarding lung cancer mortality seem to further confirm this parallel development in central European countries mentioned above (Zatoński and Jha 2000; WHO report 2002).

Epilogue: Democracy is healthier

In the 1990s, sales figures for cigarettes in Poland decreased for the first time since World War II. Tobacco industry data show that cigarette consumption fell by 10% between 1990 and 1998 (Michaels 1999). This reduction was achieved when the market was functioning normally and despite the enormously aggressive advertising policies of the tobacco companies. (In the late 1990s, the tobacco industry was spending $100 million annually on advertising) (Krajowe NTIA 1998.)

Smoking in Poland peaked at the end of the 1970s with approximately 14 million smokers (62% of adult men and 30% of adult women). It remained at this level in the 1980s, and decreased substantially in the 1990s. At present, slightly fewer than 10 million Poles smoke—about 40% of adult Polish men and a little more than 20% of adult Polish women (Zatoński 2002a).

Decreasing exposure of the Polish population to tobacco smoke has been accompanied by dramatic health improvements. In the period 1991–2001, life expectancy rose rapidly (after a 30-year period of no change) by about 4 years in men and 3 years in women (GUS [Central Statistical Office] 2002). Our epidemiological estimates indicate that an approximately third of this trend is due to reduced incidence of smoking (Zatoński et al. 1998). For the first time after the World War II morbidity in men due to lung cancer, a form of cancer affecting almost exclusively smokers, do not increase. Moreover, between 1991 and 1999 in men before the age of 65 lung cancer morbidity decreased by 20% (Fig. 13.3) (Zatoński 2002a).

References

Adriaanse, H. and Van Reek, J. (1989). Physicians' smoking and its exemplary effect. *Scand J Prim Health Care*, 7, 193–6.

Akcja Rzuć palenie razem z nami. (1999). '99 [Let's stop smoking together, The Great Polish Smoke-out 1999] Centrum Onkologii—Instytut im. Marii Skłodowskiej-Curie, Warszawa [in Polish].

Becher, H., Zatoński, W., and Jockel, K. H. (1992). Passive smoking in Germany and Poland: comparison of exposure levels, sources of exposure, validity and perception. *Epidemiology*, 3, 509–14.

Boyle, P., Gandini, S., Robertson, Ch., Zatoński, W., Fagerstrom, K., Slama, K., Kunze, M., and Gray, N. and the international smokers survey group (2000). Characteristics of smokers' attitudes towards stopping. *Eur J of Publ Health*, **10**, 3(Suppl), 5–14.

Bruthans, J. (2000). Zpráva o vývoji kardiovaskulárních onemocnění v české Republice po roce. (1989). [Report on development of morbidity from cardiovascular diseases in Czech Republic after 1989]. Alma Mater, Galén, Praha.

Brzeziński, Z., Mazur, J., and Szamotulska, K. (1998). Noworodki, niemowleta, dzieci i młodzież— podstawowe mierniki zdrowotne w 1996 roku [Newborns, infants, children and youth—basic health indicators in 1996]. Institute of Mother and Child, Warsaw [in Polish].

Djordjevic, M. V., Prokopczyk, B., and Zatoński, W. (2002). Carcinogenic tobacco-specific N-nitrosamines (TSNA) in tobacco and mainstream smoke of the leading Polish cigarettes: an international comparison. 3rd European Conference on Tobacco or Health "Closing the Gaps—Solidarity for Health", 20–22 June 2002, Warsaw, Poland.

Doll, R. (1998). Uncovering the effects of smoking: historical perspective. *Stat Methods Med Res*, **7**, 87–117.

Dz. U. Nr 10 (1996). O ochronie zdrowia przed nastepstwami używania tytoniu i wyrobów tytoniowych. Ratyfikowana przez Parlament RP dnia 9 listopada 1995 roku. [Government Gazette of the Republic of Poland, No 10 of 1996: Law on the Protection of Public Health Against the Effects of Tobacco Use. Passed by Polish Parliament on 9 November 1995] [in Polish].

Dz. U. Nr 146 (1996). Rozporzaddzenie Ministra Zdrowia i Opieki Społecznej z dnia 5 grudnia 1996 roku. [Government Gazette of the Republic of Poland, No 146 of 1996. Ordinance of Minister for Health and Social Welfare, 5 December 1996] [in Polish].

Dz. U. Nr 96 (1999). O zmianie ustawy o ochronie zdrowia przed nastepstwami używania tytoniu i wyrobów tytoniowych. Ratyfikowana przez Parlament RP 5 listopada 1995. [Government Gazette of the Republic of Poland, No 96 of 1999. On Changes to the Law on the Protection of Public Health Against the Effects of Tobacco Use. Passed by Polish Parliament on 5 November 1999] [in Polish].

Fagerström, K. O., Boyle, P., Kunze, M., and Zatoński W. (2001). The anti-smoking climate in EU countries and Poland. *Lung Cancer*, **32**(1), 1–5.

Fagerström, K. O., Kunze, M., Schoberberger, P., Breslau, N., Hughes, J. R., Hurt, R. D., Puska, P., Ramström, L., and Zatonski, W. (1996). Nicotine dependence versus smoking prevalence: comparisons among countries and categories of smokers. *Tobacco Control*, **5**, 52–6.

Feachem, R. (1994). Health decline in Eastern Europe. *Nature*, **367**, 313–14.

Forey, B., Hamling, J., Lee, P., and Wald, W. (2002). International smoking statistics. In: A collection of historical data from 30 economically developed countries. Oxford University Press.

Główny Urzad Statystyczny (1997). Stan zdrowia ludności Polski w 1996 r. Raport przygotowany na podstawie ankietowego badania stanu zdrowia ludności, przeprowadzonego w 1996 r. [Health of Polish population in 1996. The report based on a survey regarding health of Polish population, carried out in 1996]. Zakład Wydawnictw Statystycznych, Warszawa [in Polish].

Główny Urzad Statystyczny (2002). Trwanie życia w 2001 r. Informacje i opracowania statystyczne, Warszawa [Central Statistical Office: Life tables of Poland 2001. Information and statistical papers] [in Polish].

Jaworski, J. M., Przewoźniak, K., and Zatoński, W. (2000). The Great Polish Smoke-out 1991–1999: the biggest most successful health promotion in Poland. In: 11th World Conference on Tobacco and Health "Promoting a Future Without Tobacco". August 6–11, 2000, Chicago, Illinois, USA. Abstracts, vol. 3, 806.

Kaczmarczyk-Chałas, K., Gdulewicz, T., and Szadkowska-Stańczyk, I. (1984). Nawyk palenia tytoniu w środowisku lekarzy w Polsce [Smoking habits among Polish physicians]. *Pol. Tyg. Lek.*, **42**, 1395–8 [in Polish].

Krajowe Stowarzyszenie Przemysłu Tytoniowego [National Association of Tobacco Industry— NTIA]. (1998). Reklama papierosów. Fakty [Tobacco Advertising. Facts] [in Polish].

Lewith, F. (1983). Guidelines for the conduct of tobacco smoking surveys in the general population. Doc. No. WHO/SMO/83.4. World Health Organization.

Mazur, J., Woynarowska, B., and Kowalewska, A. (2000). Palenie tytoniu. Zdrowie młodzieży szkolnej w Polsce [Tobacco smoking: Health of school-aged children in Poland]. Katedra Biomedycznych Podstaw Rozwoju i Wychowania, Wydział Pedagogiczny UW, Warszawa [in Polish].

Michaels, D. (1999). Targeting Poles who smoke like chimneys: Activists make headway in fight against tobacco use. The Wall Street Journal, April 8.

Murray, C. and Lopez, A. (1994). Global and regional cause-of-death patterns in 1990. *Bulletin of the World Health Organization*, **72**(3), 447–80.

Oleś, O. (1983). The extent of tobacco use in Poland. *World Smoking and Health*, **8**, 38–42.

Peto, R., Darby, S., Deo, H., Silcocs, P., Whitley, E., and Doll, R. (2000). Smoking, smoking cessation and lung cancer in the UK since 1950: combination of national statistics with two case–control studies. *Br Med J*, **321**, 323–9.

Peto, R., Lopez, A., Boreham, J., Thun, M., and Heath C., Jr (1994). Mortality from tobacco in developed countries 1950–2000. Oxford University Press, Oxford.

Przewoźniak, K., Leppanen, A., and Zatoński, W. (1987). Substancje szkodliwe w dymie polskich i fińskich papierosów w 1983 roku. Analiza porównawcza [Harmful substances in the smoke of Polish and Finnish cigarettes, 1983: comparative analysis]. *Pol. Tyg. Lek.*, **27**, 886–888 [in Polish].

Przewoźniak, K. and Zatoński W. (2000). Decline in smoking prevalence among Polish physicians. In: 11th World Conference on Tobacco or Health "Promoting a Future Without Tobacco". August 6–11, 2000, Chicago, Illinois, USA. Abstracts, Vol. 1, 89.

Roemer, R. A brief history of legislation to control the tobacco epidemic. In: this book Statistical Yearbooks (1963–2001). Central Statistical Office, Warsaw [in Polish].

Szamotulska, K., Przewoźniak, K., Porębski, M., and Zatoński, W. (2000). Infant mortality in Poland in the nineties. II. Decrease of the prevalence of low birth weight—change in behavior: smoking. Abstract book of the 2nd Conference on Health Status of Central and Eastern European Populations After Transition, June 5–7, 2000, Warsaw, Poland. Cancer Center and Institute, Warsaw: 183.

Thun, M. J. and Henley, S. J. (1997). The great studies of smoking and disease in the twentieth century. In: this book Tobacco or health: a global status report. World Health Organization, Geneva.

WHO European country profiles on tobacco control 2001 (2002). Who Regional Office for Europe, Copenhagen.

World Bank (1996). The transition in Central and Eastern Europe. World Bank Technical Paper No. 341, Washington.

Zatoński, W. (1995). The health of the Polish population. *Public Health Rev Israel*, **23**, 139–56.

Zatoński, W. (2002a). Democracy is healthier. A health miracle on the Vistula. *Cancer Center and Institute of Oncology*, Warsaw.

Zatoński, W. (2002b). Obstacles, action and outcome—the Polish experience. *Int J Cancer*, Supplement 13, Abstract book 18th UICC International Cancer Congress, 30 June–5 July, Oslo, Norway, 28–9.

Zatoński, W. Case study of Poland's experience in tobacco control. World Bank Publications [in print].

Zatoński, W. Gaining governmental support: the case of Poland. *J Clin Psychiatry* [in print*c*].

Zatoński, W. Health warnings: case of Poland [WHO Publications, in print*b*].

Zatoński, W. and Becker, N. (1988). Atlas of cancer mortality in Poland 1975–1979. Springer-Verlag, Berlin.

Zatoński, W. and Boyle, P. (1996). Commentary. Health transformations in Poland after 1988. *J Epidemiol Biostat*, **4**, 183–97.

Zatoński, W. and Jha P. (2000). The health transformation in Eastern Europe after 1990: a second look. Cancer Center and Institute of Oncology, Warsaw.

Zatoński, W., McMichael, A. J., and Powles, J. W. (1998). Ecological study of reasons for sharp decline in mortality from ischaemic heart disease in Poland since 1991. *Br Med J*, **316**, 1047–51.

Zatoński, W. and Przewoźniak, K. (1987). Zawartość substancji szkodliwych w polskich papierosach w 1985 roku [Content of harmful substances in Polish cigarettes in 1985]. *Pneum Pol* **7–8**, 377–81 [in Polish].

Zatoński, W. and Przewoźniak, K. (1988). Zawartość substancji szkodliwych w polskich papierosach w 1986 roku [Content of harmful substances in Polish cigarettes in 1986]. *Zdrowie Publ.* **3**, 145–50 [in Polish].

Zatoński, W. and Przewoźniak, K. (1992). Zdrowotne nastepstwa palenia tytoniu w Polsce [Health consequences of tobacco smoking in Poland]. Ariel, Warszawa [in Polish].

Zatoński, W. and Przewoźniak, K. (1996). Palenie tytoniu w Polsce: postawy, nastepstwa zdrowotne i profilaktyka [Tobacco smoking in Poland: attitudes, health consequences and prevention]. Centrum Onkologii—Instytut im. Marii Skłodowskiej-Curie, Warszawa [in Polish].

Zatoński, W., Smans, M., Tyczyinski, J., and Boyle, P. (1996). (in collaboration with: Becker N., Didkowska J., Friedl H. P., Holub J., Peter Z., Plesko I., Roman V., Stabenow R., Tzvetansky Ch.). Atlas of cancer mortality in Central Europe. IARC Scientific Publications No. 134. International Agency for Research on Cancer, Lyon.

Chapter 14

The epidemic in India

Prakash C. Gupta and Cecily S. Ray

The introduction of tobacco

Tobacco was introduced in India during the late sixteenth-century into the kingdom of Adil Shah, with its capital at Bijapur, presently in Karnataka. The Ambassador of the Mogul Emperor Akbar in Delhi, after a visit to Bijapur, brought for him tobacco and jewel-encrusted European style pipes. The appreciation at court was marred only by the Emperor's physicians who forbade him to inhale the smoke, since tobacco was an unknown substance. A compromise was reached wherein the smoke was to be first passed through water for purification, resulting in invention of hookah. Hookah smoking became popular in parts of India where a strong Mogul influence prevailed; it was especially favoured among the aristocratic and elite classes, mainly in North India. Ornately crafted in engraved silver, brass, or other precious materials and decorated with enamel or jewels, the hookah became a status symbol. Paintings of the Mogul period show both men and women smoking hookahs. The lower classes began to make them out of common woods and coconut shells and as hookah was often shared, hookah smoking became associated with social acceptance, brotherhood, and equality. A common expression for social boycott in north India is to stop sharing the hookah and water from the village well.

In 1617, Emperor Jehangir, Akbar's son, decided that tobacco use produced adverse physical and mental effects on his subjects and tried to stop its use by declaring that any user would have his lips slit, but the practice continued nevertheless (Bhonsle *et al.* 1992).

Well before the introduction of tobacco smoking in India, the inhalation and smoking of aromatic herbs was practiced as a form of therapy. When tobacco smoking was introduced, it was assigned medicinal qualities—as a calmative, relaxant, and stimulant. Aromatic substances were often added to tobacco smoked through hookah. A conical clay pipe, known as a *chilum*, traditionally used for smoking narcotics, began to be used for tobacco smoking as well (Bhonsle *et al.* 1992). Tobacco was often used to stave off hunger during travel and sustain long hours of work (Sanghvi 1992).

Evolution of tobacco use

Smoking

Tobacco began to be smoked in many ways, besides in hookah and chilum. The *hookli* is an European-style pipe with a clay bowl and stem (sometimes of wood) about 7–10 cm long, commonly used in western India for smoking sun-dried tobacco. The habit of smoking a rolled tobacco leaf, tied with a thread, known as a *chutta*, was documented as early as 1670 on the east coast of India, where women commonly smoke them in reverse, i.e. with the glowing end inside the mouth. The *dhumti*, a large, cone-shaped roll of tobacco in a jack fruit leaf (*Artocarpus integrefolia L.*), is mainly used in the Konkan region, including Goa, and it, too, is often smoked in reverse by women. Reverse smoking is supposed to be convenient while doing household work and tending to children. It also generates extreme heat in the mouth, thought to be good for toothache and the smoke is believed to mask halitosis. Girls learn to imitate the habit when asked by their mothers to light up for them. Some men too practise reverse smoking. The most popular smoking product in India today is the *bidi*, first documented in 1711 and mainly smoked by men (Bhonsle *et al.* 1992; Sanghvi 1992).

Smokeless tobacco

In addition to smoking, tobacco began to be used in a wide variety of ways in India. It found its way into betel quid (*paan*) at the Mogul court, where it was served from ornate boxes. Betel quid consists of a leaf of the *Piper betle* vine smeared with slaked lime (aqueous calcium hydroxide paste), pieces of the nut of the *Areca catechu* palm and, frequently, spices. The practice of chewing betel quid had reached India by the first century or earlier, through contacts with the South Pacific Islands (Gode 1961). Chewing tobacco in betel quid soon became the most popular form of smokeless tobacco use.

Other smokeless tobacco preparations containing areca nut and slaked lime were developed. *Mainpuri* tobacco, popular in Uttar Pradesh, contains tobacco with slaked lime, finely cut areca nut, camphor, and cloves. *Mawa*, a relatively new preparation containing thin shavings of areca nut with some tobacco and slaked lime, is popular in Gujarat among youth. *Gutkha*, a dry preparation containing areca nut, slaked lime, catechu, condiments, and powdered tobacco (waste), originally available custom-mixed from pan vendors, later began to be industrially manufactured and sold in sachets and tins. It has been widely advertised since 1975 and is now very popular. Gutkha, like mawa, contains both tobacco and areca nut, making it highly addictive. The same mixture without tobacco is called *pan masala*. Offering pan masala to others is advertised as an act of hospitality, brotherhood, and equality, just like the traditional offering of betel quid to guests.

Various combinations of tobacco, spices, molasses, and lime were developed for use in betel quid or separately. Raw tobacco is sold as bundles of long strands in Kerala. *Hogesoppu* is a leaf tobacco used by women in Karnataka. *Kaddipudi* are cheap 'powdered sticks' of raw tobacco used in Karnataka. Bricks and blocks of powdered tobacco mixed with jaggery (solid molasses) are also used. *Gundi* and *kadapan* are mixtures of coarsely powdered, cured tobacco, coriander seeds, other spices and aromatic, resinous oils, used in Gujarat, Orissa and West Bengal. *Kiwam*, used mainly in North India, is a thick paste of boiled tobacco mixed with powdered spices like saffron, cardamom, aniseed, and musk, also available as granules or pellets. *Pattiwala* is sun-dried, flaked tobacco, used with or without lime, mainly in north India. North Indian tobacco and slaked lime preparations include *zarda*, coarsely cut tobacco, boiled till dry with slaked lime, with added colouring and flavouring agents, often expensive ones like saffron and cardamom. Zarda is sold in small packets and tins, used alone or in betel quid. *Khaini*, a mixture of sun-dried tobacco and slaked lime, is placed in the mandibular or labial groove and sucked slowly for 10–15 minutes, occasionally overnight.

The nasal use of dry snuff, introduced by the Europeans and once fairly common, has all but died out. Snuff-like preparations became especially popular with women due to misconception that they were good for teeth and gums (Bhonsle *et al.* 1992). *Masheri* or *mishri*, is a powdered black-roasted tobacco preparation used mainly in Goa and Maharashtra; *bajjar* is a dry snuff commonly used in Gujarat; *gudhaku* or *gul* is a moist form of powdered tobacco and molasses from eastern India; creamy snuff or tobacco toothpaste, advertised as antibacterial, became popular in western parts of India; and, tobacco water, i.e. water through which tobacco smoke has been passed, is sold for gargling in Manipur and Mizoram.

With globalization, the Swedish *snus* is being marketed in large cities of India under a brand name, Click.

Tobacco production

During the seventeenth century, the Portuguese traders imported tobacco for sale in India, using the income to buy Indian cotton textiles for Portugal. After displacing the Portuguese in India, the British imported American tobacco to India to finance foreign trade. This lasted until the American Revolution in 1776, after which the East India Company began growing tobacco as a cash crop. The area under tobacco cultivation tripled during 1891–1921 (Sanghvi 1992).

Bidi making began as a small-scale activity in rural areas. Different kinds of leaves were tried as a wrapper until the early 1890s when leaves of the tendu tree, also called temburni (*Diospyros melanoxylon*), growing mainly in the forests of Madhya Pradesh, were found to be the best suited. The oldest bidi manufacturing firm was established around 1887 and by 1930 the bidi industry had spread across the country. Some of the firms became very large, although the process of manufacturing by hand-rolling has remained the same (Chauhan 2001). Bidi manufacture, by far the most labour intensive of all tobacco industries, enjoys government protection, as bidis are made mostly at home by women.

The first Indian cigarette factory was established in 1906, by the Imperial Tobacco Company (Bhonsle 1992). From 1920 onwards, the growing urban market for cigarettes grew with the urban populace. Phillip Morris also entered India and several smaller Indian cigarette companies emerged.

In 1938, the British Raj in India established a cigarette tobacco research station at Guntur, Andhra Pradesh, from where scientific inputs began to be provided for tobacco production. After independence in 1947, the Indian Government continued this practice through the Central Tobacco Research Institute at Rajahmundry, Andhra Pradesh (Chari and Rao 1992). Tobacco is currently a highly subsidized sector: farmers receive subsidies on water, electricity and fertilisers as well as price support. Revenues to the Government from tobacco products constitute about 10% of total excise revenues and nearly 5% of agricultural exports from India.

India's tobacco production grew with the population from 1949 to 1997 as shown in Fig. 14.1. For long the world's third largest tobacco producer after China and the United States, India is currently the second largest producer after China, but produces only about 3.3% of the world's Flue Cured Virginia (FCV) or cigarette tobacco, according to the Tobacco Board (2000). Exports amount to about one-fourth of tobacco produced in India (especially FCV) and a small portion of tobacco used in India is imported. Less than one-fifth of tobacco consumed in India is used in cigarettes, the largest proportion goes into bidi manufacture and smokeless products (about 40% each), and the rest, into minor smoking products.

Tobacco use

During 1950–55, the annual per capita adult consumption of tobacco in India was around 900 g, which declined to 700 g by the late 1980s, small values compared to developed country standards. It is currently increasing by about 3% per year (PriceWaterhouse 2000). Until the end of the 1940s, tobacco was used mostly for

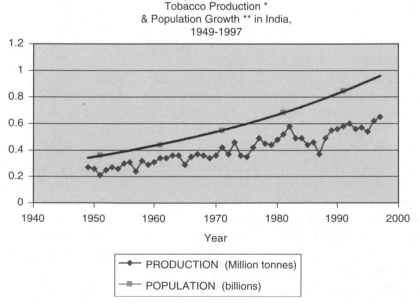

Fig. 14.1 Tobacco Production and Population Growth in India, 1949–1997. (*Moon-Stone Group 2000; **National Census figures, Visaria 2000.)

hookah smoking and for chewing. Thereafter, bidi and cigarette smoking increased tremendously with bidis becoming the predominant tobacco habit, (Sanghvi 1992). In recent years India has been witnessing a resurgence of smokeless tobacco consumption in industrially manufactured forms, especially amongst the young. By far most tobacco products consumed are produced in the country.

Prevalence in the general population

Surveys conducted by the National Sample Survey Organisation (NSSO) during 1999–2000 found that at least one person in 62% of households consumed tobacco. These data indicate that the north-eastern states have the highest prevalence of tobacco use, other northern states the next highest, and the southern states the lowest. The exception in the north is Punjab, showing the lowest prevalence, because of a high proportion of Sikhs, whose religion forbids tobacco use. The lower income groups generally prefer smokeless tobacco, the low to middle income groups favour bidis and higher income groups prefer cigarettes, in order of the cost of the product.

The most accurate information on tobacco use prevalence comes from house-to-house surveys carried out in individual areas. In these studies, conducted over a 40-year time span in different parts of India, the percentage using tobacco among men (>15 years age) ranged from 19 to 86% and among women from 7 to 77% (Table 14.1). Overall, tobacco use prevalence is higher in rural areas. Gender-wise, chewing habits are practiced about equally by men and women, while most smokers are men. The prevalence of chewing in men varied from 11 to 55% and in women from 10 to 39%. Smoking prevalence varied from 8 to 77% in men and 2 to 12% in women with some exceptions.

In a few regional pockets where certain indigenous forms of smoking have been practiced, women may smoke at equal or higher rates compared with men (Table 14.1). In one study in rural Srikakulam, Andhra Pradesh, 'reverse' chutta smoking was practiced by 59% of women and 35% of men. In rural Darbhanga, Bihar, smoking was practiced by nearly 11.4% of men and 21.8% of women—mainly hookah smokers (Mehta *et al.* 1971). Also, in an area of Orissa 85% of women smoked chuttas, compared to 30% of men (Jindal and Malik 1989). Among school personnel in rural and urban Bihar, 47.4% of men and 31% of women reported smoking (Sinha *et al.* 2002).

In a few areas, like Mumbai, both men and women tobacco users prefer chewing (Gupta 1996). In some parts of Gujarat, like Bhavnagar and Ahmedabad, chewing of a new product called mawa became very popular among young men during the 1980s and '90s. During a survey carried out in 1993–94 in Bhavnagar, the prevalence of mawa use was 19%, whereas in 1969 it was around 4.7% (Mehta *et al.* 1971; Sinor *et al.* 1992; Gupta 2000).

Overall, tobacco use in India is inversely related to educational level except for cigarette smoking (Gupta 1996). For example, nearly a third of highly educated men in Delhi and Chandigarh reported smoking (Bhattacharjee 1994; Sarkar *et al.* 1990).

Table 14.1 Tobacco use prevalence among adults from population-based studies in rural and urban India

Area	Population type	Reference	Sample size	% Tobacco users		
				Men	**Women**	**Overall**
Rural						
Maharashtra & Karnataka	Village	Khanolkar (1959)	9996	84	a	a
Uttar Pradesh	Village	Khanolkar (1959)	12 637	82	a	a
Andhra Pradesh	Village	Khanolkar (1959)	7249	86	a	a
Mainpuri, Uttar Pradesh	Village	Wahi (1968)	34 997	82	21	57
Bhavnagar, Gujarat	Village	Mehta et al. (1969)	10 071	71	15	44
Ernakulam, Kerala	Village	Mehta et al. (1969)	10 287	81	39	59
Srikakulam, Andhra Pradesh	Village	Mehta et al. (1969)	10 169	81	67	74
Singbhum, Bihar	Village	Mehta et al. (1969)	10 048	81	33	56
Darbhanga, Bihar	Village	Mehta et al. (1969)	10 340	78	51	64
Pune, Maharashtra	Village	Mehta et al. (1972)	101 761	62	49	64
Punjab	Village	Mohan et al. (1986)	24 villages	19	Very small	b
Goa	Village	Vaidya et al. (1992)	29 713	33	20	27
Bihar schools	School personnel	Sinha et al. (2002)	637	78	77	77
60 rural			Smokeless:	59	53	57
40 urban			Smoking:	47	31	43
Urban						
Bombay	Policemen	Mehta et al. (1961)	4734	76.5	a	a
Ahmedabad	Mill workers	Malaowalla et al. (1976)	57 518	b	b	85 (mostly men)
Mumbai	Lower SES group	Gupta (1996)	99 598	69	57.5	b
Delhi	All SES groups	Narayan et al. (1996)	13 558	45 c	7 c	b
Delhi	Mid-high SES group	Bhattacharjee et al. (1994)	508	31 c	a	a

a Women were not interviewed in these areas. b Not reported. c Only Smoking habits were assessed. SES = Socio-Economic Status.

Prevalence among youth

While smoking continues to be a threat, an easily observable trend among youth in India today is an increasing use of smokeless tobacco. One-third to one-half of children under the age of ten years in rural areas of different states experiment with smoking or smokeless tobacco in some form (Vaidya *et al.* 1992; Kapoor *et al.* 1995; Krishnamurthy *et al.* 1997). Despite Punjab's tradition of low tobacco use, Punjabi youth today are falling prey to gutkha, as shown in a recent survey of rural school-going teenagers in five villages, where two-thirds regularly used it (Kaur and Singh 2002). The popularization of gutkha in urban and rural areas of Gujarat, urban Bihar and Maharashtra has also been documented (Gupta and Ray 2002). In recent surveys conducted in secondary schools in Mumbai, about one-fifth of boys used gutkha in the eighth, ninth, and tenth standards (aged about 13–15 years). In a municipal school, 9% of girls in ninth standard used gutkha and in a private one, 5% of girls in seventh, eighth, and ninth standards used it. Surveys of street boys in Mumbai have shown that most start chewing gutkha and smoking bidis by the age of eight years.

Global Youth Tobacco Surveys of representative samples of 13–15-year-old students have been completed in eleven states in India so far. Between 4.5% to 86.1% students reported current use of tobacco. A large proportion of children are exposed to second hand smoke at home and outside. Even at this young age, most smokers reported wanting to quit and many had made unsuccessful attempts. Only a small percentage reported having been taught in school about the dangers of tobacco.

Among college students in Maharashtra State, at least one-fifth reported using some form of tobacco. Cigarette smoking was reported by 10.6%, tobacco chewing by 6.7%, pan masala by 9.9%, and gutkha by 9.6%—many had more than one habit. Awareness of the ill effects of tobacco was generally low, especially for smokeless products (IIans 1998). A high prevalence (20–80%) has been observed among medical and dental students, raising a concern that in future they may not provide appropriate professional advice to tobacco users.

Reasons for tobacco use

There are a wide variety of reasons why people use tobacco. Among lower socio-economic strata, people often use it to suppress hunger. In rural areas, people believe that tobacco has medicinal properties to cure or palliate common discomforts, like toothache, headache, and stomachache. Children copy the behaviour of their parents and other elders. People are largely unaware of the dangers posed by tobacco. Young working boys start smoking because they see others smoking and local shopkeepers give bidis to young boys to attract them for work. Labourers use smoking as a pretext to take a break from work.

The most common reason amongst children of the urban poor is their film hero who smokes. In higher socio-economic classes, children may smoke due to peer pressure, as a status symbol, family influence and advertising. Advertisements on television, although banned on government channels, continue to be broadcast on cable and satellite channels. These, as well as ads on public buses and in print media influence tobacco use especially gutkha, among children. Fun and enjoyment are among the most common reasons given by school and college students for using various addictive substances. The easy availability and low cost of most tobacco products are also important factors.

Burden due to tobacco

Premature mortality

Three cohort studies in different parts of India showed that tobacco users experienced a significantly higher mortality compared to non-users. Using conservative estimates (relative risk for men 1.4 and for women 1.3) and prevalence of tobacco use (60% in men and 15% in women), it was estimated that about 630 000 deaths, i.e. 12.6% of overall deaths, were attributable to tobacco use in 1986 (Gupta 1989). A later study by Indian Council for Medical Research (ICMR) estimated that in 1996 the total number of tobacco-related deaths was 800 000 (ICMR 2001). Newer information suggests that relative risk of overall mortality due to tobacco use is higher than previously estimated (Gupta and Mehta 2000). Also two-thirds of tuberculosis deaths (Gajalakshmi and Peto 2001) could be attributed to smoking (relative risk 4.5). Incorporating newer information would further increase the number of deaths attributable to tobacco use quite substantially.

Disease risks

In various studies, the relative risks of cancers of the different sites of the upper alimentary and respiratory tracts have varied from 2.5–6.2 in chewers and 2.2–11.8 in smokers and 6.2–31.7 in those who both chew and smoke. The relative risk for smokers developing myocardial infarction and coronary artery disease (CAD) have varied from 2 to 3 fold. A four-fold prevalence of chronic obstructive lung disease (COLD) was found in smokers (Notani *et al.* 1989). An Expert Committee constituted by the ICMR used the more conservative risk estimates to calculate the number of avoidable cases of the three major disease groups due to tobacco use in 1999 (ICMR 2001):

+ Incident cancers of the upper alimentary and respiratory tract amounted to nearly 163 500 cases.
+ Prevalent CAD cases attributable to smoking amounted to 4.45 million.
+ Prevalent cases of COLD attributable to smoking amounted to 39.2 million.

Financial costs

In a study on costs of tobacco-related cancers, the direct (medical and non-medical, like travel and lodging) and indirect costs, like loss of income due to absenteeism during treatment and premature death were assessed. A cohort of 195 cancer patients was followed for three years from 1990. The average cost per cancer patient, discounted at the 1999 level, amounted to Indian Rupees (INR) 350 000, with direct costs amounting to 13% of total cost. Curative intent of treatment was associated with higher expenditures. The cost of 163 500 incident tobacco-related cancers diagnosed in 1999, thus amounted to INR 57.225 billion (US Dollars 1.34 billion).

Cost information was collected for one year on 500 patients of CAD, 423 of COLD, and 28 patients of both CAD and COLD. The average yearly per capita costs in 1999 terms for CAD and COLD respectively amounted to INR 29 000 and INR 23 300 (USD 679 and USD 546), with direct costs accounting for 57% and 19% respectively. The national cost of all CAD cases due to tobacco in 1999 was estimated at INR 129.05 billion and that of COLD at INR 91.336 billion (USD 3.02 billion and USD 2.14 billion, respectively).

Thus during 1999, the three major diseases put together, cancers, CHD, and COLD, cost the country INR 277.6 billion or about USD 6.5 billion (ICMR 2001). For comparison, in 1998, total excise revenues from tobacco corresponded to INR 55.40 billion or USD 1.29 billion, and the nationwide sale value of all tobacco products was INR 244 billion or around USD 6 billion (ICMR 2001; Reserve Bank of India 1999; PriceWaterhouse 2000). Clearly the economic benefit of tobacco to the country is unable to outweigh the costs accrued due to the diseases it causes.

Interventions

Primary prevention

Sporadic attempts have been made by NGOs to conduct educational campaigns through various media. Two recent ones have been conducted in Mumbai and Delhi. In Mumbai, the Preventive Oncology Department of the Tata Memorial Centre, a cancer diagnosis and treatment centre, organized an anti-tobacco campaign in July–August, 2002, through college students volunteering in the National Social Service Scheme. After being informed of the harmful effects of tobacco use, the students developed street plays on the topic. They performed these plays in schools and public places. In Delhi, a controlled anti-tobacco intervention among adolescent students of 30 schools was conducted to raise their awareness and involve them in activities like peer interaction within and between schools, family discussions, a signature campaign in the community, and an appeal to the Prime Minister. The post-test showed that students in the intervention group were significantly less likely than controls to have been offered, received, experimented with, or have intentions to use tobacco.

Efforts in persuading illiterate villagers to stop or reduce their tobacco use have been attempted in rural areas. A large, controlled, educational intervention trial in tobacco users with 10 years of annual follow-ups was conducted during 1967–88 in three areas of India. Personal communication with visual aids after oral examination addressed factors for decision-making on tobacco use. Messages through personal communication were reinforced by documentaries, slides, posters, exhibitions, folk-dramas, radio messages, and newspaper articles (Gupta *et al.* 1986). The educational intervention was helpful in reducing tobacco use and in significantly increasing quit rates in two areas assessed after five and ten years of follow up (9% and 14.3% in Ernakulam and 17% and 18.4% in Srikakulam) (Gupta *et al.* 1992).

In another intervention study conducted in Karnataka, after a five-year interval, quit rates in men and women respectively were 26.5% and 36.7% (Anantha *et al.* 1995).

Legislation

From April 1976, a warning on cigarette packets and advertisements ('Cigarette smoking is injurious to health') was made mandatory under the Cigarette (Regulation of Production, Supply & Distribution) Act of 1975. The advertising of tobacco products was prohibited in government-controlled electronic media (television and radio) and government publications. In 1990, the Government of India issued an Executive Order prohibiting smoking in select public places like hospitals, educational institutions, domestic flights, air-conditioned trains and buses and suburban trains (Luthra *et al.* 1992). In June 1999, Indian Railways, operating under the Government of India, banned the sale of tobacco on railway platforms. Two small states, Delhi and Goa, promulgated their own tobacco control laws banning outdoor tobacco advertisements and smoking in public places.

It is well known that raising the price of items like alcohol and tobacco decreases their consumption. Over eighty per cent of total tobacco excise revenue in India comes from cigarettes. From early 1990s, bidis have begun to be taxed albeit at very low level. Many smokeless tobacco products, which are becoming increasingly popular, are taxed at a low level but evasion is rampant. There is a great scope to control tobacco use through higher taxation.

Several litigations relating to tobacco control have been filed by individuals and non-governmental organizations. The most successful one was filed in Kerala by a woman who stated that she found it difficult to commute in a bus in which her co-passengers smoked. As a result, in July 1999, the Kerala High Court imposed a ban on smoking in public places. Several other litigations are pending on issues like sports sponsorship and advertising campaigns by tobacco companies, and a case has been filed by a politician in the Supreme Court requesting compensation for the hazardous effects of tobacco on the health of citizens. As a consequence the Supreme Court issued a directive banning smoking in enclosed public places.

As a result of a case filed in the Rajasthan High Court by a manufacturer of tobacco tooth powder against an amendment to the Drugs and Cosmetics Act, 1940, prohibiting tobacco in dental care products, the Central Committee on Food Standards recommended a ban on smokeless tobacco products. This has not been implemented but several states have recently taken a major step in banning the sale, manufacture, and storage of gutkha under Prevention of Food Adulteration Act as gutkha is classed as a food product.

Although tobacco control legislation in India is not very advanced at this time, there has recently been a considerable use of litigation and of existing laws towards advancing tobacco control.

Summary and conclusions

With an initial introduction into Indian royal courts by the Portuguese, tobacco use spread quickly throughout society, taking on many indigenously developed forms to suit local tastes. The British colonisers promoted tobacco as a cash crop and as an industry. The independent Indian Government continued to support tobacco as a revenue earner and employment generator. Among the middle classes, socially, smoking is not well accepted especially by women and adolescents. The poor and uneducated have little awareness of health effects of tobacco, especially smokeless tobacco. Tobacco use, especially smoking is more prevalent among men than women, except in some small regions. The youth have shown eagerness to experiment with new tobacco products like mawa and gutkha alongside more traditional products. Young children are prone to take up tobacco use, especially in rural areas and among the urban poor. Intervention studies have demonstrated that it was possible to reduce tobacco use through education. National legislative action to combat tobacco menace has remained weak so far, although in recent years several states and judiciary seem to have taken a lead.

References

Anantha, N., Nandakumar, A., Vishwanath, N., Venkatesh, T., Pallad, Y. G., Manjunath, P., *et al.* (1995). Efficacy of an anti-tobacco community education program in India. *Cancer Causes and Control,* **6**, 119–29.

Bhattacharjee, J., Sharma, R. S., and Verghese, T. (1994). Tobacco smoking in a defined community of Delhi. *Indian Journal of Public Health,* **38**, 22–6.

Bhonsle, R. B., Murti, P. R., and Gupta, P. C. (1992). Tobacco habits in India. In: *Control of tobacco-related cancers and other diseases, International Symposium, 1990* (ed. P. C. Gupta, J. E. Hamner III, and P. R. Murti), pp. 25–46. Oxford University Press, Bombay.

Chari, M. S. and Rao, B. V. K. (1992). Role of Tobacco in the national economy: past and present. In: *Control of tobacco-related cancers and other diseases, International Symposium, 1990* (ed. P. C. Gupta, J. E. Hamner III, and P. R. Murti), pp. 57–76. Oxford University Press, Bombay.

Chauhan, Y. (2001). History and struggles of Beedi workers in India. All India Trade Union Congress, New Delhi.

Gajalakshmi, V. and Peto, R. (2002). Smoking and TB mortality in the Chennai retrospective 'case-control' study. In: *Proceedings of the International Scientific Expert Meeting on the Possible Causality between Smoking and Tuberculosis, November 17–18, 2000, Thiruvananthapuram, Kerala, India* (I. Dhillon, P. C. Gupta, and S. Asma).

Gode, P. K. (1961). Studies in Indian Cultural History. *Indological Series 9, Institute Publication, No. 189.* Hoshiarpur: Vishveshvaranand Vedic Research Institute. Vol. I, pp. 111–90.

Gupta, P. C. (1989). An assessment of excess mortality caused by tobacco usage in India. In: *Tobacco and health: The Indian scene, Proceedings of the UICC workshop, 'Tobacco or Health', April 15–16, 1987* (ed. L. D. Sanghvi and P. P. Notani), pp. 57–62. Tata Memorial Centre, Bombay.

Gupta, P. C. (1996). Survey of sociodemographic characteristics of tobacco use among 99,598 individuals in Bombay, India using handheld computers. *Tob. Control*, **5**, 114–20.

Gupta, P. C. (2000). Oral cancer and tobacco use in India: A new epidemic. In: *Tobacco the growing epidemic—Proceedings of the 10th World Conference on Tobacco or Health, 24–28 August 1997*, pp. 20–1. Beijing, China.

Gupta, P. C. and Mehta, H. C. (2000) A cohort study of all-cause mortality among tobacco users in Mumbai, India. Bulletin of the World Health Organization, **78**(7), 877–83.

Gupta, P. C., Mehta, F. S., Pindborg, J. J., Aghi, M. B., Bhonsle, R. B., Daftary, D. K., *et al.*. (1986). Intervention study for primary prevention of oral cancer among 36 000 Indian tobacco users. *Lancet*, **i**, 1235–9.

Gupta, P. C., Mehta, F. S., Pindborg, J. J., Bhonsle, R. B., Murti, P. R., Daftary, D. K., and Aghi, M. B. (1992). Primary prevention trial of oral cancer in India: A 10-year follow-up study. *Journal of Oral Pathology and Medicine*, **21**, 433–9.

Gupta, P. C. and Ray, C. (2002). Tobacco and youth in the South East Asian region. *The Indian Journal of Cancer*, **39**, 5–35.

Hans, G. (1998). Prevention of cancer in youth with particular reference to intake of paan masala and gutkha, NSS Unit, TISS, Mumbai, India.

Indian Council for Medical Research (2001). Report of the expert committee on the economics of tobacco use. Department of Health, Ministry of Health and Family Welfare, Government of India, New Delhi. pp. 9–19, 39–45, 89, 152.

Jindal, S. K. and Malik, S. K. (1989). Tobacco Smoking and Non-neoplastic Respiratory Disease. In: *Tobacco and health: The Indian scene, Proceedings of the UICC workshop, 'Tobacco or Health', April 15–16, 1987* (ed. L. D. Sanghvi and P. P. Notani), pp. 30–36. Tata Memorial Centre, Bombay.

Kapoor, S. K., Anand, K., and Kumar, G. (Jul–Aug 1995). Prevalence of tobacco use among school and college going adolescents of Haryana. *Indian Journal of Paediatrics*, **62**, 461–6.

Kaur, S. and Singh, S. (Jan. 2002). Cause for concern in Punjab villages. High levels of Gutkha intake among students. *Lifeline*, **7**, 3–4.

Khanolkar, V. R. (1959). Oral Cancer in India. *Union International Contra Cancrum Acta*, **15**, 67–77.

Krishnamurthy, S., Ramaswamy, R., Trivedi, U., and Zachariah, V. (Oct 1997). Tobacco use in rural Indian children. *Indian Journal of Paediatrics*, **34**, 923–7.

Luthra, U. K., Sreenivas, G. R., Menon, G. R., Prabhakar, A. K., and Chaudhry, K. (1992). Tobacco control in India: Problems and solutions. In: *Control of tobacco-related cancers and other diseases, International Symposium, 1990* (ed. P. C. Gupta, J. E. Hamner III, and P. R. Murti), pp. 241–8. Oxford University Press, Bombay.

Malaowalla, A. M., Silverman, S., Mani, N. J., Bilimoria, K. F., and Smith, L. W. (1976). Oral cancer in 57,518 industrial workers of Gujarat, India, a prevalence and follow-up survey. *Cancer*, **37**, 1882–6.

Mehta, F. S., Gupta, P. C., Daftary, D. K., Pindborg, J. J., and Choksi, S. K. (1972). An epidemiologic study of oral cancer and precancerous conditions among 101,761 villagers in Maharashtra, India. *International Journal of Cancer*, **10**, 134–41.

Mehta, F. S., Pindborg, J. J., Gupta, P. C., and Daftary, D. K. (1969). Epidemiologic and histologic study of oral cancer and leukoplakia among 50,915 villagers in India. *Cancer*, **24**, 832–49.

Mehta, F. S., Pindborg, J. J., Hamner, J. E., Gupta, P. C., Daftary, D. K., and Sahiar, B. E., *et al.* (1971). Report on investigations of oral cancer and precancerous conditions in Indian rural populations, 1966–1969. Munksgaard, Copenhagen.

Mehta, F. S., Sanjana, M. K., Shroff, B. C., and Doctor, R. H. (1961). Incidence of leukoplakia among 'Pan' (betel leaf) chewers and bidi smokers: A study of a sample survey. *Indian Journal of Medical Research*, **49**, 393–9.

Mohan, D., Sundaram, K. R., and Sharma, H. K. (May 1986). A study of drug abuse in rural areas of Punjab (India). *Drug and Alcohol Dependence*, **17**, 57–66.

Moon-Stone Group (2000). *Tobacco, All India area, production and yield of tobacco.* Hyderabad: Moonstone Group. indiancommodity.com/statistic/tobaco.htm—Accessed August 16th, 2002.

Narayan, K. M., Chadha, S. L., Hanson, R. L., Tandon, R., Shekhawat, S., Fernandes, R. J., and Gopinath, N. (Jun 1996). Prevalence and patterns of smoking in Delhi: Cross sectional study. *British Medical Journal*, **312**, 1576–9.

Notani, P. N., Jayant, K., and Sanghvi, L. D. (1989). Assessment of morbidity and mortality due to tobacco usage in India. In: *Tobacco and health: The Indian scene, Proceedings of the UICC workshop, 'Tobacco or Health', April 15–16, 1987* (ed. L. D. Sanghvi and P. P. Notani), pp. 63–78. Tata Memorial Centre, Bombay.

Pricewaterhouse (2000). *The Tobacco Industry – India.* Selangaor Dural Ehsani: British American Tobacco, Malaysia. Batmalaysia.com-Corporateinformation-investorRelations—The TobaccoIndustry-India Final Report.pdf.url—Accessed August 16th, 2002.

Reserve Bank of India (1999). Report on Currency & Finance for 1998–99—New Directions and Handbook of Statistics on the Indian Economy, Mumbai.

Sanghvi, L. D. (1992). Challenges in tobacco control in India: a historical perspective. In: *Control of tobacco-related cancers and other diseases, International Symposium, 1990* (ed. P. C. Gupta, J. E. Hamner III, and P. R. Murti), pp. 47–55. Oxford University Press, Bombay.

Sarkar, D., Dhand, R., Malhotra, A., Malhotra, S., and Sharma, B. K. (Jan–Mar 1990). Perceptions and attitude towards tobacco smoking among doctors in Chandigarh. *Indian Journal of Chest Diseases and Allied Sciences*, **32**, 1–9.

Sinha, D. N., Gupta, P. C., Pednekar, M. S., Jones, J. T., and Warren, C. V. (2002). Tobacco use among school personnel in Bihar, India. *Tobacco Control*, **11**, 82–5.

Sinor, P. N., Murti, P. R., Bhonsle, R. B., and Gupta, P. C. (1992). Mawa chewing and oral submucous fibrosis in Bhavnagar, Gujarat, India. In: *Control of tobacco-related cancers and other diseases, International Symposium, 1990* (ed. P. C. Gupta, J. E. Hamner III, and P. R. Murti), pp. 107–12. Oxford University Press, Bombay.

Tobacco Board (2000) *About US.* Tobacco Board, Ministry of Commerce, Government of India, AP, India. indiantobacco.com/aboutus.htm—Accessed August 16th, 2002.

Vaidya, S. G., Vaidya, N. S., and Naik, U. D. (1992). Epidemiology of tobacco habits in Goa, India. In: *Control of tobacco-related cancers and other diseases, International Symposium, 1990* (ed. P. C. Gupta, J. E. Hamner III, and P. R. Murti), pp. 315–22. Oxford University Press, Bombay.

Visaria, P. (2002). Population policy in India, performance and challenges. *The National Medical Journal of India*, **15**, Suppl. 1, 6–18.

Wahi, P. N. (1968). Epidemiology of oral and oropharyngeal cancer. *Bulletin of the World Health Organisation*, **38**, 495–521.

Chapter 15

Tobacco in Africa: More than a health threat

Yussuf Saloojee

Tobacco control has not been assigned a high status as a public health concern in most of sub-Saharan Africa (SSA). Social and economic factors are therefore the main determinants of tobacco use on the continent. Urbanization, increased literacy, the entry of women into the workforce and higher disposable incomes are among factors facilitating the adoption of consumer patterns similar to those in higher-income countries, including increased cigarette smoking.

'Across Africa the total lifestyle is starting to change' claims the head of the advertising agency Saatchi Africa, Eric Franc. 'There is a stronger move towards the western lifestyle as the pace of urbanization increases. People becoming more aware of luxury goods and consumer items they never had before' (Koenderman 2002). Cigarettes, beer, soft drinks, cellular phones, and banking are the products most prominently advertised in African markets.

On the other hand, the World Bank warns that the rapid spread of HIV/AIDS, dwindling aid and investment flows, and weak commodity prices threaten to undo the development gains achieved from 1970 to 1995 (World Bank 2002). Reduced economic growth will diminish business opportunities for the transnational tobacco companies.

Africa cannot continue to ignore tobacco control issues if it is to avoid the 'epidemiological trap' with diseases of lifestyle adding to the toll of disease caused by poverty. This chapter presents an overview of tobacco use, trade, and health policy in SSA.

Tobacco use in sub-Saharan Africa

Due to low consumer purchasing power SSA has the lowest rates of cigarette consumption in the world. In 1963, it is estimated that fewer than 400 cigarettes per adult (aged 15+) per year were sold in this region; by 1995, consumption had risen to 480 (compared to a global average of about 1325) (World Health Organization 1999).

Disposable income is a major determinant of cigarette consumption levels—there is positive relationship between gross national product (GNP) and average cigarette consumption per adult (Fig. 15.1). Cigarette usage is greatest in upper-middle income countries like Mauritius and South Africa and least in low-income countries such as Ethiopia and Guinea-Bissau (World Bank 2001).

It is estimated that about 21 per cent of adults in the region smoke cigarettes, compared to a global average of 33%. The prevalence of smoking is relatively low mainly because few women smoke cigarettes. Smoking prevalence appears to be highest in Nairobi (Kenya), Conakry (Guinea), and Namibia with high proportions of both men and women smoking. In several countries (Burkina Faso, Lesotho, Zimbabwe, Cote d'Ivoire, Nigeria) fewer than 2% of women report that they smoke, while more than half of all men smoke in Tanzania, Uganda, Guinea, Namibia, and Kenya (World Bank 2000) (Fig. 15.2).

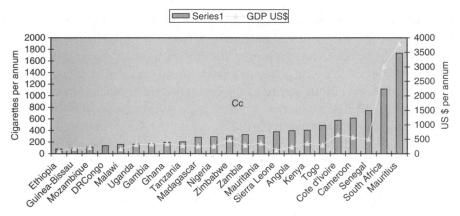

Fig. 15.1 Cigarette consumption per adult and GDP per capita, 1999.

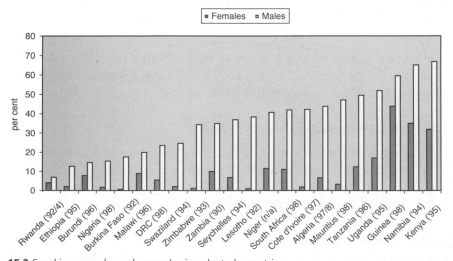

Fig. 15.2 Smoking prevalence by gender in selected countries.

In assessing tobacco use in Africa it is important to include both smoked and smoke-less tobacco (snuff, toombak). In Senegal, for instance, although 32 per cent of adults use some form of tobacco only 4.6 per cent smoke manufactured cigarettes (Corrao *et al.* 2000). Similarly, in South Africa, as many women use snuff as smoke cigarettes (about 10 per cent).

The Global Youth Tobacco Survey (GYTS) (National Center for Disease Prevention and Health Promotion 2002)—a series of school-based surveys conducted between 1999 and 2001 in selected countries—confirm that a diversity of tobacco products are used in the region. The surveys reveal that tobacco use is common among 13–15-year-olds, with about one in five school children regularly using tobacco at the time of the survey. Manufactured cigarettes were not the main form of tobacco used—only one in twelve children were current cigarette smokers. The gap between male and female tobacco use was surprisingly small (Table 15.1).

The data on the prevalence of tobacco use in Africa should be regarded with caution, as information is not available for many countries and even when available it is fre-quently not nationally representative. Most surveys of smoking behaviour usually only cover the major cities or selected sub-regions. The need for accurate information on the use of tobacco and its health consequences in Africa has long been recognized (Sasco 1990) but little has been done to address this need.

Tobacco and health

The existing African per capita cigarette consumption rate is the same as that in the industrialized countries in the 1920s. As a result, SSA is the only region of the world in which primary prevention of the tobacco epidemic is possible. Currently, tobacco use is not a major cause of death on the continent. AIDS, malaria, tuberculosis, maternal and perinatal conditions, and measles remain the major killers.

Table 15.1 Tobacco and cigarette use among school children in selected African countries

Country (city/region)	Current tobacco user (%)			Current cigarette user (%)		
	All	Males	Females	All	Males	Females
Ghana (national)	19.3	19.5	18.8	4.8	5.3	3.8
Kenya (national)	13.0	15.8	10.0	7.2	10.1	4.2
Mali (Bamako)	31.2	44.9	12.6	11.2	11.4	10.1
Malawi (Lilongwe)	18.2	21.1	14.7	6.2	9.1	2.8
Nigeria (Cross River State)	22.1	23.9	17.0	9.1	9.7	5.7
Zimbabwe (Manicaland)	22.0	23.0	20.0	11.4	12.6	9.7

It is estimated that in 1998, two million of the eight million deaths in Africa occurred beyond the age of 30, and that about 125 000 of these could be attributed to smoking (World Health Organization 1999). In contrast to some developed countries where tobacco causes 1 in every 5 or 6 deaths, in Africa it causes only 1 in every 64 deaths.

However, this may be an underestimate. The health consequences of tobacco use may not be fully apparent in Africa because insufficient data are available to demonstrate its effects. For instance, analyses of death certificate data in South Africa found that smoking increased the risk of dying from TB by 60% (Sitas 2000). As TB causes over half-a-million deaths each year in SSA, this suggests that smoking may contribute to more deaths in Africa than was previously supposed.

Although information is scanty, the available data indicates that the rates for lung cancer are intermediate to low in Africa compared to developed countries. The rate, however, is increasing in populations that have smoked tobacco for prolonged periods. Age-standardized lung cancer rates per 10 00 000 in Harare, Zimbabwe are 24.6, in Mali 4.8, and in Gambia 1. This compares to rates of 64.3/100 000 in the UK.

If African countries follow the same trend as in developed countries, its tobacco epidemic can be expected to peak in the middle of the next century. Very rarely do we have the ability to predict an epidemic that far into the future and the knowledge to prevent it now.

Tobacco control

The past two years have seen remarkable support from the African region for the Framework Convention of Tobacco Control (FCTC)—an international treaty that is due to be concluded in 2003 and which will set global standards for action and co-operation in controlling tobacco. Representatives of governments—together with non-governmental organizations as observers—have met regularly in Geneva, and regionally in Johannesburg, Algiers, and Abidjan to discuss the policies that should be included in the FCTC.

African governments have formed a common front, pressing both for progressive regulatory measures (advertising bans, tax increases, restrictions on smoking in public places, anti-smuggling measures, etc.) and for provisions to assist in providing alternative livelihoods for tobacco workers. The common front included both tobacco growing and non-tobacco growing countries.

The African position is perhaps summed up by Uganda's agriculture minister, Dr Kibirige Sebunya, who stated: 'As a government we are concerned about the ill-health caused by tobacco, but at the same time we cannot ignore the economic and social benefits the crop brings to our country.' He pledged support for the FCTC provided 'tobacco farmers are facilitated to produce an equally viable alternative crop to plug the gap that would be created if tobacco was to be eliminated from the country's economy' (New Vision 2002).

The fear that tobacco control policies will cause economic harm is 'largely unfounded' according to U.N. Secretary-General Kofi Annan (Arieff 2002). A WHO report estimates that the number of smokers worldwide would grow from the current 1.28 billion to 1.34 billion by 2050 even if tobacco control policies met their most optimistic goals.

'As the absolute number of smokers grows—because of global population increases— this will ensure a large enough market to keep the current generation of tobacco farmers in business,' Annan said in a new report to the U.N. Economic and Social Council.

Countries like Zimbabwe and Malawi need to diversify away from tobacco, less because of the fears of falling demand due to tobacco control policies and more because any economy which is highly dependent on a single crop or export is highly vulnerable. The environmental, health, and social consequences of tobacco growing are other reasons for moving away from tobacco growing (see next section). Finally, the tobacco and pharmaceutical industries are investing heavily in developing 'cleaner' nicotine delivery systems to replace the cigarette. These technologically advanced products will use less tobacco, or may even be tobacco-free, and may represent the most significant threat to the viability of tobacco farming yet.

By 1999, about half the governments in SSA had taken some steps to regulate tobacco. Some 20 countries have enacted laws regulating smoking in public places, 16 require health warnings on tobacco products and 10 have total or strong partial bans on tobacco advertising and promotion. However, apart from South Africa, Botswana, Mauritius, and Mali most countries have not passed comprehensive tobacco control laws and the legislation is weak.

South Africa has made the most progress in regulating tobacco, with consumption falling by 33% between 1990 and 2000. The South African Parliament prohibited all tobacco advertising, sponsorship, and promotions in 1999. No advertisement may contain trademarks, logos, brand names, or company names of tobacco products. The law also bans smoking in all enclosed places, including workplaces, and the free distribution of tobacco products, and awards or prizes to induce the purchase of tobacco. The government has also increased tobacco excise taxes for 'health reasons', so as to discourage consumption (Saloojee 2000).

In 1996, Mali prohibited the advertising of tobacco products in most media, and smoking in public places and requires health warnings and ingredient disclosure on cigarette packs. Mauritius enacted similar legislation in 1995.

Tobacco taxes and smuggling

One of the most cost-effective ways to control tobacco, especially in low-income countries, is to raise the price of cigarettes through increasing tobacco taxes. The World

Bank estimates that an increase of 10 per cent in the price of a pack of cigarettes across all SSA countries would persuade 3 million smokers in the region to quit smoking and prevent 0.7 million premature deaths from diseases caused by smoking. The calculations are based on 1995 population estimates (World Bank 1999).

Every tobacco tax decision is therefore a health decision, and maintaining the price of tobacco above the rate of increase in real incomes is an important public health goal. Between 1990 the real price of cigarettes in eight African countries increased by an average of 2.14 per cent annually, which is well below the rate of increase in countries with progressive tobacco control policies like France (9.25%), Hong Kong (8.63%), or Australia (6.54%) (Guindon *et al.* 2002).

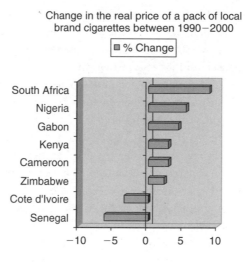

Change in the real price of a pack of local brand cigarettes between 1990–2000

The rate of tobacco taxes in African countries is also low compared to the European Union (EU). The EU adopted a directive in 1992 that fixed a minimum tax level of at least 70% of the retail price of a pack of cigarettes. In 10 African countries, for which data was available, in 1999, the average tax was 46% of the retail price (Table 15.2). The rate was lowest in Nigeria (32%) and highest in Ghana (66%) (World Bank 2000).

An increase in tobacco taxes would not only reduce consumption but would increase revenues for cash-strapped governments. If part of these new revenues were spent on health services there would be a double benefit for health—from reduced tobacco consumption and increased health spending.

In most countries there is probably a discrepancy between taxes on cigarettes and other tobacco products, with the latter being taxed at a lower rate. This differential

Table 15.2 Cigarette taxes as percentage of retail price in 1999

	Tax as percentage of retail price
Nigeria	32
Cameroon	33
Senegal	36
Cote d'Ivoire	37
South Africa	38
Malawi	40
Zimbabwe	53
Uganda	61
Kenya	64
Ghana	66

should be reduced so as to discourage switching from higher priced to lower priced tobacco products. The policy objective should be to reduce all tobacco consumption and not just cigarette use.

The tobacco industry recognizes the implications that higher taxes and prices have on their sales volumes, and has strongly opposed these through various strategies, including smuggling, price-collusion, and fixing market share.

The tobacco industry

Cigarette manufacturing: All the major transnational tobacco manufacturers and leaf companies operate in SSA, with British American Tobacco (BAT), Imperial Tobacco, and Altadis the dominant players.

BAT is the leading manufacturer in the region with a monopoly in Zambia, Zimbabwe, Ghana, Sierra Leone, Malawi, and Uganda, and a near monopoly in the Democratic Republic of Congo (95% share of market), South Africa (95% share), and Nigeria (91% share).

The second largest cigarette maker in the region is Tobaccor which has 90% of share in 8 markets—Ivory Coast, Burkina Faso, Senegal, Gabon, Congo, the Central African Republic, Chad, and Madagascar. UK-based cigarette maker, Imperial Tobacco, acquired a 75% share in Tobaccor in May 2001—paying US$ 250 million to Bollare, the French conglomerate.

Tobacco growing: Since the late 1970s, commercial growing of tobacco has shifted predominantly to low-income countries, primarily because of lower-production costs due to the availability of cheap labour and easy access to natural resources (i.e., wood-fuel and fresh pest-free soils).

The cigarette manufacturers and major leaf buying companies have encouraged tobacco growing to ensure a ready supply of tobacco leaf at lower prices. In Tanzania, the leaf merchant, Dimon, has contracted 30 000 farmers providing them with seed, fertiliser, and financial and technical assistance. BAT has contracted 50 000 farmers in Uganda and 10 000 farmers in Kenya.

Between 1989/91 and 1995 the area under tobacco cultivation in Africa south of the equator increased by 18% to 291 000 ha and crop yield was up by 27% (Geist 1988). The increase was even greater in Zimbabwe, Malawi, and Tanzania, the largest African producers, with the land under cultivation going up by 28% and production by 37%.

SSA countries produced a total of about 500 000 tons of tobacco annually accounting for 7% of global production. About 228 000 tons are produced in Zimbabwe and 99 000 tons by Malawi (the world's leading producer of Burley leaf). Other important producers in the region include South Africa (30 000 tons), Tanzania (25 000), Uganda (23 000), Kenya (18 000), and Cote d'Ivoire (12 000).

The Zimbabwean and Malawian economies are highly dependent upon tobacco, earning 30% and 70%, respectively of their total foreign earnings from the crop. Zimbabwe is ranked sixth and Malawi eighth among the world's leading tobacco producers.

The massive increase in global tobacco leaf production together with a limited number of buyers has resulted in a decline in leaf prices. Between 1985 and 2000, the real price of flue-cured tobacco fell by 37 per cent to US$ 1221 per ton.

The transnational manufacturers purchase 85–95% of the tobacco exported from the developing world and it is the companies that set leaf prices. The industry journal, Tobacco International has noted that the limited number of leaf buyers in countries like Malawi 'has led to reduced competition—especially when one company is purchasing more than 50 per cent of the crop.' (Kille 1998). In 1998, the then chairman of the International Tobacco Growers Association, Richard Tate was moved to complain: 'By switching prices on and off in successive seasons, the buyers are endangering long-term stability of supply ... We have all been surprised and shocked at the buyers' short-sighted behaviour, which has severely affected all the regional markets.'

Leaf prices slumped across all African markets in 1988 with prices falling by as much as 40% in Zimbabwe. In 2000, Malawi again experienced a harsh shock when average auction price tumbled by 35%, down from US$ 1.56 in 1999 to US$ 1.01 per kg. The 2000 season opened with the historic low price of US 10 cents per kg at the opening of the Lilongwe floors in Malawi.

In recent years, both Malawi and Zimbabwe witnessed protests by farmers over low auction prices resulting in regular delays in the opening or temporary closure of the auctions.

The decline in price in Malawi in 2000 was also in part due to the quality of tobacco sold, as farmers used less fertilizer following a hike in the price of chemical fertilizers. The President of the Tobacco Association of Malawi (TAMA) is reported as saying: 'Escalating costs of farm inputs and labour makes it difficult for many small-scale tobacco farmers to grow tobacco profitably. Many have failed to repay fertiliser and other input loans.'

Variable market prices and a diminishing rate of return have encouraged some farmers to begin moving away from tobacco. Other reasons for diversifying away from tobacco include:

*The environmental effects of heavy pesticide use associated with tobacco growing, and deforestation in countries where tobacco is cured with fuel wood. A medium to serious degree of tobacco-related deforestation exists in southern and eastern Africa (Malawi, Zimbabwe, Zambia, Tanzania, Uganda, Burundi, Ethiopia) and west Africa (Togo, Nigeria). In southern Africa an estimated 140 000 hectares of woodlands are cleared annually to supply fuelwood to cure tobacco, accounting for 12 per cent of the deforestation in the region (Geist 1988).

Furthermore, replacing indigenous forests with largely monoculture plantations of fast-growing foreign species like eucalyptus, which draws heavily on underground water resources, causes biodiversity losses in both flora and fauna.

* Tobacco threatens food security in the region, with Kenya, Malawi, and Zimbabwe all having to import maize to meet domestic requirements. Small-scale farmers complain that growing tobacco requires intensive labour for long periods so that they do not have the time to grow traditional food crops like maize, beans, and cassava—nor do they earn enough to buy sufficient food for their families (Kariuk 1998).

* The International Confederation of Free Trade Unions has complained that child labour in tobacco-growing areas continues unabated. It states that, 'more than twenty per cent of the workforce on commercial plantations, especially tobacco plantations, are children. Much child labour on these commercial plantations is hidden because the tenant farming system encourages the whole family to work. Many children are kept from school in order to contribute to the family growing effort, and smaller children are often kept from school in order to perform the domestic tasks that the parents and older siblings are not available to perform. The ILO [International Labour Organization] estimates that over 440 000 children between the ages of 10 and 14 are economically active in Malawi, which constitutes over thirty per cent of this age group.' (afrol News 2002)

The greatest stumbling block to tobacco control in SSA is the widely held perception of the importance of tobacco to its economies. The hundreds of thousands of small-scale farmers in the region barely eke out a living but they remain trapped in tobacco growing because they are in debt and have little incentive to grow other crops. These farmers need urgent supportive interventions. Firstly, they require financial assistance to offset loan; and secondly, they require production and marketing support for growing other crops.

Compared to the marketing machine driving tobacco use the resources for discouraging tobacco use are meager. There is a gross mismatch between the resources needed by governments and NGO's for tobacco control and those actually available. Enabling farmers to reduce their dependence on the tobacco crop and assisting NGOs in challenging the forces promoting tobacco use will benefit not only health but also the environment.

References

Afrol News (2002). 'Malawi slammed on workers' conditions' February 2002, http://www.afrol.com/News2002/maw2002_labour.htm

Arieff, I. (2002), *U.N. Sees More Smokers Despite Anti-Tobacco Drive.* Reuters, June 13.

Campbell, D. and Maguire, K. (2001). 'Clarke company faces new smuggling claims', *The Guardian*, August 22, http://www.guardian.co.uk/guardianpolitics/story/0,3605,540558,00.html

Corrao, M. A., Guindon, G. E., Sharma, N., and Shookoohi D. F. (ed.) (2000). *Tobacco control country profiles*, American Cancer Society, Atlanta, GA.

Geist, H. (1998). 'How tobacco farming contributes to tropical deforestation', in I. Abedian. R. van der Merwe, N. Wilkins, and P. Jha (eds), *The Economics of Tobacco Control.* Cape Town.

Guindon, G. E., Tobin, S., and Yach, D. (2002). 'Trends and affordability of cigarette prices: ample room for tax increases and related health gains', *Tobacco Control*, 11, 35–43.

Kariuk, J. (1998). 'Tobacco cultivation threatens food security in Kenya', *Panos Features*, December 20.

Kille, T. (1998). 'Big domination', *Tobacco International*, September.

Koenderman, T. (2002). 'From Beer to Banking: Interest is rising.' *Adfocus. Supplement to the Financial Mail*, South Africa, May 20.

National Center for Disease Prevention and Health Promotion (2002). Global Youth Tobacco Survey (GYTS). http://www.cdc.gov/tobacco/global/gyts

New Vision (2002). *Tobacco tops $30m,* June 20.

Saloojee, Y. (2000). '*Tobacco Control in South Africa*', South African Health Review. Health Systems Trust. Durban. http://www.hst.org.za/sahr

Sasco, A. J. (1990). 'Africa—a desperate need for data', *Tobacco Control.*

Sitas, F. (2000). (Personal communication), National Cancer Registry.

World Bank (1999). *Curbing the epidemic: governments and the economics of tobacco control.* Series: Development in practice. Washington D.C.: The World Bank, http://www!.worldbank.org/tobacco/reports.htm

World Bank (2000). *Tobacco in Kenya in the African context.* October, http://worldbank.org

World Bank (2001). *Economics of Tobacco for the African (AFR) Region.* June 20, http://worldbank.org

World Bank (2002). 'African Development Indicators 2002', *World Bank Publications,* Washington DC.

World Health Organization (1999). The World Health Report 1999. *Combating the tobacco epidemic.* Geneva. World Health Organization.

Part 5

Tobacco and health.
Global burden

Chapter 16

The future worldwide health effects of current smoking patterns

Richard Peto and Alan D Lopez

Worldwide, there are only two or three major causes of death whose effects are now increasing rapidly: tobacco and HIV (and, perhaps, obesity). If current smoking patterns persist, there will be about 1 billion deaths from tobacco during the twenty-first century, as against 'only' about 0.1 billion (100 million) during the whole of the twentieth century. About half of these deaths will be in middle age (35–69) rather than old age—and, those killed by tobacco in middle age lose, on average, more than 20 years of non-smoker life expectancy (Box A).

There are two main reasons for this large increase in tobacco deaths. First, the world population in middle and old age will increase. Second, the proportion of the deaths in middle and old age that is caused by tobacco will increase substantially over the next few decades, due to the delayed effects of the large increase in cigarette smoking among young adults over the past few decades (Doll *et al.* 1994; Peto *et al.* 1994, 1999; Murray and Lopez 1996; World Health Organization 1996, 1997). Among cigarette smokers,

Box A: Hazards for the persistent cigarette smoker: 1990s British and American evidence (Doll *et al.* 1994, 2004; Peto *et al.* 1994, 2000)

- ◆ **HALF are killed:** Among persistent cigarette smokers (those who start in early adult life and do not give up), about 50% will eventually be killed by tobacco.

- ◆ **A quarter killed in MIDDLE age (35–69):** Half those killed by tobacco are still in middle age, losing on average about 20–25 years of life.

- ◆ **Stopping smoking works:** Even in middle age, smokers who stop before they have developed some serious disease avoid MOST of their subsequent risk of death from tobacco: smokers who stop before middle age avoid almost all their risk.

the risk of death from tobacco in middle or old age is really substantial (about 1 in 2) only for those who start smoking in early adult life (Doll and Peto 1981; Peto et al. 1986, 1994; Doll et al. 1994, 2004). Hence, when there is a large upsurge in cigarette smoking among the young adults in a particular country, this will produce a large upsurge in tobacco deaths half a century later; the numbers of deaths from tobacco around the year 2000 were strongly influenced by the numbers of young adults who took up smoking around 1950, while the numbers of young adults who took up smoking around the year 2000 will strongly influence the numbers of deaths from tobacco around the year 2050 (and beyond).

The main increase in cigarette use by young adults took place during the first half of the twentieth century for men in developed countries, but it took place during the second half of the century for women in developed countries and for men in developing countries (Doll et al. 1994; Peto et al. 1994; World Health Organization 1997). Thus far, relatively few women in developing countries have begun to smoke.

For men in developed countries the epidemic of tobacco deaths may already be about as large as it will ever be, with tobacco now responsible for about one-third of all male deaths in middle age (Peto et al. 1994). Continuing increases in male tobacco deaths in developed countries such as Greece or Portugal are offset by recent decreases elsewhere, e.g., the UK. For women in most developed countries, however, the epidemic still has far to go—indeed, in many European countries such as France or Spain the main increase in tobacco deaths is only just beginning, although in the United States the proportion of deaths in middle age that is due to tobacco is now almost as great in women as in men (Peto et al. 1994).

In North America, taking both sexes together, US cigarette consumption per adult was 1, 4, and 10 per day in 1910, 1930, and 1950, after which it remained relatively constant for some decades. As a delayed result of this pre-1950 increase in cigarette consumption, the proportion of all US deaths at ages 35–69 attributed to tobacco rose from 12% in 1950 to 33% in 1990 (Peto et al. 1994).

In China, which is the largest and best studied of the developing countries (Liu et al. 1998; Niu et al. 1998; Peto et al. 1999), the increase in male cigarette consumption and in tobacco deaths both lag almost exactly 40 years behind the US. At present, few of the young women in China become smokers, but adult Chinese male cigarette consumption averaged 1, 4, and 10 per day in 1952, 1972, and 1992, with no further increase during the past few years, and the proportion of Chinese male deaths at ages 35–69 attributed to tobacco was measured to be 12% in 1990 and is projected to be about 33% in 2030. Two-thirds of the young men in China become persistent smokers, and about half of those who do so will eventually be killed by the habit: so, about one-third of all the young men in China will eventually be killed by tobacco, if current smoking patterns persist.

China, with 20 per cent of the world's population, produces and consumes about 30% of the world's cigarettes, and a large nationwide study has now shown that China already suffers almost a million deaths a year from tobacco, a figure that is likely to at least double by 2025. The Chinese study consisted of two parts, one retrospective (Liu *et al.* 1998) (ascertaining the smoking habits of adults who had recently died) and one prospective (Niu *et al.* 1998) (which will continue for decades, monitoring the long-term growth of the epidemic). In recent years large retrospective and prospective studies have been, or are being, established in China, India, Latin America, and elsewhere, to monitor the current and future hazards not only in developed but also in various developing populations: results from China (Liu *et al.* 1998; Niu *et al.* 1998), and from India (Gupta and Mehta 2000; Gajalakshmi *et al.* 2003), show that the hazards in some developing countries are already substantial.

Worldwide, there are now about 4–5 million deaths a year caused by tobacco, 2 million in developed and 2–3 million in developing countries. But, these numbers reflect smoking patterns several decades ago, and worldwide cigarette consumption has increased substantially over the past half century (World Health Organization 1997). On current smoking patterns, about 30% of young adults become persistent smokers and relatively few give up (except in selected populations, such as educated adults in parts of western Europe and North America).

The main diseases by which smoking kills people are substantially different in America (where vascular disease and lung cancer predominate) (Peto *et al.* 1994), in China (where chronic obstructive pulmonary disease predominates, causing even more tobacco deaths than lung cancer) (Liu *et al.* 1998; Niu *et al.* 1998), and in India (where half the world's tuberculosis deaths take place, and the ability of smoking to increase the risk of death from TB may well be of particular importance) (Gupta and Mehta 2000; Gajalakshmi *et al.* 2003). But, there is no good reason to expect the overall 50% risk of death from persistent cigarette smoking to be very different in different populations.

There are already a billion smokers, and by 2030 about another billion young adults will have started to smoke. On current smoking patterns, worldwide mortality from tobacco is likely to rise from about 4–5 million deaths a year around AD 2000 to about 10 million a year around 2030 (i.e. 100 million per decade) (Peto *et al.* 1994), and will rise somewhat further in later decades. So, tobacco will cause about 150 million deaths in the first quarter of the century and 300 million in the second quarter. Predictions for the third and, particularly, the fourth quarter of the next century are inevitably somewhat speculative, but if over the next few decades about 30% of the young adults become persistent smokers and about half are eventually killed by their habit, then about 15% of adult mortality in the second half of the century will be due to tobacco (implying more than half a billion tobacco deaths in 2050–2099).

These numbers of tobacco deaths before 2050 cannot be greatly reduced unless a substantial proportion of the adults who have already been smoking for some time give up the habit. For, a decrease over the next decade or two in the proportion of children who become smokers will not have its main effects on mortality until the third quarter of the century (Box B).

Box B: Effects of adult smokers quitting on tobacco deaths before 2050, and of young people not starting on tobacco deaths after 2050 (Doll *et al.* 1994, 2004; Peto *et al.* 1994, 2000)

- ◆ **Quitting:** If many of the adults who now smoke were to give up over the next decade or two, halving global cigarette consumption per adult by the year 2020, then this would prevent about one-third of the tobacco deaths in 2020 and would almost halve tobacco deaths in the second quarter of the century. Such changes would avoid about 20 or 30 million tobacco deaths in the first quarter of the century and would avoid about 150 million in the second quarter.

- ◆ **Not starting:** If, by progressive reduction over the next decade or two in the global uptake rate of smoking by young people, the proportion of young adults who become smokers were to be halved by 2020, then this would avoid hundreds of millions of the deaths from tobacco after 2050. It would, however, avoid almost none of the 150 million deaths from tobacco in the first quarter of the century, and would probably avoid "only" about 10 or 20 million of the 300 million deaths from tobacco in the second quarter of the century.

The calculations in Box B show that quitting by adult smokers offers the only realistic way in which widespread changes in smoking status can prevent large numbers of tobacco deaths over the next half century. Widely practicable ways of helping large numbers of young people not to become smokers could avoid hundreds of millions of tobacco deaths in the middle and second half of the century, but not before, whereas widely practicable ways of helping large numbers of adult smokers to quit (preferably before middle age, but also in middle age: Box A) might well avoid one or two hundred million tobacco deaths in the first half of the century. The strategies that are relevant to young people may well be of little relevance to adults, and vice versa, so over-emphasis on either at the expense of the other would be inappropriate. In particular, it is often wrongly supposed that it is impossible to get large numbers of adult smokers to quit, but the experience of several countries over the past few decades shows that decreases can occur both in the proportion who start and in the proportion who continue to smoke.

Britain, which is now experiencing the most rapid decrease in the world in pre-mature deaths from tobacco, shows that quite large improvements are possible (Peto *et al.* 1994, 2000). From 1965 to 1995 annual UK cigarette sales fell by half, and there was a threefold reduction in the machine-measured tar delivery per cigarette (and hence a moderate reduction in the hazard per smoker: Doll and Peto 1981; Peto 1986). Over the same period, annual UK tobacco deaths in middle age decreased from 80 000 to 30 000, and they are still falling rapidly (Peto *et al.* 1994, 2000). (For lung cancer, the

UK male death rate at ages 35–69 has been decreasing at the rate of 40% per decade in recent years.) (Peto *et al.* 2000). Moreover, as those now in middle age progress into old age over the next decade or two, UK mortality in old age from tobacco should also decrease substantially.

Unfortunately, however, although there have been substantial decreases in the prevalence of smoking in some developed populations, there have been large increases elsewhere, particularly in Chinese males, over the past few decades (Liu *et al.* 1998; Peto *et al.* 1999), and it is difficult to see how worldwide cigarette consumption can be halved over the next decade or two. Hence, the 100 million tobacco deaths in the twentieth century are likely to be followed, if present smoking patterns persist, by about 1 billion tobacco deaths in the twenty-first century.

Acknowledgement

This research involved collaboration with J. Boreham, Z.-M. Chen, R. Collins, R. Doll, V. Gajalakshmi, P.C. Gupta, B.-Q. Liu, and G. Mead, and support from the UK Medical Research Council, Cancer Research UK and British Heart Foundation.

This article is also published in: Critical Issues in Global Health, edited by C. Everett Koop *et al.* (Peto and Lopez 2001). Any part of it can be reproduced without seeking copyright permission.

References

Doll, R. and Peto, R. (1981). The causes of cancer: quantitative estimates of avoidable risks of cancer in the United States today. *J Natl Cancer Inst*, **66**, 1193–308 (Republished by Oxford University Press as a monograph in 1983).

Doll, R., Peto, R., Wheatley, K., Gray, R., and Sutherland, I. (1994). Mortality in relation to smoking: 40 years' observations on male British doctors. *Br Med J*, **309**, 901–11.

Doll, R., Peto, R., Boreham, J., and Sutherland, I. (2004). Mortality in relation to smoking: 50 years' observations on male British doctors. *Br Med J*, in press.

Gajalakshmi, V., Peto, R., Kanaka, T. S., and Jha, P. (2003). Smoking and morality from tuberculosis and other diseases in India: retrospective study of 43 000 adult male deaths and 35 000 controls. *Lancet*, **362**, 507–15.

Gupta, P. C. and Mehta, H. C. (2000). Cohort study of all-cause mortality among tobacco users in Mumbai, India. *Bull WHO*, **78**, 877–83.

Liu, B. Q., Peto, R., Chen, Z. M., Boreham, J., Wu, Y. P., Li, J. Y., *et al.* (1998). Emerging tobacco hazards in China: 1. Retrospective proportional mortality study of one million deaths. *Br Med J*, **317**, 1411–22.

Murray, C. J. L. and Lopez, A. D. (1996). *The global burden of disease: a comprehensive assessment of mortality and disability from diseases, injuries, and risk factors in 1990, and projected to 2020.* Harvard University Press, Cambridge, MA.

Niu, S. R., Yang, G. H., Chen, Z. M., Wang, J. L., Wang, G. H., He, X. Z., *et al.* (1998). Emerging tobacco hazards in China: 2. Early mortality results from a prospective study. *Br Med J*, **317**, 1423–4.

Peto, R. (1986). Influence of dose and duration of smoking on lung cancer rates, pp 23–33. In: *Tobacco: A growing international health hazard. IARC scientific publication no. 74* (ed. D. Zaridze and R. Peto). International Agency for Research on Cancer (IARC), Lyon.

Peto, R., Lopez, A. D., Boreham, J., Thun, M., and Heath, C. Jr. (1994). *Mortality from smoking in developed countries 1950–2000: Indirect estimates from national vital statistics.* Oxford University Press. (Second edition in press, 2004, and available on <www.ctsu.ox.ac.uk>.)

Peto, R., Chen, Z. M., and Boreham, J. (1999). Tobacco—the growing epidemic. *Nature Medicine*, 5, 15–17.

Peto, R., Darby, S., Deo, H., Silcocks, P., Whitley, E., and Doll, R. (2000). Smoking, smoking cessation, and lung cancer in the UK since 1950. *Br Med J*, 321, 323–9.

Peto, R. and Lopez, A. D. (2000). Future worldwide health effects of current smoking patterns. In: *Critical issues in global health* (ed. C.E. Koop, C.E. Pearson, and M.R. Schwarz). Jossey-Bass, San Francisco.

World Health Organization (1997). Tobacco or Health: A Global Status Report. World Health Organization, Geneva.

World Health Organization (1996). *Investing in health research and development.* World Health Organization, Geneva.

Chapter 17

Passive smoking and health

Jonathan M. Samet

Overview

Evidence on the health effects of tobacco smoking, both active and passive, and of using smokeless tobacco has been central in driving initiatives to control tobacco use. In some countries, the evidence on passive smoking has had particularly powerful consequences in shaping public policy in recent decades, as strategies have been implemented to protect nonsmokers from involuntarily inhaling tobacco smoke in public places, workplaces, and their homes. This chapter provides an overview and introduction to the now-vast data on the adverse health consequences of passive smoking, covering the risks to passive smokers, including the fetus, infants and children, and adults. Since the 1980s, the evidence has been periodically examined and synthesized in various governmental reports, which should be used by those seeking comprehensive summaries to supplement this chapter; the most recent include the report prepared by the Environmental Protection Agency of the state of California in the United States (National Cancer Institute 1999), the United Kingdom's Scientific Committee on Tobacco (Scientific Committee on Tobacco and Health & HSMO 1998), the World Health Organization (WHO 1999), and the International Agency for Research on Cancer (IARC 2002). Samet and Wang (2000) have also recently and comprehensively reviewed the literature. A report of the U.S. Surgeon General on the topic is also anticipated.

Although there were writings on the dangers to health of tobacco use centuries ago, the body of research evidence that constitutes the foundation of our present understanding of tobacco as a cause of disease dates to approximately the mid-twentieth century. Even earlier, case reports and case series had called attention to the likely role of smoking and chewing tobacco as a cause of cancer. The rise of diseases that had once been uncommon, such as lung cancer and coronary heart disease, was noticed early in the twentieth century and motivated clinical and pathological studies to determine if the increases were 'real' or an artifact of changing methods of detection. By mid-century, there was no doubt that the increases were real and the focus of research shifted to the causes of the new epidemics of 'chronic diseases,' such as lung cancer and coronary heart disease.

The epidemiological studies that were implemented to find the causes of these new epidemics quickly linked active cigarette smoking to cancers of the lung and other organs, coronary heart disease, and 'emphysema and chronic bronchitis,' now termed chronic obstructive pulmonary disease (COPD). The studies were observational, that is comparing risks of disease in those who smoked with those who did not, and were primarily of the cohort (following smokers and nonsmokers and measuring the rate at which disease develops in the two groups) and case-control (designs comparing rates of smoking in persons with the disease under study and in controls who are similar but do not have the disease). Surveys, or cross-sectional studies, were also carried out, particularly to compare rates of lung disease in smokers and nonsmokers. These same designs were subsequently used to investigate the risks of passive smoking.

By the 1960s, there was strong evidence that active smoking was a powerful cause of disease. For example, the risk of lung cancer in men who smoked was increased 10-fold or more compared to men who had never smoked, and the risk increased with the number of cigarettes smoked and the duration of smoking (US Department of Health Education and Welfare 1964). These initial observations quickly sparked complementary laboratory studies on the mechanisms by which tobacco smoking causes disease. The multidisciplinary approach to research on tobacco has been key in linking active and passive smoking to various diseases; the observational evidence has been supported with an understanding of the mechanisms by which smoking causes disease. By 1953, for example, Wynder and colleagues (1953) had shown that painting the skin of mice with the condensate of cigarette smoke caused tumors. In combination with the emerging epidemiologic evidence on smoking and lung cancer, this observation was sufficiently powerful to be followed by the US tobacco industry's dramatic response of establishing the Tobacco Industry Research Committee, later to become the Tobacco Research Council, and to initiate a campaign to discredit the emerging scientific evidence. This same tactic is still being used by the tobacco industry for research on passive smoking.

By the late 1950s and early 1960s, the mounting evidence on active smoking received formal review and evaluation by government committees, leading to definitive conclusions on causation in the early 1960s. In the United Kingdom, the 1962 report of the Royal College of Physicians (Royal College of Physicians of London 1962) concluded that smoking was a cause of lung cancer and bronchitis and a contributing factor to coronary heart disease. In the United States, the 1964 report of the Advisory Committee to the Surgeon General concluded that smoking was a cause of lung cancer in men and of chronic bronchitis (US Department of Health Education and Welfare 1964). This conclusion was based in a systematic and comprehensive evaluation of evidence and application of criteria for judgment as to the causality of association. The criteria included the association's consistency, strength, specificity, temporal relationship, and coherence. By law, a U.S. Surgeon General's report was subsequently required annually and new conclusions have been reached periodically with regard to the diseases caused by smoking. The Royal College of Physicians has also continued to release periodic reports, as have other organizations. These reports and other expert syntheses of the evidence have proved to be effective tools for translating the findings on smoking, both active and passive, and disease into policy.

The issue of passive smoking and health has a briefer history. Some of the first epidemiological studies on second-hand smoke or environmental tobacco smoke (ETS) and health were reported in the late 1960s (Cameron 1967; Colley and Holland 1967; Cameron *et al.* 1969). Prior to that point, there had been scattered case reports, the Nazi government had campaigned against smoking in public, and one German physician, Fritz Lickint, used the term 'passive smoking' in his 1939 book on smoking (Proctor 1995). In the 1960s, the initial investigations focused on parental smoking and lower respiratory illnesses in infants; studies of lung function and respiratory symptoms in children soon followed (US Department of Health and Human Services 1986; Samet and Wang 2000). The 1971 report of the U.S. Surgeon General raised concern about possible adverse effects of passive smoking (US Department of Health Education and Welfare 1971).

The first major studies on passive smoking and lung cancer in nonsmokers were reported in 1981, a cohort study in Japan and a case–control study in Athens (Hirayama 1981*a, b*; Trichopoulos *et al.* 1981), and by 1986 the evidence supported the conclusion that passive smoking was a cause of lung cancer in non-smokers, a conclusion reached by the International Agency for Research on Cancer (IARC), the U.S. Surgeon General, and the U.S. National Research Council (IARC 1986; US Department of Health and Human Services 1986). The evidence on child health and passive smoking was also reviewed in 1986 by the U.S. Surgeon General and the U.S. National Research Council (Table 17.1). A now-substantial body of evidence has continued to identify new diseases and other adverse effects of passive smoking, including increased risk for coronary heart disease (Table 17.1) (California Environmental Protection Agency 1997; Scientific Committee on Tobacco and Health & HSMO 1998; WHO 1999; Samet and Wang 2000).

In Australia and New Zealand, the United Kingdom, some countries of Scandinavia, and the United States, for example, the evidence of harm to nonsmokers from breathing secondhand smoke has led to the implementation of national and local policies and regulation to restrict smoking in public places and workplaces (National Cancer Institute 1999; Corrao *et al.* 2000). In the state of California in the U.S., all workplaces, including bars and restaurants, are now smokefree. Smoking is no longer permitted on international airplane flights. There are abundant successful examples of using the scientific evidence on passive smoking as the foundation for effective public policies for reducing exposure.

Toxicology of tobacco smoke

Tobacco smoke is generated by the burning of a complex organic material, tobacco, along with the various additives and paper, at a high temperature, reaching about

Table 17.1 Adverse effects from exposure to tobacco smoke

Health effect	SG 1984[a]	SG 1986[b]	EPA 1992[c]	CalEPA 1997[d]	UK 1998[e]	WHO 1999[f]	IARC 2002[g]
Increased prevalence of respiratory illnesses	Yes/a	Yes/a	Yes/c	Yes/c	Yes/c	Yes/c	
Decrement in pulmonary function	Yes/a	Yes/a	Yes/a	Yes/a		Yes/c	
Increased frequency of bronchitis, pneumonia	Yes/a	Yes/a	Yes/a	Yes/c		Yes/c	
Increase in chronic cough, phlegm		Yes/a				Yes/c	
Increased frequency of middle ear effusion		Yes/a	Yes/c	Yes/c	Yes/c	Yes/c	
Increased severity of asthma episodes and symptoms			Yes/c	Yes/c		Yes/c	
Risk factor for new asthma			Yes/a	Yes/c			
Risk factor for SIDS			Yes/a	Yes/c	Yes/a	Yes/c	
Risk factor for lung cancer in adults		Yes/c	Yes/c	Yes/c	Yes/c		Yes/c
Risk factor for heart disease in adults				Yes/c	Yes/c	Yes/a	

Yes/a = association.

Yes/c = cause.

[a]US Dept of Health and Human Services 1984.

[b]US Dept of Health and Human Services 1986.

[c]US Environmental Protection Agency 1992.

[d]California Environmental Protection Agency 1997.

[e]Scientific Committee on Tobacco & Health & HSMO 1998.

[f]World Health Organization 1999.

[g]IARC 2002.

a thousand degrees centigrade in the burning coal of the cigarette (US Department of Health Education and Welfare 1964). The resulting smoke, comprising numerous gases and also particles, includes myriad toxic components that can cause injury through inflammation and irritation, asphyxiation, carcinogenesis, and other mechanisms. Some examples are carbon monoxide, cyanide, radioactive polonium, benzo-(a)-pyrene, oxides of nitrogen, acrolein, benzene, and particles. Active smokers inhale mainstream smoke (MS), the smoke drawn directly through the end of the cigarette. Passive smokers inhale smoke that is often referred to as secondhand smoke or ETS, comprising a mixture of mostly sidestream smoke (SS) given off by the smoldering cigarette and some exhaled MS. Sidestream smoke is generated at lower temperatures than MS, and consequently concentrations of many toxic compounds are greater in SS than MS. However, SS is rapidly diluted following its generation as it disperses into the air. Concentrations of tobacco smoke components in secondhand smoke are far below the levels of MS inhaled by the active smoker, but there are qualitative similarities between secondhand smoke and MS (US Department of Health and Human Services 1986; IARC 2002).

Both active and passive smokers absorb tobacco smoke components through the lung's airways and alveoli and many of these components, such as the gas carbon monoxide, then enter into the circulation and are distributed systemically. There is also uptake of such components as benzo-(a)-pyrene directly into the cells that line the upper airway and the lung's airways. Some of the carcinogens undergo metabolic transformation into their active forms and evidence now indicates that metabolism-determining genes may affect susceptibility to tobacco smoke (Nelkin *et al.* 1998). The genitourinary system is exposed to toxins in tobacco smoke through the excretion of compounds in the urine, including carcinogens. The gastrointestinal tract is exposed through direct deposition of smoke in the upper airway and the clearance of smoke-containing mucus from the trachea through the glottis into the esophagus. Not surprisingly, tobacco smoking has proved to be a multisystem cause of disease.

There is a substantial scientific literature on the mechanisms by which tobacco smoking causes disease. This body of research includes characterization of many components in smoke, some having well-established toxicity, such as nicotine, hydrogen cyanide, benzo-(a)-pyrene, carbon monoxide, and nitrogen oxides. The toxicity of smoke has been studied by exposing animals to tobacco smoke and smoke condensate, in cellular and other laboratory systems for evaluating toxicity, and by assessing smokers for evidence of injury by tobacco smoke, using biomarkers such as tissue changes and levels of damaging enzymes and cytokines. The data from these studies amply document the powerful toxicity of tobacco smoke. The mechanisms of disease causation by tobacco smoke include changes in the genetic material of cells that leads to malignancy; inflammatory injury to the cells lining the surfaces, such as the lung's airways where smoke deposits, and to more distant sites, such as the blood vessels, that are affected by circulating tobacco smoke components; impairment of the body's defense mechanisms; and specific effects reflecting pharmacologic consequences of specific components, e.g. nicotine, and reduction of oxygen-carrying capacity from carbon monoxide in tobacco smoke.

Exposure to secondhand smoke

Environmental tobacco smoke concentrations

Tobacco smoke is a complex mixture of gases and particles that contains myriad chemical species (US Department of Health Education and Welfare, US Environmental Protection Agency (EPA), and National Center for Health Statistics 1979; US Department of Health and Human Services 1984; Guerin *et al.* 1992; Jenkins *et al.* 2000). Not surprisingly, tobacco smoking in indoor environments increases levels of respirable particles, nicotine, polycyclic aromatic hydrocarbons, carbon monoxide (CO), acrolein, nitrogen dioxide (NO_2), and many other substances. Tables 17.2 and 17.3 provide a summary of data from a number of recent studies (Hammond 1999). The extent of the increase in concentrations of these markers varies with the number of smokers, the intensity of smoking, the rate of exchange between the indoor air space and with the outdoor air, and the use of air-cleaning devices. Ott (1999) has used mass balance models to characterize factors influencing concentrations of tobacco smoke indoors. Using information on the source strength (i.e. the generation of emissions by cigarettes) and on the air exchange rate, researchers can apply mass balance models to predict tobacco smoke concentrations. Such models can be used to estimate exposures and to project the consequences of control measures.

Several components of cigarette smoke have been measured in indoor environments as markers of the contribution of tobacco combustion to indoor air pollution. Particles, a nonspecific marker, have been measured most often because both side-stream and mainstream smoke contain high concentrations of particles in the respirable size range (National Research Council and Committee on Passive Smoking 1986; US Department of Health and Human Services 1986). Other, more specific markers have also been measured, including nicotine, solanesol, and ultraviolet light (UV) absorption of particulate matter (Jenkins *et al.* 2000). Nicotine can be measured with active sampling methods and also using passive diffusion badges (Leaderer and Hammond 1991; Jenkins *et al.* 2000). Studies of levels of secondhand smoke components have been conducted largely in public buildings; fewer studies have been conducted in homes and offices (National Research Council 1986; US Department of Health and Human Services 1986).

The contribution of various environments to personal exposure to tobacco smoke varies with the time–activity pattern, namely the distribution of time spent in different locations. Time–activity patterns may heavily influence lung airway exposures in particular environments for certain groups of individuals. For example, exposure in the home predominates for infants who do not attend day care (Harlos *et al.* 1987).

Table 17.2 Occupational ETS exposures in non-office settings (nonsmokers only)

Company type	Year sampled	Number of samples	Mean	Standard deviation	Geometric mean	Concentration of nicotine, µg/m³		
						Minimum	Median	Maximum
Smoking allowed								
Specialty chemicals	1991–92	8	0.60	0.91	0.24	<0.05	0.46	2.78
Railroad workers (personal)	1983–84	152	0.80	3.30	0.18	<0.1	0.10	38.10
Tool manufacturing	1991–92	13	1.59	1.05	1.16	0.15	1.85	3.40
Textile finishing B	1991–92	11	1.74	1.69	1.10	0.31	0.93	5.09
Labels and paper products	1991–92	1	2.31				2.31	
Die manufacturer	1991–92	12	2.70	1.27	2.46	1.23	2.41	5.42
Sintering metal	1991–92	12	2.88	2.59	2.11	0.62	2.24	9.72
Newspaper B	1991–92	5	2.96	1.37	2.68	1.23	2.78	4.63
Miscellaneous	<1990	282	4.30	11.80	1.70	<1.6	<1.6	126.00
Textile finishing, A	1991–92	11	4.33	8.82	1.77	0.46	1.39	30.71
Flight attendants (personal)	1988	16	4.70	4.00	2.32	0.10	4.20	10.50
Fire fighters A[a]	1991–92	16	5.39	3.81	4.08	1.20	4.84	13.42
Fire fighters B	1991–92	24	5.83	6.77	3.83	0.71	3.65	27.50
Barber shop (personal)	1986–87	2	8.80			4.00		13.70
Hospital (personal)	1986–87	5	24.80	22.80	16.80	6.30	10.00	53.20
Smoking restricted								
Work clothing	1991–92	9	0.17	0.32	0.06	<0.05	<0.05	0.93
Filtration products	1991–92	10	0.32	0.87	0.08	<0.05	<0.05	2.78
Film and imaging	1991–92	6	0.82	0.83	0.39	<0.05	0.70	2.16

Table 17.2 (Continued) Occupational ETS exposures in non-office settings (nonsmokers only)

Company type	Year sampled	Number of samples	Mean	Standard deviation	Geometric mean	Concentration of nicotine, µg/m³		
						Minimum	Median	Maximum
Fiber optics	1991–92	13	1.34	2.79	0.63	0.20	0.64	10.57
Newspaper A	1991–92	4	4.86	6.65	2.62	0.93	1.85	14.81
Valve manufacturer	1991–92	10	5.80	7.85	3.62	1.16	3.26	27.31
Rubber products	1991–92	2	5.85	5.36	4.18	2.06	5.85	9.64
Smoking prohibited								
Infrared and imaging systems	1991–92	1	<0.05				<0.05	
Hospital products	1991–92	5	0.08	0.17	<0.05	<0.05	<0.05	0.39
Weapons systems	1991–92	12	0.08	0.20	<0.05	<0.05	<0.05	0.63
Aircraft components	1991–92	12	0.20	0.18	0.13	<0.05	0.21	0.61
Radar communications components	1991–92	13	0.31	0.36	0.14	<0.05	0.26	1.08
Computer chip equipment	1991–92	10	0.51	0.33	0.41	0.15	0.39	1.08

Source: Hammond 1999.

[a] Omits one data point, 101 µg/m³.

Table 17.3 Nicotine concentrations in homes

	Year sampled	Number of samples	Mean	Standard deviation	Concentration of nicotine, $\mu g/m^3$		
					Minimum	Median	Maximum
North Carolina homes (weekly)	1988	13	1.50	1.10	1.00	1.40	4.40
Personal (each sampled 3×)	1988	15					
Males (personal)[a] (16 h)	1993–94	86	2.13			1.29	>8.08
New York homes (weekly)	1986	47	2.20		0.10	1.00	9.40
Females (personal)[a] (16 h)	1993–94	220	2.93			1.14	>7.81[b]
North Carolina homes 14 h (5 p.m. to 7 a.m.)	1986	13	3.74			c. 3.3	6.5
Minnesota homes (weekly)	CI & CA 1989–	25	5.80		0.10	3.00	28.60

Source: Hammond (1999).

[a]16-h average; 'away from work.'

[b]Ninety-fifth percentile, as given in paper.

For adults residing with nonsmokers, the workplace may be the principal location where exposure takes place. A nationwide study assessed exposures of nonsmokers in 16 metropolitan areas of the United States (Jenkins *et al.* 1996). This study, involving 100 persons in each location, was directed at workplace exposure and included measurements of respirable particulate matter and other markers. The results showed that in 1993 and 1994, exposures to secondhand smoke in the home were generally much greater than those in the workplace, because of workplace smoking restrictions.

The contribution of smoking in the home to indoor air pollution has been demonstrated by studies using personal monitoring and monitoring of homes for respirable particles. In one of the early studies, Spengler *et al.* (1981) monitored homes in six US cities for respirable particle concentrations over several years and found that a smoker of one pack of cigarettes daily contributed about 20 $\mu g/m^3$ to 24 h indoor particle concentrations. Because cigarettes are not smoked uniformly over the day, higher peak concentrations must occur when cigarettes are actually smoked and also when the nonsmoker is in close proximity to the smoker. Spengler *et al.* (1985) measured the personal exposures to respirable particles sustained by nonsmoking adults in two rural Tennessee communities. The mean 24-h exposures were substantially higher for those exposed to smoke at home: 64 $\mu g/m^3$ for those exposed versus 36 $\mu g/m^3$ for those not exposed. These measurements indicate the strength of burning cigarettes as a source of indoor air pollution.

In several studies, homes have been monitored for nicotine, which is a vapor-phase constituent of ETS. In a study of ETS exposure of day-care children, average nicotine concentration during the time that the ETS-exposed children were at home was 3.7 $\mu g/m^3$; in homes without smoking, the average was 0.3 $\mu g/m^3$ (Henderson *et al.* 1989). Coultas *et al.* (1990) measured 24 h nicotine and respirable particle concentrations in 10 homes on alternate days for a week and then on five more days during alternate weeks. The mean levels of nicotine were comparable to those in the study of Henderson *et al.* (1989), but some 24 h values were as high as 20 $\mu g/m^3$. Nicotine and respirable particle concentrations varied widely in the homes.

The Total Exposure Assessment Methodology (TEAM) study, conducted by the U.S. Environmental Protection Agency, provided extensive data on concentrations of 20 volatile organic compounds in a sample of homes in several communities (Wallace and Pellizzari 1987). Indoor monitoring showed increased concentrations of benzene, xylenes, ethylbenzene, and styrene in homes with smokers compared to homes without smokers.

More extensive information is available on levels of ETS components in public buildings and workplaces of various types (Hammond 1999) (Table 17.2). Monitoring in locations where smoking may be intense, such as bars and restaurants, has generally shown elevations of particles and other markers of smoke pollution where smoking is taking place (National Research Council 1986; US Department of Health and Human Services 1986). For example, Repace and Lowrey (1980) in an early study used a portable piezobalance to sample aerosols in restaurants, bars, and other locations. In the places sampled, respirable particulate levels ranged up to 700 $\mu g/m^3$, and the levels varied with the intensity of smoking. Similar data have been reported for the office environment (National Research Council 1986; US Department of Health and Human Services 1986; National Cancer Institute 1999; Jenkins *et al.* 2000). Recent studies indicate low concentrations in many workplace settings, reflecting declining smoking prevalence in recent years and changing practices of smoking in the workplace. Using passive nicotine samplers, Hammond (1999) showed that worksite smoking policies can sharply reduce ETS exposure.

Transportation environments may also be polluted by cigarette smoking. Contamination of air in trains, buses, automobiles, airplanes, and submarines has been documented (National Research Council 1986; US Department of Health and Human Services 1986). A National Research Council report (National Research Council 1986) on air quality in airliners summarized studies for tobacco smoke pollutants in commercial aircraft. In one study, during a single flight, the NO_2 concentration varied with the number of passengers with a lighted cigarette. In another study, respirable particles in the smoking section were measured at concentrations five or more times higher than in the nonsmoking section. Peaks as high as 1000 $\mu g/m^3$ were measured in the smoking section. Mattson *et al.* (1989) used personal exposure monitors to assess nicotine exposures of passengers and flight attendants. All persons were exposed to nicotine, even if seated in the nonsmoking portion of the cabin. Exposures were much greater in the smoking than in the nonsmoking section and were also greater in aircraft with recirculated air. Fortunately, with the banning of tobacco smoking on all domestic flights in 1987 and on all flights into and out of the United States in 1999, the issue has for the most part been resolved, as reflected in the National Research Council's 2002 updated report (National Research Council 2002).

Health effects of passive smoking

Overview

Evidence on the health risks of passive smoking comes from epidemiologic studies, which have directly assessed the associations of measures of secondhand smoke exposure with disease outcomes. Judgments about the causality of associations between secondhand smoke exposure and health outcomes are based not only on this epidemiologic evidence, but also on the extensive evidence derived from epidemiologic and toxicologic investigation on the health consequences of active smoking. To date, the evidence has supported causal conclusions on a range of acute and chronic adverse effects in children and adults (Table 17.1). This paper provides an overview of the now extensive data on adverse health effects of passive smoking on women and children, drawing on various synthesis reports and other reviews (Samet and Wang 2000). The evidence is reviewed separately for adults and children.

In interpreting this evidence, a principal competing explanation to causality for associations between secondhand smoke exposure and disease risk is confounding; that is, the association between secondhand smoke exposure and disease risk reflects the action of another factor, besides secondhand smoke exposure, which is correlated with secondhand smoke exposure and also a risk factor for the outcome of concern. Critics of the evidence have repeatedly raised concerns about confounding, citing such factors as diet for lung cancer and socioeconomic status for respiratory illnesses in children. The various syntheses of evidence have given close attention to the issue of confounding and have concluded that confounding alone cannot explain the observed findings.

Concerns related to misclassification of active smoking status and also to the extent of exposure to secondhand smoke have also been raised. Misclassification of active smoking status has been offered as one potential explanation for the association of lung cancer with secondhand smoke exposure, particularly as assessed by the smoking status of the spouse (Lee 1986, 1988). Since smokers tend to marry smokers, any misreporting of active smoking status would tend to introduce a positive association of lung cancer risk with spouse smoking, given the much higher risk for lung cancer in active smokers compared with never smokers. The potential for this source of bias to explain the observed association of spouse smoking with lung cancer risk in never smokers has been examined quantitatively and set aside by, for example, the U.S. Environmental Protection Agency in its risk assessment (US Environmental Protection Agency 1992) and Hackshaw *et al.* (1997) in their meta-analysis. Exposure to secondhand smoke is inevitably assessed with some misclassification with the extent of error depending on the exposure setting. In general, random misclassification is anticipated, which tends to reduce the strength of association. Thus, estimates of risk of exposure to secondhand smoke may tend to be underestimates.

Adverse effects of secondhand smoke exposure on children

Overview. The evidence on passive smoking and children was most recently reviewed by the World Health Organization in its 1999 consultation (WHO 1999); the conclusions were comparable to those of prior reviewing groups on the effects of passive smoking on children (Table 17.1). Exposure to secondhand smoke was found to be a cause of slightly reduced birth weight, lower respiratory illnesses, chronic respiratory symptoms, middle ear disease, and reduced lung function. Maternal smoking was characterized as a major cause of sudden infant death syndrome (SIDS), but there was inconclusive evidence on the risk from postnatal exposure to secondhand smoke versus *in utero* exposure. The conclusions of the other recent reports, those from the California Environmental Protection Agency, published as a National Cancer Institute monograph in 1999 (National Cancer Institute 1999), and the United Kingdom's Scientific Committee on Tobacco (Scientific Committee on Tobacco and Health & HSMO 1998), were similar (Table 17.1). The specific adverse effects are considered briefly below.

Fetal effects. Researchers have demonstrated that active smoking by mothers during pregnancy results in a variety of adverse health effects in children, postulated to result predominantly from transplacental exposure of the fetus to tobacco smoke components and reduced oxygen delivery (US Department of Health and Human Services 2001). Maternal smoking during pregnancy reduces birth weight (US Department of Health and Human Services 2001) and increases risk for SIDS, an association considered causal in the recent WHO consultation and by the United Kingdom's Scientific Committee on Tobacco (Scientific Committee on Tobacco and Health & HSMO 1998). Secondhand smoke exposure of nonsmoking mothers is associated with reduced birth weight as well, although the extent of the reduction is far less than that for active maternal smoking during pregnancy. In a meta-analysis, the summary estimate of the reduction of birth weight associated with paternal smoking was only 28 g (Windham *et al.* 1999), compared with about 200 g for maternal smoking.

Health effects on the child postnatally, resulting from either secondhand smoke exposure to the fetus or to the newborn child, include SIDS, and adverse effects on neuropsychologic development and physical growth. A number of components of secondhand smoke may produce these effects, including nicotine and carbon monoxide. Possible longer-term health effects of fetal secondhand smoke exposure include increased risk for childhood cancers of the brain, leukemia, and lymphomas, among others. In the WHO consultation (WHO 1999), the evidence on postnatal secondhand smoke exposure and risk of SIDS was found to be insufficient to support a causal conclusion. A meta-analysis of the evidence on childhood cancer through the time of the 1999 consultation, subsequently reported elsewhere, did not show a significant association of secondhand smoke exposure with overall risk for childhood cancer or for leukemia (Boffetta *et al.* 2000).

Perinatal health effects. These health effects include reduced fetal growth, growth retardation, and congenital abnormalities. In most studies, paternal smoking status has been used as the exposure measure to assess the association between secondhand smoke exposure and these nonfatal perinatal health effects. Low birth weight was first reported in 1957 to be associated with maternal smoking (Simpson 1957), and maternal cigarette smoking during pregnancy is considered to be causally associated with low birth weight (US Department of Health and Human Services 1989). Recent studies report lower birth weight for infants of nonsmoking women passively exposed to tobacco smoke during pregnancy (Martin and Bracken 1986; Rubin *et al.* 1986).

Other nonfatal perinatal health effects possibly associated with secondhand smoke exposure are growth retardation and congenital malformations, and a few studies assessed fatal perinatal health effects. Martin and Bracken (1986) demonstrated a strong association with growth retardation in their 1986 study, and several more recent studies provide support (Zhang *et al.* 1992; Roquer *et al.* 1995). The few studies conducted to assess the association between paternal smoking and congenital malformations (Seidman *et al.* 1990; Savitz *et al.* 1991; Zhang *et al.* 1992) have demonstrated risks ranging from 1.2 to 2.6 for those exposed compared with those nonexposed. These studies are too limited to support any conclusions.

Postnatal health effects. Secondhand smoke exposure due to maternal or paternal smoking may lead to postnatal health effects, including increased risk for SIDS, reduced physical development, decrements in cognition and behavior, and increased risk for childhood cancers. For cognition and behavior, evidence is limited and is not considered in this review. There is more extensive information available on maternal smoking during pregnancy and subsequent neurocognitive development (US Department of Health and Human Services 2001; US Department of Health and Human Services & Centers for Disease Control and Prevention 2003).

SIDS. SIDS refers to the unexpected death of a seemingly healthy infant while asleep. Although maternal smoking during pregnancy has been causally associated with SIDS, these studies measured maternal smoking after pregnancy, along with paternal smoking and household smoking generally. In the WHO consultation, the evidence on passive smoking (i.e. postbirth) and SIDS was considered to be inconclusive, although there was some indication of increased risk (WHO 1999). Since most women who smoke during pregnancy continue to do so after delivery, researchers cannot separate the effects of exposure from maternal smoking before and after delivery and the evidence on paternal smoking, constituting exposure to secondhand smoke alone, is inconclusive.

Cancers. Secondhand smoke exposure has been evaluated as a risk factor for the major childhood cancers. The evidence is limited and does not yet support conclusions about the causal nature of the observed associations. In the meta-analysis conducted for the WHO consultation (Boffetta *et al.* 2000), the pooled estimate of the relative risk for any childhood cancer associated with maternal smoking was 1.11 (95 per cent confidence interval (CI): 1.00, 1.23) and that for leukemia was 1.14 (95 per cent CI: 0.97, 1.33).

Lower respiratory tract illnesses in childhood. Lower respiratory tract illnesses are extremely common during childhood. Studies of involuntary smoking and lower respiratory illnesses in childhood, including the more severe episodes of bronchitis and pneumonia, provided some of the earliest evidence on adverse effects of secondhand smoke (Colley *et al.* 1974; Harlap and Davies 1974). Presumably, this association represents an increase in the frequency or in the severity of illnesses that are infectious in etiology and not a direct response of the lung to the toxic components of secondhand smoke. Effects of exposure to tobacco smoke *in utero* on the airways may also play a role in the effect of postnatal exposure on risk for lower respiratory illnesses. Infants of mothers who smoke during pregnancy have evidence of damage to their airways during gestation on lung function testing shortly after birth, and this damage may increase the likelihood of having a more severe infection (Samet and Wang 2000). The evidence indicates that the airways of the exposed infants are functionally narrowed and have a higher degree of nonspecific responsiveness.

Investigations conducted throughout the world have demonstrated an increased risk of lower respiratory tract illness in infants with parents who smoked (Strachan and Cook 1997). These studies indicate a significantly increased frequency of bronchitis and pneumonia during the first year of life of children with parents who smoked. Strachan and Cook (1997) reported a quantitative review of this information, combining data from 39 studies. Overall, the approximate increase in illness risk was 50 per cent if either parent smoked, with an odds ratio for maternal smoking somewhat higher, at 1.72 (95 per cent CI: 1.55, 1.91). Although the health outcome measures varied somewhat among the studies, the relative risks associated with involuntary smoking were similar, and dose–response relations with extent of parental smoking were demonstrable. Although most of the studies have shown that maternal smoking rather than paternal smoking underlies the increased risk of lower respiratory tract illness, studies from China show that paternal smoking alone can increase incidence of lower respiratory illness (Yue Chen et al. 1986; Strachan and Cook 1997). In these studies, an effect of passive smoking has not been readily identified after the first year of life. During the first year of life, the strength of its effect may reflect higher exposures consequent to the time–activity patterns of young infants, which place them in proximity to cigarettes smoked by their mothers.

Respiratory symptoms and illness in children. Data from numerous surveys demonstrate a greater frequency of the most common respiratory symptoms: cough, phlegm, and wheeze in the children of smokers (US Department of Health and Human Services 1986; Cook and Strachan 1997; National Cancer Institute 1999). In these studies, the subjects have generally been schoolchildren, and the effects of parental smoking have been examined. Thus, the less prominent effects of passive smoking, in comparison with the studies of lower respiratory illness in infants, may reflect lower exposures to secondhand smoke by older children who spend less time with their parents.

Cook and Strachan (1997) have conducted a quantitative summary of the relevant studies, including 41 of wheeze, 34 of chronic cough, seven of chronic phlegm, and six of breathlessness. Overall, this synthesis indicates increased risk for respiratory symptoms for children whose parents smoke (Cook and Strachan 1997). There was even increased risk for breathlessness (OR = 1.31, 95 per cent CI: 1.08, 1.59). Having both parents smoke was associated with the highest levels of risk.

Childhood asthma. Exposure to secondhand smoke might cause asthma as a long-term consequence of the increased occurrence of lower respiratory infection in early childhood or through other pathophysiologic mechanisms, including inflammation of the respiratory epithelium (Samet et al. 1983; Tager 1988). The effect of secondhand smoke may also reflect, in part, the consequences of *in utero* exposure. Assessment of airways responsiveness shortly after birth has shown that infants whose mothers smoke during pregnancy have increased airways responsiveness, a characteristic of asthma, compared with those whose mothers do not smoke (Young et al. 1991). Maternal smoking during pregnancy also reduces ventilatory function measured shortly after birth (Hanrahan *et al.* 1992). These observations suggest that *in utero* exposures from maternal smoking may affect lung development and may increase risk for asthma and also for more severe lower respiratory illnesses, as reviewed above.

While the underlying mechanisms remain to be identified, the epidemiologic evidence linking secondhand smoke exposure and childhood asthma is mounting (Cook and Strachan 1997; National Cancer Institute (NCI) 1999). The synthesis by Cook and Strachan (1997) shows a significant excess of childhood asthma if both parents smoke or the mother smokes (Table 17.4). Evidence also indicates that involuntary smoking worsens the status of those with asthma. For example, Murray and Morrison (1986, 1989) evaluated asthmatic children followed in a clinic in Canada. Level of lung function, symptom frequency, and responsiveness to inhaled histamines were adversely affected by maternal smoking. Population studies have also shown increased airways responsiveness for secondhand smoke-exposed children with asthma (O'Connor *et al.* 1987; Martinez *et al.* 1988). The increased level of airway responsiveness associated with secondhand smoke exposure would be expected to increase the clinical severity of asthma. In this regard, exposure to smoking in the home has been shown to increase the number of emergency room visits made by asthmatic children (Burnett *et al.* 1997). Asthmatic children with mothers who smoked are more likely to use asthma medications (Weitzman *et al.* 1990), a finding that confirms the clinically significant effects of secondhand smoke on children with asthma. Guidelines for the management of asthma all urge reduction of secondhand smoke exposure at home (US Department of Health and Human Services *et al.* 1997; National Institutes of Health 2002).

Lung growth and development. During childhood, measures of lung function increase, more or less parallel to the increase in height. On the basis of the primarily cross-sectional data available at the time, the 1984 report of the Surgeon General (US Department of Health and Human Services 1984) concluded that the children of parents who smoked in comparison with those of nonsmokers had small reductions of lung function, but the long-term consequences of these changes were regarded as unknown. On the basis of further longitudinal evidence, the 1986 report (US Department of Health and Human Services 1986) concluded that involuntary smoking reduces the rate of lung function growth during childhood. Evidence from cohort studies has continued to accumulate (Samet and Lange 1996; National Cancer Institute 1999). The WHO consultation noted the difficulty of separating effects of *in utero* exposure from those of childhood secondhand smoke exposure because most mothers who smoke while pregnant continue to do so after the birth of their children (WHO 1999).

Secondhand smoke and middle-ear disease in children. Numerous studies have addressed secondhand smoke exposure and middle-ear disease. Positive associations between secondhand smoke and otitis media have been consistently demonstrated in studies of the prospective cohort design, but not as consistently in case–control studies.

Table 17.4 Summary of pooled random effects odds ratios with 95% confidence intervals

| | Either parent smokes | | | One parent smokes | | | Both parents smoke | | | Mother only smokes | | | Father only smokes | | |
	OR	(95% CI)	(*n*)	OR	(95% CI)	(*n*)	OR	(95% CI)	(*n*)	OR	(95% CI)	(*n*)	OR	(95% CI)	(*n*)
Asthma	1.21	(1.10–1.34)	(21)	1.04	(0.78–1.38)	(6)	1.50	(1.29–1.73)	(8)	1.36	(1.20–1.55)	(11)	1.07	(0.92–1.24)	(9)
Wheeze[a]	1.24	(1.17–1.31)	(30)	1.18	(1.08–1.29)	(21)	1.47	(1.14–1.90)	(11)	1.28	(1.19–1.38)	(18)	1.14	(1.06–1.23)	(10)
Cough	1.40	(1.27–1.53)	(30)	1.29	(1.11–1.51)	(15)	1.67	(1.48–1.89)	(16)	1.40	(1.20–1.64)	(14)	1.21	(1.09–1.34)	(9)
Phlegm[b]	1.35	(1.13–1.62)	(6)	1.25	(0.97–1.63)	(5)	1.46	(1.04–2.05)	(5)						
Breathless-ness[b]	1.31	(1.08–1.59)	(6)												

Source: Cook and Strachan (1997).

Note: Number of studies in parentheses.

[a]Excluding EC study, in which the pooled odds ratio was 1.20.

[b]Data for phlegm and breathlessness restricted as several comparisons are based on fewer than five studies.

This difference in findings may reflect the focus of the cohort studies on the first two years of life, the peak age of risk for middle ear disease. The case–control studies, on the other hand, have been directed at older children who are not at lower risk for otitis media. Exposure to secondhand smoke has been most consistently associated with recurrent otitis media and not with incident or single episodes of otitis media. In their 1997 meta-analysis, Cook and Strachan (1997) found a pooled odds ratio of 1.40 (95 per cent CI: 1.08, 2.04) for recurrent otitis media if either parent smoked, 1.38 (95 per cent CI: 1.23, 1.55) for middle-ear effusions, and 1.21 (95 per cent CI: 0.95, 1.53) for outpatient or inpatient care for chronic otitis media or 'glue ear.'

The US Surgeon General's Office (US Department of Health and Human Services 1986), the National Research Council (National Research Council 1986), and the US Environmental Protection Agency (1992) have all reviewed the literature on secondhand smoke and otitis media and have concluded that there is an association between secondhand smoke exposure and otitis media in children. The evidence to date supports a causal relation, as noted by the WHO consultation (WHO 1999).

Health effects of involuntary smoking on adults

Lung cancer. In 1981, reports were published from Japan (Hirayama 1981*a*) and from Greece (Trichopoulos *et al.* 1981) that indicated increased lung cancer risk in non-smoking women married to cigarette smokers. Subsequently, this still-controversial association has been examined in many investigations conducted in the United States and other countries around the world, including a substantial number of studies in Asia. The association of involuntary smoking with lung cancer derives biologic plausibility from the presence of carcinogens in sidestream smoke and the lack of a documented threshold dose for respiratory carcinogenesis in active smokers (US Department of Health and Human Services 1982; IARC 1986). Moreover, genotoxic activity, the ability to damage DNA, has been demonstrated for many components of secondhand smoke (Claxton *et al.* 1989; Lofroth 1989; Weiss 1989). Experimental exposure of nonsmokers to secondhand smoke leads to their excreting 4-(methylnitrosamino)-1-(3-pyridyl)-1-butanol (NNAL), a tobacco-specific carcinogen, in their urine. Nonsmokers exposed to secondhand smoke in their homes also excrete higher levels of this carcinogen (Anderson *et al.* 2001). Nonsmokers, including children, exposed to secondhand smoke also have increased concentrations of adducts of tobacco-related carcinogens, that is detectable binding of the carcinogens to DNA of white blood cells, for example (Maclure *et al.* 1989; Crawford *et al.* 1994).

The early report by Hirayama (1981*a*) was based on a prospective cohort study of 91 540 nonsmoking women in Japan. Standardized mortality ratios for lung cancer increased significantly with the amount smoked by the husbands. The findings could not be explained by confounding factors and were unchanged when follow-up of the study group was extended (Hirayama 1984). On the basis of the same cohort, Hirayama also reported significantly increased risk for nonsmoking men married to wives who smoked 1–19 cigarettes and 20 or more cigarettes daily (Hirayama 1984). In 1981, Trichopoulos *et al.* (1981) also reported increased lung cancer risk in nonsmoking women married to cigarette smokers. These investigators conducted a case–control study in Athens, Greece, which included cases with a diagnosis other than for orthopedic disorders. The positive findings reported in 1981 were unchanged with subsequent expansion of the study population (Trichopoulos *et al.* 1983). By 1986, the evidence had mounted, and the three synthesis reports published in that year concluded that secondhand smoke was a cause of lung cancer (IARC 1986; National Research Council 1986; US Department of Health and Human Services 1986).

In 1992, the US Environmental Protection Agency (US Environmental Protection Agency 1992) published its risk assessment of secondhand smoke as a carcinogen. The Agency's evaluation drew on the toxicologic evidence on secondhand smoke and the extensive literature on active smoking. A meta-analysis of the 31 studies published to that time was central to the decision to classify secondhand smoke as a class A carcinogen, i.e., a known human carcinogen. The meta-analysis considered the data from the epidemiologic studies by tiers of study quality and location and used an adjustment method for misclassification of smokers as never-smokers. Overall, the analysis found a significantly increased risk of lung cancer in never-smoking women married to smoking men; for the studies conducted in the United States, the estimated relative risk was 1.19 (90 per cent CI: 1.04, 1.35).

The meta-analysis included pooled estimates by geographic region. The data from China and Hong Kong were notable for not showing the increased risk associated with passive smoking that was found in other regions (US Environmental Protection Agency 1992). The epidemiologic characteristics of lung cancer in women in this region of the world have been distinct with a relatively high proportion of lung cancers in nonsmoking women. Explanations for this pattern have centered on exposures to cooking fumes and indoor air pollution from coal-fueled space heating.

The 1997 meta-analysis by Law *et al.* (1997) included 37 published studies. The excess risk of lung cancer for smokers married to nonsmokers was estimated as 24 per cent (95 per cent CI: 13 per cent, 36 per cent). Adjustment for potential bias, including misclassification of some smokers as never smokers, and confounding by diet did not alter the estimate. This meta-analysis supported the conclusion of the United Kingdom's Scientific Committee on Tobacco and Health (Scientific Committee on Tobacco and Health & HSMO 1998) that secondhand smoke is a cause of lung cancer. More recently, the International Agency for Research on Cancer (IARC 2002) reviewed more than 50 studies, finding a similar increase in risk.

Secondhand smoke and coronary heart disease (CHD). Causal associations between active smoking and fatal and nonfatal CHD outcomes have long been demonstrated (US Department of Health and Human Services 1989). The risk of CHD in active smokers increases with the amount and duration of cigarette smoking and decreases relatively quickly with cessation. Active cigarette smoking is considered to: (1) increase the risk of cardiovascular disease by promoting atherosclerosis; (2) increase the tendency to thrombosis; (3) cause spasm of the coronary arteries; (4) increase the likelihood of cardiac arrhythmias; and (5) decrease the oxygen-carrying capacity of the blood (US Department of Health and Human Services 1990). Glantz and Parmley (1991) summarized the pathophysiologic mechanisms by which passive smoking might increase the risk of heart disease. It is biologically plausible that passive smoking could also be associated with increased risk for CHD through the same mechanisms considered relevant for active smoking, although the lower exposures to smoke components of the passive smoker have raised questions regarding the relevance of the mechanisms cited for active smoking.

Epidemiologic data first raised concern that passive smoking may increase risk for CHD with the 1985 report of Garland *et al.* (1985), based on a cohort study in southern California. There are now more than 20 studies on the association between environmental tobacco smoke and cardiovascular disease. These studies assessed both fatal and nonfatal cardiovascular heart disease outcomes, and most used self-administered questionnaires to assess secondhand smoke exposure. They cover a wide range of populations, both geographically and racially. While many of the studies were conducted within the United States, studies were also conducted in Europe (Scotland, Italy, and the United Kingdom), Asia (Japan and China), South America (Argentina), and the South Pacific (Australia and New Zealand). The majority of the studies measured the effect of secondhand smoke exposure due to spousal smoking; however, some studies also assessed exposures from smoking by other household members or occurring at work or in transit. Only one study included measurement of exposure biomarkers.

While the risk estimates for secondhand smoke and CHD outcomes vary in these studies, they range from null to modestly significant increases in risk, with the risk for fatal outcomes generally higher and more significant. In their 1997 meta-analysis, Law *et al.* (1997) estimated the excess risk from secondhand smoke exposure as 30 per cent (95 per cent CI: 22 per cent, 38 per cent) at age 65 years. The findings were similar in a meta-analysis of 18 studies reported by He *et al.* (1999). The overall increase in risk associated with passive exposure was 25 per cent and the risk increased with duration and level of smoking. The California Environmental Protection Agency (National Cancer Institute 1999) recently concluded that there is an overall excess risk of 30 per cent for CHD due to exposure from secondhand smoke. The American Heart Association's Council on Cardiopulmonary and Critical Care has also concluded that environmental tobacco smoke both increases the risk of heart disease and is 'a major preventable cause of cardiovascular disease and death' (Taylor *et al.* 1992). This conclusion was echoed in 1998 by the Scientific Committee on Tobacco and Health in the United Kingdom (Scientific Committee on Tobacco and Health & HSMO 1998).

Respiratory symptoms and illnesses in adults. Only a few cross-sectional investigations provide information on the association between respiratory symptoms in nonsmokers and involuntary exposure to tobacco smoke. These studies have primarily considered exposure outside the home. Consistent evidence of an effect of passive smoking on chronic respiratory symptoms in adults has not been found (Lebowitz and Burrows 1976; Schilling *et al.* 1977; Comstock *et al.* 1981; Schenker *et al.* 1982; Euler *et al.* 1987; Hote *et al.* 1989; Kauffmann *et al.* 1989). Several studies suggest that passive smoking may cause acute respiratory morbidity, i.e., illnesses and symptoms (Ostro 1989; Robbins *et al.* 1993; Dayal *et al.* 1994; Riboli *et al.* 1995; Eisner *et al.* 1998). Neither epidemiologic nor experimental studies have established the role of secondhand smoke in exacerbating asthma in adults (Weiss *et al.* 1999). The acute responses of asthmatics to secondhand smoke have been assessed by exposing persons with asthma to tobacco smoke in a chamber. This experimental approach cannot be readily controlled because of the impossibility of blinding subjects to exposure to secondhand smoke. However, suggestibility does not appear to underlie physiologic responses of asthmatics to secondhand smoke (Shephard *et al.* 1979). Of three studies involving exposure of unselected asthmatics to secondhand smoke (Shephard *et al.* 1979; Dahms *et al.* 1981; Hargreave *et al.* 1981), only one showed a definite adverse effect. Stankus *et al.* (1988) recruited 21 asthmatics who reported exacerbation with exposure to secondhand smoke. With challenge in an exposure chamber at concentrations much greater than is typically encountered in indoor environments, seven of the subjects experienced a more than 20 per cent decline in FEV_1.

Lung function in adults. With regard to involuntary smoking and lung function in adults, exposure to passive smoking has been associated in cross-sectional investigations with reduction of several lung function measures. However, the findings have not been consistent, and methodological issues constrain interpretation of the findings. A conclusion cannot yet be reached on the effects of secondhand smoke exposure on lung function in adults. However, further research is warranted because of widespread exposure in workplaces and homes.

Conclusion

In about three decades, we have progressed from the first studies on passive smoking and health to definitive evidence that passive smoking causes disease. The evidence includes not only epidemiological studies, but studies with biomarkers documenting that tobacco smoke inhaled by nonsmokers delivers doses of toxic components and metabolites to target organs. There are also animal studies and extensive data on patterns of exposure. The strength of the evidence and its public health implications have been a strong force for motivating tobacco control policy.

References

Anderson, K. E., Carmella, S. G., Ye, M., Bliss, R. L., Le, C., Murphy, L., and Hecht, S. S. (2001). Metabolites of a tobacco-specific lung carcinogen in nonsmoking women exposed to environmental tobacco smoke. *J. Natl. Cancer Inst.*, **93**(5), 378–81.

Boffetta, P., Tredaniel, J., and Greco, A. (2000). Risk of childhood cancer and adult lung cancer after childhood exposure to passive smoke: A meta-analysis. *Environ. Health Perspect.*, **108**(1), 73–82.

Burnett, R. T., Cakmak, S., Brook, J. R., and Krewski, D. (1997). The role of particulate size and chemistry in the association between summertime ambient air pollution and hospitalization for cardiorespiratory diseases. *Environmental Health Perspectives*, **105**(6), 614–20.

California Environmental Protection Agency (Cal EPA) and Office of Environmental Health Hazard Assessment (1997). *Health effects of exposure to environmental tobacco smoke*. California Environmental Protection Agency.

Cameron, P. (1967). The presence of pets and smoking as correlates of perceived disease. *Journal of Allergy*, **67**(1), 12–5.

Cameron, P., Kostin, J. S., Zaks, J. M., Wolfe, J. H., Tighe, G., Oselett, B., *et al.* (1969). The health of smokers' and nonsmokers' children. *Journal of Allergy*, **43**(6), 336–41.

Claxton, L. D., Morin, R. S., Hughes, T. J., and Lewtas, J. (1989). A genotoxic assessment of environmental tobacco smoke using bacterial bioassays. *Mutation Research*, **222**(2), 81–99.

Colley, J. R. and Holland, W. W. (1967). Social and environmental factors in respiratory disease. A preliminary report. *Archives of Environmental Health*, **67**(1), 157–61.

Colley, J. R. T., Holland, W. W., and Corkhill, R. T. (1974). Influence of passive smoking and parental phlegm on pneumonia and bronchitis in early childhood. *Lancet*, **2**(7888), 1031–4.

Comstock, G. W., Meyer, M. B., Helsing, K. J., and Tockman, M. S. (1981). Respiratory effects of household exposures to tobacco smoke and gas cooking. *American Review of Respiratory Disease*, **124**, 143–8.

Cook, D. G. and Strachan, D. P. (1997). Health effects of passive smoking. 3. Parental smoking and prevalence of respiratory symptoms and asthma in school age children. *Thorax*, **52**(12), 1081–94.

Corrao, M. A., Guindon, G. E., Sharma, N., and Shokoohi, D. F. (2000). *Tobacco control country profiles*. American Cancer Society, Atlanta, GA.

Coultas, D. B., Samet, J. M., McCarthy, J. F., and Spengler, J. D. (1990). Variability of measures of exposure to environmental tobacco smoke in the home. *American Review of Respiratory Disease*, **142**, 602–6.

Crawford, F. G., Mayer, J., Santella, R. M., Cooper, T. B., Ottman, R., Tsai, W. Y., *et al.* (1994). Biomarkers of environmental tobacco smoke in preschool children and their mothers. *Journal of the National Cancer Institute*, **86**(18), 1398–402.

Dahms, T. E., Bolin, J. F., and Slavin, R. G. (1981). Passive smoking: Effects on bronchial asthma. *Chest*, **80**(5), 530–4.

Dayal, H. H., Khuder, S., Sharrar, R., and Trieff, N. (1994). Passive smoking in obstructive respiratory disease in an industrialized urban population. *Environmental Research*, **65**(2), 161–71.

Eisner, M. D., Yelin, E. H., Henke, J., Shiboski, S. C., and Blanc, P. D. (1998). Environmental tobacco smoke and adult asthma. The impact of changing exposure status on health outcomes. *American Journal of Respiratory and Critical Care Medicine*, **158**, 170–5.

Euler, G. L., Abbey, D. E., Magie, A. R., and Hodgkin, J. E. (1987). Chronic obstructive pulmonary disease symptom effects of long-term cumulative exposure to ambient levels of total suspended particulates and sulfur dioxide in California Seventh-Day Adventist residents. *Archives of Environmental Health*, **42**(4), 213–22.

Garland, C., Barret-Connor, E., Suarez, L., Criqui, M. H., and Wingard, D. L. (1985). Effects of passive smoking on ischemic heart disease mortality of nonsmokers: A prospective study. *American Journal of Epidemiology*, **121**(5), 645–50.

Glantz, S. A. and Parmley, W. W. (1991). Passive smoking and heart disease: Epidemiology, physiology, and biochemistry. *Circulation*, **83**, 1–12.

Guerin, M. R., Jenkins, R. A., and Tomkins, B. A. (1992). *The chemistry of environmental tobacco smoke: Composition and measurement*. Lewis Publishers, Inc., Chelsea, Michigan.

Hackshaw, A. K., Law, M. R., and Wald, N. J. (1997). The accumulated evidence on lung cancer and environmental tobacco smoke. *British Medical Journal*, **315**(7114), 980–8.

Hammond, S. K. (1999). Exposure of U.S. workers to environmental tobacco smoke. *Environmental Health Perspectives*, **107**(Suppl 2), 329–40.

Hanrahan, J. P., Tager, I. B., Segal, M. R., Tosteson, T. D., Castile, R. G., Van Vunakis, H., *et al.* (1992). The effect of maternal smoking during pregnancy on early infant lung function. *American Review of Respiratory Disease*, **145**, 1129–35.

Hargreave, F. E., Ryan, G., Thomson, N. C., O'Bryne, P. M., Latimer, K., Juniper, E. F., and Dolovich, J. (1981). Bronchial responsiveness to histamine or methacholine in asthma: Measurement and clinical significance. *Journal of Allergy and Clinical Immunology*, **68**, 347–55.

Harlap, S. and Davies, A. M. (1974). Infant admissions to hospital and maternal smoking. *Lancet*, **1**, 529–32.

Harlos, D. P., Marbury, M., Samet, J. M., and Spengler, J. D. (1987). Relating indoor NO_2 levels to infant personal exposures. *Atmospheric Environment*, **21**(2), 369–78.

He, J., Vupputuri, S., Allen, K., Prerost, M. R., Hughes, J., and Whelton, P. K. (1999). Passive smoking and the risk of coronary heart disease—A meta-analysis of epidemiologic studies. *New England Journal of Medicine*, **340**(12), 920–6.

Henderson, R. W., Reid, H. F., Morris, R., Wang, O. L., Hu, P. C., Helms, R. W., *et al.* (1989) Assessing environmental tobacco smoke exposure of pre-school children in homes by monitoring air particles, mutagenicity, and nicotine. *Measurement of toxic and related air pollutants*. Environmental Protection Agency/Air and Waste Management Association International Symposium. Raleigh, NC, Air and Waste Management Association, Pittsburgh, PA, pp. 611–6.

Hirayama, T. (1981*a*). Non-smoking wives of heavy smokers have a higher risk of lung cancer: A study from Japan. *Br Med J (Clin Res Ed)*, **282**(6259), 183–5.

Hirayama, T. (1981*b*). Passive smoking and lung cancer. *British Medical Journal*, **282**, 1393–4.

Hirayama, T. (1984). Cancer mortality in nonsmoking women with smoking husbands based on a large-scale cohort study in Japan. *Preventive Medicine*, **13**(6), 680–90.

Hote, D. J., Gillis, C. R., Chopra, C., and Hawthorne, V. M. (1989). Passive smoking and cardiorespiratory health in a general population in the west of Scotland. *British Medical Journal*, **299**, 423–7.

International Agency for Research on Cancer (IARC) (1986). IARC Monographs on the Evaluation of the Carcinogenic Risk of Chemicals to Humans: Tobacco Smoking [Monograph 38]. Lyon, France, World Health Organization, IARC.

International Agency for Research on Cancer (IARC) (2002). Tobacco smoke and involuntary smoking. [Monograph 83]. Lyon, France, International Agency for Research on Cancer.

Jenkins, M. A., Clarke, J. R., Carlin, J. B., Robertson, C. F., Hopper, J. L., Dalton, M. F., *et al.* (1996). Validation of questionnaire and bronchial hyperresponsiveness against respiratory physician assessment in the diagnosis of asthma. *International Journal of Epidemiology*, **25**(3), 609–16.

Jenkins, R. A., Guerin, M. R., and Tomkins, B. A. (2000). *The chemistry of environmental tobacco smoke: Composition and measurement* (2nd edn). Lewis Publishers, Boca Raton.

Kauffmann, F., Dockery, D. W., Speizer, F. E., and Ferris, B. G., Jr. (1989). Respiratory symptoms and lung function in relation to passive smoking: a comparative study of American and French women. *International Journal of Epidemiology*, **18**(2), 334–44.

Law, M. R., Morris, J. K., and Wald, N. J. (1997). Environmental tobacco smoke exposure and ischaemic heart disease: an evaluation of the evidence. *British Medical Journal*, **315**(7114), 973–80.

Leaderer, B. P. and Hammond, S. K. (1991). Evaluation of vapor-phase nicotine and respirable suspended particle mass as markers for environmental tobacco smoke. *Environmental Science and Technology*, **25**, 770–7.

Lebowitz, M. D. and Burrows, B. (1976). Respiratory symptoms related to smoking habits of family adults. *Chest*, **69**(1), 48–50.

Lee, P. N. (1986). Misclassification as a factor in passive smoking risk [letter]. *Lancet*, **86**(8511), 867.

Lee, P. N. (1988). *Misclassification of smoking habits and passive smoking*. Springer Verlag, Berlin.

Lofroth, G. (1989). Environmental tobacco smoke: Overview of chemical composition and genotoxic components. *Mutation Research*, **222**(2), 73–80.

Maclure, M., Katz, R. B., Bryant, M. S., Skipper, P. L., and Tannenbaum, S. R. (1989). Elevated blood levels of carcinogens in passive smokers. *American Journal of Public Health*, **89**(10), 1381–4.

Martin, T. R. and Bracken, M. B. (1986). Association of low birth weight with passive smoke exposure in pregnancy. *American Journal of Epidemiology*, **124**(4), 633–42.

Martinez, F. D., Antognoni, G., Macri, F., Bonci, E., Midulla, F., DeCastro, G., and Ronchetti, R. (1988). Parental smoking enhances bronchial responsiveness in nine-year-old children. *American Review of Respiratory Disease*, **138**, 518–23.

Mattson, M. E., Boyd, G., Byor, D., Brown, C., Callahan, J. F., Corle, D., *et al.* (1989). Passive smoking on commercial airline flights. *Journal of the American Medical Association*, **261**, 867–72.

Murray, A. B. and Morrison, B. J. (1986). The effect of cigarette smoke from the mother on bronchial responsiveness and severity of symptoms in children with asthma. *Journal of Allergy and Clinical Immunology*, **77**(4), 575–81.

Murray, A. B. and Morrison, B. J. (1989). Passive smoking by asthmatics: Its greater effect on boys than on girls and on older than on younger children. *Pediatrics*, **84**(3), 451–9.

National Cancer Institute (NCI) (1999). Health effects of exposure to environmental tobacco smoke. The report of the California Environmental Protection Agency. Monograph 10. [NIH Pub. No. 99-4645]. Bethesda, MD, U.S. Department of Health and Human Services, National Institutes of Health, National Cancer Institute. Smoking and Tobacco Control.

National Institutes of Health (NIH) and National Heart, L. a. B. I. N. (2002). *Global initiative for asthma. Global strategy for asthma management and prevention*. NIH, Bethesda, MD, NIH Pub. No. 02-3659.

National Research Council (NRC) and Committee on Air Quality in Passenger Cabins of Commercial Aircraft (2002). *The airliner cabin environment and the health of passengers and crew*. National Academy Press, Washington, D.C.

National Research Council (NRC) and Committee on Airliner Cabin Environment Safety Committee (1986). *The airliner cabin environment: Air quality and safety*. National Academy Press, Washington, D.C.

National Research Council (NRC) and Committee on Passive Smoking (1986). *Environmental tobacco smoke: Measuring exposures and assessing health effects*. National Academy Press, Washington, D.C.

Nelkin, B. D., Mabry, M., and Baylin, S. B. (1998). Lung cancer. In: *The genetic basis of human cancer* (ed. B. Vogelstein and K. W. Kinzler), pp. 671–9. McGraw-Hill, New York.

O'Connor, G. T., Weiss, S. T., Tager, I. B., and Speizer, F. E. (1987). The effect of passive smoking on pulmonary function and nonspecific bronchial responsiveness in a population-based sample of children and young adults. *American Review of Respiratory Disease*, **135**, 800–4.

Ostro, B. D. (1989). Estimating the risks of smoking, air pollution, and passive smoke on acute respiratory conditions. *Risk Anal*, **9**(2), 189–96.

Ott, W. R. (1999). Mathematical models for predicting indoor air quality from smoking activity. *Environmental Health Perspectives*, **107**(Suppl 2), 375–81.

Proctor, R. N. (1995). *Cancer wars. How politics shapes what we know and don't know about cancer.* Basic Books, New York.

Repace, J. L. and Lowrey, A. H. (1980). Indoor air pollution, tobacco smoke, and public health. *Science*, **208**, 464–72.

Riboli, E., Haley, N. J., Tredaniel, J., Saracci, R., Preston-Martin, S., and Trichopoulos, D. (1995). Misclassification of smoking status among women in relation to exposure to environmental tobacco smoke. *European Respiratory Journal*, **8**, 285–90.

Robbins, A. S., Abbey, D. E., and Lebowitz, M. D. (1993). Passive smoking and chronic respiratory disease symptoms in non-smoking adults. *International Journal of Epidemiology*, **22**(5), 809–17.

Roquer, J. M., Figueras, J., Botet, F., and Jimenez, R. (1995). Influence on fetal growth of exposure to tobacco smoke during pregnancy. *Acta Paediatr*, **84**, 118–21.

Royal College of Physicians of London (1962). *Smoking and Health. Summary of a report of the Royal College of Physicians of London on smoking in relation to cancer of the lung and other diseases.* Pitman Medical Publishing Co., LTD, London.

Rubin, D. H., Krasilnikoff, P. A., Leventhal, J. M., Weile, B., and Berget, A. (1986). Effect of passive smoking on birth-weight. *Lancet*, **2**(8504), 415–7.

Samet, J. M. and Lange, P. (1996). Longitudinal studies of active and passive smoking. *American Journal of Respiratory and Critical Care Medicine*, **154**(6 Pt 2), S257–S265.

Samet, J. M., Tager, I. B., and Speizer, F. E. (1983). The relationship between respiratory illness in childhood and chronic airflow obstruction in adulthood. *American Review of Respiratory Disease*, **127**, 508–23.

Samet, J. M. and Wang, S. S. (2000). Environmental tobacco smoke. In: *Environmental toxicants: human exposures and their health effects*, (2nd edn) (ed. M. Lippmann) Van Nostrand Reinhold Company, Inc., New York, pp. 319–75.

Savitz, D. A., Schwingl, P. J., and Keels, M. A. (1991). Influence of paternal age, smoking, and alcohol consumption on congenital anomalies. *Teratology*, **44**(4), 429–40.

Schenker, M. B., Samet, J. M., and Speizer, F. E. (1982). Effect of cigarette tar content and smoking habits on respiratory symptoms in women. *American Review of Respiratory Disease*, **125**, 684–90.

Schilling, R. S., Letai, A. D., Hui, S. L., Beck, G. J., Schoenberg, J. B., and Bouhuys, A. H. (1977). Lung function, respiratory disease, and smoking in families. *American Journal of Epidemiology*, **106**(4), 274–83.

Scientific Committee on Tobacco and Health & HSMO (1998). *Report of the scientific committee on tobacco and health.* The Stationary Office, 011322124x.

Seidman, D. S., Ever-Hadani, P., and Gale, R. (1990). Effect of maternal smoking and age on congenital anomalies. *Obstetrics and Gynecology*, **76**(6), 1046–50.

Shephard, R. J., Collins, R., and Silverman, F. (1979). 'Passive' exposure of asthmatic subjects to cigarette smoke. *Environmental Research*, **20**(2), 392–402.

Simpson, W. J. (1957). A preliminary report on cigarette smoking and the incidence of prematurity. *American Journal of Obstetrics and Gynecology*, **73**(4), 808–15.

Spengler, J. D., Dockery, D. W., Turner, W. A., Wolfson, J. M., and Ferris, B. G., Jr. (1981). Long-term measurements of respirable sulfates and particles inside and outside homes. *Atmospheric Environment*, **15**, 23–30.

Spengler, J. D., Treitman, R. D., Tosteson, T., Mage, D. T., and Soczek, M. L. (1985). Personal exposures to respirable particulates and implications for air pollution epidemiology. *Environmental Science and Technology*, **19**, 700–7.

Stankus, R. P., Menan, P. K., Rando, R. J., Glindmeyer, H., Salvaggio, J. E., and Lehrer, S. B. (1988). Cigarette smoke-sensitive asthma: Challenge studies. *Journal of Allergy and Clinical Immunology*, **82**(3 Pt 1), 331–8.

Strachan, D. P. and Cook, D. G. (1997). Health effects of passive smoking. 1. Parental smoking and lower respiratory illness in infancy and early childhood. *Thorax*, **52**(10), 905–14.

Tager, I. B. (1988). Passive smoking-bronchial responsiveness and atopy. *American Review of Respiratory Disease*, **138**, 507–9.

Taylor, A. E., Johnson, D. C., and Kazemi, H. (1992). Environmental tobacco smoke and cardiovascular disease: A position paper from the council on cardiopulmonary and critical care, American Heart Association. *Circulation*, **86**(2), 1–4.

Trichopoulos, D., Kalandidi, A., and Sparros, L. (1983). Lung cancer and passive smoking: Conclusion of Greek study. *Lancet*, **2**, 677–8.

Trichopoulos, D., Kalandidi, A., Sparros, L., and MacMahon, B. (1981). Lung cancer and passive smoking. *International Journal of Cancer*, **27**(1), 1–4.

US Department of Health and Human Services (USDHHS) (1982). *The health consequences of smoking: Cancer. A report of the Surgeon General*, U.S. Department of Health and Human Services, Public Health Service, Office on Smoking and Health, Washington, D.C., DHHS Publication No. (PHS) 82-50179.

US Department of Health and Human Services (USDHHS) (1984). *The health consequences of smoking—chronic obstructive lung disease. A report of the Surgeon General*. U.S. Government Printing Office, Washington, D.C.

US Department of Health and Human Services (USDHHS) (1986). *The health consequences of involuntary smoking: A report of the Surgeon General*. U.S. Government Printing Office, Washington, D.C., DHHS Publication No. (CDC) 87-8398.

US Department of Health and Human Services (USDHHS) (1989). *Reducing the health consequences of smoking. 25 years of progress. A report of the Surgeon General*. U.S. Government Printing Office, Washington, D.C.

US Department of Health and Human Services (USDHHS) (1990). *The health benefits of smoking cessation. A report of the Surgeon General*, U.S. Government Printing Office, Washington, D.C.

US Department of Health and Human Services (USDHHS) (2001). *Women and smoking. A report of the Surgeon General*, US Department of Health and Human Services, Rockville, MD.

US Department of Health and Human Services (USDHHS) and Centers for Disease Control and Prevention (CDC) (2003). *Smoking and Health. A Report of the U.S. Surgeon General*, US Department of Health and Human Services, Bethesda, MD.

US Department of Health and Human Services (USDHHS), Public Health Service, National Institutes of Health (NIH), and National Heart, L. a. B. I. N. (1997). *Practical guide for the diagnosis and management of asthma*. NIH, 97-4053.

US Department of Health Education and Welfare (DHEW) (1964). *Smoking and health. Report of the Advisory Committee to the Surgeon General*. U.S. Government Printing Office, Washington, DC, DHEW Publication No. [PHS] 1103.

US Department of Health Education and Welfare (DHEW) (1971). *The health consequences of smoking. A report of the Surgeon General: 1971.* U.S. Government Printing Office, Washington, DC, DHEW Publication No. (HSM) 73-8704.

US Department of Health Education and Welfare (DHEW), US Environmental Protection Agency (EPA), and National Center for Health Statistics (1979). *Changes in cigarette smoking and current smoking practices among adults: United States, 1978.* U.S. Government Printing Office, Washington, D.C., Advance Data 52.

US Environmental Protection Agency (EPA) (1992). *Respiratory health effects of passive smoking: Lung cancer and other disorders.* U.S. Government Printing Office, Washington, D.C., EPA/600/006F.

Wallace, L. A. and Pellizzari, E. D. (1987). Personal air exposures and breath concentrations of benzene and other volatile hydrocarbons for smokers and nonsmokers. *Toxicol Lett,* **35**(1), 113–6.

Weiss, B. (1989). Behavior as an endpoint for inhaled toxicants. In: *Concepts in inhalation toxicology,* (ed. R. O. McClellan and R. F. Henderson), pp. 475–93. Hemisphere Publishing, New York.

Weiss, S. T., Utell, M. J., and Samet, J. M. (1999). Environmental tobacco smoke exposure and asthma in adults. *Environ Health Perspect.,* **107** (Suppl 6), 891–5.

Weitzman, M., Gortmaker, S., Walker, D. K., and Sobol, A. (1990). Maternal smoking and childhood asthma. *Pediatrics,* **85**(4), 505–11.

Windham, G. C., Eaton, A., and Hopkins, B. (1999). Evidence for an association between environmental tobacco smoke exposure and birthweight: a meta-analysis and new data. *Paediatric and Perinatal Epidemiology,* **13**(1), 35–7.

World Health Organization (1999). *International consultation on environmental tobacco smoke (ETS) and child health. Consultation Report.* World Health Organization, Geneva.

Wynder, E. L., Graham, E. A., and Croninger, A. B. (1953). Experimental production of carcinoma with cigarette tar. *Cancer Research,* **13**, 855–64.

Young, S., Le Souef, P. N., Geelhoed, G. C., Stick, S. M., Turner, K. J., and Landau, L. I. (1991). The influence of a family history of asthma and parental smoking on airway responsiveness in early infancy. *New England Journal of Medicine,* **324**(17), 1168–73.

Yue Chen, B. M., Wan-Xian, L. I., and Shunzhang, Y. (1986). Influence of passive smoking on admissions for respiratory illness in early childhood. *British Medical Journal,* **293**, 303–6.

Zhang, J., Savitz, D. A., Schwingl, P. J., and Cai, W. W. (1992). A case-control study of paternal smoking and birth defects. *International Journal of Epidemiology,* **21**(2), 273–8.

Chapter 18

Adolescent smoking

John P. Pierce, Janet M. Distefan, and David Hill

Introduction

It is over forty years since the public health community came to the consensus that smoking tobacco, particularly cigarettes, caused lung cancer. Despite widespread dissemination of the likely health consequences, cigarette smoking is still a prevalent behavior in all developed countries and is a rapidly increasing behavior in developing countries. There is an extensive literature on quitting studies indicating that, for many smokers, successful quitting is one of the hardest lifestyle changes to achieve. Given this, many argue that the majority of the emphasis should be on preventing initiation of smoking in the first place. This chapter focuses on influences encouraging young people to become smokers.

Trends in who initiates smoking

Cigarette smoking can be considered the epidemic of the twentieth century. In 1900, cigarette smoking was rare, with total cigarette sales at 54 cigarettes per person in the United States. Over the next half century, the prevalence of smoking rose rapidly, with sales peaking in 1963 at 4345 cigarettes per person (FTC 2000). The peak of cigarette smoking for men was seen in those who were born between 1915 and 1930, of whom 70 per cent were addicted. Importantly, all of the men in this highest smoking prevalence cohort were over 20 years of age when the first evidence was published in scientific journals demonstrating that smoking caused lung cancer in men. The highest prevalence of cigarette smoking for women was observed in those who were born between 1935 and 1950, of whom 45 per cent were addicted (Burns *et al.* 1997). Importantly, cigarette smoking among women was a very rare event prior to 1925 at the start of the first cigarette advertising campaign that specifically targeted women (Pierce and Gilpin 1995). Notably, women in the highest prevalence birth cohorts were all exposed to cigarette advertising targeted to them throughout their teenage years.

In all of these early birth cohorts, the vast majority of people who started to smoke did so between the ages of 14 and 25 years, with the peak starting ages being 18–24 years (Lee *et al.* 1993). However, throughout the latter half of the twentieth century, this uptake pattern changed dramatically. At the end of the twentieth century, the vast majority of those who started smoking regularly were between the ages of 14 and 19 years, with the peak starting age group being 14 and 17 years. Among both genders, the initiation rates among 18–21 and 22–24 year olds have continuously declined since the public health consensus that smoking caused disease in 1964 (Gilpin *et al.* 1994).

A study of trends across birth cohorts in the proportion of adolescents who started smoking as 14–17-year-olds adds further evidence implicating cigarette advertising and promotions as a major factor in adolescent smoking (Table 18.1). The incidence of initiation in 14–17-year-old males increased considerably during both World Wars I and II, by 71 and 62 per cent, respectively, when cigarettes became viewed as important in helping soldiers be better fighters by 'soothing the nerves' and were freely distributed to the armed forces (Pierce and Gilpin 1995). As noted above, 14–17-year-old females did not smoke before the first 'Reach for a Lucky instead of a sweet' advertisements in 1925. During the period 1925–30, initiation rates of 14–17-year-old females increased dramatically by 280 per cent (Pierce *et al.* 1994). Thereafter, the rates progressively increased with each birth cohort through 1950. In 1967, the tobacco industry launched a series of cigarettes with advertising campaigns announcing that they were specifically designed for women, the most well known of which was the Virginia Slims cigarette. Coincident with the starting of these campaigns, the uptake of smoking among girls, particularly those who would not proceed to higher education, jumped dramatically by 41 per cent for the period 1967–73 (Pierce *et al.* 1994).

In 1971, Congress enacted a ban on all broadcast advertising of cigarettes in the United States. Shortly thereafter, the initiation rate in all 14–17 year olds started a 12-year decline (CDCP 1998). The tobacco industry's reaction to this decline in adolescent smoking was to progressively increase tobacco advertising and promotional expenditures. By the mid-1980s, the decline in adolescent smoking was halted. Thereafter, the tobacco industry increased its advertising and promotional expenditures almost exponentially. This was associated with a rapid increase in the uptake of smoking through 1996 that was confined almost completely to the 14–17-year-old age group.

This volatility in trends in the uptake of smoking among adolescents demonstrates that it is possible to rapidly impact the rate of smoking initiation. The question is what

Table 18.1 Events associated with marked change in incidence of initiation among 14–17-year-old adolescents

Historical event	Period	Targeted audience	% Change in incidence of initiation
World war I	1916–18	Males	71%
Lucky strike campaign	1925–30	Females	280%
World war II	1941–45	Males	62%
Virginia slims campaign	1967–73	Females	41%

Source: Pierce and Gilpin (1995).

would be the impact of this on population prevalence? Obviously, smoking prevalence cannot be maintained if there is no initiation to replace those who successfully quit or who die. The rapidity of the effect on prevalence of smoking in the population can be seen from the experience of United States physicians. At the time of the consensus that smoking caused lung cancer, approximately half the physicians and medical students smoked. However, the report appeared to have a huge effect on medical students; by the early 1980s, only 2 per cent of students in US medical schools in the United States were smoking (Pierce and Gilpin 1994). On the other hand, successful quitting among physicians increased only slowly, in a pattern very similar to other highly educated people in the society. However, within 20 years, the rapid and sustained decline in smoking initiation led to a 6 per cent prevalence of smoking among US physicians (USDHHS 1989).

Studying trends in smoking uptake also provides valuable information on the likely impact of different health promotion messages aimed at discouraging adolescents from smoking. Between 1950 and 1964, there was a barrage of news media coverage on the health consequences of smoking that was associated with many smokers quitting (Pierce and Gilpin 2001). However, there was no discernable effect on initiation rates of people aged 14–24 years. However, after the public health consensus that smoking caused disease in 1964, there has been a continual decline in the proportion of never-smoking adults (aged 18–24 years) who initiated smoking. This effect of the dissemination of the health consequences of smoking in reducing the incidence of initiation in young adults has been replicated in many countries. This declining pattern was not observed among 14–17-year-old adolescents in the United States or anywhere else.

What is the process by which someone becomes a smoker?

Longitudinal studies of adolescents in the late 1980s and 1990s have shown that, at the end of elementary school, children are generally committed never smokers, that is, they do not envisage that there is any way that they will become a smoker. However, for many this certainty does not last, and they eventually become unwilling to rule out smoking in all situations, which we have defined as becoming susceptible to smoking. Susceptible smokers indicate that their decision depends on the particular situation they are in and many would describe themselves as curious about smoking. A series of studies have demonstrated that susceptible never smokers are at twice the risk of smoking of committed never smokers (Pierce *et al.* 1996; Unger *et al.* 1997; Jackson 1998).

Many studies have shown that the more experience a person has with smoking, the greater the likelihood they will be a continuing smoker. Indeed, each increase in the level of experience increases the probability of future smoking. However, this probability decreases with time since the last smoking experience. What people expect they will do in the future is also important. If an adolescent is certain that they will not try a cigarette again, then their risk level is reduced (Choi *et al.* 2001). These variables can be put together to create a continuum for assessing the probability of future smoking for any individual at any point in time.

We use three age-specific indices to identify where a community or population is on this uptake continuum. The first is the proportion of the group who are committed never smokers. In the United States, the main movement out of the committed never-smoking group occurs between the ages of 10 and 14 years. The second marker is the proportion of adolescents who have experimented with smoking, even a few puffs. The modal age of experimentation in the United States is between 12 and 14 years. There is thought to be an important age window for completing experimentation during the teenage years that influences the probability of later daily smoking. The marker used to indicate completion of the experimentation phase is having smoked at least 100 cigarettes in one's lifetime, which is the accepted definition of an adult smoker in the United States. It has been estimated that 50 per cent of adolescents who reach at least 100 cigarettes will still be smoking at age 35 years (Pierce and Gilpin 1996). Interestingly, previously secret tobacco industry documents obtained through the US lawsuits have indicated that the tobacco industry felt that brand loyalty occurred generally after smoking as little as 200 cigarettes of the same brand. Despite this research and concerns relating to recall bias, the traditional measure of adolescent smoking is a period prevalence measure, the proportion who have smoked in the previous 30 days.

How strong is genetics in determining who will become a smoker?

In 1958, the famous statistician, Sir Ronald Fisher, argued that it was possible that people who were genetically at risk to develop cancer were the same people who were genetically at risk to start smoking (Fisher 1958). Given the overwhelming evidence supporting a causal association between smoking and lung cancer, this argument was not at all persuasive in the public policy debate of the time. However, it did raise the issue that there is probably a genetic component to smoking initiation. There has now been considerable research on identical twins, some who have been raised apart. These studies allow the separation of the social environmental influences from genetic influences, and have generally found that there is an important genetic influence on who becomes a smoker. However, the genetic influence is not related to the development of a susceptibility to smoking. Instead, people respond differently to exposure to nicotine, with some appearing to be genetically predisposed to become dependent. In a series of different studies, it appears that a relatively constant 30–50 per cent of experimenters go on to become addicted smokers. As there is a lot of research in this area at the present time, we can expect the knowledge base in this area to expand rapidly in the next decade.

How do friends who smoke effect initiation?

One of the most consistent findings in research on adolescent smoking is that nonsmokers who have friends who smoke soon become smokers themselves (USDHHS 1994).

Indeed, the majority of early smoking experiences occur in social settings with cigarettes obtained from a friend, often in the company of a best friend (Bauman *et al.* 1984).

Peer groups are particularly important in the early adolescent years (Steinberg 2002). At the start of adolescence, there is a sharp increase in the amount of time spent with peers, most often without adult supervision. Brown (1990) noted that adolescents in schools quickly start to identify with one of a series of large, reputation-based collectives of similarly stereotyped individuals, even if they don't spend much time with them. In the United States, commonly used labels for these different collectives include 'jocks', 'brains', 'druggies', 'populars', 'nerds', etc. Identifying with one of these collectives locates the teen within the school social structure. To identify with a particular collective, an adolescent will often need to follow the dress code of the collective and to adhere to lifestyle and behavior preferences of the collective, which includes choice of friends (Brown *et al.* 1993). These collectives serve as the reference group for the adolescent and a source of identity. Adolescents judge one another on the basis of the company they keep, the clothes they wear, the music they listen to, the language that they use, and the places in which they 'hang out'. It is the desire/need of the adolescent to be seen to belong to one of these collectives that provides the 'peer pressure' on adolescents. This is particularly strong in the middle school years, where, typically, the number of peer collectives is limited. It isn't until high school that the collectives become more differentiated and permeable, and thus there is less pressure to conform.

Clearly, if a middle school adolescent is seeking to identify with a collective that has smoking as a condoned lifestyle, then the likelihood of the adolescent starting to smoke will increase significantly. Adolescents do choose the collective they wish to identify with, thus they can influence the type of 'peer pressure' to which they will be subject. However, in the recent studies of the progress toward smoking by committed never smokers, the influence of peers has been somewhat muted (Pierce *et al.* 1998, 2002). This suggests that adolescents who have been influenced to become curious about smoking may seek out peers or friends who smoke as a way of obtaining the first cigarette.

What is the role of parents as an influence on initiation?

Numerous studies have demonstrated that parents and parenting practices are one of the major influences on how an adolescent adjusts in society (Steinberg 2002). A series of studies have identified high levels of responsiveness (good bidirectional communication and support) and demandingness (setting limits and ceding independence with evidence of responsibility) as the most important factors in appropriate adolescent socialization (Baumrind 1978). Contrary to some people's belief, adolescents generally share the value system of their parents. Thus, parenting which comprises high levels of both responsiveness and demandingness, which is considered recommended parenting, can influence adolescent behavior in many ways, including which 'collective' the adolescent associates with at school.

When parents value not smoking, recommended parenting can be expected to be associated with a much lower level of adolescent smoking. This appears to be the situation in most of the United States in the early twenty-first century, and many studies indicate that recommended parenting practices are associated with a halving of the use of nonsanctioned substances, including cigarettes (Mounts and Steinberg 1995; Jackson et al. 1994, 1998; Pierce et al. 2002). One way this appears to be achieved is by reducing the probability that the adolescent has best friends who smoke (Pierce et al. 2002).

Measures of the importance of not smoking in the parental value system include whether or not the parents smoke themselves, their attitudes and behavior toward other smokers, whether they have a smoke-free home, and the adolescent's expectations of how parents will respond to him or her smoking. Within the tobacco control literature, the measure of parental influence most emphasized has been parental smoking behavior. While many studies have shown that parental smoking increases the probability of adolescent smoking, there is a growing literature on studies that do not report such an association. Differences in effect would be expected between adolescents who interpret parent smoking as evidence of the difficulty of overcoming a nicotine addiction compared to those who interpret it as evidence that smoking has some real advantages (such as weight or stress control).

How can advertising and promotions entice adolescents to start smoking?

Advertising and promotions have the goal of building sales and profits for a company. A tobacco company's sales can be increased if current smokers change brands, however, the future of the industry requires a continuing supply of new smokers. Over the past century, every time a tobacco company advertising campaign was acclaimed as innovative and successful, adolescent smoking increased (Pierce et al. 1994, 1996).

Ray (1982) uses a farming analogy to explain the different tasks of advertising and promotion. The farmer must invest in seeds, plant them, and nurture them before he can reap a crop and sell it to make a profit. To be successful, the farmer needs to balance the amount of sowing and nurturing that he does with the amount of reaping that can be done. Advertising and publicity, as well as some promotional efforts, aim at building the product franchise. Therefore, they can be considered to be in the 'sowing' category. The goals of these types of communication for the tobacco industry are to build awareness of the brand, to increase the proportion of the population who see a benefit to smoking, and to have a positive (or not so negative) feeling toward smoking. Image marketing attempts to associate values with the product (i.e. the cigarette) that the target group would like to have, nearly always through visual imagery. Thus, by buying Marlboro cigarettes, adolescents present a symbol to others that they have reached independence. The initial goal is to build curiosity to try smoking (equivalent to susceptibility to smoking).

Once people are susceptible to smoking, converting them to smoking a particular brand is the goal of 'reaping' activities. The first goal of the tobacco industry is to ensure that cigarettes are fairly easily accessible and at a low cost to the person who is susceptible to smoking. Pricing, package design, and promotions (such as two-for-one and free gift with purchase) are activities that can be described as in the 'reaping' category. One of the secret industry documents outlined a 'reaping' strategy that had as its goal getting the young person to smoke 200 cigarettes, claimed as sufficient to achieve brand loyalty in a new smoker (Young and Rubicam 1990).

The tobacco industry documents outline that they evaluate their advertising campaigns using the standard 'hierarchy of effects' approach. This approach assumes that the adolescent initially needs to be exposed to the message, with the goal of saturation exposure. The 'hierarchy of effects' model of advertising takes account of the fact that not everyone who sees an advertising message will be receptive to it. An individual's level of receptivity to an advertising campaign can be measured. We classify people who label an ad as one of their favorites as moderately receptive. Companies that have been successful in branding their product with an image that resonates with the target audience frequently use brand-extenders such as tee-shirts or tote bags. The person who is willing to wear the image of the product on a piece of clothing, for example, is classified as highly receptive to the marketing campaign.

Using the hierarchy of effects approach to evaluating tobacco advertising, there is very strong evidence that vast majority of adolescents are not only exposed to cigarette advertising but are well aware of the images of the advertised cigarette brands. The vast majority of adolescents understand that cigarette advertising promotes one of the following benefits of smoking: smoking is enjoyable; it helps people relax; it helps people feel comfortable in social situations; it helps people stay thin; it helps people with stress; helps them overcome boredom; and, the 'in-crowd' are smokers. Further, the majority of United States adolescents (even as young as 12–14 years) have a favorite cigarette advertisement. Around 30 per cent of 15–17-year-old adolescents are willing to wear a tee-shirt displaying the brand image used to advertise a cigarette. These results place cigarettes at the top of the products that have good advertising penetration with adolescents.

There are now four separate longitudinal studies in the United States (Pierce *et al.* 1998, 2002; Biener and Siegel 2000; Sargent *et al.* 2000) that have shown that the more receptive an adolescent is to cigarette advertising and promotions (using the above hierarchy of effects) the higher the probability that they will experiment with smoking and become dependent on it. The most recent of these studies indicates that receptivity to tobacco industry advertising can undermine the effectiveness of good parenting in protecting adolescents from starting to smoke (Pierce *et al.* 2002).

Public health approaches to reduce smoking initiation

In the United States and in many other countries, there is strong public support for using the public sector to discourage adolescents from starting to smoke. Four of the major approaches used are: the conduct of counter advertising campaigns, increases in cigarette price through increases in state excise taxes on cigarettes, and increasing enforcement of regulations and laws forbidding merchants to sell cigarettes to minors and school programs.

Can a mass media campaign lead to a reduction in initiation rates?

The first population-based antismoking mass media campaign occurred in the late 1960s and was associated with a marked decline in the per capita consumption of cigarettes (Warner 1977). During the 1980s the Office on Smoking and Health in the United States ran a sporadic national mass media program through public service announcements (Pierce *et al.* 1992) and many of these productions targeted adolescent smoking. The first statewide antismoking mass media campaigns started in Australia in 1983 using health consequences messages in paid media. These were demonstrated to effectively reduce adult-smoking prevalence (Dwyer *et al.* 1986; Pierce *et al.* 1990). While adolescents were a target of some of the early campaigns, effective changes in adolescent smoking behavior were not demonstrated.

Clear evidence that mass media antismoking campaigns could affect youth smoking was demonstrated with the Florida Tobacco Control Program (Bauer *et al.* 2000). The Florida 'Truth' campaign sought to engage youth in a movement that included questioning tobacco industry public messages. This program achieved extremely high awareness among 12–17 year olds (92%). More than 10 000 youth signed up for an action program. Over 2 years, this program achieved dramatic changes in youth smoking across all levels of the smoking uptake continuum in both middle and high schools. The level of committed never smokers increased from 67 to 76 per cent in middle schools. The level of experimentation decreased by 25 per cent and the prevalence of current smokers dropped by more than one-third in middle school and by 18 per cent in high school. These changes are unprecedented, and this program is the model for the American Legacy National antismoking program that began in the United States in 1999 with money supplied by the tobacco industry in their legal settlement agreement with the Attorneys General of the various states.

What is the effect of price on initiation?

Econometric studies abound demonstrating that smoking behavior is heavily influenced by cigarette price, as predicted by standard economic theory. The price elasticity of demand is the phrase used to describe the estimated impact of a change in price on subsequent consumption. Most studies estimate that a 10 per cent increase in price will reduce overall per capita consumption among the overall population by between 2 and 5 per cent. Several studies of adolescents suggest that they are more than twice and possibly three times as responsive to price changes than are adults, as would be expected from their lower level of disposable income (Chaloupka and Grossman 1996; Lewit *et al.* 1997). Further, as expected, the effect of price in reducing adolescent smoking is mainly seen on those who purchase cigarettes. As discussed earlier, initial experimentation usually involves cigarettes supplied from social sources and evidence supports the hypothesis that price changes will have a considerably lower impact on the proportion of adolescents who experiment than on subsequent purchasing behavior (Gruber 2000; Tauras *et al.* 2000; Emery *et al.* 2001).

It is important to remember that the public health approach is limited to setting the excise tax, while the tobacco industry sets the price as part of their marketing strategy. Indeed, a major component of the advertising and promotional budget is the use of retail value added items that can selectively reduce the actual price that an individual pays for cigarettes. Many of these promotions are focused on the small convenience store, the source of cigarettes for the majority of adolescent smokers and potential smokers.

Does accessibility of cigarettes matter?

During the twentieth century world wars, cigarettes became perceived as essential to the United States war effort and were provided to all soldiers both in their ration packs and on street corners by the Red Cross. This made access to cigarettes relatively easy for 14–17-year-old males. As presented earlier in Table 18.1, these two periods were associated with rapid increases in the initiation of smoking by these adolescents.

In the last 20 years, public policy on reducing teens' access to cigarettes has focused on effectively barring sales of cigarettes to minors. Limiting the ability of minors to purchase cigarettes or other tobacco products is a seemingly practical and politically popular measure (in the United States) aimed at curbing teen smoking, by making it difficult for adolescents to purchase cigarettes. Whether this strategy actually limits teens' access to cigarettes is controversial. Several studies have shown that such laws have minimal impact on teen perceptions that cigarettes are accessible to them or on teen smoking (Chaloupka and Grossman 1996; Rigotti *et al.* 1997). However, there may be a threshold effect. Analyses of the impact of California's strong enforcement of laws banning tobacco sales to minors have demonstrated a major reduction in the perceived accessibility of cigarettes and that, for the first time, perceived ease of access of cigarettes predicts later smoking behavior (Gilpin *et al.* 2001).

What influence do schools have on initiation?

School smoking prevention efforts have the potential to influence adolescent smoking in several ways. A study from Australia indicates that many adolescents start smoking regularly at school (Hill and Borland 1991). The implementation and enforcement of smoke-free school policies limits the opportunity for teens to smoke. Further, the existence and enforcement of these policies promote norms against smoking as an acceptable behavior for everyone, including teachers, who are important role models for adolescents. Finally, antismoking curricula can provide vital information on the health dangers and the addictive nature of cigarettes.

For decades, schools have played a central role in educational efforts aimed at smoking prevention (USDHHS 1989, 1994; Hansen 1992; Glynn 1993). It is recognized that such programs have the best chance of success in the setting of comprehensive community-based tobacco control programs (Glynn 1993). If tobacco policies are not consistently enforced in schools, they can convey a mixed message to students (Bowen *et al.* 1995). However, Pentz *et al.* (1989) showed that, when consistently enforced and coupled with cessation education, school-smoking policies are associated with decreased smoking prevalence among adolescents.

By the time adolescents have reached high school, students routinely have had smoking prevention education classes that discuss the health dangers of smoking. The level of smoking experience of the adolescent is associated with how effective they perceive these classes to be. In California, a majority of adolescents who have smoked do not credit the classes with influencing their peers against smoking (Gilpin *et al.* 2001). Therefore, such classes likely have minimal personal impact as well.

Compliance with smoke-free school policies is associated with decreased levels of exposure to smoking at school, including teachers' smoking and increased levels of students who think that the classes on the health effects of smoking are effective. General acceptance of school smoking bans for everyone at school may be a factor in reducing adolescent smoking.

References

Bauer, U. E., Johnson, T. M., Hopkins, R. S., and Brooks, R. G. (2000). Changes in youth cigarette use and intentions following implementation of a tobacco control program: Findings from the Florida Youth Tobacco Survey, 1998–2000. *JAMA*, **284**, 723–8.

Bauman, K. E., Fisher, L. A., Bryan, E. S., and Chenoweth, R. L. (1984). Antecedents, subjective expected utility and behavior: A panel study of adolescent cigarette smoking. *Addict. Behav.*, **9**, 121–36.

Baumrind, D. (1978). Parental disciplinary patterns and social competence in children. *Youth and Society*, **9**, 239–75.

Biener, L. and Siegel, M. (2000). Tobacco marketing and adolescent smoking: More support for a causal inference. *Am. J. Pub. Health*, **90**, 407–11.

Brown, B. (1990). Peer groups. In: *At the threshold: the developing adolescent* (ed. S. Feldman and G. Elliott). Harvard University Press, Cambridge, MA, pp. 171–96.

Brown, B. B., Mounts, N., Lamborn, S. D., and Steinberg, L. (1993). Parenting practices and peer group affiliation in adolescence. *Child Development*, **64**, 467–82.

Bowen, D. J., Kinne, S., and Orlandi, M. (1995). School policy in COMMIT: A promising strategy to reduce smoking by youth. *J. School Health*, **65**, 140–4.

Burns, D., Garfinkel, L., and Samet, J. M. (1997). Introduction, summary, and conclusions. In: *Smoking and tobacco control, Monograph 8.* National Cancer Institute, pp. 1–11.

Centers for Disease Control and Prevention (CDCP) (1998). Incidence of initiation of cigarette smoking—United States, 1965–1996. *MMWR, 47,* 837–40.

Chaloupka, F. and Grossman, M. Price (1996). *Tobacco control policies and youth smoking.* National Bureau of Economic Research, Cambridge, MA.

Choi, W. S., Gilpin, E. A., Farkas, A. J., and Pierce, J. P. (2001). Determining the probability of future smoking among adolescents. *Addiction, 96,* 313–23.

Dwyer, T, Pierce, J. P., Hannam, C. D., and Burke, N. (1986). Evaluation of the Sydney 'Quit For Life' Anti-Smoking Campaign. Part II. Changes in smoking prevalence. *Medical Journal of Australia,* **144,** 344–7.

Emery, S., White, M. M., and Pierce J. P. (2001). Does cigarette price influence adolescent experimentation? *Journal of Health Economics, 20,* 261–70.

Fisher, R. A. (1958). Cancer and smoking. *Nature,* **182,** 596.

FTC (US Federal Trade Commission) (2000). Cigarette Report for 2000. Issued 2002. (http://www.ftc.gov/bcp/menu-tobac.htm). Accessed July 20, 2002.

Gilpin, E. A., Lee, L., Evans, N., and Pierce, J. (1994). Smoking initiation rates in adults and minors: United States, 1944–1988. *American Journal of Epidemiology,* **140,** 535–43.

Gilpin, E. A., Emery, S. L., Farkas, A. J., Distefan, J. M., White, M. M., and Pierce, J. P. (2001). *The California tobacco control program: A decade of progress, 1989–1999.* University of California, San Diego, La Jolla, CA.

Glynn, Thomas, J. (1993). Improving the health of U.S. children: The need for early interventions in tobacco use. *Prev. Med., 22,* 513–9.

Gruber, J. (2000). Youth smoking in the US: Prices and policies. National Bureau of Economic Research Working Paper, No. 7506.

Hansen, W. B. (1992). School-based substance abuse prevention: A review of the state of the art in curriculum, 1980–1990. *Health Educ. Res., 7,* 403–30.

Hill, D. and Borland R. (1991). Adults' accounts of onset of regular smoking: Influences of school, work, and other settings. *Public Health Reports,* **106,** 181–5.

Jackson, C., Henriksen, L., and Foshee, V. A. (1998). The Authoritative Parenting Index: Predicting health risk behaviors among children and adolescents. *Health Education and Behavior,* **25,** 319–37.

Jackson, C., Bee-Gates, D. J., and Henriksen, L. (1994). Authoritative parenting, child competencies, and initiation of cigarette smoking. *Health Education Quarterly,* **21,** 103–16.

Jackson, C. (1998). Cognitive susceptibility to smoking and initiation of smoking during childhood: A longitudinal study. *Preventive Medicine,* **27,** 129–34.

Lee, L. L., Gilpin, E. A., and Pierce, J. P. (1993). Changes in the patterns of initiation of cigarette smoking in the United States: 1950, 1965, and1 980. *Cancer Epidemiol. Biomarkers Prev.,* **2,** 593–7.

Lewit, E. M., Hyland, A., *et al.* (1997). Price, public policy, and smoking in young people. *Tob Control,* (Suppl 2), S17–24.

Mounts, N. S. and Steinberg, L. D. (1995). An ecological analysis of peer influence on adolescent grade point average and drug use. *Developmental Psychology,* **31,** 915–22.

Pentz, M. A., Brannon, B. R., Charlin, V. L., Barrett, E. J., MacKinnon, D. P., and Flay, B. R. (1989). The power of policy: The relationship of smoking policy to adolescent smoking. *Am. J. Pub. Health,* **79,** 857–62.

Pierce, J. P., Macaskill, P., and Hill, D. (1990). Long term effectiveness of Mass Media Led Anti-Smoking Campaigns in Australia. *American Journal of Public Health*, **80**(5), 565–9.

Pierce, J. P., Anderson, M., Romano, R. M., Meissner, H. I., and Odenkirchen, J. C. (1992). Promoting smoking cessation in the United States: Effect of public service announcements of the Cancer Information Service Telephone Line *Journal of the National Cancer Institute*, **84**(9), 677–83.

Pierce, J. P., Lee, L., and Gilpin, E. A. (1994). Smoking initiation by adolescent girls, 1944 through 1988 in association with targeted advertising. *JAMA*, **271**, 608–11.

Pierce, J. P. and Gilpin, E. A. (1994). Trends in physicians' smoking behavior and patterns of advice to quit. In: *Tobacco and the clinician: Interventions for medical and dental practice, smoking and tobacco control, Monograph No. 5*. National Institutes of Health, National Cancer Institute, pp. 12–23.

Pierce, J. P. and Gilpin, E. A. (1995). A historical analysis of tobacco marketing and the uptake of smoking by youth in the United States: 1890–1977. *Health Psychology*, **14**, 500–8.

Pierce, J. P., Choi, W. S., Gilpin, E. A., Farkas, A. J., and Merritt, R. K. (1996). Validation of susceptibility as a predictor of which adolescents take up smoking in the U.S. *Health Psychology*, **15**, 355–61.

Pierce, J. P. and Gilpin, E. (1996). How long will today's new adolescent smokers be addicted to cigarettes? *American Journal of Public Health*, **86**, 253–6.

Pierce, J. P., Choi, W., Gilpin, E. A., Farkas, A. J., and Berry C. C. (1998). Tobacco industry promotion of cigarettes and adolescent smoking. *JAMA*, **279**, 511–15.

Pierce, J. P. and Gilpin, E. A. (2001). News media coverage of smoking and health is associated with changes in population rates of smoking cessation but not initiation. *Tobacco Control*, **10**, 145–53.

Pierce, J. P., Distefan, J. M., Jackson, C., White, M. M, and Gilpin, E. A. (2002). Does tobacco marketing undermine the influence of recommended parenting in discouraging adolescents from smoking? *Am. J. Prev. Med.*, **23**, 73–81.

Ray, M. L. (1982). *Advertising and communication management*. Prentice Hall, Englewood Cliffs, NJ.

Rigotti, N. A., DiFranza, J. R., Chang, Y., Tisdale, T., Kemp, B., and Singer, D. (1997). The effect of enforcing tobacco sales laws on adolescents' access to tobacco and smoking behavior. *New Engl. J. Med.*, **337**, 1044–51.

Sargent, J. D., Dalton, M., Beach, M., Bernhardt, A., Heatherton, T., and Stevens, M. (2000). Effect of cigarette promotions on smoking uptake among adolescents. *Prev. Med.*, **30**, 320–7.

Steinberg, L. (2002). *Adolescence*. (6th edn) McGraw-Hill, New York.

Tauras, J. A., Johnston, L. D., and O'Malley, P. M. (2000). An analysis of teenage smoking initiation: the effects of government intervention. Impact Teen/YES! Research Paper No. 2.

Unger, J. B., Johnson, C. A., Stoddard, J. L., Nezami, E., and Chou, C. P. (1997). Identification of adolescents at risk for smoking initiation: Validation of a measure of susceptibility. *Addictive Behaviors*, **22**, 81–91.

US Department of Health and Human Services (1989). Reducing the health consequences of smoking: 25 years of progress. A report of the surgeon general. USDHHS, Centers for Disease Control and Prevention, National Center for Chronic Disease Prevention and Health Promotion, Office on Smoking and Health, Atlanta, GA. DHHS Pub. No. (CDC) 89-8411.

US Department of Health and Human Services (1994). Preventing tobacco use among young people: A report of the surgeon general. USDHHS, Centers for Disease Control and Prevention, National Center for Chronic Disease Prevention and Health Promotion, Office on Smoking and Health, Atlanta, GA.

Warner, K. E. (1977). The effects of the anti-smoking campaign on cigarette consumption. *American Journal of Public Health*, **67**, 645–50.

Young and Rubicam (1990). Mangini Document No. RJR472678.

Chapter 19

Tobacco and women

Amanda Amos and Judith Mackay

The epidemic

The global picture

Smoking is still seen mainly as a male problem, since in most countries smoking prevalence is lower among women than men. Yet, it is currently estimated that there are already about 200 million women in the world who smoke, and in addition, there are others who chew tobacco (WHO 1999). Approximately 15% of women in developed countries and 8% of women in developing countries smoke, but because most women live in developing countries, there are numerically more women smokers in developing countries. Unless effective, comprehensive and sustained initiatives are implemented to reduce smoking uptake among young women and increase cessation rates among women, the prevalence of female smoking in developed and developing countries could rise to 20% by 2025 (Lopez A., personal communication 1997). This would mean that by 2025 there could be 532 million women smokers. Even if prevalence levels do not rise, the number of women who smoke will increase because the population of women in the world is predicted to rise from the current 3.1 billion to 4.2 billion by 2025. Thus, while the epidemic of tobacco use among men is in slow decline, the epidemic among women will not reach its peak until well into the twenty-first century. This will have enormous consequences not only for women's health and economic well being but also that of their family.

The prevalence of smoking and smoking-related diseases in countries across the world varies markedly by gender and socio-economic status. Women have traditionally started smoking later and consumed fewer numbers of cigarettes than men. Thus, the patterning of smoking among and between women and men differs according to the stage of the smoking epidemic which countries inhabit (Fig. 19.1).

Developed countries

Currently, about 15% of women aged 15 years and above in developed countries smoke cigarettes, almost 80 million women. In the earlier decades of the smoking epidemic in developed countries, smokers were much more likely to be male than female. In the past four decades, however, the pattern in many of these countries has changed dramatically. Drawing on a widely used four-stage model of the global smoking

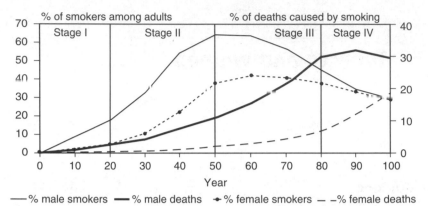

Fig. 19.1 A model of the cigarette epidemic. (Source: Lopez *et al.* 1994.)

epidemic (Fig. 19.1), some countries in southern Europe (e.g. Portugal) and some developed countries in Asia and the Western pacific (e.g. Japan) can be located currently at stage 2 with smoking rates peaking at between 50% and 80% among men while the trend among women is rising. Stage 3 countries have a longer history of widespread smoking and include many southern, central, and eastern European countries (e.g. Italy, Spain, Greece). In these countries prevalence rates among men are decreasing but cigarette smoking is either still increasing among women or has not shown any decline. Women's smoking rates typically peak at 35–45%.

Stage 4 countries have the longest history of cigarette smoking (e.g. the USA, UK, Canada, Australia, Finland, Germany) and in these countries cigarette smoking is declining among both women and men (Graham 1996; Cavelaars *et al.* 2000). However, the gap in smoking between women and men in these countries has also greatly decreased. Indeed, in Sweden smoking rates in women are now higher than in men. This has been due to a combination of a narrowing in the gap between uptake rates of smoking in girls and boys, and relatively lower cessation rates in cigarette smoking women compared to men. In several of these countries (e.g. UK, Sweden, Austria, Denmark, Finland, Germany) (Wold *et al.* 2000), smoking rates among young girls are higher than those among boys. In addition, smoking in these countries has now become highly concentrated among the poorer and more disadvantaged sections of the population. This reflects relatively lower uptake rates and higher quit rates in more affluent groups. In these countries smoking is therefore an increasingly important cause of inequalities in health.

Another cause for concern in developed countries is that the speed of transition from one stage of the epidemic to the next seems to be getting faster, in part due to tobacco companies targeting of young women in countries undergoing rapid social and economic change. In Lithuania, for example, smoking among women doubled over a five year period in the 1990s and increased by fivefold amongst the youngest groups (Amos and Haglund 2000). In Sweden, one of Lithuania's neighbours, where women started to smoke in large numbers in the 1950s, it took almost 20 years for the female prevalence to double. Between 1993 and 1997, rates of smoking among 12–25 year-old young women in former East Germany nearly doubled from 27% to 47%. In contrast rates among young men showed a less steep increase from 38% to 45%, and there was little change in smoking rates among the same age group in former West Germany (Corrao *et al.* 2000).

Developing countries

Most women live in developing countries, where currently only between 2 and 10% smoke cigarettes, although in some regions, such as South Asia, women more commonly chew tobacco. Therefore most of these countries are at stage 1 or stage 2 of the epidemic, with much higher rates of smoking in men compared to women. Typically, rates of smoking are highest among well-educated, affluent, urban young women. Although smoking prevalence among women in these countries is generally lower than in developed countries, this is no cause for complacency as it does not reflect health awareness, but rather social and religious traditions and women's low economic resources. Also in many developing countries, such as China, there is evidence that the age of first smoking is becoming younger. The numbers of women smokers in developing countries will inevitably increase because:

- the female population will rise from the present 3.1 to 4.2 billion by 2025, so even if the prevalence remains low, the absolute numbers of smokers will increase

- the spending power of girls and women is increasing so that cigarettes are becoming more affordable

- the social and cultural constraints which previously prevented many women smoking are weakening in some places

- the tobacco companies are targeting women with well-funded, alluring marketing campaigns, linking smoking with emancipation and glamour

- many gender specialists, women's organizations, women's magazines, models, film and pop stars, and other female role models have not yet acted on the basis that smoking is a women's issue, or their need to take an appropriate role

- women-specific health education and quitting programmes are rare

- governments in developing countries may be less aware of the harmfulness of tobacco use and are preoccupied with other health issues; where they are concerned with smoking, they focus on the higher levels of male smoking. In fact, no developing country is addressing the emerging female epidemic to the extent the problem warrants.

Regional cameos (Table 19.1)

Africa. Data are available for only a minority of African countries (Mackay and Eriksen 2002). Some of these studies were undertaken on a select group, such as students or urban dwellers, and therefore may not represent the national picture. Smoking rates vary, but overall it is estimated that about 10% of African women smoke. This ranges from less than 2% in Nigeria, Ivory Coast, and Zimbabwe to 11% in South Africa. Studies from the few countries where more than one survey has been undertaken show a rising trend, especially in urban areas (Elegbeleye and Femi-Pearse 1976). Smoking patterns and trends may also differ considerably by ethnic group. For example, in South Africa 59% of coloured women smoked in 1995 compared to 10% of black women and 7% of Indians (WHO 1997). Rates of smoking have declined among white South African women but are increasing among black women.

Americas. Rates of smoking in women vary considerably between the 36 countries. In the USA and Canada rates among women peaked at over 30% and are now declining. In contrast, low rates of female smoking are reported in Caribbean countries. Prevalence in women varies from 6% in Paraguay to 39% in Venezuela (Mackay and Eriksen 2002). Rates of female smoking can vary considerably by ethnic group. While in the USA smoking rates among white women have been consistently higher than those among Black women, a study in Trinidad and Tobago found that there was a higher prevalence among women of European origin (14%) than among women of African (7%) or Indian origin (8%).

South East Asia. The prevalence of cigarette smoking is generally very low among women. Only 3% of women smoke manufactured cigarettes but in several countries other forms of tobacco use by women have been integrated into cultural practices for several decades. In several areas of India, for example, 50–60% of women chew tobacco, and rural women smoke the kretek, dhumti, khi yo, ya muan, chilum, and water pipe, and 'reverse smoke' bidis and chutta, with the lighted end inside the mouth (Aghi *et al.* 1988). Very high rates of tobacco smoking are found in women in Nepal.

Western Pacific. Although the overall smoking rate across these 31 countries is estimated to be less than 10%, there are wide variations. For example, in some parts of Papua New Guinea 80% of women smoke, and rates are also high among women in the Pacific Islands (Tuomilehto *et al.* 1986). Only 4% of women in China smoke (Chinese Academy of Preventive Medicine 1999) and 3% in Hong Kong (Hong Kong CSD 1998), Malaysia, and Thailand. Tobacco chewing is uncommon. China deserves special mention because of its size. The prevalence of smoking remains high among older women in cities such as Beijing and Tianjin. Although a substantial minority of women born before 1940 became smokers by age 25, only about 2% of those born since 1950 have done so. In two large nationwide surveys, the prevalence of smoking among women aged 15–24 was 0.5% both in 1984 and in 1996 (Chinese Academy of Preventive Medicine 1999). However, it is still possible that the number of young women becoming smokers will increase. Surveys have reported 10% of young women smoking in selected small areas in China (Liu *et al.* 1998).

Eastern Mediterranean. Smoking in women is often considered vulgar, improper, even immoral. Only 2% of Egyptian women smoke compared with 35% of men

Table 19.1 Prevalence of cigarette smoking among women in selected countries

	Prevalence (%)	Date of survey
Americas		
Bolivia	18	1998
Brazil	29	1995
Honduras	11	1988
Jamaica	13	1990
Mexico	18	1998
Trinidad and Tobago	8	1986
USA	22	1999
Europe		
Denmark	29	1999/2001
France	30	2000
Germany	31	1999/2001
Poland	25	1999/2001
Portugal	7	1995/6
Spain	25	1997
Russia	10	1997/8
UK	26	1999/2001
Africa		
Algeria	7	1997/8
Ivory Coast	2	1977
Lesotho	1	1992
South Africa	11	1998
Nigeria	2	1998
Swaziland	2	1994
Zaire	25	1990
Eastern Mediterranean		
Bahrain	6	1998
Bangladesh	24	2001
Egypt	2	1998
Sudan	1	2000
Tunisia	8	1997
South-East Asia		
India	3	1998/9
Indonesia	4	1998
Nepal	29	2001
Thailand	3	1999
Western Pacific		
Australia	18	2001
China	4	1996
Hong Kong	3	2000
Japan	13	1998
Malaysia	4	1996
New Zealand	25	2001
Singapore	3	1998

Source: Corrao *et al.* (2000), Mackay and Eriksen (2002).

(Mackay and Eriksen 2002). In the Gulf region, about 8% of women smoke in contrast to 33% of men. The highest reported female smoking prevalence is 29% in Yemen (Mackay and Eriksen 2002). However, surveys may significantly underestimate smoking prevalence among women in these countries as, due to religious and cultural reasons, women may be reluctant to admit to their smoking.

Europe. Prevalence rates in some countries in central and eastern Europe (Czech Republic, Hungary, Poland, and Bulgaria) are now similar to those in western Europe, about 20–30% and are increasing. In countries such as Russia, where it is less acceptable for women to smoke in public places, the rates are generally lower, around 10–15%.

Health effects of tobacco use

Active tobacco use

Because the health effects of smoking only become fully evident 40–50 years after the widespread uptake of smoking (Fig. 19.1), we have yet to see the full global impact of smoking on women's health. This also means that most of what is known about the health effects of smoking has come from studies of cigarette smoking in developed countries which have tended to focus more on men than women. However, it is now clear that women around the world who smoke, as with male smokers, have markedly increased risks of many cancers, particularly lung cancer, heart disease, stroke, emphysema, and other fatal diseases. Indeed there is now evidence that the health effects of smoking for women may be even more serious than those for men. Smoking currently kills around half a million women in the world each year and this number is increasing rapidly (WHO 1999). Between 1950 and 2000, around 10 million women died from tobacco use. It is estimated that over the next 30 years, tobacco-attributable deaths among women will more than double (Jacobs 2001).

In countries which have the longest history of widespread female smoking, such as the USA and UK, smoking is now the single most important preventable cause of premature death in women, accounting for at least a third of all deaths between the ages 35 and 69 (Amos 1996). It is also a major cause of inequalities in health among women (Gaunt-Richardson *et al.* 1999; USSG 2001). In the USA, as in the UK and Japan, lung cancer has now overtaken breast cancer as the leading cause of cancer deaths in women. Death rates from lung cancer among white women in the United States increased by 600% between 1950 and 2000 (USSG 2001). In 1950 lung cancer accounted for only 3% of all female cancer deaths, whereas in 2000 it accounted for an estimated 25%. WHO has identified the epidemic in lung cancer among women as most worrying health trend in Europe (WHO 1999). The number of women developing lung cancer in Europe doubled during the last half of the twentieth century. In developed countries cardiovascular diseases are the major cause of death among women. As in men, women who smoke have a greater risk of developing these diseases. Nor are the serious effects confined to older women. The relative risk for coronary heart disease associated with smoking is higher among younger than older women (Ernster 2001).

In most developing countries the impact of smoking on women's health is currently much lower than in many developed countries because they are at an earlier stage of the epidemic. For example, in China, the risks for those who smoke have been found to be much the same for women and men, but because smoking has been low among women, only 2.7% of the deaths of women aged 35–69 are attributed to smoking compared with 13.0% of those of men (Liu *et al.* 1998). Also the impact on women's health can vary depending on the type of tobacco use in these countries. For example, in India where betel quid chewing is common among women, oral cancer is more common among women than breast cancer (Jacobs 2001).

In addition to the health risks that women share with men, women face particular problems linked to tobacco use (RCP 1992; Ernster 2001; Jacobs 2001; USSG 2001). These include:

- Cancer: Female-specific cancers, such as cancer of the cervix.
- Coronary heart disease: increased risk with use of oral contraceptives.
- Menstruation: Irregular cycles, higher incidence of painful cramps (dysmenorrhea).
- Menopause: Women who smoke tend to enter menopause at age 49—1–2 years before nonsmokers. This places them at a greater risk for heart disease and osteoporosis, including hip fractures (SG), as well as an increased incidence of hot flushes.
- Pregnancy: Smoking in pregnancy causes increased risks of spontaneous abortion (miscarriage), ectopic pregnancy, low birth weight, higher perinatal mortality, long-term effects on growth/development of the child. Many of these problems affect not only the health of the fetus, but also the health of the mother. For example, a miscarriage with bleeding is dangerous for the mother, especially in poor countries where health facilities are inadequate or nonexistent.
- Infertility: Smoking is also linked to infertility and delays in conceiving.

However, many women are unaware of these risks, even in countries such as the USA. For example, a US study found a serious lack of knowledge among women regarding gender-specific health risks of smoking (Roth and Taylor 2001). The study surveyed female hospital employees, who represented a wide span of age, socio-economic, and educational backgrounds, as to their awareness of reproductive health risks associated with smoking. While nearly all were aware of increased complications in pregnancy (91%), only a minority knew of the increased risk of miscarriage (39%), and even fewer knew of the increased risk of ectopic pregnancy (27%), cervical cancer (24%), and infertility (22%).

Environmental tobacco smoke

Environmental Tobacco Smoke (ETS), or passive smoking, has a negative impact on women's general and reproductive health, causing many illnesses, including lung cancer and heart disease (Samet and Yang 2001; USSG 2001). As the majority of smokers in the world are men, women are at particular risk from ETS at home. As the majority of people who work outside the home in the world are also male, women working in these workplace settings may also be exposed to passive smoking.

Women's own smoking may impact on the health of her family. As well as women's smoking during pregnancy having an impact on the health of the fetus, smoking by the father (or other close adult) can cause complications during pregnancy, such as low birth weight. Smoking, especially by the mother or father, around a baby or child also increases the risk of childhood chest infections and worsening of asthma, and can have long-term effects on growth/development (RCP 1992). Children of smokers are also more likely to become smokers themselves.

Economic impact of tobacco use on women

Tobacco use results in a net loss of US $200 billion per year to the global economy, with half of these losses occurring in low-income countries. There are immeasurable personal, social, and economic costs to women, particularly those living in poverty, in low-income countries and in rural settings. Women tend to have fewer resources than men and are more likely to be poor lone parents. More than 70% of the estimated 1.3 billion people living in poverty are women (Hunter 2001). There are also considerable impacts of the cost of smoking on other aspects of the family budget such as expenditure on diet.

Smoking and socio-economic status

Recent international comparisons of the variation in cigarette smoking by educational level (a proxy indicator of socio-economic status) show that in mature smoking economies (i.e. stage 4 countries) higher smoking prevalence is associated with lower educational attainment (Cavelaars *et al.* 2000). In these countries, over the past few decades, higher uptake rates and lower quit rates among lower socio-economic groups have resulted in smoking becoming overwhelmingly associated with social and material disadvantage, with rates highest in areas of low income and multiple deprivation. In the UK, for example, over 60% of female smokers experience one or more of four forms of disadvantage (low-skilled worker or tenant or social security claimant or lone mother), whereas over 60% of female nonsmokers experience none of these disadvantages (Graham 1998). Similarly in the US, smoking prevalence is nearly three times higher among women with 9–11 years of education (30.9%) than among women with 16 or more years of education (10.6%) (USSG 2001). In the US, Canada, New Zealand, and Australia, the highest female smoking rates are found among native and aboriginal populations, which characteristically experience high levels of disadvantage and depri-vation (Greaves 1996; Carrao *et al.* 2000). In these countries, therefore, smoking is both a direct and indirect cause of inequality in women's health and their wider social and economic well being. Directly, it impacts on women's health and consequently their economic productivity and prosperity. Indirectly, expenditure on tobacco means less resources are available for other essential household requirements.

Purchasing cigarettes

The economic impact of purchasing cigarettes can have a considerable effect on per-sonal and family income. This may be more serious for women, given their initial lower earning power. In particular, it will hit poor women the hardest irrespective of whether cigarettes are purchased by men and/or women in a family. Women who smoke a pack of 20 cigarettes daily in Hong Kong spend approximately US$ 1500 per annum on the habit. In China, research carried out in the outskirts of Shanghai showed that farmers spend more on cigarettes and wine than on grains, pork, and fruits. Another study on 2716 households in Minhang district showed that smokers spent an average of 60% of their personal income and 17% of household income on cigarettes (Gong *et al.* 1995). In Bangladesh smoking is twice as high among the poor as the wealthy (Efroymson *et al.* 2001). Average male smokers spend more than twice as much on cigarettes as per capita expenditure on clothing, housing, health, and education combined. An esti-mated 10.5 million Bangladeshis who are currently malnourished could have an ade-quate diet if money spent on tobacco was spent on food instead. In Vietnam, a survey showed that the average smoker spends as much on cigarettes in one month as spent on health care in one year, or which could have bought 169 kg of rice, more than enough to feed one person for one year (Thuy 1998). The impact on diet is not only restricted to developing countries. In the UK, for example, family diet has been shown to be adversely affected among smokers on low income (Jarvis 1997) (Box 19.1).

Health costs

By 2025 the transmission of the tobacco epidemic from rich to poor countries will be well advanced, with 85% of the world's smokers living in developing countries (Lopez A., personal communication 1997). Health care facilities will be hopelessly inadequate to cope with this epidemic, especially among women. Also, as smokers (in addition to earlier death) have significantly higher rates of illness, they incur higher health care costs and also loss of income. This will impact particularly on women as they usually have to care for family smokers when they are ill. Structural adjustment and the global financial crisis have severely increased health costs for women and children.

Tobacco taxation

Despite the addictive components of tobacco, there is strong evidence that smokers' demand for tobacco is strongly affected by price. Higher taxes reduce cigarette

BOX 19.1: A PACK OF MARLBORO IS EQUAL TO ...

% of Daily Income:

66.3%—China

62.5%—Moldova

62%—Pakistan

60%—Papua New Guinea (BAT's Benson and Hedges)

56%—Ghana

56%—Bangladesh (15% of average income of the wealthiest 5% of the population)

30%—Romania

28%—Bulgaria

14%—France

6%—US (using Marlboro price in Oregon)

Source: Global Partnerships (2001)

consumption (Townsend *et al.* 1994; USDHHS 1998) and postpone initiation of smoking (Lewit *et al.* 1997). For example, tax increases in Canada between 1982 and 1993 led to a steep increase in the real price of cigarettes and consumption fell considerably. When tax was reduced in an attempt to counter smuggling, consumption rose sharply again until a subsequent tax increase in 1995, when consumption levelled off (World Bank 1999). Increases in the price of tobacco appears to have a disproportionately greater impact on low- and middle-income countries than in high-income countries, and among lower socio-economic groups in high-income countries (Townsend *et al.* 1994).

There has been very little economic research on gender sensitivity to price in developing countries. Research from developed countries is somewhat conflicting (Jacobs 2001). In the US, for example, it has been found that men, particularly young men, are most sensitive to price (Lewit *et al.* 1981; Lewit and Coate 1982). While most British research has concluded that women are more price sensitive than men. Price was found to have a significant effect on the prevalence of smoking in women in the lowest socio-economic groups where prevalence is highest. However, the number of cigarettes smoked by women on low income seemed not to vary with price changes in the expected way. It has been suggested that while they may respond more than other groups to price increases by quitting, those who continue to smoke, will smoke cheaper, smaller, hand-rolled, or smuggled cigarettes rather than reduce the number of cigarettes smoked (Jacobs 2001; Wiltshire *et al.* 2001).

Thus, despite their overall positive effects, policies to increase tobacco taxation can be seen as regressive, penalising female smokers within the very poorest group of society which is least able to find a way out of addiction. Therefore, nonprice measures in conjunction with price measures may be more effective in helping women to quit (Jacobs 2001). In addition, interventions and public policies relevant to smoking should take account of the needs of the poorest female smokers. For example, a proportion of tobacco tax revenues could be hypothecated to address both the dimensions of disadvantage that bind women to smoking as well as providing specifically targeted smoking interventions (Marsh 1997; Graham 1998; Gaunt-Richardson *et al.* 1999; INWAT Europe 2000).

Smoking cessation

Our understanding of smoking cessation among women is mainly drawn from research carried out in countries with the longest history of smoking, in particular the US and UK. In these countries the decline in cigarette smoking has been faster in men than women. This may in part be due to some men changing from smoking cigarettes to cigar and/or pipes. However, several studies have suggested that women may indeed find it more difficult to quit smoking than men, and that as well as similarities, there may be important differences between men and women as to the reasons why they smoke which have implications for policy and practice.

The reasons why women seem to find it more difficult to quit than men are not well understood (Hunter 2001). It is likely to be due to a combination of biological, psychological, and social factors. There is increasing evidence that while most smokers are addicted to nicotine, factors other than nicotine may be more important in reinforcing smoking among women than men. For example, cessation studies with nicotine replacement therapy (NRT) have consistently reported lower quit rates in women compared to men (Perkins *et al.* 1999). Similarly, studies of self-quitters have found that women were less likely to quit initially or to remain abstinent at follow up. British data show that, despite a similar desire to quit, women feel more dependent on their smoking than men (Bridgwood *et al.* 2000). Women are more likely to say that they would find it very hard to go without smoking for a whole day than men who smoke the same amount.

Social and environmental factors are believed to be a more important influence on the smoking behaviour of women than men. For example, British and Canadian qualitative sociological research has shown how the social circumstances of disadvantage play an important part in reinforcing smoking among women (Graham 1993; Greaves 1996). This research illustrates how smoking is one mechanism which women use to cope with living and caring in disadvantaged circumstances. That is, smoking may constitute an important source of pleasure and satisfaction for women in caring roles by helping them to deal with frustration, stress, boredom, and material insecurity.

This research has made important inroads into our understanding of the difficulties of quitting for low-income mothers and to the development of new approaches to tackle this issue (Gaunt-Richardson *et al.* 1999).

Thus, while in many developed countries men and women smokers show similar levels of motivation to quit, many women appear to face additional barriers to quitting, particularly those living in disadvantaged circumstances such as low-income mothers. It is becoming more widely accepted therefore that tailored approaches to cessation are needed which address the particular personal, social, and cultural factors that make it difficult for women to quit successfully (Gaunt-Richardson *et al.* 1999; INWAT Europe 2000; Amos 2001; Samet and Yoon 2001). These programmes and services need to be accessible to women throughout the life course and should be integrated into quality and affordable health services. However, the true potential of such programmes will only be fully realized when the wider social and economic factors that bind women to smoking, their life circumstances, are also addressed by action at national and international levels.

The tobacco industry

A recent review of the marketing of tobacco to women concluded that 'selling tobacco products to women currently represents the single largest product marketing opportunity in the world' (Kaufman and Nichter 2001). And it is clear from tobacco companies own internal documents and proclamations that they are seizing this opportunity with gusto by manipulating various aspects of the marketing mix (product, price, packaging, and promotion) to make their products more appealing and accessible to girls and women around the world. While tobacco companies have only started marketing tobacco relatively recently to women in developing countries, they can draw on over 80 years experience of successful marketing to women in countries like the US and UK (Amos 1996; Joossens and Sasco 1999; Amos and Haglund 2000; Kaufman and Nichter 2001; USSG 2001).

Developed countries

The development of cheap mass produced cigarettes at the end of the nineteenth century greatly affected tobacco consumption. However, although cigarette smoking became increasingly popular among men, smoking was seen by many as a dirty habit that corrupted both men and women. The tobacco companies responded by employing the new modern marketing methods to help spread their message (Amos and Haglund 2000). Although women often featured in promotional materials their role was to entice male rather than female customers. There is little evidence that tobacco companies directly targeted women to any significant extent at this time or attempted to challenge the dominant social stigma attached to female smoking.

World War 1 was a watershed in both the emancipation of women and the spread of smoking among women. During the war many women not only took on 'male' occupations but also started to wear trousers, play sports, cut their hair short, and smoke. Subsequently, attitudes towards women smoking began to change, and more women started to use the cigarette as a weapon in challenging traditional ideas about female behaviour. The cigarette became a symbol of new roles and expectations of women's behaviour. But it's questionable whether smoking would have become as popular among women as it did if tobacco companies had not seized on this opportunity in the 1920s and 1930s to exploit ideas of liberation, power, and other important values for women to recruit them to the cigarette market. Smoking was repositioned as being respectable, sociable, fashionable, stylish, feminine, and an aid to slimming.

The Lucky Strike campaign 'Reach for Lucky instead of a Sweet' of 1925 was one of the first media campaigns targeted at women. The message was highly effective and made Lucky Strike the best selling brand. Another important element in the marketing campaign was to challenge the social taboo against women smoking in public. In 1929 there was the much publicized event in the Easter Sunday Parade in New York where Great American Tobacco hired several young women to smoke their 'torches of freedom' (Lucky Strikes) as they marched down Fifth Avenue protesting against women's inequality. This event generated widespread newspaper coverage and provoked a national debate. Tobacco companies also needed to ensure that women felt confident about smoking in public. While to some extent they tackled this by using images of women smoking in cigarette advertisements, they also ensured that Hollywood stars were well supplied with cigarettes and often paid them to give endorsements in advertisements. Philip Morris even went so far as to organize a lecture tour in the US giving women lessons in cigarette smoking. Within 20 years of starting to target women, over half the young women (16–35 years) in Britain, for example, had become smokers.

Since starting to target women in North America and northern Europe in the 1920s and 1930s, the tobacco industry has become more sophisticated in its marketing strategies, developing a diverse range of messages, products, and brands to appeal to different segments of the female market. Such marketing messages, and the way that they have been reflected in and reinforced by the mass media such as films and magazine, has led to the cultural meaning of women's smoking changing from being a symbol of being *bought* by men (prostitute), to being *like* men (lesbian/mannish), to being able to *attract* men (glamorous/heterosexual) (Greaves 1996). To this could also be added its symbolic value of freedom, i.e. being *equal* to men (feminism) and to being your *own woman* (emancipation).

New markets

In the latter decades of the twentieth century up to today, tobacco companies have been seizing the opportunities presented by often very rapid cultural, economic, social, and political change to promote the 'liberating' symbolic value of smoking to women (Amos and Haglund 2000). For example, in Spain after the fall of the Franco regime, ads for Kim in the 1980s promoted the slogan 'Asi, como soy' (It's so me). More recently,

West ads in Spain have shown women in traditionally male occupations such as fighter pilots. Some of the most blatant targeting of young women has occurred in the former socialist countries of central and eastern Europe, which are now exposed to the commercial forces of 'free' markets. Here cigarettes are promoted as a potent symbol of Western freedom, as in Czech Republic 'West—the taste of now'. Young women are encouraged to join men in their western male leisure pursuits. In Germany in the 1990s, young women have become a prime target for cigarette ads, and many of which have promoted smoking as synonymous with western images of modern emancipated womanhood (Poetschke-Langer and Schunk 2001). Cigarette advertisements were among the first to appear on Berlin wall with slogans such as 'Test the West'. More recently, West has been advertised in women's magazines as being the 'taste' and 'power' of now. It is therefore not surprising that between 1993 and 1997, rates of smoking among young women in former East Germany nearly doubled from 27% to 47%. In addition, the desire to quit among 12–25-year-old smokers declined from two-thirds to less than half over this period (Corrao *et al.* 2000).

The marketing of cigarettes as both a passport to and symbol of emancipation, independence and success is not restricted to countries in the West. A 1990 editorial in Tobacco Reporter noted the growth opportunities represented by women as 'Women are becoming more independent and, consequently, adopting less-traditional lifestyles. One symbol of their newly discovered freedom may well be cigarettes' (Zimmerman 1990). Thus we have seen in Japan Virginia Slims advertisements urging women to 'Be you'. Capri advertisements have encouraged them to have their own opinions and have featured 'real-life' European female role models such as a dress designer stating that 'The dress I design represents my own way of life'. Virginia Slims has shown a pair of Caucasian male and female rugby players with the by-line 'the locker rooms are separate but the playground and the goal are common'. A recent survey found that smoking among Japanese women in their twenties more than doubled between 1986 and 1999, from 10% to 23%.

Developing countries

UPBEAT. Amid the gloomy environment, Tobacco Reporter continued to look for the positive in Asia. And guess what! There are reasons for optimism; 'The situation does not fundamentally change the underlying strengths of the *market*,' an Indonesian source assures us. Rising per-capita consumption, a growing population and an increasing acceptance of women smoking continue to generate new demand.

Tobacco Reporter editorial about the Asian market (Tuinstra 1998).

Until the 1980s, there was relatively little tobacco promotion in developing countries. The national monopolies did not, in general, promote their products, or did so only minimally. But from the 1980s, when young women in some countries were starting to become more independent and were copying western fashion and trends, the trans-national tobacco industry introduced tobacco advertisements into developing countries.

Many of these initial advertisements were very 'masculine' like the Marlboro cowboy, but gradually a whole range of advertisements were produced, moving from 'men-only' advertisements; through 'neutral' advertisements showing, for example, a pleasant mountain scene or a blue lagoon; advertisements where both men and women appeared, for example, enjoying the outdoors in a group; to women-only advertisements.

By the mid-1980s, examples of these latter advertisements specifically targeting women were beginning to emerge, in particular advertisements for Virginia Slims. Smoking was promoted as being glamorous, sophisticated, fun, romantic, sexually attractive, healthy, sporty, sociable, relaxing, calming, emancipated, feminine, rebellious, and an aid to slimming. Designer cigarettes then appeared: in 1989, the Yves St. Laurent brand of cigarettes was launched in Malaysia and other countries throughout Asia, with elegant packing appealing to women. Some of the monopolies and national companies, such as in Indonesia, then began to copy promotion targeting women. The tobacco industry used seductive but false images of health, emancipation, slimness, modernity, glamour, sophistication, fun, romance, sexual attractiveness, health, sport, sociability, femininity, and rebelliousness. Concurrently, feminized cigarettes appeared—long, extra-slim, low-tar, light-coloured, menthol.

In South Africa, for example, Benson and Hedges started to produce advertisements which feature young black women. One advertisement showed a young dark-skinned woman in aerobics gear smoking a cigarette with a young black male. In another a black woman wearing traditional headgear was shown seated with a black man accepting a cigarette from a white man. The copy line was 'Share the feeling, share the taste'. In the Middle East a recent Gauloise advertisement featured a young woman in western dress with the copyline 'Always Freedom' (Simpson 2001).

Not only do these advertising images and messages echo those seen in the 1930s advertisements in the US and UK, but so do other elements of the social marketing strategies. This was seen recently in Sri Lanka where, in a modern version of the 1929 New York Easter Parade march, the Ceylon Tobacco Company hired young women to drive around in 'Players Gold Leaf' cars handing out free cigarettes and promotional items (Seiman and Mehl 1998). These women also handed out free merchandise at popular shopping malls and university campuses. In a country where only one per cent of women smoke, this seemed to be part of a wider strategy to challenge the social taboo that respectable women in Sri Lanka should not smoke and certainly not in the street.

Other forms of marketing

Other forms of marketing are also being targeted at women. For example, tobacco companies have now produced a range of brands aimed at women. Most notable are the 'women-only' brands such as Kim, Virginia Slims, Capri, Vogue, MS, and More. These are feminized cigarettes—long, extra-slim, low-tar, light-coloured, menthol.

In India in 1990 the Golden Tobacco Company attempted to target women with a new brand, 'MS Special Filter' (Gupta and Ball 1990). Advertisements featured Indian women in Western clothing and affluent settings, symbols of liberation for Indian women who are gaining financial and professional independence. More recently, a new cigarette brand Just Black, was launched in Goa, India with the advertising featuring a young, fair-skinned woman leaning against a large black motor cycle while holding a tennis racket (Kaufman and Nichter 2001). Tobacco industry documents have revealed that this brand and campaign was developed to appeal to a new generation of image conscious young people and to shock their parents. In China the first ever brands to be developed by the Chinese tobacco industry are aimed at women (Hui 1998). Some companies have also produced special gift packs and offers designed to appeal to women. In Taiwan, tobacco companies launched gift packs for the Lunar New Year, with the Yves St. Laurent luxurious gift pack containing two cartons of cigarettes plus one crystal item. The 555 gift packs had either a tea set or an ashtray and the Virginia Slim Lights gift packs stylish lighters suitable for women smokers. In Australia there have been Alpine fashion key rings, bags, and silk underwear.

Tobacco companies also sponsor popular sport and leisure events in an attempt to reach young women. Although it is mainly men's sports that are sponsored in developing countries, these are watched by many women. For example, 46% of spectators at the Hong Kong Salem Tennis in 1993 were women. Michael Chang, who plays regularly in Marlboro and Salem tennis events in China, Japan, the Republic of Korea, and Hong Kong, enjoys idol status with many teenage girls throughout Asia. There are sponsored women's events. In 1989, British-American Tobacco Co decided to add the Viceroy Women Football Competition on to the final match of Viceroy Cup in Hong Kong. In 1995, Benson and Hedges ran whole page advertisements in newspapers in Malaysia featuring a female climber Lum Yuet Mei, suspended from a rock face, provocatively saying 'Tonight cling on to me as I attempt to conquer the amazing Dolomite cliffs' in an advertisement entitled 'She took the challenge and realized her golden dream.' Malaysia is the prime example in the world of brand-stretching— for example, travel holidays and bistros. R.J. Reynolds has designed 'Salem Attitude' clothing stores for the Asian market specifically to circumvent restrictions on tobacco promotion (Kaufman and Nichter 2001).

Arts sponsorship provides the tobacco industry with culture, glamour, and respectability, sponsoring events that appeal to women as well as men. Events in Asia include Peter Ustinov (Hong Kong 1992); Tony Bennett Jazz concerts (Thailand 1993); Central Ballet of China (1994); Andrew Lloyd Webber's 'The Phantom of the Opera' sponsored by Philip Morris (Hong Kong 1995); ASEAN Arts Awards (Asia 1994). In New Zealand there are the Benson and Hedges Fashion Design Awards.

Events and activities popular with the young also receive sponsorship. Admission to films and pop or rock concerts has been either free, or through the exchange of empty cigarette packets for free tickets (Taiwan 1988; Hong Kong 1994). American singers, such as Jewel and Madonna, who would not promote tobacco in the US, have allowed their names to be associated with cigarettes in other countries. Film stars such as Sylvester Stallone have accepted money from the tobacco industry for product placement in their films.

Action

Tobacco control strategies targeted at decreasing smoking uptake and increasing cessation are much more cost-effective than treating patients with lung cancer and other tobacco-related illnesses. There is therefore an urgent need to develop effective gender-sensitive and gender-specific tobacco control strategies, and to allocate sufficient funds for tobacco control programmes that reach women and girls (INWAT Europe 2000). Public policy, legislation, research, and education therefore need to be geared specifically towards preventing girls from initiating smoking and helping women quit (Jacobs 2001). Over the past 10 years there has been a growing recognition, at both the international and national levels, of the growing impact of smoking on women's health around the world. However, action on this issue has tended to be restricted to those countries with the longest history of female cigarette smoking.

International level

WHO

The previous Director General of WHO, Dr Gro Harlem Brundtland, recognized the importance of tobacco as a women's issue. WHO has brought more women into the organization, and given high priority to strengthening global action on women and tobacco issues, for example:

◆ WHO has secured funding for a major initiative on women and tobacco currently underway in the Southern African Development Commission (14 Southern African countries).

◆ An international meeting on Women and Tobacco took place in Kobe, Japan in November 1999. This drew in, for the first time, women's organizations beyond the traditional tobacco control groups, culminating in The Kobe Declaration on Women and Tobacco.

◆ In the Western Pacific Region, all three 5-year Action Plans on Tobacco or Health since 1990 have emphasized the importance of preventing a rise in smoking among women as a high priority.

WHO is also working with many UN organizations, such as UNICEF, IMF, World Bank, and others to form partnerships to reduce the epidemic.

The World Bank

The World Bank's report 'Curbing the Epidemic' marked the first time a major financial institution had supported policies designed to reduce tobacco demand

(World Bank 1999). The document argues that tobacco control is good for the wealth as well as the health of nations; that it does not lead to loss of taxes or jobs; and that tobacco control measures (e.g. price increases, advertising bans, smoke-free areas, health education, pharmaceutical assistance in quitting) are cost-effective in both industrialized and developing countries. Men and women are not specifically indexed, but the findings have relevance to both.

International NGOs

The International Network of Women Against Tobacco (INWAT) was founded in 1990 to address the issues around tobacco and women. It has members in about 60 countries. Other NGOs involved with tobacco maintain a gender awareness, like the International Union Against Cancer (UICC), the International Union Against Tuberculosis and Lung Disease (IUATLD), the World Heart Federation, the Framework Convention Alliance and The International Non-Government Coalition Against Tobacco (INGCAT). They encourage their member organizations to take a public stand on tobacco, and some fund projects, research, and meetings. GLOBALink, the internet network based at the UICC Headquarters in Geneva, links tobacco control advocates all over the world, and has a specific website devoted to tobacco and women.

International conferences

The tenth World Conference on Tobacco or Health in Beijing in 1997, pioneered gender equity in World Conferences. Fifty per cent of all committee members, chairs, and invited speakers were women. When funding was offered to developing countries for two delegates, it was suggested that one be a female. Each speaker was asked to incorporate the twin themes of 'developing countries' and 'women' into his or her presentation on whatever topic. In 1998 the European Union, through Europe Against Cancer, organized the first European conference on women and tobacco in Paris.

Regional level

APACT

The Asia Pacific Association for the Control of Tobacco (APACT), first established by Dr David Yen in Taipei, organizes biennial regional meetings. Delegates from the poorer countries find the smaller regional meetings more supportive than the large, international conferences, and it facilitates delegates, especially women, speaking out.

INWAT Europe

The INWAT Europe Development Project was a pilot project funded by the European Union (Europe Against Cancer) from 1997 to 2002. It aims to contribute to reducing tobacco use among women in Europe by developing a strong, effective, and sustainable network which raises awareness about this issue, promoting communication and exchange of information and support, and developing consensus on a women centred tobacco control strategy for Europe. A key element of the project was an expert seminar held in 1999 which brought together leading experts in the field of gender and health, and tobacco control (INWAT Europe 2000). The report on the seminar identified three main areas for future action:

- Research and policy frameworks for establishing coherent tobacco control policies for women, taking into account the important intersections between gender, socio-economic status, and age.

- The importance of linking women's tobacco control with other organizations and pressure groups concerned with the general status of women in society.

- Proposals whereby INWAT could become a resource for promoting women-specific tobacco control to a higher priority status in Europe, drawing on its extensive network and the high quality expertise of its members.

National level

At national level, governments have a central and crucial role in tobacco control, especially in the area of legislation and tobacco tax increases. Without government leadership and commitment, tobacco control measures—especially in developing countries—are unlikely to succeed. Because the full impact of tobacco-related deaths is not yet apparent in developing countries, many governments are still not convinced of the degree of the harmfulness of smoking. They are preoccupied with other problems, such as high infant mortality, communicable diseases, economic difficulties, or political conflict, they lack funds, and have little experience in dealing with the tactics of the transnational tobacco companies. In addition, they may be reluctant to act because of the mistakenly perceived economic 'benefits' of tobacco.

The lead government ministry is the Ministry of Health, but with the issue of tobacco and women, women's commissions or ministries should be active. There is no government department that does not have some role. Many developing countries have implemented tobacco control programmes, including legislation, far ahead of many western countries, and without any severe economic consequences. For example, legislation in Singapore, Fiji, Mongolia, Hong Kong, South Africa, Thailand, and Vietnam is far ahead of many western countries. Many tobacco control measures cost little other than political will—for example, legislation requiring health warnings on cigarette packets; or the creation of smoke-free areas in government buildings, public areas, transport, or schools. However, many tobacco control programmes in both developed and developing countries continue to take a gender neutral or gender blind approach.

NGOs, including women's groups, can:

- lobby, advise, or pressure governments to make sure that all legislation and other tobacco control action is gender sensitive

- make sure that ministries or commissions on women address tobacco as a woman's issue and uphold the principle of women's right to health as a basic human right, building on the progress made at the Fourth World Conference on Women and the Convention to Eliminate All Forms of Discrimination Against Women (CEDAW)

- demand a total ban on direct and indirect advertising, promotion, and sponsorship by the tobacco industry, especially that targeting women
- ask for increased public funding for research and advocacy on women and girls and tobacco
- promote women's leadership in tackling tobacco
- lobby women's magazines to better inform women about the issue
- recruit the entertainment industry, especially female movie and popstars
- counter the claims of the tobacco industry that tobacco is a freedom for women
- assist with cessation
- join the International Network of Women Against Tobacco (INWAT).

Individual women can act in an exemplar role by not smoking themselves, by discouraging their own children from starting smoking, and by encouraging their partners, parents, children, and co-workers to quit.

Research gaps

Developing more effective tobacco control programmes for women, particularly in developing countries, is hampered by the lack of research on women and smoking. Recent national and international reviews on women and smoking have identified a range of research questions, including biomedical, social, economic, policy, intervention, and evaluation, which need addressing. For example, the INWAT Europe seminar outlined key research questions in relation to:

- understanding the determination of tobacco use among women across the life-course and in different countries
- a biomedical research agenda which looked at the impact of smoking in relation to sex-specific biological factors (developmental and reproductive) across the life-course, including nicotine addiction
- extending and deepening current understanding of the effectiveness and cost-effectiveness of tobacco control policies, particularly by providing a gender-sensitive perspective that takes into account socio-economic status.

Similarly, the Kobe report on women and tobacco identified the need for 'prospectively designed research studies to further elucidate the complexity of the relationships between failure to quit, nicotine withdrawal symptoms, level of addiction to nicotine, cigarette smoking relapse, depression, alcohol use, eating, and fear of weight gain in girls and women' (Hunter 2001). Among the other research issues highlighted was the importance of researching the differential impact of tobacco control polices and the health consequences of such policies on girls, women, and women from ethnic minorities, particularly in developing countries, given that the burden of the tobacco epidemic is shifting to these population groups (Jacobs 2001). More recently, the major research funding councils in Canada in 2001 supported a national expert seminar to identify research gaps and develop a multidisciplinary research agenda on teenage girls and smoking (Greaves and Cormier 2002).

Conclusion

At the beginning of the twentieth century few people could have imagined how such a stigmatized behaviour as female smoking would be transformed, through judicious marketing by the tobacco companies, into a socially acceptable and desirable behaviour in developed countries. The challenge facing us at beginning of the twenty-first century is how to stem the second wave of the tobacco epidemic, particularly in developing countries and among disadvantaged women in developed countries. There needs to be wider recognition that women's tobacco use is a global health problem and that effective women-centred tobacco control programmes should be implemented at international as well as national levels. Clearly there is a need to ban all tobacco promotion. But building support for women-centred tobacco control programmes through partnerships will also be vital to achieve success. In particular, there is a need to work with and involve both women's organizations and women themselves, and to broaden the agenda to encompass other social and economic factors that work against girls and women breaking free from this fatal addiction (INWAT Europe 2003).

References

Aghi, M., Gupta, P. C., and Mehta, F. S. (1988). Impact of intervention on the reverse smoking habit of rural Indian women. In: *Smoking and health*, (ed. M. Aoki, *et al.*). Proceedings of the 6th World Conference on Smoking and Health, *Excerpta Medica*, Amsterdam, p. 255.

Amos, A. (2001). Women, smoking and cessation—meeting the challenge. *Promoting Health*, 12, 24–5.

Amos, A. (1996). Women and smoking. *British Medical Bulletin*, 52, 74–89.

Amos, A. and Haglund, M. (2000). From social taboo to 'torch of freedom'—the marketing of cigarettes to women. *Tobacco Control*, 9, 3–8.

Bridgwood, A., Lilly, R., Thomas, M., Bacon, J., Sykes, W., and Morris, S. (2000). *Living in Britain 1998*. Stationery Office, London.

Cavelaars, A., Kunst, A., Geurts, J., Crialesi, R., Grotvedt, L., and Helmert, U., *et al.* (2000). Educational differences in smoking: international comparison. *BMJ*, 320, 1102–7.

Chinese Academy of Preventive Medicine (1999). *Smoking and health in China: 1996 National prevalence survey of smoking patterns*. China Science and Technology Press, Beijing.

Corrao, M. A., Guidon, G. E., Sharma, N., and Shokoohi, D. F. (2000). *Tobacco control country profiles*. American Cancer Society, Atlanta.

Efroymson, D., *et al.* (2001). Hungry for tobacco: an analysis of the economic impact of tobacco consumption on the poor in Bangladesh. *Tobacco Control*, 10, 212–17.

Elegbeleye, O. O. and Femi-Pearse, D. (1976). Incidence and variables contributing to the onset of cigarette smoking among secondary school children and medical students in Lagos, Nigeria. *Br. J. Prev. Soc. Med.* 30, 66–70.

Ernster, V. (2001). Impact of tobacco use on women's health. In: *Women and the tobacco epidemic—Challenges for the 21st century* (ed. J. M. Samet and S.-Y. Yoon), pp.1–16. WHO, Geneva.

Gaunt-Richardson, P., Amos, A., Howie, G., McKie, L., and Moore, M. (1999). *Women, low income and smoking—breaking down the barriers*. Edinburgh, ASH Scotland/ Health Education Board for Scotland.

Global Partnerships (2001). Global partnerships for Tobacco Control, Essential Action Survey, www.essential.org/tobacco.

Gong, L. Y., Koplan, J. P., Feng, W., Chen, C. H., Zheng, P., and Harris, J. R. (1995). Cigarette smoking in China. *JAMA*, **274**, 1232–4.

Graham, H. (1996). Smoking prevalence among women in the European Community 1950–1990. *Social Science and Medicine*, **43**, 243–54.

Graham, H. (1993). *When life's a drag*. HMSO, London.

Graham, H. (1998). Promoting health against inequality: using research to identify targets for intervention—A case study of women and smoking. *Health Education Journal*, **57**, 292–302.

Greaves, L. (1996) *Smokescreen—Women's smoking and social control*. Fernwood Publishing, Halifax.

Greaves, L. and Cormier, R. (2002). Teenage Girls and Smoking: A Research Agenda. British Coloumbia Centre of Excellence for Women's Health, Vancouver.

Gupta, P. C. and Ball, K. (1990). India: a tobacco tragedy. *Lancet*, **335**, 594–5.

Hunter, S. M. (2001). Quitting. In: *Women and the tobacco epidemic—challenges for the 21st century* (ed. J.M. Samet and S.-Y. Yoon), pp. 121–46. WHO, Geneva.

Hong Kong Census and Statistics Department. (1998). *General Household Survey 1993*. Census and Statistics Department, Hong Kong Special Administrative Region.

Hui, L. (1998). *Chinese smokers take to slim cigarettes*. World Tobacco, July 11.

INWAT Europe (2000). *Part of the solution? Tobacco control policies and women*. Health Development Agency/Cancer Research Campaign, London. www.inwat.org.

INWAT Europe (2003). Searching for the solution: Women, smoking and inequalities in Europe. Health Development Agency, London.

Jarvis, J. M. (1997). Health behaviour interventions in the context of lifestyles and influences: Cigarette smoking and inequalities. MRC/ESRC meeting on health behavioural interventions, London, April 30–May 1.

Jacobs, R. (2001). Economic policies, taxation and fiscal measures. In: *Women and the tobacco epidemic—challenges for the 21st century* (ed. J.M. Samet and S.-Y. Yoon), pp. 177–200. WHO, Geneva.

Joossens, L. and Sasco, A. J. (1999) *Some like it 'light'—women and smoking in the European Union*. European Union Europe Against Cancer/ENSP, Brussels.

Kaufman, N. and Nichter, M. (2001). The marketing of tobacco to women: global perspectives. In: *Women and the tobacco epidemic—challenges for the 21st century* (ed. J.M. Samet and S.-Y. Yoon), pp. 69–98. WHO, Geneva.

Lewit, E. M., Hyland, A., Kerrebrock, N., and Cummings, K. M. (1997). Price, public policy, and smoking in young people. *Tobacco Control*, **6**(Suppl 2), S17–24.

Lewit, E. M., Coate, J. L., and Grossman, M. (1981). The effects of government regulation on teenage smoking. *J. Law Econ.*, **24**, 545–69.

Lewit, E. M., and Coate, J. L. (1982). The potential for using excise taxes to reduce smoking. *J. Health Econ.*, **1**, 121–45.

Liu, B.-Q., Peto, R., Chen, Z.-M., Boreham, J., Wu, Y.-P., Li, J.-Y., *et al.* (1998). Emerging tobacco hazards in China: 1. Retrospective proportional mortality study of one million deaths. *British Medical Journal*, **317**, 1411–22.

Lopez, A. D., Collishaw, N. E., and Piha, T. (1994). A descriptive model of the cigarette epidemic in developed countries. *Tobacco Control*, **3**, 242–7.

Marsh, A. (1997). Tax and spend: A policy to help poor smokers. *Tobacco Control*, **6**, 5–6.

Mackay, J. and Eriksen, M. (2002). *The tobacco atlas*. WHO, Geneva.

Perkins, K. A., Donny, E., and Caggiula, A. R. (1999) Sex differences in nicotine effects and self-administration: review of human and animal evidence. *Nicotine and Tobacco Research*, **1**, 301–15.

Poetschke-Langer, M. and Schunk, S. (2001). Germany: tobacco industry paradise. *Tobacco Control*, **10**, 300–3.

Samet, J. M. and Yang G. (2001). Passive smoking, women and children. In: *Women and the tobacco epidemic—challenges for the 21st century* (ed. J.M. Samet and S.-Y. Yoon), pp. 17–48. WHO, Geneva.

Samet, J. M. and Yoon, S.-Y. (2001). *Women and the tobacco epidemic- challenges for the 21st century*. WHO, Geneva,

Seimon, T. and Mehl, G. L. (1998). Strategic marketing to young people in Sri Lanka: 'Go ahead—I want to see you smoke it now'. *Tobacco Control*, **7**, 429–33.

Roth, L. K. and Taylor, H. S. (2001). Risks of smoking to reproductive health: Assessment of women's knowledge. *American Journal of Obstetrics and Gynecology*, **184**, 934–9.

Royal College of Physicians (1992). Passive smoking and health of fetus. *Chapter 1 in Smoking and the Young*. RCP, London.

Simpson, D. (2001). Gauloises: to Oxford and the Middle East. *Tobacco Control*, **10**, 92–3.

Thuy, T. T. (1998). Activities for tobacco control in Vietnam. 4th Working Group on TOH, Manila, Philippines, Nov 1998.

Townsend, J., Roderick, P., and Cooper, J. (1994). Cigarette smoking by socio-economic group, sex and age: effects of price, income and health publicity. *British Medical Journal*, **309**, 923–7.

Tuinstra, T. (1998). *The end of the tunnel*. Tobacco Reporter, Summer, 4.

Tuomilehto, J., Zimmet, P., Taylor, R., Bennet, P., Wolf, E., and Kankaapaa, J. (1986). Smoking rates in Pacific islands. *Bulletin of the World Health Organization*, **64**, 447–56.

US Department of Health and Human Services (USDHHS) (1998). Responses to increases in cigarette prices by race/ethnicity, income and age groups—United States, 1976–1993. *MMWR*, **47**, 605–9.

USSG (2001). *Women and smoking: A report of the surgeon general*. Department of Health and Human Services. www.cdc.gov/tobacco/sgr_forwomen.htm

Wiltshire, S., Bancroft, A., Amos, A., and Parry, O. (2001). 'They're doing people a service'— qualitative study of smoking, smuggling and social deprivation. *British Medical Journal*, **323**, 203–7.

Wold, B., Holstein, B., Griesbach, D., and Currie, C. (2000). *Control of adolescent smoking*. University of Bergen Research Centre for Health Promotion, Bergen.

World Bank (1999). *Curbing the epidemic*. Governments and the economics of tobacco control. The World Bank, Washington DC.

WHO (1999). *Report of the WHO international conference on tobacco and health. Kobe—making a difference in tobacco and health*, WHO, Geneva.

WHO (1997). *Tobacco or health—A global status report*. WHO, Geneva. http://www.cdc.gov/tobacco/who/whofirst.htm

Zimmerman, C. (1990). Growth is the watchword for the Asian tobacco industry. *Tobacco Reporter*, **117**, 4.

Part 6

Tobacco and cancer

Chapter 20

Cancer of the prostate

Fabio Levi and Carlo La Vecchia

Prostate cancer is the fourth site for cancer incidence worldwide in men, and the third in developed countries after lung and colon-rectum (Parkin *et al.* 1999). Considerable changes in incidence rates from prostate carcinoma have been observed in the USA, the European Union, and in most other developed countries, suggesting that an epidemic of this neoplasm occurred in the late 1980s or early 1990s, followed by a fall in rates. A critical appraisal of the descriptive epidemiology of prostate cancer indicates, however, that most trends were likely attributable to changes in diagnostic procedures (mainly, the introduction of prostate-specific antigen–PSA–blood test), rather than substantial changes in risk-factor exposure (Levi *et al.* 2000).

The descriptive epidemiology of prostate cancer is in any case inconsistent with a major role of tobacco on prostate cancer risk, given its time trends and geographic pattern. Thus, while mortality rates from lung and other tobacco-related neoplasms have substantially changed in various countries following the spread of cigarette smoking in subsequent generations, only minor long-term changes have been observed in prostatic cancer mortality rates.

Nonetheless, a possible relation between prostate cancer and cigarette smoking has been considered in several studies (Schwartz *et al.* 1961; Hammond 1966; Kahn 1966; Weir and Dunn 1970; Wynder *et al.* 1971; Kolonel and Winkelstein 1977; Schuman *et al.* 1977; Williams and Horm 1977; Hirayama 1979; Niijima and Koiso 1980; Rogot and Murray 1980; Mishina *et al.* 1985; Whittemore *et al.* 1985; Carstensen *et al.* 1987; Checkoway *et al.* 1987; Ross *et al.* 1987, 1990; Honda *et al.* 1988; Yu *et al.* 1988; Mills *et al.* 1989; Newell *et al.* 1989; Oishi *et al.* 1989; Severson *et al.* 1989; Elghany *et al.* 1990; Fincham *et al.* 1990; Hsing *et al.* 1990, 1991; Slattery *et al.* 1990; Mills and Beeson 1992; Slattery and West 1993; Talamini *et al.* 1993; Doll *et al.* 1994; Hayes *et al.* 1994; Hiatt *et al.* 1994; Tavani *et al.* 1994; Van der Gulden *et al.* 1994; De Stefani *et al.* 1995; McLaughlin *et al.* 1995; Siemiatycki *et al.* 1995; Adami *et al.* 1996; Andersson *et al.* 1996; Coughlin *et al.* 1996; Ilic *et al.* 1996; Pawlega *et al.* 1996; Cerhan *et al.* 1997; Key *et al.* 1997; Lumey *et al.* 1997; Rodriguez *et al.* 1997; Rohan *et al.* 1997; Giovannucci *et al.* 1999; Parker *et al.* 1999; Sung *et al.* 1999; Villeneuve *et al.* 1999; Lotufo *et al.* 2000; Lund Nilsen *et al.* 2000; Putnam *et al.* 2000; Giles *et al.* 2001; Sharpe and Siemiatycki 2001). Among these, only two case–control (Schuman *et al.* 1977; Honda *et al.* 1988) and four prospective studies (Kahn 1966; Rogot and Murray 1980; Hsing *et al.* 1990, 1991; Hiatt *et al.* 1994; McLaughlin *et al.* 1995; Rodriguez *et al.* 1997) showed a positive relation between prostate cancer and tobacco smoking. This relationship, if real, may be mediated by hormonal factors, since male cigarette smokers have elevated levels of serum testosterone and androstenedione (Dai *et al.* 1988). However, one review on the health effects of cigarette smoking (IARC 1986) and two other on major risk factors for prostate cancer (Nomura and Kolonel 1991; Boyle *et al.* 1997) did not support the association between cigarette smoking and increased risk for prostate cancer.

The main results from case–control studies are given in Table 20.1. Among the 30 case–control studies that examined the role of cigarette smoking on prostate cancer (Schwartz *et al.* 1961; Wynder *et al.* 1971; Kolonel and Winkelstein 1977; Schuman *et al.* 1977; Williams and Horn 1977; Niijima and Koiso 1980; Mishina *et al.* 1985; Checkoway *et al.* 1987; Ross *et al.* 1987; Honda *et al.* 1988; Yu *et al.* 1988; Newell *et al.* 1989; Oishi *et al.* 1989; Elghany *et al.* 1990; Fincham *et al.* 1990; Slattery *et al.* 1990; Slattery and West 1993; Talamini *et al.* 1993; Hayes *et al.* 1994; Tavani *et al.* 1994; Van der Gulden *et al.* 1994; De Stefani *et al.* 1995; Siemiatycki *et al.* 1995; Andersson *et al.* 1996; Ilic *et al.* 1996; Pawlega *et al.* 1996; Key *et al.* 1997; Lumey *et al.* 1997; Rohan *et al.* 1997; Sung *et al.* 1999; Villeneuve *et al.* 1999; Giles *et al.* 2001), only two reported a positive association (Schuman *et al.* 1977; Honda *et al.* 1988). The study by Honda *et al.* (1988), based on 216 cases and 212 controls, showed a moderate positive relation between prostate cancer and cigarette smoking (smokers vs. nonsmokers: RR = 1.9, 95% confidence interval (CI), 1.2–3.0) and a significant direct trend only in the highest level of smoking duration. The study by Schuman *et al.* (1977) also showed some association with cigarette smoking when comparison was made with population controls only, but it was too small (40 cases) to be informative. Furthermore, a study of 345 cases and 1346 hospital controls from the Netherlands (Van der Gulden *et al.* 1994) found a direct association with ever smoking, but no dose, nor duration–risk relationship. Moreover, these results also contrast with other case–control studies (Williams and Horm 1977; Mishina *et al.* 1985; Ross *et al.* 1987; Slattery *et al.* 1990; Elghany *et al.* 1990; Fincham *et al.* 1990; Slattery and West 1993; Hayes *et al.* 1994; Siemiatycki *et al.* 1995; Key *et al.* 1997) which, using population controls, did not show any meaningful association between tobacco smoking and prostate cancer. However, a large Canadian population-based case–control study (Villeneuve *et al.* 1999) found a modest and inconsistent inverse association with various measures of cigarette smoking.

Thus, most case–control studies found no association between smoking and prostate cancer, with a few reporting direct or other inverse associations, which appear to be attributable to the play of chance, in the absence of any causal association.

Among 22 prospective studies (Hammond 1966; Kahn 1966; Weir and Dunn 1970; Hirayama 1979; Rogot and Murray 1980; Whittemore *et al.* 1985; Carstensen *et al.* 1987; Mills *et al.* 1989; Severson *et al.* 1989; Hsing *et al.* 1990, 1991; Ross *et al.* 1990;

Table 20.1 Summary of results of case–control studies on prostate cancer in relation to cigarette smoking

Investigator(s)	Location	No. of subjects	Major findings
Schwartz et al. 1961	Paris, France	139 cases 139 hospital controls	No association. 79% and 73% of smokers among cases and controls, respectively
Wynder et al. 1971	New York, U.S.	300 cases 400 hospital controls	No association. 40% and 39% of cigarette smokers among cases and controls, respectively
Kolonel and Winkelstein 1977	New York, U.S.	176 cases 269 hospital controls	No significant association.[a] Ever smokers: OR = 1.1 (noncancer controls), OR = 1.0 (cancer controls)
Schuman et al. 1977	Minneapolis, U.S.	40 cases 43 hospital 35 neighborhood controls	Direct association, when neighborhood, but not hospital controls, were used
Williams and Horm 1977	U.S. (Third Nat. Cancer controls survey)	257 cases 1116 population controls	No association. No of cigarette smoked: 1-400/year, OR = 0.7; 401-800/year, OR = 0.7; >800/year, OR = 0.9.
Niijima and Koiso 1980	Japan	187 cases 200 hospital controls	No association
Mishina et al. 1985	Kyoto, Japan	111 cases 100 population controls	No significant association.[a] Ever smokers: RR = 1.6
Checkoway et al. 1987	Chapel Hill, U.S.	40 cases 64 hospital controls	No association
Ross et al. 1987	Los Angeles, U.S.	284 cases (142 blacks and 142 whites) 284 population controls (142 blacks and 142 whites)	No association.[a] Ever smokers: Whites, RR = 1.1; Blacks, RR = 0.9
Honda et al. 1988	California, U.S.	216 cases 212 population controls	Ever smokers: RR = 1.9; years of smoking: >40, RR = 2.6
Yu et al. 1988	U.S.	1162 cases (989 whites and 161 blacks) 3124 hospital controls (2791 whites and 320 blacks)	No significant association.[a] Whites: ex-smokers OR = 0.9; current smokers OR = 1.0. Blacks: ex-smokers OR = 1.4; current smokers OR = 1.7

Table 20.1 (continued) Summary of results of case–control studies on prostate cancer in relation to cigarette smoking

Investigator(s)	Location	No. of subjects	Major findings
Newell et al. 1989	Houston, U.S.	103 cases 220 hospital controls	No association
Oishi et al. 1989	Kyoto, Japan	117 cases 296 hospital controls	No significant association. Current smokers: OR=0.6; former smokers: OR=1.4
Fincham et al. 1990	Alberta, Canada	382 cases 625 population controls	No association.[a] Ex-smokers: RR = 0.8; current smokers RR = 0.9
Slattery et al. 1990	Utah, U.S.	385 cases 679 population controls	No association
Slattery and West 1993; Elghany et al. 1990	Utah, U.S.	720 cases 1364 population controls	57% and 58% of ever smokers among cases and controls
Talamini et al. 1993; Tavani et al. 1994	Northern Italy	281 cases 599 hospital controls	No significant association.[a] Ever-smokers: OR=0.8
Hayes et al. 1994	Atlanta, Detroit, New Jersey, U.S.	981 cases (502 whites, 479 blacks) 1315 population controls (721 whites, 594 blacks)	Whites: current: OR=1.2; former-smokers, OR=1.2. Blacks: current: OR=1.0; former-smokers: RR=1.1
Van der Gulden et al. 1994	The Netherlands	345 cases 1346 hospital controls	Significant direct association. Ever-smokers: OR=2.1. No relation with amount, duration, or age started smoking
De Stefani et al. 1995	Uruguay	156 cases 302 hospital (cancer) controls	No significant association.[a] Ever-smoker: OR=0.7; ex-smokers: OR=0.6; current: OR=0.8
Siemiatycki et al. 1995; Sharpe and Siemiatycki 2001	Montreal, Canada	449 hospital cases 1266 population controls	No significant association[a]. Ever-(cigarette) smokers: OR=1.1

Reference	Country	Cases/Controls	Results
Andersson et al. 1996	Sweden	256 cases / 252 population controls	Current-smokers: OR=1.8. No dose–response trend
Ilic et al. 1996	Serbia, Yugoslavia	101 cases / 202 hospital controls	No significant difference in smoking habits or in the number or type of smoking
Pawlega et al. 1996	Poland	76 cases / 152 controls	No association
Key et al. 1997	UK	328 cases / 328 population controls	No significant association. Current smokers: OR=1.1; former-smokers: OR=1.1
Lumey et al. 1997	US	1097 cases / 3250 hospital controls	No association. Current smoker: OR=0.9; ex-smokers: OR=0.9; No dose–response trend
Rohan et al. 1997	Canada	408 cases / 407 population controls	Direct association. Current-smokers: OR=1.4; ex-smokers: OR=1.7
Sung et al. 1999	Taiwan	90 cases / 180 hospital controls	46% and 40% of smokers in cases and controls, respectively. Ever-smokers: OR=1.3
Villeneuve et al. 1999	Canada	1623 cases / 1623 population controls	Nonsignificant inverse association
Giles et al. 2001	Australia	1476 cases / 1409 population controls	No association.[a] Ever-smoker: OR=1.0; ex-smoker: OR=1.0; current smoker: OR=0.8

[a]Never smokers as reference category; RR, relative risk; OR, odds ratio.

Mills and Beeson 1992; Doll *et al.* 1994; Hiatt *et al.* 1994; McLaughlin *et al.* 1995; Adami *et al.* 1996; Coughlin *et al.* 1996; Cerhan *et al.* 1997; Rodriguez *et al.* 1997; Giovannucci *et al.* 1999; Parker *et al.* 1999; Lotufo *et al.* 2000; Lund Nilsen *et al.* 2000; Putnam *et al.* 2000), four (Kahn 1966; Rogot and Murray 1980; Hsing *et al.* 1990, 1991; Hiatt *et al.* 1994; McLaughlin *et al.* 1995, Rodriguez *et al.* 1997) showed some positive relation with cigarette smoking (Table 20.2). Hsing *et al.* (1991) and McLaughlin *et al.* (1995) in the US Veterans Cohort Study found a significantly elevated relative risk among cigarette smokers (RR = 1.18; 95% CI, 1.09–1.28), particularly among heavy smokers (OR = 1.51 in smokers of 40 or more cigarettes per day compared with non-smokers). Hsing *et al.* (1990) in a report on a Lutheran Brotherhood cohort study reported significantly elevated relative risk among persons who smoked any type of tobacco (RR = 1.8; 95% CI, 1.1–2.9), as well as among users of smokeless tobacco (RR = 2.1; 95% CI, 1.1–4.1). No clear dose–response relation was however found. Likewise, the data of the Cancer Prevention Study II (CPSII; Rodriguez *et al.* 1997) showed an elevated risk (RR = 1.34; 95% CI, 1.16–1.56) of fatal prostate cancer in cigarette smokers, with a stronger association below age 60, but no trend in risk with number of cigarettes smoked nor duration of smoking. The conclusion was that smoking may adversely affect survival in prostatic cancer patients (Rodriguez *et al.* 1997). Positive results came from the U.S. Kaiser Permanente Study (Hiatt *et al.* 1994) based on 238 cases.

Another prospective study from Norway (Lund Nilsen *et al.* 2000) found a weak positive association with number of cigarettes smoked, and a cohort study of Iowa men (Parker *et al.* 1999; Putnam *et al.* 2000), including only about 100 prostate cancer cases, showed a nonsignificant association with number of cigarettes. Likewise, the MRFIT (Coughlin *et al.* 1996) cohort showed a significant excess risk for smokers versus nonsmokers, in the absence of any dose–risk relation (i.e. RR was 1.5 for smokers of < 15 cigarettes/day, but 1.2 for smokers of > 45 cigarettes/day).

In contrast, no association between smoking and prostate cancer was evident from the British Physicians (Doll *et al.* 1994), the U.S. Health Professionals' (Giovannucci *et al.* 1999) and the Physicians' Health Study (Lotufo *et al.* 2000).

This pattern of risk would suggest that the relation between smoking and prostate cancer diagnosis or death may not be causal, but attributable to other socioeconomic or lifestyle correlates of smoking (IARC 1986; Dai *et al.* 1988; Nomura and Kolonel 1991; La Vecchia *et al.* 1992; Boyle *et al.* 1997), which are likely to be less relevant in studies conducted in health conscious populations like doctors or health professionals. A major problem of cohort studies, in fact, is often the limited number of covariates available in order to allow for potential confounding.

The report by Giles *et al.* (2001), based on a uniquely large case–control study, provides further evidence on an absence of excess risk of prostate cancer among current or former smokers, including those who smoked the highest number of cigarettes for the longest period of time. There is also a lack of material influence of smoking on prostate

Table 20.2 Summary of results of cohort studies on prostate cancer in relation to cigarette smoking

Investigator(s) (reference)	Location	No. of subjects	Major findings
Hammond 1966	U.S.	440 558 (319 cases)	No association
Kahn 1966; Rogot and Murray 1980; Hsing et al. 1991	U.S. (Veterans)	293 916 (4607 cases)	Ex-smokers: RR = 1.1; current smokers: RR = 1.2; No. of cigarettes smoked: 10–20/day, RR = 1.2; 21–39/day, RR = 1.2; > 39/day, RR = 1.5
Weir and Dunn 1970	California, U.S.	68 153 (37 cases)	No association.[a] Ever smokers: RR = 0.8; <1/2 pk/day, RR = 0.6; 1 pk/day, RR = 1.0; >1 pk/day, RR = 0.8
Hirayama 1979	Japan	122 261 (63 cases)	No association. Age-standardized death rate per 100 000 (6.1) among nonsmokers, (3.7) ex-smokers, (5.8) current smokers
Whittemore et al. 1985	U.S. (college alumni)	47 271 (243 cases)	No association
Carstensen et al. 1987	Sweden	25 129 (193 cases)	No association.[a] Ex-smokers: RR = 1.0; No. of cigarettes smoked: 1–7/day, RR = 1.1; 8–15/day, RR = 0.8; >15/day, RR = 0.9
Mills et al. 1989	California, U.S.	14 000 (180 cases)	No association.[a] Ex-smokers: RR = 1.2; current smokers: RR = 0.5
Severson et al. 1989	Honolulu, Japan	7999 (174 cases)	No association.[a] Ex-smokers: RR = 0.9; current smokers: RR = 0.9
Hsing et al.1990	Minnesota, U.S. (Lutheran)	17 633 (149 cases)	Positive association.[a] Ever used any form of tobacco: RR = 1.8; current smokers: RR = 2.0
Ross et al. 1990	U.S., California	5105 (138 cases)	No association.[a] Current-smokers: RR = 0.9; former-smokers: RR = 0.8
Mills and Beeson 1992	U.S., California (7th Day Adventists)	14 000 (180 cases)	No association. Current-smokers: RR = 1.0. No relation with amount or duration of smoking
Doll et al. 1994	U.K. (physicians)	34 440 (568 cases)	RR = 0.8,1.1,1.2 in subsequent levels of smoking
Hiatt et al. 1994	U.S., California (Kaiser Perman)	43 432 (238 cases)	Positive association. Compared to never smokers, ≤ 20 cig/day, RR = 1.0; >20 cig/day, RR = 1.9 (95% CI 1.2–3.1)
McLaughlin et al. 1995	U.S. (Veterans)	293 916 (3124 deaths)	Positive association.[a] Ex-smokers, RR = 1.1. 1–9 cig/day, RR = 1.1; 10–20 cig/day, RR = 1.2; 21–39 cig/day, RR = 1.2; 21–39 cig/day, RR = 1.2; ≥40 cig/day, RR = 1.5

Table 20.2 (continued) Summary of results of cohort studies on prostate cancer in relation to cigarette smoking

Investigator(s) (reference)	Location	No. of subjects	Major findings
Adami et al. 1996	Sweden	135 006 (2368 cases)	Current-smokers, RR = 1.1; ex-smokers, RR = 1.1. No trend with amount or duration of smoking
Coughlin et al. 1996	U.S. (MRFIT)	348 874 (826 cases)	Positive association. No. of cigarettes smoked, 1–15 cig/day, RR = 1.5; 16–25 cig/day, RR = 1.3; 26–35 cig/day, RR = 1.2; 36–45 cig/day, RR = 1.5; >45 cig/day, RR = 1.2
Rodriguez et al. 1997	U.S. (Cancer Prevention Study II)	450 279 (1748)	Positive association with current smoking for fatal cancers. Ever-smokers, RR = 1.0; current cigarettes. only smokers, RR = 1.3; former cigarettes. only smokers, RR = 1.0. No trend with amount or duration of smoking
Cerhan et al. 1997	Iowa, U.S.	1050 (71 cases)	63% and 58% ever smokers among cases and controls. Current, <20 cig/day, RR = 2.0; current, ≥20 cig/day, RR = 2.9. Significant dose-dependent trend
Giovannucci et al. 1999	U.S. (Health Professionals)	51 529 (1369 cases)	No association.[a] Current smokers, RR = 1.1. Impact of recent use on occurrence of fatal cancer (RR = 1.6)
Parker et al. 1999	Iowa, U.S.	1117 (81 cases)	Former-smokers, RR = 1.3; current, <20 cig/day, RR = 1.7; current, ≥20 cig/day, RR = 1.9
Lotufo et al. 2000	U.S. (Physicians' Health Study)	22 071 (996 cases)	No association.[a] Ex-smokers, RR = 1.1; current <20 cig/day, RR = 1.1; current, ≥20 cig/day, RR = 1.1. No dose- or duration-dependent trend
Lund Nilsen et al. 2000	Norway	22 895 (644 cases)	RR = 0.8, 1.1, 1.4, 1.3 for subsequent levels of cigarette smoking
Putnam et al. 2000	Iowa, U.S.	1572 (101 cases)	Nonsignificant association. Former-smokers, RR = 1.4; current, <20 cig/day, RR = 1.3; current, ≥20 cig/day, RR = 1.6

[a]Never smokers as reference category; RR, relative risk; OR, odds ratio.

cancer in younger or elderly men, with early or advanced, or moderate or high-grade neoplasms.

Together with the available evidence on this issue, the results from this study provide therefore definite evidence that cigarette smoking is not a relevant risk factor for prostate cancer, even after a long latency period. The issue of a modest association remains open to debate, but it is unclear whether such a modest association can be investigated in observational epidemiological studies, in consideration also of the need for careful allowance for confounding, since some differences in other factors (including dietary, socioeconomic, or other) may account for the apparent inconsistencies observed across studies (Wynder 1990; Colditz 1996).

These cautions notwithstanding, it is now clear, in conclusion, that tobacco smoking is not a relevant risk factor for prostate cancer.

References

Adami, H.-O., Bergstrom, R., Engholm, G., Nyrén, O., Wolk, A., Ekbom, A., Englund, A., and Baron, J. (1996). A prospective study of smoking and risk of prostate cancer. *International Journal of Cancer*, **67**, 764–8.

Andersson, S. O., Baron, L., Bergstrom, R., Lindgren, C., Wolk, A., and Adami, H. O. (1996). Lifestyle factors and prostate cancer risk: A case-control study in Sweden. *Cancer Epidemiology Biomarkers and Prevention*, **5**, 509–13.

Boyle, P., Maisonneuve, P., and Napalkov, P. (1997). Urological cancers: an epidemiological overview of a neglected problem. *Journal of Epidemiology and Biostatistics*, **2**, 125–45.

Carstensen, J. M., Pershagen, G., and Eklund, G. (1987). Mortality in relation to cigarette and pipe smoking: 16 years' observation of 25000 Swedish men. *Journal of Epidemiology and Community Health*, **41**, 166–72.

Cerhan, J. R., Torner, J. C., Lynch, C. F., Rubenstein, L. M., Lemke, J. H., Cohen, M. B., *et al.* (1997). Association of smoking, body mass, and physical activity with risk of prostate cancer in the Iowa 65+ Rural Health Study (United States). *Cancer Causes and Control*, **8**, 229–38.

Checkoway, H., Di Ferdinando, G., Hulka, B. S., and Mickey, D. D. (1987). Medical, life-style, and occupational risk factors for prostate cancer. *Prostate*, **10**, 79–88.

Colditz, G. (1996). Consensus conference: smoking and prostate cancer. *Cancer Causes and Control*, **7**, 560–2.

Coughlin, S. S., Neaton, J. D., and Sengupta, A. (1996). Cigarette smoking as a predictor of death from prostate cancer in 348,874 men screened for the Multiple Risk Factor Intervention Trial. *American Journal of Epidemiology*, **143**, 1002–6.

Dai, W. S., Gutai, J. P., Kuller, L. H., and Cauley, J. A. for the MRFIT Research Group (1988). Cigarette smoking and serum sex hormones in men. *American Journal of Epidemiology*, **128**, 796–805.

De Stefani, E., Fierro, L., Barrios, E., and Ronco, A. (1995). Tobacco, alcohol, diet and risk of prostate cancer. *Tumori*, **81**, 315–20.

Doll, R., Peto, R., Wheatley, K., Gray, R., and Sutherland, I. (1994). Mortality in relation to smoking: 40 years' observations on male British doctors. *British Medical Journal*, **309**, 901–10.

Elghany, N. A., Schumacher, M. C., Slattery, M. L., West, D. W., and Lee, J. S. (1990). Occupation, cadmium exposure, and prostate cancer. *Epidemiology*, **1**, 107–15.

Fincham, S. M., Hill, G. B., Hanson, J., and Wijayasinghe, C. (1990). Epidemiology of prostatic cancer: a case-control study. *Prostate*, **17**, 189–206.

Giles, G. G., Severi, G., McCredie, M. R. E., English, D. R., Johnson, W., Hopper, J. L., and Boyle, P. (2001). Smoking and prostate cancer: Findings from an Australian case-control study. *Annals of Oncology*, **12**, 761–5.

Giovannucci, E., Rimm, E. B., Ascherio, A., Colditz, G. A., Spiegelman, D., Stampfer, M. J., and Willett, W. C. (1999). Smoking and risk of total and fatal prostate cancer in United States Health Professionals. *Cancer Epidemiology Biomarkers and Prevention*, **8**, 277–82.

Hammond, E. C. (1966). Smoking in relation to the death rates of one million men and women. *National Cancer Institute Monograph*, **19**, 127–204.

Hayes, R. B., Pottern, L. M., Swanson, G. M., Liff, G. M., Schoenberg, J. B., Greenberg, R. S., *et al.* (1994). Tobacco use and prostate cancer in blacks and whites in the United States. *Cancer Causes and Control*, **5**, 221–6.

Hiatt, R. A., Armstrong, M. A., Klatsky, A. L., and Sidney, S. (1994). Alcohol consumption, smoking, and other risk factors and prostate cancer in a large health plan cohort in California (United States). *Cancer Causes and Control*, **5**, 66–72.

Hirayama, T. (1979). Epidemiology of prostate cancer with special reference to the role of diet. *National Cancer Institute Monograph*, **53**, 149–55.

Honda, G. D., Bernstein, L., Ross, R. K., Greenland, S., Gerkins, V., and Henderson, B. E. (1988). Vasectomy, cigarette smoking, and age at first sexual intercourse as risk factors for prostate cancer in middle-aged men. *British Journal of Cancer*, **57**, 326–31.

Hsing, A. W., McLaughlin, J. K., Schuman, L. M., Bjelke, E., Gridley, G., Wacholder, S., Co Chien, H. T., and Blot, W. J. (1990). Diet, tobacco use, and fatal prostate cancer: Results from the Lutheran Brotherhood Cohort Study. *Cancer Research*, **50**, 6836–40.

Hsing, A. W., McLaughlin, J. K., Hrubec, Z., Blot, W. J., and Fraumen, J. F., Jr. (1991). Tobacco use and prostate cancer: 26-year follow-up of US veterans. *American Journal of Epidemiology*, **133**, 437–41.

IARC Working Group on the Evaluation of the Carcinogenic Risk of Chemicals to Humans (1986). IARC Monographs on the evaluation of carcinogenic risk of chemicals to humans. *Tobacco smoking*, Vol. 38, pp. 199–298. International Agency for Research on Cancer, Lyon, France.

Ilic, M., Vlajinac, H., and Marinkovic, J. (1996). Case-control study of risk factors for prostate cancer. *British Journal of Cancer*, **74**, 1682–6.

Kahn, H. A. (1966). The Dorn study of smoking and mortality among U.S. veterans: Report on eight and one-half years of observation. *National Cancer Institute Monographs*, **19**, 1–125.

Key, T. J. A., Silcocks, P. B., Daveay, G. K., Appleby, P. N., and Bishop, D. T. (1997). A case-control study of diet and prostate cancer. *British Journal of Cancer*, **76**, 679–87.

Kolonel, L. and Winkelstein, W., Jr. (1977). Cadmium and prostatic carcinoma. *Lancet*, **2**, 566–7.

La Vecchia, C., Negri, E., Franceschi, S., Parazzini, F., and Decarli, A. (1992). Differences in dietary intake with smoking, alcohol, and education. *Nutrition and Cancer*, **17**, 297–304.

Levi, F., La Vecchia, C., and Boyle, P. (2000). The rise and fall of prostate cancer. *European Journal of Cancer Prevention*, **9**, 381–5.

Lotufo, P. A., Lee, I.-M., Ajani, U. A., Hennekens, C. H., and Manson, J. E. (2000). Cigarette smoking and risk of prostate cancer in the Physicians' Health Study (United States). *International Journal of Cancer*, **7**, 141–4.

Lumey, L. H., Pittman, B., Zang, E. A., and Wynder, E. L. (1997). Cigarette smoking and prostate cancer: No relation with six measures of lifetime smoking habits in a large case-control study among U.S. Whites. *Prostate*, **33**, 195–200.

Lund Nilsen, T. I., Johnsen, R., and Vatten, L. J. (2000). Socio-economic and lifestyle factors associated with the risk of prostate cancer. *British Journal of Cancer*, **82**, 1358–63.

McLaughlin, J. K., Hrubec, Z., Blot, W. J., and Fraumeni, J. F., Jr. (1995). Smoking and cancer mortality among U.S. veterans; a 26-year follow-up. *International Journal of Cancer*, **60**, 190–5.

Mills, P. K. and Beeson, W. (1992). Re: Tobacco use and prostate cancer: 26 year follow-up of US veterans. *American Journal of Epidemiology*, **135**, 326–7.

Mills, P. K., Beeson, W. I.., Phillips, R. L., and Fraser, G. E. (1989). Cohort study of diet, lifestyle, and prostate cancer in Adventist men. *Cancer*, **64**, 598–604.

Mishina, T., Watanabe, H., Araki, H., and Nakao, M. (1985). Epidemiological study of prostatic cancer by matched-pair analysis. *Prostate*, **6**, 423–36.

Newell, G. R., Fueger, J. J., Spitz, M. R., and Babaian, R. J. (1989). A case–control study of prostate cancer. *American Journal of Epidemiology*, **130**, 395–8.

Niijima, T. and Koiso, K. (1980). Incidence of prostatic cancer in Japan and Asia. *Scandinavian Journal of Urology and Nephrology*, **55**(suppl), 17–21.

Nomura, A. M. Y. and Kolonel, L. N. (1991). Prostate cancer: A current perspective. *Epidemiologic Reviews*, **13**, 200–27.

Oishi, K., Okada, K., Yoshida, O., Yamabe, H., Ohno, Y., Hayes, R. B., and Schroeder, F. H. (1989). Case-control study of prostatic cancer in Kyoto, Japan: Demographic and some life-style factors. *Prostate*, **14**, 117–122.

Parker, A. S., Cerhan, J. R., Putmann, S. D., Cantor, K. P., and Lynch, C. F. (1999). A cohort study of farming and risk of prostate cancer in Iowa. *Epidemiology*, **10**, 452–5.

Parkin, D. M., Pisani P., and Ferlay J. (1999). Estimates of the worldwide incidence of 25 major cancers in 1990. *International Journal of Cancer*, **80**, 827–41.

Pawlega, J., Rachtan, J., and Dyba, T. (1996). Dietary factors and risk of prostate cancer in Poland. Results of case-control study. *Neoplasma*, **43**, 61–3.

Putnam, S. D., Cerhan, J. R., Parker, A. S., Bianchi, G. D., Wallace, R. B., Kantor, K. P., and Lynch, C. F. (2000). Lifestyle and anthropometric risk factors for prostate cancer in a cohort of Iowa men. *Annals of Epidemiology*, **10**, 361–9.

Rodriguez, C., Tatham, L. M., Thun, M. J., Calle, E. E., and Heath, C. W., Jr. (1997). Smoking and fatal prostate cancer in a large cohort of adult men. *American Journal of Epidemiology*, **145**, 466–75.

Rogot, E. and Murray, J. L. (1980). Smoking and causes of death among U.S. veterans: 16 years of observation. *Public Health Reports*, **95**, 213–22.

Rohan, T. E., Hislop, T. G., Howe, G. R., Gallagher, R. P., The C.-Z., and Ghadirian, P. (1997). Cigarette smoking and risk of prostate cancer: A population-based case-control study in Ontario and British Columbia, Canada. *European Journal of Cancer Prevention*, **6**, 382–8.

Ross, R. K., Shimizu, H., Paganini-Hill, A., Honda, G., and Henderson. B. E. (1987). Case-control studies of prostate cancer in Blacks and Whites in Southern California. *Journal of the National Cancer Institute*, **78**, 869–74.

Ross, R. K., Bernstein, L., and Paganini-Hill, A. (1990). Effects of cigarette smoking on 'hormone related' diseases in a southern California retirement community. In: *Smoking and hormone-related disorders* (ed. N. Wald and J. Baron), pp. 32–54. Oxford University Press, New York.

Schuman, L. M., Mandel, J., Blackard, C., Bauer, H., Scarlett, J., and McHugh, R. (1977). Epidemiologic study of prostatic cancer: Preliminary report. *Cancer Treatment Reports*, **61**, 181–6.

Schwartz, D., Flamant, R., Lellouch, J., and Denoix, P. F. (1961). Results of a French survey on the role of tobacco, particularly inhalation, in different cancer sites. *Journal of the National Cancer Institute*, **26**, 1085–108.

Severson, R. K., Nomura, A. M. Y., Grove, J. S., and Stemmermann, G. N. (1989). A prospective study of demographics, diet, and prostate cancer among men of Japanese ancestry in Hawaii. *Cancer Research*, **49**, 1857–60.

Sharpe, C. R. and Siemiatycki, J. (2001). Joint effects of smoking and body mass index on prostate cancer risk. *Epidemiology*, **12**, 546–51.

Siemiatycki, K., Krewski, D., Franco, E., and Kaiserman, M. (1995). Associations between cigarette smoking and each of 21 types of cancer. A multi-site case-control study. *International Journal of Epidemiology*, **24**, 504–14.

Slattery, M. L., Schumacher, M. C., West, D. W., Robison, L. M., and French, T. K. (1990). Food-consumption trends between adolescent and adult years and subsequent risk of prostate cancer. *American Journal of Clinical Nutrition*, **52**, 752–7.

Slattery, M. L. and West, D. W. (1993). Smoking, alcohol, coffee, tea, caffeine, and theobromine: risk of prostate cancer in Utah (United States), *Cancer Causes and Control*, **4**, 559–63.

Sung, J. F. C., Lin, R. S., Pu, Y.-S., Chen, Y.-C., Chang, H. C., and Lai, M.-K. (1999). Risk factors for prostate carcinoma in Taiwan. A case-control study in a Chinese population. *Cancer*, **86**, 484–91.

Talamini, R., Franceschi, S., La Vecchia, C., Guarneri, S., and Negri, E. (1993). Smoking habits and prostate cancer: A case-control study in Northern Italy. *Preventive Medicine*, **22**, 400–8.

Tavani, A., Negri, E., Franceschi, S., Talamini, R., and La Vecchia, C. (1994). Alcohol consumption and risk of prostate cancer. *Nutrition and Cancer*, **21**, 25–31.

Van der Gulden, J. W. J., Verbeek, A. L. M., and Kolk, J. J. (1994). Smoking and drinking habits in relation to prostate cancer. *British Journal of Urology*, **73**, 382–9.

Villeneuve, P. J., Johnson, K. C., Kreiger, N., and Mao, Y. (1999). Risk factors for prostate cancer: results from the Canadian National Enhanced Cancer Surveillance System. The Canadian Cancer Registries Epidemiology Research Group. *Cancer Causes and Control*, **10**, 355–67.

Weir, J. M. and Dunn, J. E., Jr. (1970). Smoking and mortality: A prospective study. *Cancer*, **25**, 105–12.

Whittemore, A. S., Paffenbarger, R. S., Jr., Anderson, K., and Lee, J. E. (1985). Early precursors of site-specific cancers in college men and women. *Journal of the National Cancer Institute*, **74**, 43–51.

Williams, R. R. and Horm, J. W. (1977). Association of cancer sites with tobacco and alcohol consumption and socioeconomic status of patients: Interview study from the Third National Cancer Survey. *Journal of the National Cancer Institute*, **58**, 525–47.

Wynder, E. L. (1990). Epidemiological issues in weak associations. *International Journal of Epidemiology*, **19**(Suppl 1), S5–7.

Wynder, E. L., Mabuchi, K., and Whitmore, W. F., Jr. (1971). Epidemiology of cancer of the prostate. *Cancer*, **28**, 344–60.

Yu, H., Harris, R. E., and Wynder, E. L. (1988). Case-control study of prostate cancer and socio-economic factors. *Prostate*, **13**, 317–25.

Chapter 21

Laryngeal cancer

Paolo Boffetta

Summary

More than 160 000 new cases of laryngeal cancer are estimated to occur each year worldwide, and 89 000 people die from this disease. Tobacco smoking is the main cause of laryngeal cancer in all populations among which studies have been conducted, and at least two-thirds of cases among men and one-third of cases among women are attributable to tobacco smoking. The risk of laryngeal cancer among heavy smokers is at least 20 times higher than that of non-smokers. Both the amount of cigarettes smoked per day and the duration of smoking are important determinants of the risk; a protective effect of quitting smoking is clear after five years. Several studies have suggested a higher risk among deep inhalers; smokers of hand-rolled cigarettes and smokers of black-tobacco cigarettes have a higher risk than other smokers. An increased risk has been shown following smoking of cigar and pipe, as well as of bidi and other local tobacco products. Tobacco smoking seems to exert a stronger carcinogenic effect on the supraglottic region of the organ than on the glottis. Tobacco smoking acts synergistically with alcohol drinking in causing laryngeal cancer; a similar interaction with the carcinogenic effect of a diet poor is fruits and vegetables is probable. A genetic susceptibility to tobacco-induced laryngeal cancer is plausible, but specific factors have not yet been identified. Data on p53 mutations in laryngeal cancer are consistent with a major carcinogenic role played by tobacco. Tobacco control remains the main tool to prevent laryngeal cancer.

Epidemiology of laryngeal cancer

The incidence of laryngeal cancer in men is high (age-standardized rate 10/100 000 or more) in southern and central Europe, southern Brazil, Uruguay, and Argentina, and among blacks in the USA, while the lowest rates (<1/100 000) are recorded in southeast Asia and central Africa (Parkin *et al.* 1997). The incidence in women is below 1/100 000 in most populations. Rates have not changed markedly during the last two decades, but the interpretation of time trends is complicated by changes in diagnostic accuracy. An estimated 161 400 new cases occurred worldwide in 2000, of which 142 200 among men and 92 300 in developing countries (Ferlay *et al.* 2001). The estimated number of deaths in 2000 was 89 100 globally, of which 78 600 among men and

55 100 in developing countries. More than 90% of cancers of the larynx are squamous cell carcinomas, and the majority originate from the supraglottic and glottic parts of the organ.

In most populations, the majority of cases of laryngeal cancer are attributable to tobacco smoking, alcohol drinking, and the interaction between these two factors (see below). A protective effect is probably exerted by high intake of fruits and vegetables, although the evidence regarding specific micronutrients such as carotenoids and vitamin C is inadequate to draw a conclusion (WCRF 1997). Maté drinking has been suggested to be a risk factor in studies from Brazil and Uruguay (Austin and Reynolds 1996). Data concerning a possible effect of other food items are not consistent. Occupational exposure to mists of strong inorganic acids, sulfuric acid in particular, is an established risk factor for laryngeal cancer (IARC 1992). A possible effect has been suggested for other occupational exposures, including nickel, asbestos, and ionizing radiation, but the evidence is not conclusive (Berrino 1993). Laryngeal papillomatosis, a condition characterized by multiple benign tumours called papillomas, is caused by infection with human papillomavirus (HPV) types 6 and 11, the same types that cause genital condylomata acuminata. In children, infection occurs in both genders, during delivery; in adults, infection is common among men and may occur via orogenital sexual contact. Papillomatosis patients have an increased risk of laryngeal cancer; however, studies aimed at assessing the presence of HPV DNA have not yet provided conclusive evidence for a higher prevalence of infection in cases of laryngeal cancer than in controls. Herpes simplex virus type 1 is another virus with a possible causal role in laryngeal cancer (Austin and Reynolds 1996). There is no evidence of strong genetic factors in laryngeal carcinogenesis; however, polymorphism for enzymes implicated in the metabolism of alcohol and tobacco, such as alcohol and aldehyde dehydrogenase, are possible susceptibility factors, with relative risks in the order of 1.5–2.

Tobacco smoking

A strong association between tobacco smoking and laryngeal cancer has been reported since the 1950s (Schrek *et al.* 1950; Doll and Hill 1954; Wynder *et al.* 1955). This finding has been replicated in different populations and under different circumstances of tobacco smoking. As early as 1964, public health and scientific authorities considered that the causal association between tobacco smoking and laryngeal cancer was clearly established (USDEHW 1964). Since then, evidence has accumulated on different aspects of the carcinogenic effect of tobacco smoking on the larynx, based on data from both cohort and case–control studies. On the one hand, cohort studies, although they may be considered methodologically superior, are mainly based on mortality data and have primarily been assembled in areas with a low incidence of laryngeal cancer, such as the USA, the United Kingdom, Japan, and the Nordic countries, resulting in a relatively small number of cases, even in the largest cohorts. For example, during the

12-year follow-up of the American Cancer Society Cancer Prevention Study I, which included over one million individuals, a total of 109 deaths from laryngeal cancer was recorded among men and 22 among women (Burns *et al.* 1996). On the other hand, case–control studies are based on incident cases and have often been conducted in high-risk areas, such as southern Europe and South America.

Cigarette smoking

Among men, the risk of laryngeal cancer is increased 5–10 times among ever cigarette smokers as compared to never smokers. In population-based series, the proportion of cases who report not having smoked during their lifetime is in the order of 1–5%. In all studies that have analysed it, a positive trend was found between amount of smoking and risk of laryngeal cancer relative to that of non-smokers. Table 21.1 summarizes the results of the selected case–control studies. Additional studies provided similar results for other populations, e.g. Uruguay (De Stefani *et al.* 1995), Spain (Lopez-Abente *et al.* 1992), and Denmark (Olsen *et al.* 1985), but they did not fulfil the criteria for inclusion in Table 21.1. The heterogeneity in the results can be explained by the small number of non-smoking cases in some of the studies, by the type of tobacco smoked, by differences in the interactive effect of alcohol drinking, and possibly by differences in genetic susceptibility factors, in addition to differences in the quality of the studies and the validity of the results.

Results from cohort studies are comparable to those available from case–control studies (e.g. Doll and Hill 1954; Dorn 1959; Burch *et al.* 1981). As an example, Fig. 21.1 shows the relative risk among white men and women enrolled in the American Cancer Society Cancer Prevention Study I (Burns *et al.* 1996).

Several cohort and case–control studies reported a positive dose–response according to duration of smoking (Falk *et al.* 1989; Restrepo *et al.* 1989; Sankaranarayanan *et al.* 1990; Choi and Kahyo 1991; Lopez-Abente *et al.* 1992; Zheng *et al.* 1992; Dosemeci *et al.* 1997). For example, in the study by Zheng *et al.* (1992) from China, the odds ratios were 1.4 (95% confidence interval [CI] 0.4–4.6), 4.1 (1.6–11.1), 12.0 (4.8–30.1), and 13.2 (5.6–31.2) for less than 20 years, 20–29 years, 30–39 years, and 40 or more years of smoking.

Selected results on the effect of quitting are summarized in Table 21.2. No protective effect is apparent during the first five years after quitting, a phenomenon that can be partially explained by quitting because of early symptoms of the neoplastic lesion. After that time, however, there is strong evidence of a decrease in risk of laryngeal cancer.

A higher relative risk was suggested in several studies for deep inhalation of tobacco smoke, as compared to light or no inhalation (Restrepo *et al.* 1989; Lopez-Abente *et al.* 1992; Burns *et al.* 1996; Lewin *et al.* 1998). In a study from Uruguay, smokers of hand-rolled cigarettes had a higher risk than smokers of manufactured cigarettes (De Stefani *et al.* 1992). Studies from southern Europe and South America have consistently reported a 1.5- to 2-fold stronger risk among smokers of black-tobacco

Table 21.1 Results of selected case–control studies of tobacco smoking and laryngeal cancer

Study	Area, period, gender*	Cases**	Controls***	Categories (cig/day)	OR	95% CI	Comments
Graham et al. 1981	USA, 1957–1965, M	374, NA	H, 381, NA	0	1.0	Ref.	controls from cancer institute
				1–10	2.1	$p < 0.05$	
				11–20	4.8	$p < 0.005$	
				21–39	8.8	$p < 0.005$	
				40+	8.5	$p < 0.005$	
Burch et al. 1981	Canada, 1977–1979	204, 79%	N, 204, 77%	0	1.0	Ref.	
				1–14	3.0	1.4–6.3	
				15–24	3.4	1.7–6.8	
				25+	4.5	2.2–9.2	
Tuyns et al. 1988	Italy, Spain, France, Switzerland, 1973–1980, M	696, >80%	P, 3057, 56–75%	0	1.0	Ref.	
				1–7	2.4	1.3–4.3	
				8–15	6.7	4.2–10.7	
				16–25	13.7	8.7–21.6	
				26+	16.4	10.1–26.6	
Zheng et al. 1992	China, 1988–1990	201, 76%	P, 414, 88%	0	1.0	Ref.	
				1–9	1.6	0.5–4.9	
				10–19	7.1	3.1–16.6	
				20	12.4	4.6–33.2	
				21+	25.1	9.9–63.2	

Reference	Country, period	Controls [***]	Cases [**]	Cigarettes/day	OR	95% CI	Comments
Hedberg et al. 1994	USA, 1983–1987	P, 547, 75%	235, 81%	0	1.0	Ref.	ref. cat. includes ex-smokers >15 years
				1–19	6.3	3.1–11.8	
				20–39	10.6	6.5–18.7	
				40+	23.1	9.4–52.6	
Tavani et al. 1994	Italy, 1986–1992, M	H, 1373, NA	350, NA	0	1.0	Ref.	low exp. cat. includes ex-smokers
				1–14	3.5	2.1–6.0	
				15+	10.4	6.2–17.5	
Dosemeci et al. 1997	Turkey, 1979–1984, M	H, 829, NA	832, NA	0	1.0	Ref.	
				1–10	1.6	0.9–2.6	
				11–20	3.5	2.6–4.8	
				21+	6.6	4.2–10.3	

Selection criteria include publication after 1980; N, cases of laryngeal cancer > 200, report of odds ratios for amount of smoking, adjustment for alcohol drinking, use of never smokers as referent category.

*M if results are restricted to men, no indication if they refer to both sexes.

**Number of cases, response rate.

***Source of controls, number of controls, response rate.

NA, not available; H, hospital-based; P, population-based; N, neighbourhood.

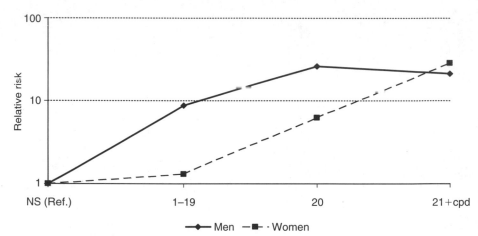

Fig. 21.1 Relative risk of laryngeal cancer by amount of smoking (American Cancer Society Cancer Prevention Study 1) (Burch *et al.* 1996).

Table 21.2 Odds ratios of laryngeal cancer among ex-smokers: results of selected case–control studies

Study*	Years since quitting	OR	95% CI
Tuyns *et al.* 1988	<1**	1.0	Ref.
	1–4	1.5	1.2–2.0
	5–9	0.5	0.3–0.8
	>9	0.3	0.2–0.4
Zatonski *et al.* 1991	<5**	1.0	Ref.
	5–10	0.8	0.3–1.8
	>10	0.3	0.1–0.6
Zheng *et al.* 1992	<2**	1.0	Ref.
	2–4	1.8	0.6–4.9
	5–9	0.6	0.2–1.5
	>9	0.6	0.3–1.2

*See Table 21.1 for details on study design.

**Including current smokers.

cigarettes as compared to blond-tobacco cigarettes (De Stefani *et al.* 1987; Tuyns *et al.* 1988; Lopez-Abente *et al.* 1992; Schlecht *et al.* 1999).

Smoking of products other than cigarettes

An increased risk of laryngeal cancer from cigar and pipe smoking was noticed in the early epidemiological studies (Wynder *et al.* 1955, 1976) and confirmed in some (Schlecht *et al.* 1999) but not all (Freudenheim *et al.* 1992) recent investigations. The magnitude of the risk is similar to that of light smokers, possibly reflecting a lower consumption of tobacco in this group of smokers. Smoking of local tobacco products, such as bidis in India (Sankaranarayanan *et al.* 1990) and yaa muan in Thailand (Simarak *et al.* 1977), also increases the risk of laryngeal cancer. In particular, the effect of bidi smoking seems to be similar to that exerted by cigarette smoking (Fig. 21.2). Use of oral snuff and chewing of tobacco-containing products have also been associated with an increased risk in Europe, North America, and India (Wynder *et al.* 1955; Jussawalla and Deshpande 1971; Lewin *et al.* 1998), although some studies did not detect an increased risk (Sankaranarayanan *et al.* 1990).

Involuntary smoking

Limited data are available on the risk of laryngeal cancer following involuntary exposure to tobacco smoke. In a study of 59 non-smoking head and neck cancer cases and matched non-smoking controls, cases had higher exposure to involuntary smoking than controls (Tan *et al.* 1997). In a further study of 26 non-smoking cases of head and neck cancer and 59 non-smoking controls, the relative risk of ever exposure to

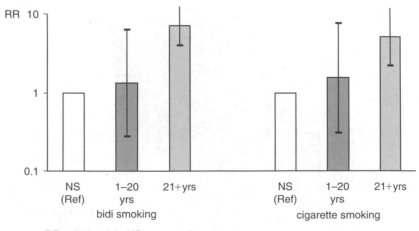

Fig. 21.2 Relative risk of laryngeal cancer from bidi and cigarette smoking—India (Sankaranarayanan *et al.* 1990).

involuntary smoking was 2.2 (95% CI 0.6–8.4) and that of heavy exposure was 4.3 (95% CI 0.8–23) (Zhang *et al.* 2000). Supportive evidence for a possible carcinogenic role of involuntary smoking on the larynx comes from the similarities of the carcinogenic effect of active smoking on the lung and the larynx, both at the epidemiological and the molecular level (Stewart and Semmler 2002). It can be concluded therefore that an increased risk of laryngeal cancer following involuntary smoking in humans is plausible, although it has not yet been demonstrated.

Interaction with other risk factors

The synergism between tobacco smoking and alcohol drinking in laryngeal carcinogenesis has been noted in the early epidemiological studies (Wynder *et al.* 1976) and analysed in many subsequent reports (Flanders and Rothman 1982; Herity *et al.* 1982; Olsen *et al.* 1985; Brownson and Chang 1987; De Stefani *et al.* 1987; Falk *et al.* 1989; Franceschi *et al.* 1990; Choi and Kahyo 1991; Zatonski *et al.* 1991; Zheng *et al.* 1992; Baron *et al.* 1993; Tavani *et al.* 1994; Burns *et al.* 1996). Figure 21.3 shows the relative risks for different combinations of tobacco smoking and alcohol drinking estimated in the largest available study (Tuyns *et al.* 1988). An independent effect of the two carcinogens is clearly shown, and the combined relative risk fits well with a multiplicative model of interaction. For example, based on the results shown in Fig. 21.3, the relative risk among heavy drinkers who are light smokers is 3.78, that of light drinkers who are heavy smokers is 11.47, and that of heavy drinkers and smokers is 43.21, which is the product

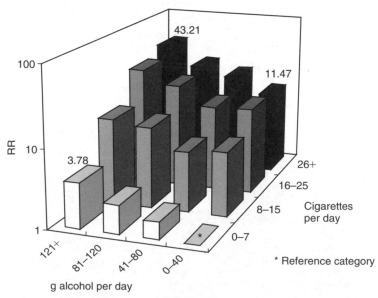

Fig. 21.3 Relative risk of laryngeal cancer among men according to alcohol and tobacco consumption. (Tuyns *et al.* 1988).

of 3.78 and 11.47. An interpretation of these results is that tobacco smoking and alcohol drinking act through independent carcinogenic mechanisms on the laryngeal mucosa.

The joint effect of tobacco smoking and dietary factors has been studied by several authors. Freudenheim *et al.* (1992) found a greater effect of high fat or retinol intake (but not of low carotenoid intake) among heavy smokers than among light smokers. De Stefani *et al.* (1995) found a similar risk from high intake of salted or fresh meat among heavy and light smokers. A similar lack of synergism was reported for low fruit intake by De Stefani *et al.* (1987), for low intake of β-carotene by Tavani *et al.* (1994), and for low intake of fruits or vegetables by Zheng *et al.* (1992). Overall, the available evidence suggests no interaction in laryngeal carcinogenesis, under a multiplicative model, between tobacco smoking and dietary factors. In one single study, an increased risk from heavy mate intake was found among heavy smokers but not among light smokers (De Stefani *et al.* 1987). No data are available on the joint effect of tobacco smoking and exposure to other known causes of laryngeal cancer, such as occupational exposures.

Susceptibility factors

Few studies are available on the smoking-related risk of laryngeal cancer in men and women separately. In most cases, this analysis was hampered by the small number of female cases (e.g. only six female cases were available in the study by Choi *et al.* 1991). In the most informative studies (e.g. Wynder and Stellman 1979), higher relative risks have been reported among women than among men for comparable amounts of smoking. Similar findings have been reported for lung cancer: although these studies might reflect an increased susceptibility to tobacco carcinogenesis among women compared to men (Haugen 2002), they should most likely be interpreted as a phenomenon due to lower rates of laryngeal cancer in non-smoking women than men, possibly reflecting the lack of effect of other environmental carcinogens.

A role of genetic polymorphism of enzymes involved in the metabolism of tobacco carcinogens in modulating tobacco-related risk of laryngeal cancer can be postulated on the basis of knowledge on mechanisms of action. No modification of the effect was suggested in a study for null polymorphism of GSTM1 and GSTT1, two detoxifying enzymes (Jourenkova *et al.* 1998). In the same population, the effect of tobacco smoking was stronger among individuals with high activity of CYP2D6, an activating enzyme, than among other individuals (Benhamou *et al.* 1996).

Effect of different sub-sites within the larynx

A number of case-control studies have provided separate estimates of the tobacco-related risk of glottic (or intrinsic laryngeal) cancer and supraglottic (or extrinsic laryngeal) cancer (Elwood *et al.* 1984; Brugere *et al.* 1986; Guenel *et al.* 1988; Tuyns *et al.* 1988; Falk *et al.* 1989; Lopez-Abente *et al.* 1992; Maier *et al.* 1992; Muscat and Wynder 1992;

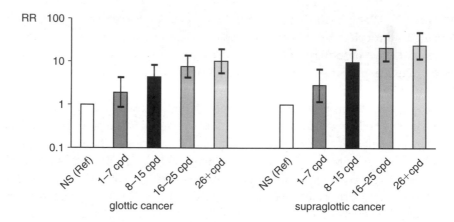

RR, relative risk; NS, non-smoker; cpd, cigarettes per day

Fig. 21.4 Relative risk of glottic and supraglottic cancer from cigarette smoking—Europe (Tuyns *et al.* 1988).

Dosemeci *et al.* 1997). Without exception, relative risks are higher for supraglottic than for glottic cancer, which is compatible with a direct contact mechanism of tobacco carcinogenicity on the organ. As an example, Fig. 21.4 reports the results of the largest available study from four European countries.

Limited data are available on the synergism between tobacco smoking and alcohol drinking on cancer in different parts of the organ (Dosemeci *et al.* 1997; Guenel *et al.* 1988): although risk estimates are often unstable due to small numbers, it is suggested that the combined effect of the two exposures on glottic cancer is compatible with a multiplicative model of interaction, while for supraglottic cancer the combined relative risks are lower than expected according to the multiplicative model, suggesting some overlap in the carcinogenic action of the two agents.

Evidence from mechanistic studies

Mutation in the p53 gene is a common genetic alteration in laryngeal cancer. A distinct pattern of mutations has been reported in cancer of the larynx, and in other tobacco-related cancers, as compared to non-tobacco related cancers. This includes a higher proportion of tumours harbouring a mutation and a higher proportion in G–T transversions, in particular at codons 157, 158, 179, and 249. These mutations likely reflect the effect of the interaction of tobacco carcinogens, such as BPDE, the active metabolite of benzo(*a*)pyrene, on the DNA (Brennan and Boffetta in press). The evidence directly linking tobacco smoking to p53 mutation in laryngeal carcinogenesis, however, is weak. Out of 171 p53 mutations reported in laryngeal cancers in the IARC p53 database (www.iarc.fr/p53/index.html), data on smoking habit were available for 73 patients, of whom only 3 were non-smokers.

Effect on survival

In two studies from Europe, mortality of laryngeal cancer cases was greater among heavy smokers than among non-smokers and light smokers (Crosignani *et al.* 1996; Boffetta *et al.* 1997). This result reflects the increased risk of other tobacco-related causes of death; however, similar results were obtained when only deaths from laryngeal cancer were considered, possibly reflecting an effect of smoking on the natural history of the neoplasm and on response to therapy.

Public health impact

Tobacco smoking greatly increases the risk of laryngeal cancer. The proportion of male cases of laryngeal cancer attributable to tobacco smoking in Europe and North America is around 80%. This proportion might be lower in men from other regions of the world where other causes of laryngeal cancer might play an important role, and in women. A study of the burden of tobacco-related cancer worldwide provided conservative estimates of 67% of cases in men and 28% in women, corresponding to 100 600 new cases each year and, assuming no effect of smoking on laryngeal cancer-specific mortality, 55 600 deaths (Parkin *et al.* 1994).

Tobacco control is the main avenue for prevention of laryngeal cancer; the evidence of an interaction between tobacco smoking and other risk factors should not be used as an argument to reduce the emphasis on avoiding and quitting smoking. As it is shown in Fig. 21.5, tobacco smoking plays by far the largest aetiological role in laryngeal carcinogenesis, either alone or in combination with other factors. The decline during the recent decades in the incidence of laryngeal cancer among men in some regions in which tobacco control has been implemented more effectively (e.g. the USA and Finland vs. Denmark, Fig. 21.6) suggests that prevention of this disease through the avoidance of its major cause is possible. As for other tobacco-related diseases, the main priorities are today among women and in the developing countries.

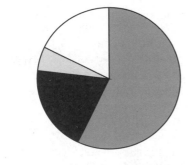

Fig. 21.5 Risk of laryngeal cancer attributable to tobacco smoking and alcohol drinking—Northern Italy (Tavani *et al.* 1994).

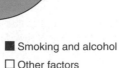

■ Smoking alone   ■ Smoking and alcohol
□ Alcohol alone   □ Other factors

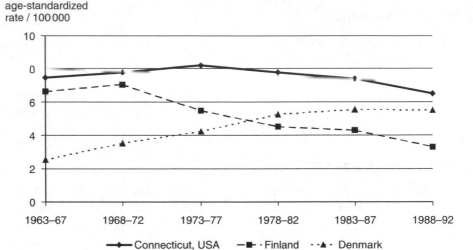

Fig. 21.6 Time trends in the incidence of laryngeal cancer among men in selected regions (Cattaruzza *et al.* 1996; Parkin *et al.* 1997).

References

Austin, D. F., and Reynolds, P. (1996). Laryngeal cancer. In: *Cancer epidemiology and prevention* (2nd edn.) (ed. D. Schottenfeld and J.F. Fraumeni, Jr), pp. 619–36. Oxford University Press, New York.

Baron, A. E., Franceschi, S., Barra, S., Talamini, R., and La Vecchia, C. (1993). A comparison of the joint effects of alcohol and smoking on the risk of cancer across sites in the upper aerodigestive tract. *Cancer Epidemiol Biomarkers Prev*, **2**, 519–23.

Benhamou, S., Bouchardy, C., Paoletti, C., and Dayer, P. (1996). Effects of CYP2D6 activity and tobacco on larynx cancer risk. *Cancer Epidemiol Biomarkers Prev*, **5**, 683–6.

Berrino, F. (1993). Occupational factors of upper respiratory tract cancers. *Prevention of respiratory diseases (Lung Biology in Health Disease, Vol 68)*. In: (ed. A. Hirsch, M. Goldberg, JP. Martin, R. Masse), pp. 81–96. Marcel Dekker, New York.

Boffetta, P., Merletti, F., Faggiano, F., Migliaretti, G., Ferro, G., Zanetti, R., *et al.* (1997). Prognostic factors and survival of laryngeal cancer patients from Turin, Italy: A population-based study. *Am J Epidemiol*, **145**, 1100–5.

Brennan, P. and Boffetta, P. Head and neck cancer. In: *Mechanistic considerations in the molecular epidemiology of cancer (IARC Scientific Publication No 157)* (ed. P. Buffler, M. Bizd, P., Boffetta, JM. Rice). International Agency for Research on Cancer, Lyon (in press).

Brownson, R. C., and Chang, J. C. (1987). Exposure to alcohol and tobacco and the risk of laryngeal cancer. *Arch Environ Health*, **42**, 192–6.

Brugere, J., Guenel, P., Leclerc, A., and Rodriguez, J. (1986). Differential effects of tobacco and alcohol in cancer of the larynx, pharynx, and mouth. *Cancer*, **57**, 391–5.

Burch, J. D., Howe, G. R., Miller, A. B., and Semenciw, R. (1981). Tobacco, alcohol, asbestos, and nickel in the etiology of cancer of the larynx: A case-control study. *J Natl Cancer Inst*, **67**, 1219–24.

Burns, D. M., Shanks, T. G., Choi, W., Thun, M. J., Heath, C. W., Jr., and Garfinkel, L. (1996). *The American Cancer Society Cancer Prevention Study I: 12-year followup of 1 million men and women (Smoking and Tobacco Control Monograph No 8)*, pp. 113-304. National Cancer Institute, Washington (DC).

Cattaruzza, M. S., Maisonneuve, P., and Boyle, P. (1996). Epidemiology of laryngeal cancer. *Oral Oncol Eur J Cancer*, **32**, 293–305.

Choi, S. Y., and Kahyo, H. (1991). Effect of cigarette smoking and alcohol consumption in the aetiology of cancer of the oral cavity, pharynx and larynx. *Int J Epidemiol*, **20**, 878–85.

Crosignani, P., Russo, A., Tagliabue, G., and Berrino, F. (1996). Tobacco and diet as determinants of survival in male laryngeal cancer patients. *Int J Cancer*, **65**, 308–13.

De Stefani, E., Correa, P., Oreggia, F., Leiva, J., Rivero, S., Fernandcz, G., *et al.* (1987). Risk factors for laryngeal cancer. *Cancer*, **60**, 3087–91.

De Stefani, E., Oreggia, F., Rivero, S., and Fierro, L. (1992). Hand-rolled cigarette smoking and risk of cancer of the mouth, pharynx, and larynx. *Cancer*, **70**, 679–82.

De Stefani, E., Oreggia, F., Rivero, S., Ronco, A., and Fierro, L. (1995). Salted meat consumption and the risk of laryngeal cancer. *Eur J Epidemiol*, **11**, 177–80.

Doll, R., and Hill, A. B. (1954). The mortality of doctors in relation to their smoking habits: A preliminary report. *Brit Med J*, **1**, 1451–5.

Dorn, H. F. (1959). Tobacco consumption and mortality from cancer and other diseases. *Public Health Rep*, **74**, 581–93.

Dosemeci, M., Gokmen, I., Unsal, M., Hayes, R. B., and Blair, A. (1997). Tobacco, alcohol use, and risks of laryngeal and lung cancer by subsite and histologic type in Turkey. *Cancer Causes Control*, **8**, 729–37.

Elwood, J. M., Pearson, J. C. G., Skippen, D. H., and Jackson, S. M. (1984). Alcohol, smoking, social and occupational factors in the aetiology of cancer of the oral cavity, pharynx and larynx. *Int J Cancer*, **34**, 603–12.

Falk, R. T., Pickle, L. W., Brown, L. M., Mason, T. J., Buffler, P. A., and Fraumeni, J. F. Jr. (1989). Effect of smoking and alcohol consumption on laryngeal cancer risk in coastal Texas. *Cancer Res*, **49**, 4024–9.

Ferlay, J., Bray, F., Pisani, P., and Parkin, D. M. (ed.) (2001). *Globocan 2000: Cancer incidence, mortality and prevalence worldwide (IARC Cancer Bases No 5)*. International Agency for Research on Cancer, Lyon.

Flanders, W. D., and Rothman, K. J. (1982). Interaction of alcohol and tobacco in laryngeal cancer. *Am J Epidemiol*, **115**, 371–9.

Franceschi, S., Talamini, R., Barra, S., Baron, A. E., Negri, E., Bidoli, E., *et al.* (1990). Smoking and drinking in relation to cancers of the oral cavity, pharynx, larynx, and esophagus in northern Italy. *Cancer Res.*, **50**, 6502–7.

Freudenheim, J. L., Graham, S., Byers, T. E., Marshall, J. R., Haughey, B. P., Swanson, M. K., *et al.* (1992). Diet, smoking, and alcohol in cancer of the larynx: A case-control study. *Nutr Cancer*, **17**, 33–45.

Graham, S., Mettlin, C., Marshall, J., Priore, R., Rzepka, T., and Shedd, D. (1981). Dietary factors in the epidemiology of cancer of the larynx. *Am J Epidemiol*, **113**, 675–80.

Guenel, P., Chastang, J-F., Luce, D., Leclerc, A., and Brugere, J. (1988). A study of the interaction of alcohol drinking and tobacco smoking among French cases of laryngeal cancer. *J Epidemiol Comm Health*, **42**, 350–4.

Haugen, A. (2002). Women who smoke: Are women more susceptiblie to tobacco-induced lung cancer? *Carcinogenesis*, **23**, 227–9.

Hedberg, K., Vaughan, T. L., White, E., Davis, S., and Thomas, D. B. (1994). Alcoholism and cancer of the larynx: A case-control study in western Washington (United States). *Cancer Causes Control*, **5**, 3–8.

Herity, B., Moriarty, M., Daly, L., Dunn, J., and Bourke, G. J. (1982). The role of tobacco and alcohol in the aetiology of lung and larynx cancer. *Br J Cancer*, **46**, 961–4.

IARC (1992). Occupational exposures to mists and vapours from sulfuric acid and other strong inorganic acids. In: *IARC Monographs on the Evaluation of Carcinogenic Risks to Humans, Vol 54, Occupational exposures to mists and vapours from strong inorganic acids; and other industrial chemicals*, pp. 41–130. International Agency for Research on Cancer, Lyon.

Jourenkova, N., Reinikainen, M., Bouchardy, C., Dayer, P., Benhamou, S., and Hirvonen, A. (1998). Larynx cancer risk in relation to glutathione 3-transferase M1 and T1 genotypes and tobacco smoking. *Cancer Epidemiol Biomarkers Prev*, **7**, 19–23.

Jussawalla, D. J. and Deshpande, V. A. (1971). Evaluation of cancer risk in tobacco chewers and smokers: An epidemiologic assessment. *Cancer*, **28**, 244–52.

Lewin, F., Norell, S. E., Johansson, H., Gustavsson, P., Wennerberg, J., Biörklund, A., *et al.* (1998). Smoking tobacco, oral snuff, and alcohol in the etiology of squamous cell carcinoma of the head and neck: A population-based case-referent study in Sweden. *Cancer*, **82**, 1367–75.

Lopez-Abente, G., Pollan, M., Monge, V., and Martinez-Vidal, A. (1992). Tobacco smoking, alcohol consumption, and laryngeal cancer in Madrid. *Cancer Detection Prev*, **16**, 265–71.

Maier, H., Gewelke, U., Dietz, A., and Heller, W- D. (1992). Risk factors of cancer of the larynx: Results of the Heidelberg case-control study. *Otolaryngol Head Neck Surg*, **107**, 577–82.

Muscat, J. E., and Wynder, E. L. (1992). Tobacco, alcohol, asbestos, and occupational risk factors for laryngeal cancer. *Cancer*, **69**, 2244–51.

Olsen, J., Sabreo, S., and Fasting, U. (1985). Interaction of alcohol and tobacco as risk factors in cancer of the laryngeal region. *J Epidemiol Comm Health*, **39**, 165–8.

Parkin, D. M., Pisani, P., Lopez, A. D., and Masuyer, E. (1994). At least one in seven cases of cancer is caused by smoking: Global estimates for 1985. *Int J Cancer*, **59**, 494–504.

Parkin, D. M., Whelan, S. L., Ferlay, J., Raymond, L., and Young, J. (ed.) (1997). *Cancer Incidence in Five Continents, Vol 7 (IARC Scientific Publications No 143)*. International Agency for Research on Cancer, Lyon.

Restrepo, H. E., Correa, P., Haenszel, W., Brinton, L. A., and Franco, A. (1989). A case–control study of tobacco-related cancers in Colombia. *Bull Pan Am Health Organ*, **23**, 405–13.

Sankaranarayanan, R., Duffy, S. W., Nair, M. K., Padmakumary, G., and Day, N. E. (1990). Tobacco and alcohol as risk factors in cancer of the larynx in Kerala, India. *Int J Cancer*, **45**, 879–82.

Schlecht, N., Franco, E. L., Pintos, J., and Kowalski, L. P. (1999). Effect of smoking cessation and tobacco type on the risk of cancers of the upper areo-digestive tract in Brazil. *Epidemiology*, **10**, 412–8.

Schrek, R., Baker, L. A., Ballard, G. P., and Dolgoff, S. (1950). Tobacco smoking as an etiologic factor in disease, I, Cancer. *Cancer Res*, **10**, 49–58.

Simarakl, S., de Jong, U. W., Breslow, N., Dahl, C. J., Ruckphaopunt, K., and Scheelings, P., *et al.* (1977). Cancer of the oral cavity, pharynx/larynx and lung in north Thailand: Case-control study and analysis of cigar smoke. *Br J Cancer*, **36**, 130–40.

Stewart, B. W., and Semmler, P. C. (2002). Sharp v Port Kembla RSL Club: Establishing causation of laryngeal cancer by environmental tobacco smoke. *Med J Aust*, **176**, 113–6.

Tan, E-H., Adelstein, D. J., Droughton, M. L., Van Kirk, M. A., and Lavertu, P. (1997). Squamous cell head and neck cancer in nonsmokers. *Am J Clin Oncol*, **20**, 146–50.

Tavani, A., Negri, E., Franceschi, S., Barbone, F., and La Vecchia, C. (1994). Attributable risk for laryngeal cancer in northern Italy. *Cancer Epidemiol Biomarkers Prev*, **3**, 121–5.

Tuyns, A. J., Esteve, J., Raymond, L., Berrino, F., Benhamou, E., Blanchet, F., *et al.* (1988). Cancer of the larynx/hypopharynx, tobacco and alcohol: IARC international case-control study in Turin and Varese (Italy), Zaragoza and Navarra (Spain), Geneva (Switzerland) and Calvados (France). *Int J Cancer*, **41**, 483–91.

USDHEW (1964). Laryngeal cancer. In: *Smoking and health: Report of the Advisory Committee to the Surgeon General of the Public Health Service*, pp. 205–12. US Department of Health, Education and Welfare, Public Health Service.

WCRF (World Cancer Research Fund) (1997). *Food, nutrition and the prevention of cancer: A global perspective*. American Institute for Cancer Research, Washington (DC).

Wynder, E. L., Bross, I. J., and Day, E. (1955). A study of environmental factors in cancer of the larynx. *Cancer*, **9**, 86–110.

Wynder, E. L., Covey, L. S., Mabuchi, K., and Mushinski, M. (1976). Environmental factors in cancer of the larynx: A second look. *Cancer*, **38**, 1591–601.

Wynder, E. L., and Stellman, S. D. (1979). Impact of long-term filter cigarette usage on lung and larynx cancer risk: A case-control study. *J Natl Cancer Inst*, **62**, 471–7.

Zatonski, W., Becher, H., Lissowska, J., and Wahrendorf, J. (1991). Tobacco, alcohol, and diet in the etiology of laryngeal cancer: A population-based case-control study. *Cancer Causes Control*, **2**, 3–10.

Zhang, Z. -F., Morgenstern, H., Spitz, M. R., Tashkin, D. P., Yu, G-P., Hsu, T. C., *et al.* (2000). Environmental tobacco smoking, mutagen sensitivity, and head and neck squamous cell carcinoma. *Cancer Epidemiol Biomarkers Prev*, **9**, 1043–9.

Zheng, W., Blot, W. J., Shu, X.-O., Gao, Y.-T., Ji, B.-T., Ziegler, R. G., *et al.* (1992). Diet and other risk factors for laryngeal cancer in Shanghai, China. *Am J Epidemiol*, **136**, 178–91.

Chapter 22

Smoking and cancer of the oesophagus

Eva Negri

It has been estimated that in the year 2000 there were in the world about 280 000 new cases of oesophageal cancer (OC) among men and 130 000 among women (Ferlay *et al.* 2001). The great majority of these cases (220 000 men and 120 000 women) occur in less developed countries. The age-standardized rate in men is twofold in less developed areas compared to more developed areas of the world (12.8/100 000 vs 6.7/100 000). In women the ratio between rates in less and more developed areas is 5 (6.2/100 000 vs 1.3/100 000).

OC incidence rates show a remarkably large geographical variation, with a difference of over 300-fold between high- and low-risk areas (Munoz and Day 1996). Very high rates have been observed in a belt starting in eastern Turkey and extending through the southern states of the former Soviet Union, Iran, and Iraq into northern China (Kmet and Mahboudi 1972; Blot 1994). Large differences in rates can be observed also within small geographical areas (Munoz and Day 1996), and rapid changes of rates over time have been observed (Negri *et al.* 1996). In North America, rates are much higher among African Americans than among whites (Munoz and Day 1996).

The vast majority of OC worldwide are squamous-cell carcinomas of the oesophagus (SCCO), and most of the epidemiologic studies on OC were based solely or chiefly on this histologic type. Increases in the incidence of adenocarcinoma of the oesophagus (ACO) have been reported in the US and other countries, and adenocarcinoma has become the most frequent cell type among US whites (Blot and McLaughlin 1999).

Squamous cell and adenocarcinoma of the oesophagus differ in geographic distribution, temporal trends and risk factors, and thus represent two separate epidemiological entities. Thus, they will be considered separately in this chapter.

Squamous-cell carcinoma of the oesophagus (SCCO)

Already in the late 1950s some studies reported an association between tobacco and cancer of the oesophagus (Hammond and Horn 1958; Dorn 1959; Tuyns *et al.* 1977), although the authors still doubted the causality of this association.

In the following years, further evidence accumulated, and in 1986 the International Agency for Research on Cancer (IARC) concluded that 'smoking is an important cause of oesophageal cancer' (IARC 1986). Several other studies published since have further confirmed this association, and in the evaluation on the carcinogenicity of tobacco done in 2002 the IARC concluded that 'tobacco smoking is causally associated with cancer of the oesophagus' (IARC 2002).

This conclusion relies on overwhelming evidence, derived from studies conducted in different areas of the world and with different designs, that—with only very rare exceptions—found higher risks of OC in smokers. Table 22.1 shows the results of selected case–control studies of OC. As it will be discussed later, alcohol consumption is an important confounder/effect modifier of the relation between smoking and risk of SCCO. Thus, only studies that present alcohol-adjusted estimates are included in the table. In most studies, the risk of smokers was 2–5 times that of never smokers, and the risk of former smokers was intermediate between the two. The causality of the association is further supported by the fact that the risk of oesophageal cancer increases with increasing daily dose and with duration of the habit in almost all studies.

Type of cigarettes. De Stefani and colleagues (1993) noted that the OR of OC were higher in studies conducted in populations smoking mainly black tobacco, as compared to those in populations smoking predominantly blond tobacco. Consistently, studies presenting ORs separately for smokers of blond and black tobacco cigarettes tended to find higher risks in black tobacco smokers. Compared to blond tobacco cigarette smoker, the risk of OC of black tobacco cigarette smokers was 2.6 and 3.6 in two studies from Uruguay (De Stefani *et al.* 1993). Smokers of hand-rolled cigarettes also tend to have higher risks of OC than smokers of commercial cigarettes (Tuyns and Esteve 1983; De Stefani *et al.* 1993; Hu *et al.* 1994; Launoy *et al.* 2000). Also high-tar cigarettes convey a higher risk of OC (La Vecchia *et al.* 1986).

Cigars and pipe smoking. Also cigar and pipe smokers have an increased risk of OC. In the study by Wynder and Bross (1961) the OR of OC of cigarette smokers was 2.8, compared to never smokers, that of cigar and pipe smokers was 6.0, and that of pipe only smokers was 9.0. Other studies also found higher risks of OC in pipe smokers compared to cigarette smokers (Tuyns and Esteve 1983; De Stefani *et al.* 1993). The studies that analysed the risk of smokers of cigars only were generally based on small numbers of cases, but they consistently found an increased risk of about fourfold for ever cigar smokers (La Vecchia *et al.* 1998; Shanks and Burns 1998).

Interaction with alcohol. Alcohol is another well-established risk factor for OC, and alcohol and tobacco act synergistically in magnifying the risk. Thus, in countries where both habits are widespread, the effect of tobacco cannot be considered separately from that of alcohol. Some studies have analysed how the joint exposure to alcohol and tobacco influences the risk of OC.

Already in 1961 Wynder and Bross noted that both factors were independently associated to oesophageal cancer risk. In 1977 Tuyns and colleagues published the results of their case–control study on cancer of the oesophagus conducted in

Table 22.1 Results from selected case–control studies on smoking and risk of squamous-cell carcinoma of the oesophagus

Reference and location	Type of controls Cases:controls	OR for current and former smokers	Dose Cutpoints	Dose OR[1]	Duration Cutpoints	Duration OR[1]
North America						
Wynder and Bross, 1961—New York, USA	Hospital 99 OC[2]:100 Co[3]		1–9[4] 10–20 21–34 ≥35	2.3 2.7 4.1 4.6		
Brown et al. 1988—Coastal South Carolina, USA	Hospital or deceased (for deceased cases) 207 OC:422 Co Men only	Current: OR=1.8 (1.0–3.0) Former (<10 yrs) 2.0 (1.0–3.7) Former (10+ yrs) 1.0 (0.5–2.1)	1–19[5] 20–29 ≥30	0.8 (0.4–2.5) 2.0 (1.1–3.4) 2.6 (1.4–4.7)	1–24 yrs 25–34 ≥35	1.4 (0.6–2.9) 1.6 (1.0–2.8) 1.8 (1.0–3.3)
Kabat et al. 1993—8 US cities	Hospital 212 SCCO[6]: 6772 Co	*Men* Current OR=4.5 (2.5–8.1) Former OR=1.3 (0.7–2.4) *Women* Current OR=6.8 (3.7–12) Former OR=2.2 (1.1–4.3)	1–20[5] 21–30 >30 1–20 >20	1.9 (1.1–3.5) 2.7 (1.3–5.4) 2.7 (1.5–5.0) 3.7 (2.0–6.7) 4.8 (2.4–9.5)		
Gammon et al. 1997—3 areas of USA	Population 221 SCCO:695 Co	Current OR=5.1 (2.8–9.2) Former OR=2.8 (1.5–4.9)	<16[5] 16–20 21–30 >30	2.7 (1.4–5.1) 3.9 (2.1–7.2) 5.3 (2.6–11) 3.9 (2.0–7.6)	<20 yrs 20–31 32–42 >42	1.8 (0.9–3.7) 2.0 (1.0–4.0) 3.3 (1.8–6.1) 5.9 (2.0–7.6)

Table 22.1 (continued) Results from selected case–control studies on smoking and risk of squamous-cell carcinoma of the oesophagus

Reference and location	Type of controls Cases:controls	OR for current and former smokers	Dose Cutpoints	Dose OR[1]	Duration Cutpoints	Duration OR[1]
South America						
Castellsagué et al. 1999—Argentina, Brasil, Paraguay, Uruguay	Hospital (5 studies) 830 SCCO:1779 Co	*Men* Current OR=5.1 (3.4–7.6) Former OR=2.8 (1.8–4.3)	1–7[5] 8–14 15–24 ≥25	2.2 (1.3–3.5) 4.1 (2.6–6.4) 5.3 (3.4–8.1) 5.0 (3.2–7.7)	1–29 yrs 30–39 40–49 ≥50	2.6 (1.7–4.2) 3.6 (2.3–5.6) 4.7 (3.0–7.2) 5.0 (3.8–9.5)
		Women Current OR=3.1 (1.8–5.3) Former OR=1.6 (0.8–3.1)	1–14[5] ≥15	2.1 (1.2–3.7) 2.8 (1.4–5.4)	1–29 yrs 30–39 ≥40	0.5 (0.8–2.9) 2.0 (0.9–4.4) 4.4 (2.2–9.0)
Europe						
Tuyns et al. 1977—Ille-et-Vilaine, France			0–9[4] 10–19 20–29 ≥30	1.0 (ref) 1.5 1.6 6.1		
Lagergren et al. 2000—Sweden	Population 167 SCCO: 820 Co	Current OR=9.3 (5.1–17) Former OR=2.5 (1.4–4.7)	1–9[5] 10–19 >19	2.3 (1.1–4.6) 2.9 (1.5–5.8) 8.8 (4.9–16)	1–20 yrs 21–35 >35	2.3 (1.1–4.6) 2.9 (1.5–5.8) 8.8 (4.9–16)
Zambon et al. 2000—Northern Italy	Hospital 275 SCCO:593 Co Men only		1–14[5] 15–24 ≥25	3.2 (1.6–6.4) 5.4 (2.8–10) 7.0 (3.2–15)	1–24 yrs 25–34 ≥35	1.5 (0.4–6.2) 2.6 (1.2–5.6) 6.4 (3.5–12)

Asia

Study	Population	Smoking status	Amount	Duration
Gao et al. 1994—Shanghai, China	Population 605 SCCO:1552 Co	Current OR=1.9* Former OR=1.6*	1–9[5]: 1.1 10–19: 1.7* 20–29: 2.5* ≥30: 4.8*	0.5–19 yrs: 0.7 20–29: 1.6* 30–39: 2.2* ≥40: 2.5*
Guo et al. 1994—Linxian, north-central China	Nested within a cohort 640 OC:3200 Co (Men only)	Ever OR=1.8 (1.4–2.4)	<10[5]: 1.8[7] (1.3–2.6) 10–19: 1.8 (1.3–2.5) ≥20: 1.9 (1.3–2.8)	<20 yrs: 1.2 (0.7–2.0) 20–39: 1.8 (1.3–2.5) ≥40: 2.1 (1.4–3.1)
Hu et al. 1994—North-east China	Hospital 196 OC:392 Co		1–10[5]: 1.7 (1.0–2.9) 11–20: 2.2 (1.3–3.7) 21–30: 1.7 (0.8–3.7) ≥31: 3.3 (1.5–7.4)	1–10 yrs: 1.5[8] (05.–5.2) 11–20: 2.1 (1.1–4.3) 21–30: 2.8 (1.6–5.0) ≥31: 3.3 (2.0–5.3)
Shankaranarayanan et al. 1991—Kerala, Southern India	Hospital 267 OC:895 Co		1–10[9]: 1.9 (0.8–4.3) 11–20: 3.9 (1.7–8.9) ≥21: 4.8 2.3–9.8)	<20[10] yrs: 2.1 (0.8–5.9) ≥20: 4.7 (2.8–7.9)
Takezaki et al. 2000—Nagoya, Japan	Outpatients 284 OC:11936 Co (Men only)	Current OR=3.5 (2.1–5.8) Former OR=1.6 (0.9–2.8)	1–19[5]: 3.1 (1.8–5.5) ≥20: 3.5 (2.1–5.9)	1–29 yrs: 2.2 (1.1–4.4) ≥30: 3.6 (2.1–6.0)

Africa

Study	Population	Smoking status	Amount	Duration
Segal et al. 1988—Soweto, South Africa	Hospital 200 OC:391 cont		0–19[4]: 1.0 (ref) 20–39: 3.0 (1.5–5.9) ≥40: 2.2 (1.3–3.7)	

Table 22.1 (continued) Results from selected case–control studies on smoking and risk of squamous-cell carcinoma of the oesophagus

Reference and location	Type of controls Cases:controls	OR for current and former smokers	Dose Cutpoints	Dose OR[1]	Duration Cutpoints	Duration OR[1]
Vizcaino et al. 1995—Bulawayo, Zimbabwe	Non-smoking or alcohol related cancers 826 OC:3007 Co Men only	Former OR=3.4 (1.9–6.2)	<15[4] ≥15	3.5 (2.7–4.5) 5.7 (3.8–8.4)		
Pacella-Norman et al. 2002—South Africa	Non-smoking or alcohol related cancers 267 OC:804 Co	Current OR=3.8 (2.3–6.1) Former OR=3.8 (2.3–6.3)	1–14[4] ≥15	3.3 (2.0–5.5) 6.0 (3.2–11)		

[1]All odds ratios presented were adjusted for age, sex (when required), plus a variable number of other potential confounders. The reference category is set to never smokers, if not otherwise specified.

[2]OC=oesophageal cancers.

[3]Co=controls.

[4]Grams of tobacco per day.

[5]Cigarettes per day.

[6]SCCO=squamous-cell oesophageal cancer.

[7]Not adjusted for alcohol. Drinking uncommon in controls, 22% of OC cases were drinkers.

[8]Not alcohol-adjusted.

[9]Cigarettes+bidi.

[10]Duration of bidi smoking.

Ille-et-Vilaine, France. This study of 200 cases of OC and 778 controls has been used in textbooks (Breslow and Day 1980) as an example of how the joint effect of two factors can affect the OR.

Figure 22.1 shows the odds ratios for the Ille-et-Vilaine study (Tuyns *et al.* 1977), modified by Doll and Peto (1981), for the combination of alcohol and tobacco. The reference category is set to those who smoke less than 10 g of tobacco per day, and drink 40 g or less alcohol per day. The risk of OC increases with dose of tobacco for each level of alcohol drinking: in non or light drinkers, the OR is 1.0 in smokers of less than 10 g of tobacco per day (reference category), 3.4 in smokers of 10–19 g/day, 3.8 in smokers of 20–29 g/day, and 7.8 in smokers of 30 or more g/day. In drinkers of 41–80 g/day the corresponding OR in subsequent categories of tobacco consumptions are 7.3, 8.4, 8.8, and 35.5; in drinkers of 81–120 g/day the OR for smoking are 11.7, 13.6, 12.4, and 87.1; and in very heavy drinkers (>120 g/day) the risk for increasing tobacco consumption categories are 49.8, 64.0, 130.7, and 149.3. Likewise, for every category of tobacco consumption, the OR increases as alcohol consumption increases. Heavy smokers and heavy drinkers have a risk of OC which is 150 times that of those who are non- or moderate smokers and non or moderate drinkers. This impressive risk would have been higher if only non-smokers had been included in the reference category. This was not possible due to lack of cases not exposed to the two factors: only 9 of the 200 cases were non-smokers, as compared to 57 expected from the control distribution, and none of them drank less than 40 g/day of alcohol. Thus, in the high-risk area of

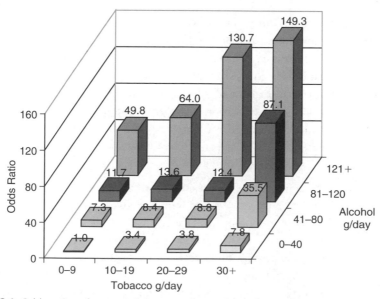

Figure 22.1 Odds ratios of cancer of the oesophagus for various combinations of alcohol and tobacco consumption. Data from Tuyns *et al.* (1977), modified by Doll and Peto (1981).

Ille-et-Vilaine, OC is a rare disease in non-smoking moderate drinkers. Further studies have confirmed that the risk of OC in heavy smokers and drinkers, compared to non- or light smokers and drinkers, is of that order of magnitude (Segal *et al.* 1988; Zambon *et al.* 2000).

Tuyns and colleagues further noted that the risks appeared to follow a multiplicative model, i.e. the risk for subjects simultaneously exposed to both alcohol and tobacco is the product of the risks of those exposed to only one factor. Breslow and Day (1980) have modeled in detail the relation between alcohol and tobacco consumption and risk of cancer of the oesophagus, using the Ille-et-Vilaine data. Also in many other studies, a multiplicative model appeared to describe the joint ORs for alcohol and tobacco satisfactorily (Zambon *et al.* 2000). Moreover, smoking may interact in a multiplicative way also with other risk factors, e.g. dietary factors.

Although oesophageal cancer is less frequent in women than in men in many countries, and most of the studies were based only or prevalently on men, smoking and drinking are also risk factors for women (Gallus *et al.* 2001).

Tobacco in alcohol non-drinkers. The few studies that investigated the effect of smoking in alcohol non-drinkers were generally based on small numbers of cases. Nevertheless, they have consistently reported that smoking is a risk factor for OC also in absence of alcohol consumption (Tuyns 1983; La Vecchia and Negri 1989; Tavani *et al.* 1996). These studies included both never and former drinkers. In a case–control study conducted in Hong Kong among never drinkers, smoking was still a risk factor for OC, and the OR for heavy smokers was increased 10-fold compared to never smokers (Cheng *et al.* 1995).

Smoking and drinking cessation. Several studies have shown that the risk is lower in ex-smokers than in current smokers, and declines steeply with time since stopping smoking (Brown *et al.* 1988; Yu *et al.* 1988; La Vecchia *et al.* 1990; Castellsagué *et al.* 1999a).

A study conducted in Italy and Switzerland provided convincing evidence that stopping consumption of both alcohol and tobacco leads to a substantial reduction of OC risk (Bosetti *et al.* 2000). After 10 or more years since stopping both habits the risk was only about one-tenth of that of current smokers and drinkers (Fig. 22.2). Similar results were found also in a combined analysis of five case–control studies conducted in South America (Castellsagué *et al.* 2000).

Attributable risks. The proportion of cases of OC attributable to smoking, and to the joint effect of alcohol and tobacco, varies widely between geographical areas. The attributable fraction depends not only from the relative risk but also from the frequency of the exposure in a population. Moreover, as shown above, the effect of smoking is magnified by alcohol (and possibly other risk factors). Thus, even the same amount of smoking may have a different impact in populations with different exposure to alcohol or other factors. In North and South America and Europe, alcohol and tobacco explain the vast majority of cases, particularly in men, where the disease is more frequent than

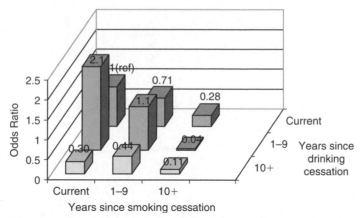

Fig. 22.2 Odds ratios of cancer of the oesophagus for various combinations of times since cessation of alcohol and tobacco consumption. Data from Bosetti *et al.* (2000).

in women (Wynder and Bross 1961; Tuyns *et al.* 1977; Negri *et al.* 1992; Castellsagué *et al.* 1999*b*). Moreover, different smoking and alcohol consumptions have been shown to account for the differences in rates between sexes or urban and rural areas (Tuyns *et al.* 1977; Negri *et al.* 1992).

In some areas of China and central Asia where the higher incidence rates of the world are observed, and rates in women are comparable to those in men, these two factors appear to play only a limited role, and nutritional deficiencies or other yet not well-identified factors may play an important role (Munoz and Day 1996). The effect of tobacco, however, is not negligible in some areas of Asia and Africa. Tobacco accounted for 50% of cases in men and 14% in women in urban Shanghai (Gao *et al.* 1994), 54% of cases in Bombay (Jayant *et al.* 1977), and 54% in men in Bulawayo, Zimbabwe (Vizcaino *et al.* 1995).

Adenocarcinoma of the oesophagus

Adenocarcinoma of the oesophagus is much less frequent, worldwide, than SCCO. There are thus fewer and smaller studies available. Most studies have been conducted in North America and Europe, and only few data from other areas of the world are available. This neoplasm resembles under many aspects to the adenocarcinoma of the gastric cardia, and cancers that occur at the oesophageal-gastric junction are difficult to attribute to one site or the other. Thus, several studies have considered adenocarcinomas of the oesophagus and gastric cardia together. There is, however, evidence that these two cancers differ as concerns their geographic distribution and risk factors (Lagergren *et al.* 1999; Corley and Buffler 2001; Eksteen *et al.* 2001). Thus, in this review we consider only studies showing separate results for adenocarcinoma of the oesophagus. Table 22.2 presents the results of selected studies of ACO according to

Table 22.2 Results from selected case–control studies on smoking and risk of adenocarcinoma of the oesophagus

Reference and location	Type of controls Cases:controls	OR for current and former smokers	Dose Cutpoints	Dose OR[1]	Duration Cutpoints	Duration OR[1]
North America						
Brown et al. 1994—3 areas of the USA	Population 174 ACO[2,3] 750 Co[4] Men only	Current OR=1.7 (0.9–3.2)	<20[5] 20–39 ≥40	1.1 (0.5–2.4) 2.4 (1.3–4.4) 2.6 (1.3–5.0)	<30 yrs 30–39 ≥40	2.5 (1.3–4.7) 2.5 (1.3–4.9) 1.6 (0.8–3.2)
Gammon et al. 1997—3 areas of USA	Population 293 ACO: 695 Co	Current OR=2.2 (1.4–3.3) Former OR=2.0 (1.4–2.9)	<16[5] 16–20 21–30 >30	1.5 (1.0–2.4) 2.2 (1.4–3.4) 3.1 (1.9–5.1) 2.1 (1.3–3.3)	<20 yrs 20–31 32–42 >42	1.4 (0.9–2.2) 1.7 (1.0–2.8) 2.9 (1.8–4.4) 2.4 (1.5–3.7)
Wu et al. 2001— Los Angeles county, USA	Population 222 ACO:1356	Current OR=2.8 (1.8–4.3) Former OR=1.5 (1.0–2.2)	Former 1–19[5] ≥20 Current 1– 20–39 ≥40	1.2 (0.8–2.0) 1.7 (1.1–2.5) 1.6 (0.7–3.3) 2.9 (1.8–4.8) 4.5 (2.3–8.7)	≤20 yrs 21–40 ≥41	1.4 (0.9–2.2) 2.1 (1.4–3.1) 2.2 (1.3–3.5)
Europe						
Levi et al. 1990—Lausanne, Switzerland	Barrett's oesophagus (BE) 30 ACO in BE: 140 Co with BE		<15[6] 15–24 >25	1.0 (0.3–.41) 0.6 (0.2–1.9) 0.9 (0.3–2.9)		
Menke-Pluymers et al. 1993—Rotterdam, The Netherlands	BE 62 ACO in BE: 96 Co with BE	Current OR=2.3[7] (p<0.05)				

Study	Study type / subjects	Smoking status	Cigarettes/day	Duration
Garidou et al. 1996—Athens, Greece	Hospital 56 ACO:200 Co		≤20[5] 1.5 (0.7–3.1) >20 2.7 (1.3–5.8)	
Cheng et al. 2000—4 regions of the UK	Population 74 ACO:74 Co Women only	Current OR=1.4 (0.5–3.7) Former OR=1.0 (0.5–1.9)		≤37.7 yrs 0.2 (0.02–2.0) 37.7–48.6 2.2 (0.4–12) ≥48.6 3.0 (0.6–16)
Lagergren et al. 2000—Sweden	Population 189 ACO:820 Co	Current OR=1.6 (0.9–2.7) Former OR=1.9 (1.2–2.9)	1–9[5] 1.2 (0.7–2.2) 10–19 1.7 (1.0–2.9) >19 1.1 (0.6–2.0)	1–20 yrs 1.8 (1.1–3.1) 21–35 1.5 (0.9–2.6) >35 2.0 (1.2–3.3)
Asia				
Gao et al. 1994—Shanghai, China	Population 55 ACO:1552 Co	Current OR=2.1 Former OR=1.8	1–9[5] 2.0 10–19 1.1 20–29 2.0 ≥30 3.5	0.5–19[1] yrs 1.8 20–29 1.0 30–39 2.0 ≥40 2.0

[1] All odds ratios presented were adjusted for age and sex (when required) and alcohol consumption (plus a variable number of other potential confounders), if not otherwise specified. The reference category is set to never smokers, if not otherwise specified.

[2] ACO=adenocarcinoma of the oesophagus.

[3] Includes oesophagogastric junction.

[4] Co=controls.

[5] Cigarettes per day.

[6] Grams of tobacco per day.

[7] Former smokers and smokers of less than 5 cigarettes/day included in the reference category.

tobacco consumption. In spite of the small number of cases in many studies, smoking is quite consistently associated to the risk of ACO, and the risk increases with increasing dose and duration. For this reason the IARC evaluation of tobacco in 2002 concluded that tobacco smoking is causally associated with adenocarcinoma of the oesophagus (IARC 2002). In contrast with SCCO, alcohol consumption does not appear to increase the risk of ACO, and thus interaction between alcohol and tobacco is not an important issue for this histologic type.

While the risk of SCCO decreases steadily after stopping smoking, Gammon *et al.* (1997) did not observe a decline in risk of ACO until 30 years after smoking cessation. They thus suggested that smoking may affect an early stage in the induction of oesophageal adenocarcinoma, whereas a later stage may be involved in SCCO. This could also partly explain the diverging trends observed for the two histologic types of oesophageal cancer in the US and some European countries.

References

Blot, W. J. (1994). Esophageal cancer trends and risk factors. 46: *Semin Oncol*, **21**, 403–10.

Blot, W. J. and McLaughlin, J. K. (1999). The changing epidemiology of esophageal cancer. *Semin Oncol*, **26** (Suppl 15), 2–8.

Bosetti, C., Franceschi, S., Levi, F., Negri, E., Talamini, R., and La Vecchia, C. (2000). Smoking and drinking cessation and the risk of oesophageal cancer. *Br J Cancer*, **83**, 689–91.

Brown, L. M., Blot, W. J., Schuman, S. H., Smith, V. M., Ershow, A. G., Marks, R. D., and Fraumeni, J. F., Jr. (1988). Environmental factors and high risk of esophageal cancer among men in coastal South Carolina. *J Natl Cancer Inst*, **80**, 1620–5.

Brown, L. M., Silverman, D. T., Pottern, L. M., Schoenberg, J. B., Greenberg, R. S., Swanson, G. M., *et al.* (1994). Adenocarcinoma of the esophagus and esophagogastric junction in white men in the United States: alcohol, tobacco, and socioeconomic factors. *Cancer Causes Control*, **5**, 333–40.

Breslow, N. E. and Day, N. E. (1980). Statistical methods in cancer research, Vol. 1: The analysis of case-control studies. International Agency for Research on Cancer, Lyon. *Sci Publ* 32.

Castellsagué, X. and Munoz, N. (1999*a*). Re: Cancer of the oral cavity and pharynx in nonsmokers who drink alcohol and in nondrinkers who smoke tobacco. *J Natl Cancer Inst*, **91**, 1336–8.

Castellsagué, X., Munoz, N., De Stefani, E., Victora, C. G., Castelletto, R., Rolon, P. A., and Quintana, M. J., (1999*b*). Independent and joint effects of tobacco smoking and alcohol drinking on the risk of esophageal cancer in men and women. *Int J Cancer*, **82**, 657–64.

Castellsagué, X., Munoz, N., De Stefani, E., Victora, C. G., Quintana, M. J., Castelletto, R., and Rolon, P. A. (2000). Smoking and drinking cessation and risk of esophageal cancer (Spain). *Cancer Causes Control*, **11**, 813–8.

Cheng, K. K., Duffy, S. W., Day, N. E., and Lam, T. H. (1995). Oesophageal cancer in never-smokers and never-drinkers. *Int J Cancer*, **60**, 820–2.

Cheng, K. K., Sharp, L., McKinney, P. A., Logan, R. F., Chilvers, C. E., Cook-Mozaffari, P., *et al.* (2000). A case–control study of oesophageal adenocarcinoma in women: A preventable disease. *Br J Cancer*, **83**, 127–32.

Corley, D. A. and Buffler, P. A. (2001). Oesophageal and gastric cardia adenocarcinomas: Analysis of regional variation using the Cancer Incidence in Five Continents database. *Int J Epidemiol*, **30**, 1415–25.

De Stefani, E., Barrios, E., and Fierro, L. (1993). Black (air-cured) and blond (flue-cured) tobacco and cancer risk. III: Oesophageal cancer. *Eur J Cancer*, **29A**, 763–6.

Doll, R. and Peto, R. (1981). The causes of cancer. *J Natl Cancer Inst*, **66**, 1191–308.

Dorn, H. F. (1959). Tobacco consumption and mortality from cancer and other diseases. *Publ Health Rep*, **74**, 581–93.

Eksteen, J. A., Latchford, A., Thomas, S. J., and Jankowski, J. A. (2001). Commentary: Regional variations in oesophageal and gastric cardiacancers—implications and practice. *Int J Epidemiol*, **30**, 1425–7.

Ferlay, J., Bray, F., Pisani, P., and Parkin, D. M. (2001). GLOBOCAN 2000: Cancer Incidence, Mortality and Prevalence Worldwide, Version 1.0. IARC CancerBase No. 5. Lyon, IARC Press.

Gallus, S., Bosetti, C., Franceschi, S., Levi, F., Simonato, L., Negri, E., and La Vecchia, C. (2001). Oesophageal cancer in women: Tobacco, alcohol, nutritional and hormonal factors. *Br J Cancer*, **85**, 341–5.

Gammon, M. D., Schoenberg, J. B., Ahsan, H., Risch, H. A., Vaughan, T. L., Chow, W. H., *et al.* (1997). Tobacco, alcohol, and socioeconomic status and adenocarcinomas of the esophagus and gastric cardia. *J Natl Cancer Inst*, **89**, 1277–84.

Gao, Y. T., McLaughlin, J. K., Blot, W. J., Ji, B. T., Benichou, J., Dai, Q., and Fraumeni, J. F. Jr. (1994). Risk factors for esophageal cancer in Shanghai, China. I. Role of cigarette smoking and alcohol drinking. *Int J Cancer*, **58**, 192–6.

Garidou, A., Tzonou, A., Lipworth, L., Signorello, L. B., Kalapothaki, V., and Trichopoulos, D. (1996). Life-style factors and medical conditions in relation to esophageal cancer byhistologic type in a low-risk population. *Int J Cancer*, **68**, 295–9.

Guo, W., Blot, W. J., Li, J. Y., Taylor, P. R., Liu, B. Q., Wang, W., *et al.*(1994). A nested case-control study of oesophageal and stomach cancers in the Linxian nutrition intervention trial. *Int J Epidemiol*, **23**, 444–50.

Hammond, E. C. and Horn, D. (1958). Smoking and death rates. Report on 44 months of follow-up of 187,783 men. *J. Am. Med. Ass.*, **116**, 1159–72 and 1294–1308.

Hu, J., Nyren, O., Wolk, A., Bergstrom, R., Yuen, J., Adami, H. O., *et al.* (1994). Risk factors for oesophageal cancer in northeast China. *Int J Cancer*, **57**, 38–46.

International Agency for Research on Cancer (1986). Tobacco smoking. In: IARC Monographs on the evaluation of the carcinogenic risk of chemicals to Human, Vol. 38. WHO, IARC, Lyon.

International Agency for Research on Cancer (2002). Tobacco smoking and tobacco smoke. In IARC monographs on the evaluation of the carcinogenic risks to Human, Vol. 83. WHO, IARC, Lyon.

Jayant, K., Balakrishnan, V., Sanghvi, L. D., and Jussawalla, D. J. (1977). Quantification of the role of smoking and chewing tobacco in oral, pharyngeal, and oesophageal cancers. *Br J Cancer*, **35**, 232–5.

Kabat, G. C., Ng, S. K., and Wynder, E. L. (1993). Tobacco, alcohol intake, and diet in relation to adenocarcinoma of the esophagus and gastric cardia. *Cancer Causes Control*, **4**, 123–32.

Kmet, J. and Mahboudi, E. (1972). Esophageal cancer in the Caspian littoral of Iran: Initial studies. *Science*, **175**, 846–53.

La Vecchia, C., Liati, P., Decarli, A., Negrello, I., and Franceschi, S. (1986). Tar yields of cigarettes and the risk of oesophageal cancer. *Int J Cancer*, **38**, 381–5.

La Vecchia, C. and Negri, E. (1989). The role of alcohol in oesophageal cancer in non-smokers, and of tobacco in non-drinkers. *Int J Cancer*, **43**, 784–5.

La Vecchia, C., Bidoli, E., Bana, S., D'Avanzo, B., Negri, E., Talamini, R., Franceschi, S. (1990). Type of cigarettes and cancers of the upper digestive and respiratory tract. *Cancer, Causes, Controls*, **1**, 69–74.

La Vecchia, C., Bosetti, C., Negri, E., Levi, F., and Franceschi, S. (1998). Cigar smoking and cancers of the upper digestive tract. *J Natl Cancer Inst*, **90**, 1670.

Lagergren, J., Bergstrom, R., Lindgren, A., and Nyren, O. (1999). Symptomatic gastroesophageal reflux as a risk factor for esophageal adenocarcinoma. *New Engl J Med* **340**, 825–31.

Lagergren, J., Bergstrom, R., Lindgren, A., and Nyren, O. (2000). The role of tobacco, snuff and alcohol use in the aetiology of cancer of the oesophagus and gastric cardia. *Int J Cancer*, **85**, 340–6

Launoy, G., Milan, C., Faivre, J., Pienkowski, P., and Gignoux, M. (2000). Tobacco type and risk of squamous cell cancer of the oesophagus in males: a French multicentre case-control study. *Int J Epidemiol*, **29**, 36–42.

Levi, F., Ollyo, J. B., La Vecchia, C., Boyle, P., Monnier, P., and Savary, M. (1990). The consumption of tobacco, alcohol and the risk of adenocarcinoma in Barrett's oesophagus. *Int J Cancer*, **45**, 852–4.

Menke-Pluymers, M. B., Hop, W. C., Dees, J., van Blankenstein, M., and Tilanus, H. W. (1993). Risk factors for the development of an adenocarcinoma in columnar-lined (Barrett) esophagus. The Rotterdam Esophageal Tumor Study Group. *Cancer*, **72**, 1155–8.

Munoz, N. and Day, N. E. (1996). Esophageal cancer. In: *Cancer epidemiology and prevention*, second edn (ed. D. Schottenfeld, F.J. Fraumeni, Jr). pp. 681–706, Oxford University Press, New York.

Negri, E., La Vecchia, C., Franceschi, S., Decarli, A., and Bruzzi, P. (1992). Attributable risks for oesophageal cancer in northern Italy. *Eur J Cancer*, **28A**, 1167–71.

Negri, E., La Vecchia, C., Levi, F., Franceschi, S., Serra-Majem, L., and Boyle, P. (1996). Comparative descriptive epidemiology of oral and oesophageal cancers in Europe. *Eur J Cancer Prev*, **5**, 267–79.

Pacella-Norman, R., Urban, M. I., Sitas, F., Carrara, H., Sur, R., Hale, M., *et al.* (2002). Risk factors for oesophageal, lung, oral and laryngeal cancers in black South Africans. *Br J Cancer*, **86**, 1751–6.

Sankaranarayanan, R., Duffy, S. W., Padmakumary, G., Nair, S. M., Day, N. E., and Padmanabhan, T. K. (1991). Risk factors for cancer of the oesophagus in Kerala, India. *Int J Cancer*, **49**, 485–9.

Segal, I., Reinach, S. G., and de Beer, M. (1988). Factors associated with oesophageal cancer in Soweto, South Africa. *Br J Cancer*, **58**, 681–6.

Shanks, T. G. and Burns, D. M. (1998). Disease consequencies of cigar smoking. Smoking and tobacco control monograph 9. Cigars, health effects and trends, pp. 105–58. National Institutes of Health DHHS Publ No 98–4302, Bhetesda (MD).

Takezaki, T., Shinoda, M., Hatooka, S., Hasegawa, Y., Nakamura, S., Hirose, K., *et al.* (2000). Subsite-specific risk factors for hypopharyngeal and esophageal cancer (Japan). *Cancer Causes Control*, **11**, 597–608.

Tavani, A., Negri, E., Franceschi, S., and La Vecchia, C. (1996). Tobacco and other risk factors for oesophageal cancer in alcohol non-drinkers. *Eur J Cancer Prev*, **5**, 313–8.

Tuyns, A. J., Pequignot, G., and Jensen, O. M. (1977). Le cancer de l'oesophage en Ille-et-Vilaine en fonction des niveaux de consommation d'alcool et de tabac. Des risques qui se multiplient. *Bull Cancer*, **64**, 45–60.

Tuyns, A. J. (1983). Oesophageal cancer in non-smoking drinkers and in non-drinking smokers. *Int J Cancer*, **32**, 443–4.

Tuyns, A. J. and Esteve, J. (1983). Pipe, commercial and hand-rolled cigarette smoking in oesophageal cancer. *Int J Epidemiol*, **12**, 110–3.

Vizcaino, A. P., Parkin, D. M., and Skinner, M. E. (1995). Risk factors associated with oesophageal cancer in Bulawayo, Zimbabwe. *Br J Cancer*, **72**, 769–73.

Wu, A. H., Wan, P., and Bernstein, L. (2001). A multiethnic population-based study of smoking, alcohol and body size and risk of adenocarcinomas of the stomach and esophagus (United States). *Cancer Causes Control*, **12**, 721–32.

Wynder, E. L. and Bross, I. J. (1961). A study of etiological factors in cancer of the esophagus. *Cancer*, **14**, 389–413.

Yu, M. C., Garabrant, D. H., Peters, J. M., and Mack, T. M. (1988). Tobacco, alcohol, diet, occupation, and carcinoma of the esophagus. *Cancer Res* **48**, 3843–8.

Zambon, P., Talamini, R., La Vecchia, C., Dal Maso, L., Negri, E., Tognazzo, *et al.* (2000). Smoking, type of alcoholic beverage and squamous-cell oesophageal cancer in northern Italy. *Int J Cancer* **86**, 144–9.

Chapter 23

Tobacco use and risk of oral cancer

Tongzhang Zheng, Peter Boyle, Bing Zhang,
Yawei Zhang, Patricia H. Owens, Qing Lan
and John Wise

Introduction

Epidemiological studies from various populations have consistently shown that tobacco smoking (including filter- and non-filter cigarettes, cigars, and pipe tobacco) increases oral cancer risk. In sum, these results indicate that: ever-smokers experience an increased risk; current smokers have a higher risk than ex-smokers; those who started smoking at younger ages have a higher risk than those that started at later ages; risk increases with amount of cigarettes smoked per day, duration of smoking, and lifetime pack-years of smoking; smokers of filter cigarettes have lower risk than smokers of unfiltered cigarettes. Epidemiological studies have also shown that other factors may also contribute to the effect of smoking on oral cancer risk. For example, alcohol consumption dramatically increases the effect of tobacco smoking on the risk of oral cancer. Similarly, xenobiotic metabolizing enzymes, involved in the metabolism of tobacco carcinogens, have a significant impact on the relationship between tobacco smoking and oral cancer risk. Overall, based on very conservative estimates, about 46% of the cancers of the oral cavity and pharynx in men and 11% in women are attributable to smoking worldwide, with considerable variation by location (Parkin *et al.* 2000).

In this review, we will summarize the results from major epidemiological studies investigating the association between oral cancer and tobacco product use, including cigarette smoking, pipe tobacco and cigar smoking, and smokeless tobacco use (snuff dipping and chewing tobacco). In most of the epidemiological studies, 'oral cancer' includes cancer of the tongue (CD9 141), mouth (ICD9 143–145), and pharynx (ICD146, 148, 149), with a few including larynx (ICD9 161). Cancer of the lip (ICD9 140), salivary glands (ICD9 142), and nasopharynx (ICD9 147) were not included in most of the epidemiological studies of oral cancer, and therefore, cancers of these sites will not be discussed in this review. These cancer sites also appear to have quite different etiological profiles and very distinct natural histories as reviewed by Boyle *et al.* (1995).

Descriptive epidemiology

Cancers of the oral cavity and pharynx combined is the sixth most common cancer site for both sexes (reviewed in Boyle *et al.* 1990*a*, 1995; La Vecchia *et al.* 1997; Franceschi *et al.* 2000). Combined these cancers account for approximately 220 000 new cases per year in men and 90 000 in women worldwide. Their incidence rates vary approximately 20-fold in both sexes across the world. At present, high incidence rates are found in southern India, Pakistan, northern France, and a few areas of central and eastern Europe, with the highest rate recorded in Bas Rhin, France (49.4/100 000 men) (Franceschi *et al.* 2000).

Men are more likely to be diagnosed with oral cancer than women. Male-to-female ratios for oral and pharyngeal cancers ranged between 4 and 20 in southern, central, and eastern Europe (Franceschi *et al.* 2000). In the United States, the rates for men are 2.5–4 times higher than those for women (Weller *et al.* 1993). Based on the SEER program, in the US, African-Americans have an overall incidence of oral cancer 13.2/100 000, 65% higher than Whites of 8.0/100 000 (Weller *et al.* 1993). The majority of these racial and gender differences in the US is attributable to the effects of tobacco and alcohol (Day 1993).

In many parts of the world (such as India, Puerto Rico, and Colombia), a steady decline in oral cancer incidence in both sexes has been observed while a stable incidence rate was observed in the USA (Franceschi *et al.* 2000). There are, however, reports that oral cancer is increasing, particularly amongst younger persons in the Nordic countries and Europe with the reasons unknown (Boyle *et al.* 1990*b*; Macfarlane *et al.* 1994).

Tobacco use and risk of oral cancer

Cigarette smoking

Oral cancer and smoking has been investigated for many years. The early studies were restricted by the methodologies of their time and have been the subject of numerous other reviews (Boyle *et al.* 1995). Accordingly, this review will focus on more recent studies using newer epidemiological methods. In fact, a large number of studies have explored the relationship of cigarette smoking and oral cancer risk over the past two decades. The methods have varied but largely consist of hospital-based case–control studies, population-based case–control studies, and prospective follow-up studies. The major findings using each method are discussed below (also see Table 23.1) with a brief presentation of the strengths and limitations of each method.

Hospital-based case–control studies:

A number of hospital-based case–control studies have been conducted and have clearly shown a strong relationship between oral cancer and cigarette smoking. In interpreting the results from these hospital-based case–control studies, a major concern is whether

Table 23.1 Tobacco use and risk of oral cancer

Author (year) country (Cases/controls)	Cancer site	Major results			Comments
		Cigarettes	Cigar/pipe	Smokeless	
Hospital-based case–control studies					
Winn DM et al. (1981) Southern United States, (255/502)	Oral cavity, pharynx	RR=4.6 (95% CI 1.6–13.4) for oral cavity; RR=9.6 (95% CI 2.5–37.0) for pharynx among non-users of snuff		RR=47.5 (95% CI 9.1– 249.5) for cancer of the gum and buccal mucosa among snuff use of 50 or more years	The study subjects were women residing in 67 counties in central North Carolina
Elwood et al. (1984), Vancouver, Canada (374/374)	Oral cavity, pharynx, larynx	OR=2.1 (95% CI 0.9–4.8) for smoking more than 50 cigarettes per day			Controls were cancer patients with tumor sites which were considered to be no strong evidence of association with smoking
Spitz et al. (1988) Houston, US (185/185)	Oral cavity, pharynx, larynx	OR=7.5 (P_{trend}<0.01) for men OR=12.0 (P_{trend}<0.01) for women for smoking 50+ pack-years	Men: Cigar: OR=2.8 (95% CI 1.5–5.5) Pipe: OR=1.8 (95% CI 1.0–3.4)	Snuff dipping: OR=3.4 (95% CI 1.0– 10.9)	Combined effects of alcohol and tobacco were more than additive, but less than multiplicative
Franco et al. (1989), Brazil (232/464)	Oral cavity	RR=6.3 for ever vs. never smokers	RR=13.9 for pipe RR=5.5 for cigar for ever vs. never smokers	Snuff dipping or tobacco chewing was not associated with oral cancer risk	The RR was 142 for those with >100 pack-years of smoking and >1000 kg of alcohol drinking. Only 9 cases and 13 controls used smokeless tobacco

Table 23.1 (continued) Tobacco use and risk of oral cancer

Author (year) country (Cases/controls)	Cancer site	Major results			Comments
		Cigarettes	Cigar/pipe	Smokeless	
Kabat et al. (1989), US (125/107)	Oral cavity	OR=2.0 (95% CI 1.0–4.0) for current vs. never			Women only anc the numbers of case: and controls were srrall
Zheng et al. (1990), Beijing, China (404/404)	Tongue and oral cavity	OR=1.6 for ever vs. never smokers	Pipe: OR=5.7 for ever vs. never in men		The combined effects of tobacco and alcohol were approximately multiplicative. Tcbacco smoking accounts for about 34% of all cases of oral cancer in this population
Talamini et al. (1990), Northern Italy (336/1652)	Oral cavity, pharynx	OR=3.8 (95% CI 0.2–58.2) for smokers of <15 cigarettes per day; OR=12.9 (95% CI 2.3–106.3) for smokers of >15 cigarettes per day			The results are for non-drinkers
La Vecchia et al. (1990), Northern Italy (741/1272)	Oral cavity, pharynx, larynx	Oral cavity/pharynx: RR=2.3 (95% CI 1.6–3.2) Larynx: RR=1.8 (95% CI 1.2–2.8)			Reference category is smokers of cigarette brands with less than 22 mg tar yield per cigarette

Reference	Site				Comments
Franceschi et al. (1990), Northern Italy (741/1272)	Oral cavity, pharynx, larynx	Oral cavity: OR=11.1 (95% CI 3.4–34.8) for ever vs. never Pharynx: OR=12.9 (95% CI 3.1–52.9) for ever vs. never Larynx: OR=4.6 (95% CI 2.2–9.6) for ever vs. never	Oral cavity: OR=20.7 (95% CI 5.6–76.3) for ever vs. never		The risk of oral cavity and pharyngeal cancer for the highest levels of alcohol and smoking was increased 80-fold relative to the lowest levels of both factors
Nandakumar et al. (1990), Bangalore, India (348/348)	Oral cavity	OR=2.1 (95% CI 1.1–4.2) for cigarette smoking		OR=17.7 (95% CI 8.7–36.1) for chewing during sleep	OR=242.6 (95% CI 52.6–1119.0) for tobacco chewing and ragi consumption
Franceschi et al. (1992), Northern Italy (206/726)	Tongue and mouth	Tongue: OR=10.5 (95% CI 3.2–34.1) for current vs. never Mouth: OR=11.8 (95% CI 3.6–38.4) for current vs. never	Mouth: OR=21.9 (95% CI 3.8–125.6)		Smokers of high tar cigarettes had a 10-fold increased risk of cancer of the tongue and 14-fold increased risk of cancer of mouth compared with non-smokers. Results are for male only.
Boffetta et al. (1992), US (359/2280)	Mouth	Floor of the mouth: OR=4.0 (95% CI 1.5–10.3) for smoking of >35 cigarettes per day Soft palate complex: OR=4.9 (95% CI 1.1–21.5) for smoking of >35 cigarettes per day	Non-significantly increased risk was observed for floor of mouth (OR=1.8), soft palate (OR=2.3), buccal mucosa (OR=1.9)		This study supports the hypothesis of the carcinogenic effect of tobacco smoke on the oral mucosa through direct contact

Table 23.1 (continued) Tobacco use and risk of oral cancer

Author (year) country (Cases/controls)	Cancer site	Major results			Comments
		Cigarettes	**Cigar/pipe**	**Smokeless**	
Negri et al. (1993), Northern Italy (439/2106)	Oral cavity and pharynx	RR=3.6 for moderate smokers vs. never smokers; RR=9.4 for heavy smokers vs. never smokers			The single factor with the highest attributable risk was smoking, which account for 81–87% of oral cancers in males and for 42–47% in females
Mashberg et al. (1993), New Jersey, US (359/2280)	Oral cavity and pharynx	OR=4.0 (95% CI 1.9–8.2) for smoking of >36 cigarettes per day	OR=3.3 (95% CI 1.5–7.0)	No increased risk was found for use of snuff (OR=0.8) or chewing tobacco (OR=1.0)	The number of subjects using snuff and chewing tobacco was small
Rao et al. (1994) India (713/635)	Lip, oral cavity (excluding base of the tongue and soft palate)	No significantly increased risk for smoking cigarettes		RR=2.8 (95% CI 2.3–3.6) for tobacco chewers compared to non-chewers	Very few subjects smoked cigarette alone
Kabat et al. (1994), US (1560/2948)	Oral cavity and pharynx	OR=3.3 (95% CI 2.4–4.3) for current vs. never in males; OR=4.3 (95% CI 3.2–5.9) for current vs. never in females		Crude OR=2.3 (95% CI 0.7–7.3) for regular chewer in men. Crude OR=34.5 (95% CI 8.5–140.1) for snuff users in women	The results for smokeless tobacco use were based on small number of subjects
Macfarlane et al. (1995), US, Italy, China (835/1300)	Oral cavity, tongue, pharynx	OR=3.8 (95% CI 2.5–5.8) for smoking of >30 pack-years in males; OR=6.2 (95% CI 3.4–11.2) for smoking of >18 pack-years in females			The risk of oral cancer increased with increasing tobacco consumption among women who never drank alcohol

Study	Site	Results	Comments
Muscat et al. (1996), US (1009/923)	Oral cavity and pharynx	OR=2.1 (95% CI 1.4–3.2) for cumulative lifetime tar intake of >6.8 kg in males; OR=4.6 (95% CI 2.5–8.7) for cumulative tar intake of >6.8 kg in females	Very few subjects used oral snuff and chewing tobacco	Oral snuff and chewing tobacco were unrelated to oral cancer risk in this study
Zheng et al. (1997), Beijing, China (111/111)	Tongue	OR=2.7 (95% CI 1.3–5.9) for current vs. never; OR=2.2 (95% CI 1.1–4.6) for ex-smokers vs. never	The number of cases and controls was small
De Stefani et al. (1998), Uruguay, US (471/471)	Oral cavity and pharynx	OR=13.4 (95% CI 6.5–27.9) for smoking of >62 pack-years vs. never smoking	The combined effect for tobacco and alcohol is supramultiplicative
Schlecht et al. (1999), Brazil (784/1578)	Mouth, pharynx, and larynx	OR=8.0 (95% CI 4.6–13.8) for smoking of >40 cigarettes per day	Pipe: OR=8.2 (95% CI 3.7–17.8) for smoking of >20 pack years Cigar: OR=3.9 (95% CI 1.5–10.4) for ever vs. never	Smoking cessation resulted in a significant risk reduction, decreasing nearly to the levels of never smokers after 20 years of abstention
Franceschi et al. (1999), Italy (638/1254)	Oral cavity and pharynx	OR=10.7 (95% CI 5.0–22.8) for smoking of ≥25 cigarettes per day	Men only

Table 23.1 (continued) Tobacco use and risk of oral cancer

Author (year) country (Cases/controls)	Cancer site	Major results			Comments
		Cigarettes	Cigar/pipe	Smokeless	
Moreno-lopez et al. (1999), Spain (75/150)	Oral cavity	OR=8.3 (95% CI 3.4–20.4) for smoking of >20 cigarettes per day			The number of cases and controls was small
La Vecchia et al. (1999), Italy (1280/4179)	Oral cavity and pharynx	OR=8.4 (95% CI 6.6–10.6) for current vs. never			Significantly reduced risk was observed for smoking cessation
Zavras et al. (2000), Greece (110/115)	Oral cavity and pharynx	OR=3.3 (95% CI 1.3–8.5) for smoking of >50 pack years during lifetime			OR was 8.3 (95% CI 2.4–29.1) for smoking >50 pack years and drinking 23 drinks per week. The number of cases and controls was small
Talamini et al. (2000), Italy (132/148)	Tongue, mouth, and pharynx	OR=14.8 (95% CI 3.1–70.4) for smoking of ≥25 cigarettes per day			The number of cases and controls was small
Garrote et al. (2001), Havana city, Cuba (200/200)	Oral cavity, pharynx	OR=20.8 (95% CI 8.9–48.3) for smoking of ≥30 cigarettes per day	OR=20.45 (95% CI 4.7–89.7) for smoking of >4 cigars/pipes per day		A supra-multiplicative effect for smoking and drinking on oral cancer risk. 82% of oral cancer cases in Cuba attributable to tobacco smoking

Population-based case–control studies

Reference	Site				Comments
Blot et al. (1988), US (1114/1268)	Oral cavity and pharynx	OR=1.9 (95% CI 1.1–3.4) for ever vs. never in males; OR=3.0 (95% CI 2.0–4.5) for ever vs. never in females	OR=1.9 (95% CI 1.1–3.4) for ever vs. never in males	OR=6.2 (95% CI 1.9–19.8) for non-smoking females	The tobacco smoking and alcohol drinking combine to account for about 75% of all oral and pharyngeal cancers in US
Tuyns et al. (1988), Italy, Spain, Switzerland, and France (1147/3057)	Larynx and pharynx	Endolarynx: RR=9.9 (95% CI 6.4–15.4) for ever vs. never. Hypopharynx/Epilarynx: RR=12.4 (95% CI 6.3–24.4) for ever vs. never			Men only. The relative risks for joint exposure to alcohol and tobacco are consistent with a multiplicative model
Merletti et al. (1989), Italy (122/606)	Oral cavity and pharynx	OR=3.9 (95% CI 1.6–9.4) for ever vs. never	Pipe: OR=3.8 (95% CI 1.1–12.6) for ever vs. never Cigar: OR=14.6 (95% CI 4.7–45.6) for ever vs. never		Attributable risks for tobacco in this population were 72% in men and 54% in women. The number of cases was small
Marshall et al. (1992), US (290/290)	Tongue, pharynx, and floor of mouth	OR=5.7 (95% CI 2.7–12.1) for smoking of >70 pack-years			The effects of cigar and pipe smoking as practiced might be much less significant than cigarette smoking in this study. The number of cases and controls were small

Table 23.1 (Continued) Tobacco use and risk of oral cancer

Author (year) country (Cases/controls)	Cancer site	Major results			Comments
		Cigarettes	Cigar/pipe	Smokeless	
Day et al. (1993), US (1065/1182)	Oral cavity, tongue and pharynx	OR=3.6 (95% CI 2.6–4.8) for ever vs. never in whites; OR=2.3 (95% CI 1.1–4.7) for ever vs. never in blacks	OR=2.2 (95% CI 1.3–4.0) for ever vs. never in whites; OR=1.8 (95% CI 0.4–8.5) for ever vs. never in blacks		Smoking–drinking interaction was generally consistent with a multiplicative enhancement of risk following joint exposure to tobacco and alcohol among both whites and blacks
Day et al. (1994), US (83/189)	Oral cavity and pharynx	OR=4.3 (95% CI 1.6–12) for current vs. never and former	OR=5.0 (95% CI 0.6–4.4) for ever vs. never		The number of cases and controls was small
Bundgaard et al. (1995), Denmark (161/483)	Oral cavity	OR=6.3 (95% CI 3.1–12.9) for smoking of >235 kg during lifetime			A multiplicative enhancement of risk for the combination of tobacco and alcohol exposure was observed in this population. The number of cases was small
Andre et al. (1995), France (299/645)	Oral cavity, pharynx, and larynx	OR=12.9 (95% CI 5.3–31.5) for smoking of ≥20 cigarettes per day			The combined effect of alcohol and tobacco appeared to follow a multiplicative model
Hung et al. (1997), Taiwan (41/123)	Oral cavity	OR=5.9 (95% CI 1.9–18.5) for smoking of ≥22.5 pack-years			Men only. The number of cases and controls was small

Study	Site	Results		Comments
Lewin et al. (1997), Sweden (605/756)	Oral cavity, pharynx, and larynx	RR=6.5 (4.4–9.5) for current vs. never	RR=1.8 (95% CI 0.9–3.7) for ex-users vs. never	The joint effect of high alcohol intake (≥0 grams per day) and current smoking was nearly multiplicative
Schwartz et al. (1998), US (284/477)	Oral cavity and pharynx	OR=2.5 (95% CI 1.5–4.3) for past smoking of ≥20 pack-years; OR=5.5 (95% CI 3.5–8.6) for current smoking of ≥20 pack-years	OR=1.0 (95% CI 0.4–2.3) for smokeless tobacco use in men	Very few subjects used smokeless tobacco in this study
Schildt et al. (1998), Sweden (410/410)	Oral cavity	OR=1.8 (95% CI 1.1–2.7) for current vs. never; Pipe: OR=2.0 (95% CI 1.1–3.4) for current vs. never	Oral snuff: OR=1.5 (0.8–2.9) for ex-users vs. never	A potential interaction between smoking and alcohol drinking
Hayes et al. (1999), Puerto Rico (342/521)	Oral cavity and pharynx	OR=3.9 (95% CI 2.1–7.1) for ever vs. never in men; OR=4.9 (95% CI 2.0–11.6) for ever vs. never in women		Cigarette smoking included cigar or pipe smoking. Joint exposure to alcohol and tobacco resulted in risks consistent with independent effects on a multiplicative scale

Table 23.1 (continued) Tobacco use and risk of oral cancer

Author (year) country (Cases/controls)	Cancer site	Major results			Comments
		Cigarettes	Cigar/pipe	Smokeless	
Prospective follow-up studies					
Hammond and Seidman (1980), US (more than 1 000 000)	Buccal, pharynx, and larynx	Mortality ratio = 6.5 for ever vs. never in men; Mortality ratio = 3.3 for ever vs. never in women	Mortality ratio = 5.1 for ever vs. never in men		
Akiba and Hirayama (1990), Japan (265 000)	Oral cavity, larynx	Oral cavity: RR = 2.5 (95% CI 1.3–5.7) for ever vs. never in men; Larynx: RR = 23.8 (95% CI 5.3–420) for ever vs. never in men			Non-significantly increased RR found in women
Chyou et al. (1995), Hawaiian, US (7995)	Upper aero-digestive tract	RR = 3.2 (95% CI 1.7–5.9) for current vs. never			Men only. The RR = 14.35 for men who drank 14 or more ounces per month and smoked more than 20 cigarettes per day compared with those who had never drunk or smoked

the control group selected represents the population that produced the cases. Indeed, in some of the hospital-based case–control studies, the control group considered included cancers thought to be unrelated to smoking and drinking, and some with benign neoplastic or non-neoplastic lesions, which may be smoking related. If it turns out that these diseases were actually associated with tobacco smoking, then, the true relationship between tobacco smoking and oral cancer risk would be underestimated. Since most of these studies showed a strong association between cigarette smoking and oral cancer risk, underestimation is less of a concern. But the variation of disease in controls in different studies is still important to note as when considered together with the relatively small sample size in some of the studies, it may explain in large part, the significant variation in the magnitude of the reported association between tobacco smoking and oral cancer risk.

In 1984, Elwood *et al.* reported an alcohol-adjusted OR of 2.8 (95% CI 1.3–6.0) for smoking 50 or more cigarettes per day when compared to never smokers. Additional adjustment for 4 other factors reduced the OR to 2.1 (95% CI 0.9–4.8). A weak association observed in this study could be due to the fact that controls were composed of various cancer patients (including cancer of the prostate, colo-rectum, skin, breast, etc.).

In a case–control study of oral cancer in Brazil, Franco *et al.* (1989) reported that tobacco smoking was, by any measure, the strongest risk factor for oral cancer in this population. The adjusted ORs for ever vs. never smokers were 6.3 (95% CI 2.4–16.3), 5.5 (95% CI 1.2–24.8), 13.9 (95% CI 4.4–44.2), and 7.0 (95% CI 2.7–18.7) for industrial brand cigarettes, cigars, pipe, and hand-rolled cigarettes, respectively. The OR for the heaviest vs. the lowest consumption categories (>100 vs. <1 pack-years) was 14.8 (95% CI 4.7–47.3). Smoking cessation also resulted in a significant risk reduction, with levels close to those of never smokers after 10 years stopping smoking. A study by Spitz *et al.* (1988) in Texas, US, also showed a linear increase in risk with increasing pack-years of cigarette smoking ($P_{trend} < 0.01$ for both males and females). In males, the OR rose from 1.8 (95% CI 0.7–4.4) for those who smoked 1–24 pack-years to 7.5 (95% CI 3.7–15.3) for those who smoked >49 pack-years when compared to non-smokers. In females, the corresponding values were 1.5 (95% CI 0.4–5.1) and 12.0 (95% CI 3.8–38.0), respectively. Site-specific analysis for males also showed a significant increase with increasing pack-years of cigarette smoking for cancer of the larynx ($P_{trend} < 0.01$), tongue ($P_{trend} < 0.01$), and floor of mouth ($P_{trend} = 0.02$), but not for orohypopharynx ($P_{trend} = 0.13$), and other oral cavity ($P_{trend} = 0.15$). A significant risk reduction was observed after 15 or more years of smoking cessation.

Zheng *et al.* (1990) conducted a case–control study of oral cancer in Beijing, China, including 404 histologically confirmed incident cases and an equal number of hospital-based controls. The study reported an alcohol-adjusted OR of 2.4 (95% CI 1.5–4.0) for male smokers when compared to never smokers. Three measures of level of exposure— cigarette equivalents smoked per day, years smoked, and lifetime pack-years of smoking—all showed highly significant exposure–response relationships ($P_{trend} < 0.001$).

Among females, while the numbers of smokers is small, the same trends as were seen among males are evident. An OR of 2.1 (95% CI 1.1–4.2) for male cigarette smokers was also reported from a case–control study in India by Nandakumar et al. (1990). The ORs were 2.2 (95% CI 1.1–4.3) for those who smoked for more than 25 years, and 2.1 (95% CI 1.0–4.4) for those who smoked more than 20 cigarettes per day. A small study from the United States by Kabat et al. (1989) also reported an alcohol-adjusted OR of 2.0 (95% CI 1.0–4.0) for current smokers. Being an ex-smoker was not found to be associated with an increased risk in this study (OR=1.0, 95% CI 0.5–2.1).

Using the data from the northern Italy study, Talamini et al. (1990) further examined the role of tobacco in non-drinkers for oral and pharyngeal cancer. They found that, among non-drinkers, ex-smokers had a risk four times that of never smokers (OR=4.1, 95% CI 0.5–93.6). For current smokers, ORs for smokers of <15 and ≥15 cigarettes per day were 3.8 (95% CI 0.2–58.2) and 12.9 (95% CI 2.3–106.3), respectively. The test for trend in risk was highly significant ($P_{trend} < 0.001$). La Vecchia et al. (1990) further examined the risk by low/medium or high tar contents of the cigarettes smoked, using only the male subjects of the study. They found that, among ever smokers, the ORs for oral and pharyngeal cancer were 8.5 (95% CI 3.7–19.4) for low to medium tar and 16.4 (95% CI 7.1–38.2) for high tar. The corresponding estimates were 4.8 (95% CI 2.3–10.1) and 7.1 (95% CI 3.2–15.6) for laryngeal cancers. A direct comparison between high vs. low tar cigarettes showed an OR 2.3 for oral cavity and pharyngeal cancers, and 3.8 for laryngeal cancer, and all these estimates were statistically significant.

Franceschi et al. (1990) reported the results from a case–control study involving cancer of the tongue and oral cavity, pharynx, and esophagus. The study found that the alcohol-adjusted ORs for current smokers of cigarettes were 11.1 for oral cavity, 12.9 for pharynx, and 4.6 for larynx. The risks increased significantly with increasing the number of cigarettes smoked per day, duration of smoking, and with younger age started smoking, however, decreased with smoking cessation.

Using the data from a case–control study in northern Italy, Negri et al. (1993) reported that, compared to non-smokers, the alcohol-adjusted ORs were 3.6 for moderate smokers, and 9.4 for heavy smokers. In another report from northern Italy, Franceschi et al. (1992) reported that, among current smokers, the risk associated with cigarette smoking was similar for cancer of the tongue (OR=10.5, 95% CI 3.2–34.1) and for cancer of the mouth (OR=11.8, 95% CI 3.6–38.4). The risks also increased significantly with increasing number of cigarette smoking and duration of smoking for both cancer sites. An early age at starting smoking led to an OR of 7.6 (95% CI 2.3–25.0) for cancer of the tongue and 11.0 (95% CI 3.3–36.4) for cancer of the mouth. Smokers of high-tar cigarettes had a 10-fold increased risk of cancer of the tongue (95% CI 2.9–33.1) and a 14-fold increased risk (95% CI 4.2–49.5) of cancer of the mouth compared with non-smokers. Ex-smokers, who had quit smoking for more than 10 years, had an OR close to unity in this study.

Mashberg et al. (1993), in a study of US veterans in New Jersey, reported that smokers of filter cigarettes had a lower risk of oral cancer than that of smokers of unfiltered cigarettes.

For smokers of unfiltered cigarettes, the ORs were 7.8 (95% CI 2.4–19.0), 7.7 (3.6–16.5), 12.3 (5.3–28.6), and 7.6 (3.5–16.8) for consumption of 6 to 15, 16 to 25, 26 to 35, and 36 or more cigarettes per day, respectively. The corresponding ORs for smokers of filtered cigarettes were 1.5 (0.5–4.2), 3.6 (1.6–7.7), 1.9 (0.7–5.0), and 2.3 (1.0–5.2), respectively. Using the same dataset, Boffetta *et al.* (1992) showed that soft palate had the highest ORs associated with tobacco smoking (OR = 4.9, 95% CI 1.1–21.5 for those smoking more than 35 cigarettes per day). A similar susceptibility to tobacco was shown for floor of the mouth (OR = 4.0, 95% CI 1.5–10.3, $P_{trend} < 0.01$ for those smoking more than 35 cigarettes per day). A stronger effect of tobacco on posterior sites of the oral cavity, such as soft palate, is consistent with the earlier studies by Hirayama (1966) and by Jussawalla and Deshpande (1971).

Kabat *et al.* (1994) reported a large hospital-based case–control study in eight US cities, involving 1560 histologically incident cases of oral and pharyngeal cancer and 2948 controls (including both cancerous and non-cancerous controls). The study found that the OR for oral cancer was significantly increased in current smokers for both males (OR = 3.3, 95% CI 2.4–4.3) and females (OR = 4.3, 95% CI 3.2–5.9). Among current smokers of both sexes the OR increased with amount of smoking, and among ever smokers the risk increased with duration of smoking. Compared to lifetime non-filter smokers, lifetime filter smokers or those who switched to filter cigarettes had a reduced risk of oral cancer. Quitting smoking was associated with a substantial reduction of cancer risk which was evident even in the first few years following cessation.

Macfarlane *et al.* (1995) also reported a higher risk of female smokers from tobacco smoking in a combined analysis of three case–control studies from China, US, and Italy. They found that, among men, the ORs were 1.7 (95% CI 1.2–2.5) for those who smoked 33 pack-years or less, and 3.8 (95% CI 2.5–5.8) for those who smoked more than 33 pack years. Among women, the corresponding ORs were 2.7 (95% CI 1.6–4.7) and 6.2 (95% CI 3.4–11.2), respectively. The large sample size of the combined analysis allowed the authors to examine the risk associated with smoking among never alcohol drinkers. They reported that, among those who never consumed alcohol, the risk of oral cancer increased with increasing consumption of tobacco and the risk again was found to be higher for females amongst whom the increases were statistically significant. Smoking cessation resulted in a significant risk reduction, those who had stopped smoking for more than 9 years had a risk half that of current smokers (OR = 0.5, 95% CI 0.3–0.7).

In a case–control study of 1009 oral cancer patients and 923 age-matched controls in the US, Muscat *et al.* (1996) not only found a significant dose-response relationship between oral cancer risk and lifetime cumulative tar intake ($P_{trend} < 0.01$) or lifetime pack-years of smoking ($P_{trend} < 0.01$), they also reported a significant gender difference in the smoking-related risks for oral cancer. For example, the adjusted OR for men, according to increasing quartile of cumulative lifetime tar consumption and relative to never smokers, was 1.0, 0.9, 1.6, and 2.1. Among women, the corresponding ORs were 1.8, 2.8, 3.2, and 4.6.

Zheng *et al.* (1997) reported a case–control study of tongue cancer in Beijing, China. They found a significantly increased risk of tongue cancer among ex-smokers (OR=2.2, 95% CI 1.1–4.6), and among current smokers (OR=2.7, 95% CI 1.3–5.9). The risk also increased with increasing tobacco smoking, as reflected by both cigarette equivalents smoked per day and lifetime pack-years of tobacco smoking. Quitting smoking was associated with a significant risk reduction for tongue cancer.

In a case–control study in Uruguay, De Stefani *et al.* (1998) reported an increased risk of squamous-cell carcinoma of the oral cavity and pharynx for ever-smokers (OR= 7.4, 95% CI 3.7–14.8), current smokers (OR=10.5, 95% CI 5.2–21.3), and former smokers (OR=4.5, 95% CI 2.2–9.2). The risk increases with the increasing intensity of smoking, smoking duration, and pack-years of smoking. An OR of 13.4 (95% CI 6.5–27.9) was observed for heavy smokers (more than 62 pack-years). Analyses by type of tobacco products showed that risk was higher for black tobacco smokers (OR=10.2, 95% CI 5.0–20.5) than for blond tobacco smokers (OR=4.5, 95% CI 2.2–9.2).

A study from Brazil by Schlecht *et al.* (1999) investigated the relationship between different types of tobacco smoking and oral cancer risk. The study found that smokers of non-filter cigarettes had an OR of 6.9 (95% CI 4.1–11.8), and smokers of filter ciga-rettes had an OR of 6.2 (3.9–10.0). Smokers of more than 40 pack-years of commercial cigarettes had an OR of 8.0 (95% CI 4.6–13.8), and smokers of more than 40 pack-years of black tobacco had an OR of 7.0 (95% CI 4.2–11.5). Current smokers were found to have an alcohol-adjusted RR of 8.1 (95% CI 4.9–13.4) compared to never smokers. As observed in other studies, smoking cessation resulted in a significant risk reduction, decreasing nearly to the levels of never smokers after 20 years of abstention.

Franceschi *et al.* (1999) also reported a dose-dependent relationship between cigarette smoking per day and oral cancer risk. The alcohol-adjusted OR was 3.3 (95% CI 1.5–7.2) for smoking 1–14 cigarettes daily, 7.7 (95% CI 3.8–15.4) for smoking 15–24 cigarettes daily, and 10.7 (95% CI 5.0–22.8) for smoking 25 or more cigarettes daily. Similarly, a dose–response relationship was observed for daily cigarette smoking by Moreno-Lopez *et al.* (2000) in Spain. The study reported that the alcohol-adjusted OR was 3.1 (95% CI 1.4–6.7) for smoking 1–20 cigarettes/day, and 8.3 (95% CI 3.4–20.4) for smoking more than 20 cigarettes daily.

A study in the south of Greece by Zavras *et al.* (2001) also reported a significantly increased risk of oral cancer among current smokers (OR=3.0, 95% CI 1.4–6.6). No increased risk, however, was observed for former smokers (OR=0.9, 95% CI 0.4–2.1). A strong dose–response relationship was observed for pack-years of tobacco smoking (P_{trend}=0.01). For those who had more than 50 pack-years of tobacco smoking, the alcohol-adjusted OR was 3.3 (95% CI 1.3–8.5) when compared to never smokers.

In a study from north-eastern Italy, Talamini *et al.* (2000) reported an OR of 2.4 (95% CI 1.0–5.8) for former smokers compared to never smokers. Among current smokers, risk increased with increasing number of cigarettes smoked per day (P_{trend} < 0.001). An alcohol-adjusted OR of 14.8 (95% CI 3.1–70.4) was observed for those who smoked 25 or more cigarettes per day.

In a combined analysis of two hospital-based case–control studies from Italy and Switzerland involving 1280 oral and pharyngeal cases and 4179 controls, La Vecchia *et al.* (1999) reported an OR of 8.4 (95% CI 6.6–10.6) for current smokers. A significantly reduced risk was observed following smoking cessation: the ORs were 6.2 for those who had stopped smoking for less than 2 years, 4.5 for those who had stopped for 3–5 years, 3.5 for those who had stopped for 6–9 years, 1.6 for those who had stopped for 10–14 years, and 1.4 for those who had stopped for 15 or more years.

Garrote *et al.* (2001) reported the results from a case–control study of tobacco smoking and risk of oral and oro-pharyngeal cancers in Cuba. A strong dose–response was reported between cigarette smoking per day and risk of oral cancer among current smokers (P_{trend} < 0.01). The alcohol-adjusted OR for smoking 30 cigarettes or more per day, compared with never smokers, was 20.8 (95% CI 8.9–48.3) among current smokers. Former smokers also had an OR of 6.3 (95% CI 3.0–13.4), but risk was significantly reduced after 10 or more years smoking cessation.

Population-based case–control studies

A potential advantage of population-based case–control study design is that controls are randomly selected from the population which produced the cases, and therefore, more likely to represent the population with regards to the major risk factors. However, the relatively higher refusal rate from potential study subjects may still hamper the interpretation of the study.

In a multicenter study in the four areas of the US, Blot *et al.* (1988) found that, compared with never smokers, cigarette smokers had twice the risk in males (OR = 1.9, 95% CI 1.3–2.9), and three times the risk in females (OR = 3.0, 95% CI 2.0–4.5). The risks of oral cancer rose with the number of cigarettes smoked per day and with the duration of cigarette smoking. Those who smoked only filter cigarettes had a 50% (95% CI 30–80) of the risk of those who smoked only non-filter cigarettes, and smoking cessation resulted in a rapid decline in risk.

In a multi-center case–control study in four European countries, Tuyns *et al.* (1988) reported a clear dose–response relationship between cigarette smoking and risk of cancer of the larynx and hypopharynx. For those who smoked more than 26 cigarettes per day, the ORs were 24.0 (95% CI 11.8–48.7) for cancer of the supraglottic, 10.2 (95% CI 5.4–19.3) for cancer of the glottic and subglottic, 9.4 (95% CI 3.2–28.0) for cancer of the epilarynx, and 20.0 (95% CI 7.9–51.0) for cancer of the hypopharynx. The study also found that earlier age started smoking carried a higher risk. Unlike the study by Merletti *et al.* (1989), the smokers of exclusively filter cigarettes in this study were found to have only half the risk of laryngeal or hypopharynx/epilarynx cancer as compared with smokers of only plain cigarettes. As reported by Schlecht *et al.* (1999) and De Stefan *et al.* (1998), smokers of black tobacco cigarettes had higher risk than smokers of blond tobacco. Smoking cessation resulted in a decrease in risk after 5 years' abstention.

Merletti *et al.* (1989) from Italy reported a four- to sixfold increased risk among subjects with medium or high tobacco consumption in both males and females. A trend in increasing risk with duration of smoking was observed in men, but not in women. As reported by Franceschi *et al.* (1990), younger age at start of smoking was found to be associated with a higher risk in this study, and smoking cessation is associated with a sharp risk reduction. Subjects smoking black cigarettes had a higher risk, while use of filter cigarettes showed no clear risk difference.

Marshall *et al.* (1992) reported the results from a case–control study in western New York, and they found that, while the risk associated with cigarette smoking did not increase in strict dose–response fashion, it was sizably and significantly elevated from those who had 21–30 pack-years of smoking (OR=2.7, 95% CI 1.2–6.0) to those who had more than 70 pack-years of smoking (OR=5.7, 95% CI 2.7–12.1).

Using data from a multicenter population-based case–control study of oral cancer risk factors in the US (1065 cases and 1182 controls), Day *et al.* (1993) examined the Black-White differences in the risk of oral cancer associated with tobacco smoking. The study found that the patterns of risk among smokers were generally similar among blacks and whites. After controlling for alcohol consumption, the risk was almost doubled for those who smoked 20–39 cigarettes per day, and tripled for those who smoked 40 or more cigarettes per day. The alcohol-adjusted OR for current smokers was higher among Whites (OR=3.6, 95% CI 2.6–4.8) than among Blacks (OR=2.3, 95% CI 1.1–4.7), but this difference was not statistically significant. The risk declined sharply with cessation of smoking for both racial groups, with little elevation in risk even for those who had quit smoking 1–9 years earlier.

Tobacco smoking was also found to be significantly associated with the risk of second cancers of the oral cavity and pharynx in a nested case–control study by Day *et al.* (1994). The effects of smoking was found to be more pronounced than those of alcohol in this study. Current smokers relative to never and former smokers had an OR of 4.3 (95% CI 1.6–12). The alcohol-adjusted ORs for smoking rose with duration and intensity of smoking. Risk, however, was significantly reduced 5 years after smoking cessation.

Bundgaard *et al.* (1995) in Denmark also reported an increased risk of oral cancer associated with increasing lifetime kilogram cigarette smoking ($P_{trend} < 0.001$) and with current daily amount of smoking ($P_{trend} < 0.001$). For those who had a lifetime consumption of cigarettes greater than 235 kg, the OR was 6.3 (95% CI 3.1–12.9). The OR was 5.8 (95% CI 3.1–10.9) for those with current consumption of more than 20 cigarettes per day.

A dose–response relationship was observed for daily grams of cigarette smoking in a case–control study by Andre *et al.* (1995) in France. The study found that those who smoked more than one packet of cigarettes a day had a risk that was 13 times higher than that of non-smokers. Subjects who smoked only non-filter cigarettes had a higher risk (OR=2.0) than those who smoked filter cigarettes, and risk decreaseed after stopping smoking.

A small study by Hung et al. (1997) in Taiwan found that, compared with non-smokers, cigarette smoking had an increased risk of oral cancer (OR=5.0, 95% CI 1.7–15.1). The risk increased with increasing lifetime pack-years of smoking: the ORs were 4.0 (95% CI 1.2–13.5) for those with less than 22.5 pack-years of smoking, and 5.9 (95% CI 1.9–18.5) for those with more than 22.5 pack-years of smoking.

In a case–control study in Sweden, Lewin et al. (1997) reported that men who smoked only cigarettes had an OR of 3.7 (95% CI 2.5–5.5). The risk was considerably lower for ex-smokers (OR=1.9, 95% CI 1.3–2.8) than for current smokers (OR=6.5, 95% CI 4.4–9.5). No increased risk was found for men who had stopped smoking for more than 20 years. There was dose-dependent excess risk associated with duration of smoking, total lifetime kilograms of tobacco smoking, and daily grams of tobacco smoking. Analysis by cancer site showed that, for men who smoked 45 years or longer, the ORs were 6.3 (95% CI 3.2–12.4) for cancer of the oral cavity, 10.1 (95% CI 4.6–22.1) for pharynx, 7.6 (95% CI 3.9–14.7) for larynx, and 5.4 (95% CI 2.7–11.0) for esophagus.

In a case–control study of oral cancer in western Washington state, USA, Schwartz et al. (1998) reported a significantly increased risk of oral cancer for both current and past cigarette smokers. For those who smoked greater than or equal to 20 pack-years of cigarettes, the OR was 2.5 (95% CI 1.5–4.3) for past smokers and 5.5 (95% CI 3.5–8.6) for current smokers.

In a case–control study of oral cancer in Sweden, Schildt et al. (1998) found a significantly increased risk of oral cancer among the current smokers (OR=1.8, 95% CI 1.1–2.7), while found no increased risk for ex-smokers (OR=1.0, 95% CI 0.6–1.6). They found, however, that OR was 1.8 (95% CI 1.2–2.8) for current smokers with more than 124.8 kg cigarette consumption. Analysis by anatomic site showed that the risk appeared to be the highest for cancer of the floor of the mouth (OR=8.0, 95% CI 1.0–64.0).

Hayes et al. (1999) conducted a case–control study in Puerto Rico and found that any cigarette use was associated with an increased risk of oral cancer among men (OR=3.9, 95% CI 2.1–7.1) and women (OR=4.9, 95% CI 2.0–11.6). Risks increased with increasing cigarette use, whether estimated by usual daily amount ($P_{trend} < 0.0001$), or by cumulative lifetime consumption ($P_{trend} < 0.0001$). As reported by Macfarlane et al. (1995) and Muscat et al. (1996), this study also reported that women seemed to have greater risk at a given amount of cigarette consumption. Unlike the study of Mashberg et al. (1993), this study did not find a reduced risk associated with smoking filter cigarettes compared to smoking non-filter cigarettes. Smoking cessation was shown to reduce the risk gradually, with the risk remaining elevated up to 19 years after smoking cessation.

Prospective follow-up studies

A prospective follow-up study is conducted based on the presence or absence of exposure of investigation without the information regarding disease status. Therefore, a follow-up study is less prone to selection bias at the start of the study. However, the losses to follow-up may still pose an issue for the interpretation of the study results, especially for diseases, such as cancers, which have long induction and latency periods.

Hammond and Seidman (1980) reported a prospective mortality study of over one million Americans in 1721 counties in 25 states in the US. The study reported that, among men, oral cancer mortality rates were 2.3/100 000 for those who never smoked regularly, 11.7/100 000 for pipe and cigar smokers, and 15.0/100 000 for cigarette smokers. Among women, the oral cancer mortality rates were 2.0/100 000 for those who never smoked regularly and 6.5/100 000 for cigarette smokers.

Another prospective cohort mortality study from Japan by Akiba and Hirayama (1990) examined the site-specific cancer risk associated with cigarette smoking, using the data from 265 000 residents of 29 public health districts in six prefectures throughout Japan. The study reported a statistically significant dose–response relationship between cigarette smoking and mortality rate for cancer of the oral cavity, larynx, esophagus, bladder, and stomach in men. Compared to never smokers, the RRs were 2.5 (95% CI 1.3–5.7) for cancer of the oral cavity and 23.8 (95% CI 5.3–420.0) for cancer of the larynx among males. Very few women smoked cigarettes in this population.

Chyou et al. (1995) reported a cohort study of upper aerodigestive tract cancer among 7995 Japanese–American men in Hawaii in which they examined the potential impact of smoking and other risk factors on the incidence of upper aerodigestive tract cancer (30 men with oral/pharyngeal cancer, 27 men with laryngeal cancer, and 35 men with esophageal cancer). The study found that current cigarette smokers at time of examination had a threefold risk for upper aerodigestive tract cancer compared with never-smokers (RR=3.2, 95% CI 1.7–5.9). A significant positive linear trend in relative risk was observed in number of cigarettes smoked per day ($P_{trend}=0.002$), and number of years of smoking ($P_{trend}=0.0006$).

Pipe and cigar smoking

Another major source of exposure to tobacco is through cigar and pipe smoking. Similar to the observations for cigarettes smoking and oral cancer risk, the vast majority of studies have identified a strong association between cigar and pipe smoking and oral cancer risk (Blot et al. 1988; Spitz et al. 1988; Franco et al. 1989; Merletti et al. 1989; Franceschi et al. 1990; La Vecchia et al. 1990, 1998; Zheng et al. 1990; Mashberg et al. 1993; Schildt et al. 1998; Hayes et al. 1999; Schlecht et al. 1999; Shapiro et al. 2000; Garrote et al. 2001). With only a few studies, such as the study by Marshall et al. (1992), reporting little or no association. In some studies, the risk of oral cancer was actually found to be higher for pipe and cigar smokers than for cigarette smokers.

For example, a case–control study by Franceschi *et al.* (1990) reported an OR of 20.7 (95% CI 5.6–76.3) for pipe and cigar smokers compared to an OR of 11.1 (95% CI 3.4–34.8) for cigarette smokers.

Zheng *et al.* (1990) reported an OR of 5.7 (95% CI 2.4–13.3) for male pipe smokers compared to 1.6 (95% CI 1.0–2.6) for male cigarette smokers in their case–control study. Franco *et al.* (1989) reported a higher risk of oral cancer for pipe smoking compared to other smoking behaviors, particularly for cancer of other parts of the mouth (ICD9 143–145).

Pipe smoking also showed a strong dose-dependent relationship with oral cancer risk in several studies (Blot *et al.* 1988; Mashberg *et al.* 1993; Schlecht *et al.* 1999). For example, the study by Schlecht *et al.* (1999) reported an OR of 6.7 (95% CI 3.1–14.8) for those who smoked 1–20 pack-years of commercial-cigarette equivalents of pipe, and 8.2 (95% CI 3.7–17.8) for those with more than 20 pack-years of commercial-cigarette equivalents of pipe smoking. Similarly, in a large case–control study, Blot *et al.* (1988) reported an OR of 1.9 (9% CI 1.1–3.4) for those exclusively smoking cigars and/or pipes, with a positive trend associated with increasing numbers of cigars/pipes smoked. The OR rose to 16.7 (95% CI 3.7–76.7) for men who smoked 40 or more cigars/week, and to 3.1 (95% CI 1.1–8.7) for those consuming 40+ pipefuls/week.

However, other studies, such as Merletti *et al.* (1989) reported a higher risk of oral cancer for cigar smokers (OR=14.6, 95% CI 4.7–45.6) than pipe smokers (OR=3.8, 95% CI 1.1–12.6) and than cigarette smokers (OR=3.9, 95% CI 1.6–9.4) among male smokers. A strong dose–response relationship has been shown between cigar smoking and risk of oral cancer. In particular, the study by Garrote *et al.* (2001) showed a strong dose–response relationship between cigar smoking and oral cancer risk ($P_{trend} < 0.01$). They found that, compared with never smokers, those who smoked <4 cigars or equivalents per day had an OR of 4.3 (95% CI 1.1–16.4), and those who smoked ≥4 cigars or equivalents per day had an OR of 20.5 (95% CI 4.7–89.7). Shanks and Burns (1998) reported a RR of 7.9 for 'ever' cigar smokers and a RR of 15.9 for heavy cigar smokers (>5 cigars per day) for oral and pharyngeal cancer risk. In a case–control study of oral and esophageal cancers involving only those who never smoked pipe tobacco or cigarettes, La Vecchia *et al.* (1998) reported an OR of 6.8 (95% CI 2.5–18.5) for ever smokers and 8.9 for smokers of more than 3 cigars per day, and 14.9 (95% CI 4.0–55.9) for current cigar smokers when compared to never cigar smokers.

In either case, pipe and cigar smoking clearly increases the risk of oral cancer. This risk seems to vary by anatomic subsite. Shapiro *et al.* (2000) found that, compared with never smokers, current cigar smokers had an RR of 4.0 (95% CI 1.5–10.3) for cancer of the oral cavity/pharynx compared to 10.3 (95% CI 2.6–41.0) for cancer of the larynx. Former smokers had an OR of 2.4 (95% CI 0.8–7.3) for cancer of the oral cavity/pharynx, but 6.7 (95% CI 1.5–30.0) for cancer of the larynx. In their case–control study of oral and esophageal cancers, La Vecchia *et al.* (1998) reported an OR 9.0 (95% CI 2.7–30.0) for oral and pharyngeal cancers, compared to 4.1 (95% CI 0.7–23.0) for esophageal cancer among ever cigar smokers. Boffetta *et al.* (1992) showed that soft palate seems to be more susceptible to cigar and pipe smoking than other sites.

Smokeless tobacco

People are also exposed to smokeless tobacco Including snuff and chewing tobacco. Snuff consists of a tobacco that has been cured and grounded into dry snuff (<10% moisture), or moist snuff (up to 50% moisture). Snuff dipping consists of taking a small amount of snuff between the gingival and the lip or the bucca mucosa, and leaving there from a few minutes to several hours. Chewing tobacco includes plug tobacco, loose-leaf tobacco, twist or roll tobacco. Chewing tobacco is held in the mouth where it can be chewed intermittently for several hours (Grasso and Mann 1998).

Since the 1980s, there has been considerable interest in the relationship between smokeless tobacco use and oral cancer risk, and several excellent reviews have summarized the major results linking smokeless tobacco use to oral cancer risk (Winn 1988, 1997; Vigneswaran *et al.* 1995; Gupta *et al.* 1996; Grasso and Mann 1998; Johnson 2001). While the IARC has concluded that 'there is sufficient evidence that oral use of snuff of the types commonly used in North America and western Europe is carcinogenic to humans' (IARC 1985), the relationship between smokeless tobacco use and oral cancer risk is not as consistent as what was observed for tobacco smoking from different populations, ranging from no increased risk from studies in Sweden (Axell *et al.* 1978; Lewin *et al.* 1997; Schildt *et al.* 1998) to an estimated 23-fold (rural women) and 61-fold (urban women) excess in risk associated with snuff use in Atlanta (Vogler *et al.* 1962).

A number of factors may have affected the observed relationship between smokeless tobacco use and oral cancer risk. For example, few studies were designed specifically to examine the relationship. Considering the low prevalence of smokeless tobacco users in most of the populations together with the small sample sizes in many studies, few studies would have the sufficient power to address the issue.

Perhaps a more important factor, which may account for the observed inconsistent association, is that smokeless tobacco products used in different countries contain very different levels of carcinogens. For example, smokeless tobacco used in Sweden is quite different from that used in India or US. In Sweden, where studies have failed to support an association between local snuff use and oral cancer risk, snuff is not fermented and contains much lower nitrosamine levels than fermented tobaccos (Johnson 2001). In India, however, processing of smokeless tobacco is done by individual farmers and small companies with little control over fermentation and curing (Vigneswaran *et al.* 1995); fermentation produces potentially carcinogenic nitrosamines. Also, in India, smokeless tobacco is often used in combination with betel leaf, areca nut, and powdered slaked lime, and these additives make the combination more genotoxic than tobacco alone. Fermentation is also used in the US, though recent improvements in tobacco agriculture and smokeless tobacco processing have resulted in substantial decline in the concentration of several important carcinogens (Brunnemann and Hoffmann 1993).

Since the levels of carcinogens in smokeless tobacco vary considerably from country to country, studies of different populations have reached very different conclusions. In the following, we will review the studies based on the country of origin of the study.

Studies in Sweden: Approximately, 15–20% of adult males use moist snuff in Sweden (Lewin *et al.* 1997). In fact, Sweden was the world's largest per capita consumer of smokeless tobacco throughout the twentieth century (Nordgren and Ramstrom 1990). Although an early study by Wynder *et al.* (1957) suggested an increased risk of oral cancer among snuff users, more recent studies from Sweden have found no relationship between use of local snuff and oral cancer risk. The population-based case–control study by Lewin *et al.* (1997) found no increased risk of head and neck cancer with ever using oral snuff. Age started using snuff, total number of years of using snuff, and total amount of snuff used in a lifetime all had little or no impact on the risk of head and neck cancer in this study.

Another recent case–control study by Schildt *et al.* (1998) also showed no increased risk of oral cancer among current snuff users regardless of tobacco smoking habits. Lifetime consumption of snuff also showed no increased risk. While ex-snuff users were found to have an increased risk, but the risk was seen only among those who were also active tobacco smokers. Users of chewing tobacco in this study (5 cases and 8 controls) also did not show an increased risk of oral cancer (OR=0.6, 95% CI 0.2–2.2).

An early retrospective follow-up study of 200 000 male snuff users in Sweden also failed to find a significantly increased risk of oral cancer (Axell *et al.* 1978). Ecological data from Sweden do not support an association between use of local snuff and oral cancer risk in this population (Lewin *et al.* 1997). Specifically, Geographic areas where consumption of oral snuff is highest, the incidence rate of head and neck cancers is low, and, areas with low consumption of snuff, the incidence for cancer of the head and neck is the highest.

Studies in the US: In the US, while the national prevalence rate of smokeless tobacco use is low (about 5% for regular use), the rates are high in some parts of the country. In North Carolina, for example, Winn *et al.* (1981) reported that 46% of the oral cancer cases and 30% of the controls were snuff users. Epidemiological studies from the US have generally indicated an increased risk of oral cancer associated with the use of oral snuff.

The most conclusive study was conducted in North Carolina by Winn *et al.* (1981). The study interviewed 232 female cases and 410 female controls, and found that smokeless tobacco use was a potent risk factor for oral cancer in this population. Among white women without a smoking habit, the oral and pharyngeal cancer cases were 4.2 times (95% CI 2.6–6.7) more likely to have used smokeless tobacco than were controls. Among women with cancer in the cheek or gums, where tissues come in direct contact with the tobacco powder, the relative risks rose from 13-fold for less than 25, and 25 to 49 year of use, to nearly 50-fold for 50 or more years of use. It is estimated that about 31% of the oral cancer in this population could be attributable to snuff dipping alone. While the study was criticized for using hospital-based controls that may not represent the population, which produced the cases with regards to the snuff use, the underlying association would actually be underestimated if the control diseases were in fact associated with the use of smokeless tobacco.

A large population-based case–control study by Blot *et al.* (1988) also reported a significantly sixfold (95% CI 1.9–19.8) increased risk of oral cancer due to use of smokeless tobacco among non-smoking females. Kabat *et al.* (1994) reported a crude OR of 34% (95% CI 8.5–140.1) for using snuff among female never smokers. An early hospital-based case–control study by Vogler *et al.* (1962) also found an increased risk of oral cancer associated with snuff use among both urban women (Crude OR = 60.8) and rural women (crude OR = 22.9). Spitz *et al.* (1988) also reported a significantly increased risk of oral cancer associated with snuff dipping among males (OR = 3.4, 95% CI 1.0–10.9).

There are also several studies of US populations that did not find an increased risk of oral cancer associated with smokeless tobacco use (Mashberg *et al.* 1993; Muscat *et al.* 1996; Schwartz *et al.* 1998). These studies, however, generally involved populations that have a very low prevalence rate for smokeless tobacco use, and none of them were designed specifically to investigate the association between smokeless tobacco use and risk of oral cancer. For example, the study by Schwartz *et al.* (1998) from western Washington State found that, out of 294 female cases and controls, only one female control subject used smokeless tobacco. Among males, prior smokeless tobacco use was reported by only 6.7% of the cases and 5.6% of the controls (OR = 1.0, 95% CI 0.4–2.3). The hospital-based case–control study by Mashberg *et al.* (1993) in New Jersey also found no increased risk of oral cancer for use of snuff (OR = 0.8, 95% CI 0.4–1.9) or chewing tobacco (OR = 1.0, 95% CI 0.7–1.4). The proportion of snuff or chewing tobacco together was found in only 14% of the cases and 11% of the controls.

Muscat *et al.* (1996) also found no increased risk of oral cancer associated with snuff use or chewing tobacco. But only 1.3% of the cases and 1.6% of the controls in males used snuff. Among women, only two cases and one control reported snuff use in this study. About 5% of the cases and controls in men and none of the women reported regularly using chewing tobacco. Sterling *et al.* (1992) evaluated the relationship between smokeless tobacco use and cancer risk based on data from the national mortality followback survey, and found no increased risk of oral or other digestive cancers associated with smokeless tobacco use, either as snuff or chewing tobacco. However, as pointed out by Johnson (2001), a number of limitations have limited the interpretation of the study results, including small number of subjects used the products, and issues related to data collection and presentation.

Studies in India: Oral cancer is the most common cancer in India, where large quantities of smokeless tobacco are used (Jayant and Deo 1986). Smokeless tobacco use is considered to be a major risk factor for the high incidence rate of oral cancer in this country. The study by Nandakumar *et al.* (1990) reported an increased risk of oral cancer among pan tobacco chewers in both males and females, and no increased risk among pan chewing without tobacco. A dose–response was observed for years of chewing, number of times of chewing per day, and period of retaining the pan in the mouth. A linear test for trend was statistically significant ($P < 0.001$) in all three instances. Compared to those with no history of chewing tobacco, the ORs were 8.5 (95% CI 4.7–15.2) for those who did not chew during sleep, and 17.7 (95% CI 8.7–36.1) for those with a history of chewing during sleep.

Rao *et al.* (1994) also reported a significant association between tobacco chewing and risk of oral cancer (OR = 3.0, 95% CI 2.3–3.7), and the risk increased with increasing frequency ($P_{trend} < 0.001$). For chewers who chewed tobacco 21–30 times per day, the OR was 10.7 times higher than that for non-chewers. Several other earlier case–control studies (Sanghvi *et al.* 1955; Wahi *et al.* 1965; Jussawalla and Deshpande 1971; Notani 1988) and follow-up studies (Bhargava *et al.* 1975; Gupta *et al.* 1980) from different parts of India have also provided unequivocal evidence between chewing tobacco and oral cancer risk, and this risk appeared to be even higher among those who began the habit at a younger age (Jayant *et al.* 1971).

Other countries: Franco *et al.* (1989) reported no association between use of smokeless tobacco, either as snuff or tobacco chewing, and risk of oral cancer in Brazil. However, the number of subjects who used tobacco in this form was small (9 cases and 13 controls). In Sudan, however, an increased risk of oral cancer was reported among those who used toombak, a coarse powder made of dried tobacco leaves, and the risk was found to be higher for anatomic sites (buccal cavity, floor of mouth, and lip) where tissues come in direct contact with the product (Idris *et al.* 1995).

Tobacco and alcohol interaction

A number of studies from different populations or racial groups have investigated the interaction between tobacco and alcohol on the risk of oral cancer, and most of them have concluded that the effects of tobacco and alcohol are certainly more than additive and seem to be consistent with multiplicative, with some suggesting a supra-multiplicative effect (Negri *et al.* 1993; De Stefani *et al.* 1998; Garrote *et al.* 2001). Studies, which presented the joint distribution of cases and controls for each combination of smoking and alcohol consumption with the corresponding ORs, have shown a sharp increase in the risk for those with the heaviest levels of consumption of both products compared to the lowest levels of consumption of both products. The OR for the highest levels of consumption of both products reached as high as 305 (Baron *et al.* 1993).

A strong interaction between tobacco and alcohol in the risk of oral cancer was observed no matter if the relationship is expressed by lifetime consumption of the products (Franco *et al.* 1989; Zheng *et al.* 1990; Bundgaard *et al.* 1994; Schidt 1998), or daily or weekly or monthly consumption of the products (Rothman and Keller 1972; Wynder *et al.* 1976; Elwood *et al.* 1984; Blot *et al.* 1988; Tuyns *et al.* 1988; Merletti *et al.* 1989; Franceschi *et al.* 1990; Day *et al.* 1993; Mashberg *et al.* 1993; Kabat *et al.* 1994; Andre *et al.* 1995; Chyou *et al.* 1995; Franceschi *et al.* 1999; Hayes *et al.* 1999; Garrote *et al.* 2001), or by cumulative tar/amount of alcohol day (Muscat *et al.* 1996), or expressed by other means (Baron *et al.* 1993; Lewin *et al.* 1997; De Stefani *et al.* 1998; Zavras *et al.* 2001).

A strong interaction between smoking and alcohol use on the risk of oral cancer is exemplified from the study by Franceschi *et al.* (1999) in Italy. In this study, the highest level of risk of oral cancer (OR = 227.8, 95% CI 54.6–950.7) was observed among those most heavily consuming both tobacco and alcohol.

Tobacco and gene interaction

It is suggested that functional polymorphisms in genes encoding tobacco carcinogen-metabolizing enzymes may modify the relationship between tobacco smoking and an individual's oral cancer risk. This is biologically plausible since the phase I enzymes (cytochromes P-450) activate many tobacco procarcinogens by forming or exposing their functional groups. For example, CYP1A1 is the major enzyme responsible for the metabolic activation of benzo-(*a*)-pyrene and other polycyclic aromatic hydrocarbons (PAHs), and CYP2E1 is the major enzyme responsible for the metabolic activation of nitrosamines. The activated carcinogens can bind covalently to DNA to form DNA adducts. Accumulation of DNA adducts at critical loci such as oncogenes or tumor suppressor genes can lead to somatic mutation and disruption of the cell cycle (Geisler and Olshan 2001).

The phase II enzymes (such as the glutathione S-transferases (GSTs) and *N*-acetyl transferase (NATs)) are involved in the detoxification of activated metabolites of carcinogens by phase I enzymes. GSTM1, for instance, metabolizes and detoxifies benzo-(*a*)-pyrene-diol epoxides (14,15), while GSTT1 detoxifies epoxides and other constituents of tobacco smoke, such as alkyl halides (16,17). Therefore, individuals who have high phase I metabolizing activities but have low or lack certain phase II metabolizing activity, may accumulate more DNA adducts, and thus have a particularly high cancer risk after exposure to tobacco smoke (13,18,19).

A few recent studies have investigated the association between tobacco smoking, genetic polymorphisms, and oral cancer risk [11,20–26]. For example, Park *et al.* (1999) reported a greater risk for those with the GSTP1 (var/var) genotype who were exposed to low levels of smoking (i.e. ≤20 pack-years, OR = 3.4, 95% CI 1.1–11) than among heavier smokers (i.e. >20 pack-years, OR = 1.4, 95% CI 0.5–4.0), suggesting GSTP1 genotype may play a role in risk for oral cancer particularly among lighter smokers. The studies by Sato *et al.* (1999, 2000) also showed that individuals with a combined genotype of Val/Val and GSTM1(–) were at an increased risk for oral squamous-cell carcinoma compared with other combined genotypes, in particular, at a low dose level of cigarette smoking. These observations are consistent with the suggestion that genetic variations in the ability to metabolize tobacco smoke carcinogens are most important in determining cancer risk at low levels of exposure, and may be less relevant at higher smoking doses where high levels of carcinogen exposure overwhelm polymorphism-induced differences in enzyme activity and/or expression (London *et al.* 1995).

It should be pointed out, however, that epidemiological results linking, smoking, gene and oral cancer risk have been inconsistent. In their recent review of 24 published studies that evaluated the risk of squamous-cell carcinoma of the head and neck in relation to GSTM1 and GSTT1 genetic polymorphisms, Geisler and Olshan (2001) reported that some of the studies reported weak-to-moderate associations and others finding no elevation in risk for the main effect of the gene. Few studies have directly evaluated the interaction with tobacco. As pointed out by Geisler and Olshan (2001) none of the studies conducted to date have been able to assess gene–environment interaction with precision due to limited statistical power. Lack of accurate and detailed measurement of exposure in many of the studies may have also contributed to the inconsistent results. It is obvious that well-designed studies with large sample size are needed to better understand the relationship between smoking, gene and risk of oral cancer.

Attributable risk

The International Agency for Research on Cancer has classified cancer of the oral cavity, pharynx, and larynx as tobacco-related cancers. A number of case–control studies have estimated the proportion of oral cancer cases attributable to tobacco smoking, but the estimated proportion depends on the validity of the estimation of the prevalence of smoking in the population and the relative risk from the exposure. A number of factors may affect the estimation: for example, hospital-based studies with patients as controls, population-based studies with high refusal rate, or lack of adequate control for major confounding factors (such as alcohol consumption). Since smoking and drinking are highly correlated, some studies calculated estimates of the population attributable risk (PAR) of oral cancer due to smoking and/or drinking rather than due to smoking alone. In most of the studies, the reported PAR from smoking did not include the impact from smokeless tobacco use, or even pipe and cigar smoking.

Parkin *et al.* (2000) have estimated that about 46% of the cancer of the oral cavity and pharynx in men and 11% of these diseases in women are attributable to smoking worldwide. Estimates vary for specific countries and are presented below.

In Italy, Merletti *et al.* (1989) estimated that 72.4% of oral cancer cases in men and 53.9% of the cases in women are attributable to smoke of more than 7 g of tobacco/day. The study by Negri *et al.* (1993) reported that, for both sexes, the single factor with the highest attributable risk was smoking, which in males accounted for 81–87% of oral cancer cases and in females for 42–47%.

In the US, Mashberg *et al.* (1993) estimated that 74% of oral cancer in this population was attributable to smoking 6 or more cigarette equivalents per day, and 97% of the disease was attributable to the combination of smoking and drinking. In a population-based case–control study of oral cancer involving 4 states in the US, Blot *et al.* (1988) estimated that 80% of the oral and pharyngeal cancer cases in men and 61% in women were attributable to smoking and alcohol drinking. Using the data from this population-based case–control study, Day *et al.* (1993) estimated that 83% of blacks and 73% of whites developed oral cancer as a result of alcohol and/or tobacco consumption, with most tumors arising from the combined effect of drinking and smoking. Almost half of all oral cancer (48%) among black men was attributed to smoking one pack or more daily in combination with heavy drinking (≥30 drinks per week). For white men, 36% of oral cancers were accounted for by this level of smoking and drinking. Tobacco and alcohol consumption account for bulk of the racial and gender differences in oral cancer in the US.

In Beijing, China, Zheng *et al.* (1990) found that tobacco smoking accounts for about 34% of all cases of oral cancer in the Chinese population (45% among males and 21% among females) and 44% of all oral squamous-cell carcinoma. In Bombay, it is estimated that 70% of oral cancer cases were attributable to smoking and chewing tobacco.

Biological plausibility

Tobacco smoke is a complex mixture of compounds. Over 300 carcinogens have been identified in cigarette smoke. Polycyclic aromatic hydrocarbons (PAHs) have long been recognized as carcinogens present in tar. There are about 20–40 ng of benz-pyrene per cigarette and substantial levels of carcinogenic metals such as hexavalent chromium (Johnson 2001). The most important and abundant carcinogenic agents in tobacco smoke are the tobacco-specific N-nitrosamines (TSNA), including nitrosonornicotine (NNN) and 4-(methylnitrosamino)-1-(3-pyridyl)-1-butanone (NNK).

About 30 carcinogens have been identified in smokeless tobacco. Again, the TSNAs are major contributors to the carcinogenic activity of these types of tobacco (Hoffman and Djordjevic 1997). TSNAs are formed exclusively from nicotine and from the minor tobacco alkaloids, primarily formed after harvesting the leaves, during drying, curing, aging, and especially during fermentation (Hoffmann *et al.* 1994; Brunnemann *et al.* 1996).

The absorbed PAHs, TSNA, and aromatic amines from tobacco use can be metabolically activated to form electrophilic intermediates, which have the ability to react with DNA to form covalently bound DNA adducts, which interfere with DNA replication and initiate the carcinogenesis process. Oral swabbing of a low concentration of a mixture of NNN plus NNK in water induces oral tumors in rats (Hoffman and Djordjevic 1997).

In vitro assays have shown that human buccal mucosa has the capability to metabolize NNK and NNN to alkyldiazohydroxides that can react with DNA as reviewed by Gupta *et al.* (1996). DNA adducts play a crucial role in tobacco-induced carcinogenesis and studies have demonstrated a positive correlation between DNA adduct levels and patient smoking status. Jones *et al.* (1993) have shown that the mean adduct levels in isolated oral tissue DNA from smokers were significantly higher than in non-smokers, and adduct levels in ex-smokers (1–12 years since cessation) were similar to those in nonsmokers.

Studies have suggested that the p53 tumor suppressor gene is a likely target for tobacco carcinogens (Jones 1998; Ralhan *et al.* 1998; Saranath *et al.* 1999; Hsieh *et al.* 2001). p53 tumor suppressor gene mutations are the most frequently found genetic errors in oral cancer (Jones 1998). Brennan *et al.* (1995) have shown that p53 mutation were more common in tumors from patients who were exposed to both tobacco and alcohol than in tumors from patients who were not exposed to these risk factors. As discussed previously, genetic polymorphism of drug-metabolizing enzymes may affect the susceptibility to oral cancer from exposure to tobacco carcinogens.

Conclusion

In 1986 an IARC Working Party concluded that there was sufficient evidence that tobacco was carcinogenic to humans and that the occurrence of malignant tumors of the upper digestive tract was causally related to the smoking of different forms of tobacco. IARC has also concluded that there is sufficient evidence that oral use of snuff of the types commonly used in North America and western Europe is carcinogenic to humans, and there was sufficient evidence that the habit of chewing betel quid containing tobacco was carcinogenic in humans (IARC 1985). More recent epidemiological studies and experimental studies further support these conclusions. There is convincing evidence that a large attributable risk can be ascribed to the joint habits of cigarette smoking and alcohol consumption.

References

Akiba, S. and Hirayama, T. (1990). Cigarette smoking and cancer mortality risk in Japanese men and women—results from reanalysis of the Six-Prefecture Cohort Study data. *Environ Health Perspect* **87**, 19–26.

Andre, K., Schraub, S., Mercier, M., and Bontemps, P. (1995). Role of alcohol and tobacco in the aetiology of head and neck cancer: A case-control study in the Doubs Region of France. *Oral Oncol, Eur J Cancer* **31B**, 301–9.

Axell, T., Mornstad, H., and Sundstrom, B. (1978). Snuff and cancer of the oral cavity: A retrospective study. *Lakartidningen* **75**, 1224–6.

Baron, A. E., Franceschi, S., Barra, S., Talamini, R., and La Vecchia, C. (1993). A comparison of the joint effects of alcohol and smoking on the risk of cancer across sites in the upper aerodigestive tract. *Cancer Epidemiol Biomark Prevent* **2**, 519–23.

Bhargava, K., Smith, L. W., Mani, N. J., Silverman, S., Malaowalla, A. M., and Billimoria, K. F. (1975). A follow-up study of oral cancer and precancerous lesions in 57,518 industrial workers of Gujarat, India. *Indian J Cancer* **12**, 124–32.

Blot, W. J., McLaughlin, J. K., Winn, D. M., Austin, D. F., Greenberg, R. S., Preston-Martin, S., *et al.* (1988). Smoking and drinking in relation to oral and pharyngeal cancer. *Cancer Res* **48**, 3282–7.

Boffetta, P., Mashberg, A., Winkelmann, R., and Garfinkel, L. (1992). Carcinogenic effect of tobacco smoking and alcohol drinking on anatomic sites of the oral cavity and oropharynx. *Int J Cancer* **52**, 530–33.

Boyle, P., Macfarlane, R., McGinn, R., Zheng, T., La Vecchia, C., Maisonneuve, P., and Scully, C. (1990a). International epidemiology of head and neck cancer. In: *Multiple Primary Tumors in the Head and Neck* (ed. N. de Vries, and J.L. Gluckman), pp. 80–138. Thieme Medical Publishers, Inc

Boyle, P., Macfarlane, G. J., Maisonneuve, P., Zheng, T., Scully, C., and Tedesco, B. (1990b). Epidemiology of mouth cancer in 1989. *J Royal Soc Med* **83**, 724–729.

Boyle, P., La Vecchia, C., Maisonneuve, P., Zheng, T., and Macfarlane, G. J. (1995). Cancer epidemiology and prevention. In: *Oxford Textbook of Oncology* (ed. U. Veronesi, M.J. Peckham, and R. Pinedo), Oxford University Press, Oxford.

Brenna, J. A., Boyle, J. O., Koch, W. M. (1995). Association between cigarette smoking and mutation of the p53 gene in squamous-cell carcinoma of the head and neck. *N Engl J Med* **332**, 712–7.

Brunnemann, K. D. and Hoffmann, D. (1993). Chemical composition of smokeless tobacco products. Monograph 2. Smokeless tobacco or health: An international perspective. NIH publication No, 93-3461:96-1.5.

Brunnemann, K. D., Prokopczyk, B., Djordjevic, M. V., and Hoffmann, D. (1996). Formation and analysis of tobacco-specific N-nitrosamines. *Crit Rev Toxicol* **26**, 121–37.

Bundgaard, T., Wildt, J., Frydenberg, M., Elbrond, O., and Nielsen, J. E. (1995). Case-control study of squamous cell cancer of the oral cavity in Denmark. *Cancer Causes Control* **6**, 57–67.

Chyou, P. H., Momura, A. M. Y., and Stemmermann, G. N. (1995). Diet, alcohol, smoking and cancer of the upper aerodigestive tract: A prospective study among Hawaii Japanese men. *Int J Cancer* **60**, 616–21.

Day, G. L., Blot, W. J., Shore, R. E., McLaughlin, J. K., Austin, D. F., and Greenberg, R. S. (1994). Second cancers following oral and pharyngeal cancers: Role of tobacco and alcohol. *JNCI* **86**, 131–7.

Day, G. L., Blot, W. J., Austin, D. F., Bernstein, L., Greenberg, R. S., Preston-Martin, S., *et al.* (1993). Racial differences in risk of oral and pharyngeal cancer: Alcohol, tobacco, and other determinants. *JNCI* **85**, 465–73.

Elwood, J. M., Pearson, J. C. G., Skippen, D. H., and Jackson, S. M. (1984). Alcohol, smoking, social and occupational factors. The aetiology of cancer of the oral cavity, pharynx and larynx. *Int J Cancer* **34**, 603–12.

De Stefani, E., Boffetta, P., Oreggia, F., Fierro, L., and Mendilaharsu, M. (1998). Hard liquor drinking is associated with higher risk of cancer of the oral cavity and pharynx than wine drinking. A case-control study in Uruguay. *Oral Oncol* **34**, 99–104.

Franco, E. L., Kowalski, L. P., Oliveira, B. V., Curado, M. P., and Pereira, R. N. (1989). Risk factors for oral cancer in Brazil: A case-control study. *Int J Cancer* **43**, 992–1000.

Franceschi, S., Levi, F., La Vecchia, C., Conti, E., Maso, L. D., Barzan, L., *et al.* (1999) Comparison of the effect of smoking and alcohol drinking between oral and pharyngeal cancer. *Int J Cancer* **83**, 1–4.

Franceschi, S., Barra, S., La Vecchia, C., Bidoli, E., Negri, E., and Talamini, R. (1992). Risk factors for cancer of the tongue and the mouth. *Cancer* **70**, 2227–33.

Franceschi, S., Talamini, R., Barra, S., Baron, A. E., Negri, E., Bidoli, E., *et al.* (1990). Smoking and drinking in relation to cancers of the oral cavity, pharynx, larynx, and esophagus in Northern Italy. *Cancer Res* **50**, 6502–7.

Franceschi, S., Bidoli, E., Herrero, R., and Munoz, N. (2000). Comparison of cancers of the oral cavity and pharynx worldwide: Etiological clues. *Oral Oncol* **36**, 106–15.

Garrote, L. F., Herrero, R., Reyes, R. O., Vaccarella, S., Anta, J. L., Ferbeye, L., *et al.* (2001). Risk factors for cancer of the oral cavity and oro-pharynx in Cuba. *Br J Cancer* **85**, 46–54.

Geisler, S. A. and Olshan, A. F. (2001). GSTM1, GSTT1, and the risk of squamous cell carcinoma of the head and neck: A Mini-HuGE review. *Am J Epidemiol* **154**, 95–105.

Grasso, P. and Mann, A. H. (1998). Smokeless tobacco and oral cancer: An assessment of evidence derived from laboratory animals. *Food Chem Toxicol* **36**, 1015–29.

Gupta, P. C., Murti, P. R., and Bhonsle, R. B. (1996). Epidemiology of cancer by tobacco products and the significance of TSNA. *Crit Review Toxicol* **26**, 183–8.

Gupta, P. C., Mehta, F. S., Daftary, D. K., Pindborg, J. J., Bhonsle, R. B., Jalnawalla, P. N., *et al.* (1980). Incidence rates of oral cancer and natural history of oral precancerous lesions in a 10-year follow-up study of India villagers. *Community Dent Oral Epidemiol* **8**, 287–93.

Hammond, E. C. and Seidman, H. (1980). Smoking and cancer in the United States. *Prevent Med* **9**, 169–73.

Hayes, R. B., Bravo-Otero, E., Kleinman, D. V., Brown, L. M., Fraumeni, J. F., Jr., Harty L. C., *et al.* (1999). Tobacco and alcohol use and oral cancer in Puerto Rico. *Cancer Causes Control* **10**, 27–33.

Hirayama, T. (1966). An epidemiological study of oral and pharyngeal cancer in Central and South-East Asia. *Bull WHO* **34**, 41–69.

Hoffman, D., Brunnemann, K. D., Prokopczyk, B., and Djordjevic, M. V. (1994). Tobacco-specific N-nitrosamines and areca-derived N-nitrosamines: Chemistry, biochemistry, carcinogenicity, and relevance to humans. *J Toxicol Environ Hlth* **41**, 1–52.

Hoffman, D. and Djordjevic, M. V. (1997). Chemical composition and carcinogenicity of smokeless tobacco. *Adv Dent Res* **11**, 322–9.

Hsieh, L. L., Wang, P. F., Chen, I. H., Liao, C. T., Wang, H. M., Chen, M. C., *et al.* (2001). Characteristics of mutations in the p53 gene in oral squamous cell carcinoma associated with betel quid chewing and cigarette smoking in Taiwanese. *Carcinogenesis* **22**, 1497–503.

Hung, H. C., Chuang, J., Chien, Y. C., Chern, H. D., Chiang, C. P., Kuo, Y. S., *et al.* (1997). Genetic polymorphisms of CYP2E1, GSTM1, and GSTT1, environmental factors and risk of oral cancer. *Cancer Epidemiol Biomark Prevent* **6**, 901–5.

Idris, A. M., Ahmed, H. M., and Malik, M. O. A. (1995). Toomak dipping and cancer of the oral cavity in the Sudan: A case-control study. *Int J Cancer* **63**, 477–80.

International Agency for Research on Cancer (1986). Monograph 38, Tobacco Smoking. International Agency for Research on Cancer, Lyon, France.

International Agency for Research on Cancer (1985). IARC monographs on the evaluation of the carcinogenic risk of chemicals to humans: Tobacco habits other than smoking: betel-quid and areca-nut chewing; and some related nitrosamines. Vol. 37, p. 116. International Agency for Research on Cancer, Lyon, France.

Jayant, K. and Deo, M. G. (1986). Oral cancer and cultural practices in relation to betel quid and tobacco chewing and smoking. *Cancer Detect Prevent* **9**, 207–13.

Jayant, K., Balakrishnan, V., and Sanghvi, L. D. (1971). A note on the distribution of cancer in some endogamous groups in Western India. *Br J Cancer* **25**, 611–9.

Johnson, N. (2001). Tobacco use and oral cancer: A global perspective. *J Dent Educat* **65**, 328–39.

Jones, A. (1998). A general review of the p53 gene and oral squamous cell carcinoma. *Ann Roy Australas Coll Dent Surg* **14**, 66–9.

Jones, N. J., McGregor, A. D., and Waters, R. (1993). Detection of DNA adducts in human oral tissue: Correlation of adduct levels with tobacco smoking and differential enhancement of adducts using the butanol extraction and nuclease P1 versions of 32p postlabeling. *Cancer Res* **53**, 1522–8.

Jussawalla, D. J. and Deshpande, V. A. (1971). Evaluation of cancer risk in tobacco chewers and smokers: An epidemiologic assessment. *Cancer* **28**, 244–52.

Kabat, G. C., Chang, C. J., and Wynder, E. L. (1994). The role of tobacco, alcohol use, and body mass index in oral and pharyngeal cancer. *Int J Epidemiol* **23**, 1137–44.

Kabat, G. C., Hebert, J. R. and Wynder, E. L. (1989). Risk factors for oral cancer in women. *Cancer Res* **49**, 2803–6.

La Vecchia, C., Franceschi, S., Bosetti, C., Levi, F., Talamini, R., and Negri, E. (1999). Time since stopping smoking and the risk of oral and pharyngeal cancers. *JNCI* **91**, 726–7.

La Vecchia, C., Bosetti, C., Negri, E., Levi, F., and Franceschi, S. (1998). Cigar smoking and cancers of the upper digestive tract. *JNCI* **90**, 1670.

La Vecchia, C., Bidoli, E., Barra, S., D'Avanzo, B., Negri, E., Talamini, R., *et al.* (1990). Type of cigarette and cancers of the upper digestive and respiratory tract. *Cancer Causes Control* **1**, 69–74.

La Vecchia, C., Tavani, A., Franceschi, S., Levi, F., Corrao, G., and Negri, E. (1997). Epidemiology and prevention of oral cancer. *Oral Oncol* **33**, 302–12.

Lewin, F., Norell, S. E., Johansson, H., Gustavsson, P., Wennerberg, J., Biorklund, A., Rutqvist, L. E. (1997). Smoking tobacco, oral snuff, and alcohol in the etiology of squamous cell carcinoma of the head and neck. *Cancer* **82**, 1367–75.

London, S. J., Daly, A. K., Cooper, J., Navidi, W. C., Capenter, C., Idle, J. R., *et al.* (1995). Polymorphism of gluathione S-transferase M1 and lung cancer risk among African Americans and Caucasians in Los Angeles County, California. *JNCI* **87**, 1246–53.

Macfarlane, G. J., Boyle, P., Evstifeeva, T. V., Robertson, C., and Scully, C. (1994). Rising trends of oral cancer mortality among males worldwide: The return of an old public health problem. *Cancer Causes Control* **5**, 259–65.

Macfarlane, G. J., Zheng, T., Marshall, J. R., Boffetta, P., Niu, S., Brasure, J., *et al.* (1995). Alcohol, tobacco, diet and risk of oral cancer: A pooled analysis of three case-control studies. *Oral Oncol, Eur J Cancer* **31B**, 181–7.

Marshall, J. R., Graham, S., Haughey, B. P., Shedd, D., O'Shea, R., Brasure, J., *et al.* (1992). Smoking, alcohol, dentition and diet in the epidemiology of oral cancer. *Oral Oncol, Eur J Cancer* **28B**, 9–15.

Mashberg, A., Boffetta, P., Winkelman, R., and Garfinkel, L. (1993). Tobacco smoking, alcohol drinking, and cancer of the oral cavity and oropharynx among U.S. veterans. *Cancer* **72**, 1360–75.

Merletti, F., Boffetta, P., Cicone, G., Msshberg, A., and Terracini, B. (1989). Role of tobacco and alcoholic beverages in the etiology of cancer of the oral cavity/oropharynx in Torino, Italy. *Cancer Res* **49**, 4919–24.

Moreno-Lopez, L. A., Esparza-Gomez, G. C., Gonzalez-Navarro, A., Cerero-Lapiedra, R., Gonzalez-Henandez, M. J., and Dominguez-Rojas, V. (2000). Risk of oral cancer associated with tobacco smoking, alcohol consumption and oral hygiene: A case-control study in Madrid, Spain. *Oral Oncol* **36**, 170–4.

Muscat, J. E., Richie, J. P., Thompson, S., and Wynder, E. L. (1996). Gender differences in smoking and risk for oral cancer. *Cancer Res* **56**, 5192–7.

Nandakumar, A., Thimmasetty, K. T., Sreeramareddy, N. M., Venugopal, T. C., Rajanna, Vinutha, A. T., *et al.* (1990). A population-based case-control investigation on cancers of the oral cavity in Bangalore, India. *Br J Cancer* **62**, 847–51.

Negri, E., La Vecchia, C., Franceschi, S., and Tavani, A. (1993). Attributable risk for oral cancer in Northern Italy. *Cancer Epidemiol Biomark Prevent* **2**, 189093.

Nordgren, P. and Ramstrom, L. (1990). Moist snuff in Sweden: Tradition and evolution. *Br J Addict* **85**, 1107–12.

Notani, P.N. (1988) Role of alcohol in cancers of the upper alimentary tract: Use of models in risk assessment. *J Epidemiol Commun Hlth* **42**, 187–92.

Park, J. Y., Schantz, S. P., Stern, J. C., Kaur, T., and Lazarus, P. (1999). Association between glutathione S-transferase π genetic polymorphisms and oral cancer risk. *Pharmacogenetics* **9**, 497–504.

Parkin, D. M., Pisani, P., and Masuyer, E. (2000). Tobacco-attributable cancer burden: a global review. In: *Tobacco: The Growing Epidemic*, Proceedings of the Tenth World Conference on Tobacco or Health (ed. R. Lu, J. Mackay, S. Niu, and R. Peto), 24–28 August 1997, Springer-Verlag London Limited, Beijing, China. pages 81–84.

Ralhan, R., Nath, N., Agarwal, S., Mathur, M., Wasylyk, B., and Shukla, N. K. (1998). Circulating p53 antibodies as early markers of oral cancer: Correlation with p53 alterations. *Clin Cancer Res* **4**, 2147–52.

Rao, D. N., Ganesh, B., Rao, R. S., and Desai, P. B. (1994). Risk assessment of tobacco, alcohol and diet in oral cancer—A case-control study. *Int J Cancer* **58**, 469–73.

Rothman, K. and Keller, A. (1972). The effect of joint exposure to alcohol and tobacco on risk of cancer of the mouth and pharynx. *J Chron Dis* **25**, 711–6.

Sanghvi, L. D., Rao, K. C. M., and Khanolkar, V. R. (1955). Smoking and chewing tobacco in relation to cancer of the upper alimentary tract. *BMJ* I, 1111–4.

Saranath, D., Tandle, A. T., Teni, T. R., Dedhia, P. M., Borgens, A. M., Parikh, D., *et al.* (1999). p53 inactivation in chewing tobacco-induced oral cancers and leukoplakias from India. *Oral Oncol* **35**, 242–50.

Sato, M., Sato, T., Izumo, T., and Amagasa, T. (2000). Genetically high susceptibility to oral squamous cell carcinoma in terms of combined genotyping of CYP1A1 and GSTM1 genes. *Oral Oncol* **36**, 267–71.

Sato, M., Sato, T., Izumo, T., and Amagasa, T. (1999). Genetic polymorphism of drug-metabolizing enzymes and susceptibility to oral cancer. *Carcinogenesis* **20**, 1927–31.

Schildt, E. B., Eriksson, M., Hardell, L., and Maonuson, A. (1998). Oral snuff, smoking habits and alcohol consumption in relation to oral cancer in a Swedish case-control study. *Int J Cancer* **77**, 341–6.

Schlecht, N. F., Franco, E. L., Pintos, J., and Kowalski, L. P. (1999). Effect of smoking cessation and tobacco type on the risk of cancers of the upper aero-digestive tract in Brazil. *Epidemiology* **10**, 412–8.

Schwartz, S. M., Daling, J. R., Doody, D. R., Wipf, G. C., Carter, J. J., Madeleine, M. M., *et al.* (1998). Oral cancer risk in relation to sexual history and evidence of human papillomavirus infection. *JNCI* **90**, 1626–36.

Shanks, T. G. and Burns, D. M. (1998). Disease consequences of cigar smoking. Smoking and Tobacco Control Monograph 9 Cigars. Health effects and trends. Bethesda (MD), pp. 105–158. National Institutes of Health, Report No: DHHS Publ No. (NIH) 98-4302.

Shapiro, J. A., Jacobs, E. J., and Thun, M. J. (2000). Cigar smoking in men and risk of death from tobacco-related cancers. *JNCI* **92**, 333–7.

Spitz, M. R., Fueger, J. J., Goepfert, H., Hong, W. K., and Newell, G. R. (1988). Squamous cell carcinoma of the upper aerodigestive tract. *Cancer* **61**, 203–8.

Sterling, T. D., Rosenbaum, W. L., and Weinkam, J. J. (1992). Analysis of the relationship between smokeless tobacco and cancer based on data from the national mortality followback survey. *J Clin Epidemiol* **42**, 223–31.

Talamini, R., Vaccarella, S., Barbone, F., Tavani, A., La Vecchia, C., *et al.* (2000). Oral hygiene, dentition, sexual habits and risk of oral cancer. *Br J Cancer* **83**, 1238–42.

Talamini, R., Franceschi, S., Barra, S., and La Vecchia, C. (1990). The role of alcohol in oral and pharyngeal cancer in non-smokers and of tobacco in non-drinkers. *Int J Cancer* **46**, 391–3.

Tuyns, A. J., Esteve, J., Raymond, L., Berrino, F., Benhamou, E., Blanchet, F., *et al.* (1988). Cancer of the larynx/hypopharynx, tobacco and alcohol: IARC International case-control study in Turin and Varese (Italy), Zaragoza and Navarra (Spain), Geneva (Switzerland) and Calvados (France). *Int J Cancer* **41**, 483–91.

Vigneswaran, N., Dent, M., Tilashalski, K., Rodu, B., and Cole, P. (1995). Tobacco use and cancer. *Oral Surg Oral Med Oral Pathol Oral Radiol Endod* **80**, 178–82.

Vogler, W. R., Lioyd, J. W., and Milmore, B. K. (1962). A retrospective study of etiological factors in cancer of the mouth, pharynx, and larynx. *Cancer* **15**, 246–58.

Wahi, P. N., Kehar, U., and Lahiri, B. (1965). Factors influencing oral and oropharyngeal cancers in India. *Br J Cancer* **19**, 642–60.

Weller, E. A., Blot, W. J., and Feigal, E. (1993). Oral cavity and pharynx. In: *SEER Cancer Statistics Review: 1973–1990* (ed. B.A. Hiller, L.A.G. Ries, B.F. Hankey, C.L. Kosary, A. Harras, S.S, Devesa, B.K. Edwards), pp. XIX.1–15. National Cancer Institute. NIH Pub. No 932789.

Winn, D. M., Blot, W. J., Shy, C. M., Pickle, L. W., Toledo, A., and Fraumeni, J. F. Jr. (1981). *New Engl J Med* **304**, 745–9.

Winn, D. M. (1988). Smokeless tobacco and cancer: The epidemiologic evdence. *CA-A Cancer J Clin* **38**, 236–43.

Winn, D. M. (1997). Epidemiology of cancer and other systemic effects associated with the use of smokeless tobacco. *Adv Dent Res* **11**, 313–21.

Wynder, E. L., Covey, L. S., Mabuchi, K., and Mushinski, M. (1976). Environmental factors in cancer of the larynx. *Cancer* **38**, 1591–601.

Wynder, E. L., Hultberg, S., Jacobsson, F., and Bross, I. J. (1957). Environmental factors in cancer of the upper alimentary tract: A Swedish study with special reference to Plummer-Vinson (Paterson-Kelly) syndrome. *Cancer* **10**, 470–87.

Zavras, A. I., Douglass, C. W., Joshipura, K., Wu, T., Laskaris, G., Petridou, E., *et al.* (2001). Smoking and alcohol in the etiology of oral cancer: Gender-specific risk profiles in the south of Greece. *Oral Oncol* **37**, 28–35.

Zheng, T., Holford, T., Chen, Y., Jiang, P., Zhang, B., and Boyle, P. (1997). Risk of tongue cancer associated with tobacco smoking and alcohol consumption: A case-control study. *Oral Oncol* **33**, 82–5.

Zheng, T., Boyle, P., Hu, H., Duan, J., Jiang, P. J., Ma, D. Q., *et al.* (1990). Tobacco smoking, alcohol consumption and risk of oral cancer: A case-control study in Beijing, People's Republic of China. *Cancer Causes Control* **1**, 173–9.

Chapter 24

Smoking and stomach cancer

David Zaridze

Incidence and mortality from stomach cancer is declining practically in all countries. Nevertheless stomach cancer remains the second most common cause of death from cancer in the world, accounting for about one million cases annually (Parkin *et al.* 1999). Incidence and mortality from stomach cancer are high in Japan, Korea, China, Russia, in Columbia, and other countries of South America, and are low in North America and western Europe (Pisani and Pisani 1999). Decline in the incidence of stomach cancer is accompanied by increase in cancer of the gastric cardia (Devesa *et al.* 1998; Botterweck *et al.* 2000).

Helicobacter pylori infection is causally associated with stomach cancer (IARC 1994). It has been shown-that type of food storage, namely the lack of refrigeration is a major risk factor for stomach cancer (World Cancer Research Fund 1997; Zaridze *et al.* 2002). Diets low in fruits and vegetables decrease the risk of stomach cancer (Nomura *et al.* 1990; Kabat *et al.* 1993; World Cancer Research Fund 1997; De Stefani *et al.* 1998; Terry *et al.* 1998; Mathew *et al.* 2000; Zaridze *et al.* 2002), while high salt intake has been claimed to increase the risk (Nomura *et al.* 1990; World Cancer Research Fund 1997; Zaridze *et al.* 2002). Alcohol consumption and especially consumption of liquors has been found to increase the risk of gastric cancer and especially cancer of the gastric cardia (Agudo *et al.* 1992; Hansson *et al.* 1994; Kabat *et al.* 1993; Gammon *et al.* 1997; De Stefani *et al.* 1998; Lagergren *et al.* 2000; Zaridze *et al.* 2000).

Smoking has been found to be associated with an increase in the risk of stomach cancer in many cohort and case–control studies reported from Asia, America, and Europe. Thirteen cohort studies found a statistically significant association between smoking and the risk of stomach cancer, relative risks ranging from 1.4 to 2.6 in current smokers. These studies include American Cancer Society study (Hammond 1966), U.S. Veteran's cohort (Kahn 1966), Japanese cohort (Hirayma 1982), British doctors cohort study (Doll *et al.* 1994), cohort of male Japanese physicians (Kono *et al.* 1987), six prefecture study in Japan (Akiba and Hirayama 1990), cohort of American men of Japanese ancestry (Nomura *et al.* 1990, 1995), cohort of American men of Scandinavian and German descent (Kneller *et al.* 1991), cohort study of inhabitants of Aichi prefecture in Japan (Kato *et al.* 1992*a*), cohort of inhabitants of five areas of Norway (Tverdal *et al.* 1993), cardiovascular risk factor study from Iceland (Tulinius *et al.* 1997), cohort of residents of Taiwan (Liaw and Chen 1998), Cancer Prevention Study II (Chao *et al.* 2002). In four cohort studies the increase in the risk associated with smoking was statistically not significant (Kato *et al.* 1992*b*; Guo *et al.* 1994; Engeland *et al.* 1996; Yuan *et al.* 1996). Three studies did not find any association between smoking and stomach cancer (Chen *et al.* 1997; Nordlund *et al.* 1997; Terry *et al.* 1998).

In seven of the positive cohort studies dose–response relationships were observed between intensity, and/or duration of smoking and the risk of cancer of the stomach. Statistically significant trends between number of cigarettes smoked per day and the risk of stomach cancer were observed in a 16-year follow-up report of Japanese six prefecture study (P for trend < 0.01) (Akiba and Hirayma 1990), a 20-year follow-up report of the cohort of US Veterans (P for trend < 0.01) (McLaughlin *et al.* 1995), in a 20-year follow-up report of the cohort of American men of Scandinavian and German origin (P for trend 0.01) (Kneller *et al.* 1991), in a 40-year follow-up report of the cohort of British doctors (P for trend < 0.01) (Doll *et al.* 1994), and in the cohort of inhabitants of Taiwan (P for trend < 0.06) (Liaw and Chen 1998). In Cancer Prevention Study II there was a statistically significant trend between number of cigarettes smoked per day and the risk of stomach cancer among current smoking women (P for trend $= 0.04$) and among ex-smoker men (P for trend $= 0.06$). The association between duration of smoking and the risk of stomach cancer were reported by Nomura *et al.* (1990), MacLaughlin *et al.* (1995), Liaw and Chen (1998), and Chao *et al.* (2002), with a statistically significant trend between number of years smoked and the increase in relative risk. Age started smoking was significantly associated with the risk of stomach cancer in the cohort of American men of Japanese ancestry (P for trend < 0.0001) (Nomura *et al.* 1995), in the cohort of the inhabitants of Taiwan (P for trend < 0.02) (Liaw and Chen 1998) and among men in Cancer Prevention Study II (P for trend $= 0.03$) (Chao *et al.* 2002). Cumulative exposure to smoking expressed as number of pack-years of smoking has also been found to influence the risk of stomach cancer (Kneller *et al.* 1991; Chao *et al.* 2002). Cancer Prevention Study II examined the effect of cessation on the risk of gastric cancer. Among men there was a dose–response relationship between age-quit smoking (P for trend $= 0.0015$), number of years since smoking cessation (P for trend $= 0.0015$), and relative risk of gastric cancer (Chao *et al.* 2002).

It should be noted that in most if not all studies the cohorts were followed passively and the information on smoking habit of cohort members was based only on the interview at the initial survey, while many cohort members could change their smoking habit during the long follow-up period. Therefore the risk of stomach cancer associated with smoking in these cohort studies could be underestimated due to misclassification of former smokers as current smokers.

About 40 case–control studies investigated the association between tobacco smoking and stomach cancer. One of them was a retrospective mortality case-referent study (Liu *et al.* 1998). Nineteen studies were population-based and the rest hospital-based case–control studies. In most studies relative risks were adjusted for different variables, such as sex, age, SES, education, income, diet, namely consumption of fruits and vegetables, alcohol consumption.

Thirty-one case–control studies reported a statistically significant increase in the risk of stomach cancer among smokers (Hoey *et al.* 1981; Correa *et al.* 1985; Risch *et al.* 1985; Hu *et al.* 1988; You *et al.* 1988; De Stefani *et al.* 1990; Kato *et al.* 1990; Lee *et al.* 1990; Wu-Williams *et al.* 1990; Dockerti *et al.* 1991; Saha 1991; Yu and Hsieh 1991; Hoshiyama and Sasaba 1992; Kabat *et al.* 1993; Hansson *et al.* 1994; Inoue *et al.* 1994; Siemiaticky *et al.* 1995; Yu *et al.* 1995; Gajalakshmi and Shanta 1996; Ji *et al.* 1996; Zang *et al.* 1996; Gammon *et al.* 1997; De Stefani *et al.* 1998; Liu *et al.* 1998; Chow *et al.* 1999; Innoue *et al.* 1999; Ye *et al.* 1999; Lagergren *et al.* 2000; Mathew *et al.* 2000; Zaridze *et al.* 2000; Wu *et al.* 2001).

In 10 case–control studies smoking was found not to have any influence on the risk of stomach cancer (Hanszel *et al.* 1972, 1976; Armijo *et al.* 1981; Jedrychowski *et al.* 1986, 1993; Buatti *et al.* 1989; Ferraroni *et al.* 1989; Boeing *et al.* 1991; Agudo *et al.* 1992; Gao *et al.* 1994).

Twenty-one studies have shown statistically significant dose–response trend between number of cigarettes smoked per day and/or duration of smoking and/or age start smoking and/or pack-years smoked and the risk of gastric cancer (Hu *et al.* 1988; You *et al.* 1988; De Stefani *et al.* 1990; Kato *et al.* 1990; Lee *et al.* 1990; Wu-Williams *et al.* 1990; Yu and Hsieh 1991; Kabat *et al.* 1993; Hansson *et al.* 1994; Yu *et al.* 1995; Gajalakshmi and Shanta 1996; Ji *et al.* 1996; Zhang *et al.* 1996; Gammon *et al.* 1997; De Stefani *et al.* 1998; Liu *et al.* 1998; Ye *et al.* 1999; Lagergren *et al.* 2000; Mathew *et al.* 2000; Zaridze *et al.* 2000; Wu *et al.* 2001). For example, a population-based case–control study from China which included 1124 stomach cancer cases and 1452 community controls (Ji *et al.* 1996) showed statistically significant dose–response relationship between numbers of cigarettes smoked per day and risk of stomach cancer (*P* for trend = 0.0002), with highest risk observed in men who smoked 20–29 cigarettes per day (RR = 1.77, 95% CI 1.35–2.33); statistically significant trend in the risk was observed for duration of smoking (*P* for trend = 0.002), with highest risk seen in men who smoked for more than 40 years (RR = 1.64, 95% CI 1.21–2.24) and for cumulative lifelong exposure to smoking expressed as pack-years smoked (*P* for trend = 0.0002), with highest risk estimates in the highest exposure group (RR = 1.68, 95% CI 1.22–2.30). Statistically significant dose–response relationships between duration of smoking (*P* for trend < 0.001), pack-years smoked (*P* for trend < 0.001), age at start smoking (*P* for trend < 0.01), and relative risks of stomach cancer were observed in hospital-based case–control study from Uruguay which included 330 male cases and 622 controls drawn from the same hospitals as cases (De Stefani *et al.* 1998). In the population-based study in USA (Gammon *et al.* 1997) statistically significant dose–response was observed for number of cigarettes smoked per day (*P* for trend < 0.05), duration of smoking in years (*P* for trend < 0.05), and cumulative exposure to tobacco smoke, or pack-years (*P* for trend < 0.05).

Cessation of smoking affected the risk of cancer of the stomach. In the population-based case–control study from Sweden which included 338 cases of stomach cancer and 678 community controls (Hansson et al. 1994), there was a statistically significant association between number of years since quitting and the risk of stomach cancer (P for trend = 0.02). In the study of De Stefani et al. (1998) relative risk of stomach cancer among men who gave up smoking 10–14 years ago was 1.0 (95% CI 0.5–2.1), while in those who gave up smoking 1–4 years ago relative risk was 2.4 (95% CI 1.3–3.6), and in current smokers was 2.6 (95% CI 1.6–4.1). In the study reported by De Stefani et al. in 1990, quitting for more than 10 years resulted in the decrease of relative risk (RR = 0.6, 95% CI 0.3–1.0) in comparison with individuals who gave up smoking 1–4 years ago (P for trend = 0.028).

Several case–control studies presented results separately for gastric cardia (or for adenocarcinoma of distal oesophagus and gastric cardia) and distal stomach (Wu-Williams et al. 1990; Kabat et al. 1993; Zhang et al. 1996; Gammond et al. 1997; De Stefani et al. 1998; Ye et al. 1999; Zaridze et al. 2000; Wu et al. 2001). In all these studies effects of smoking on the risk have been seen for cancers of both sites. In some studies association was somewhat stronger for distal stomach (Wu-Williams et al. 1990; Zhang et al. 1996; Wu et al. 2001), in others with cancer of the gastric cardia (Kabat et al. 1993; Zaridze et al. 2000). Dose–response relationship was observed between number of cigarettes smoked per day, duration of smoking, pack-years of smoking, age started smoking, and the risk of cancer of the gastric cardia (Zhang et al. 1996; Gammon et al. 1997; De Stefani et al. 1998; Ye et al. 1999; Zaridze et al. 2000; Wu et al. 2001) and distal stomach (Gammon et al. 1997; De Stefani et al. 1998; Zheng et al. 1996; Wu et al. 2001). Case–control study from Sweden reported similar trends in relative risk of stomach cancer related to number of cigarettes smoked per day—for cancer of the distal stomach (P for trend = 0.005) and gastric cardia (P for trend = 0.04), duration of smoking—for cancer of the distal stomach (P for trend = 0.002) and gastric cardia (P for trend = 0.03).

Smoking cessation significantly decreased the risk of cancer of gastric cardia. In a population-based case–control study reported from Sweden which included 262 cases of cancer of gastric cardia and 820 community controls, the increase in numbers of years since smoking cessation was associated with statistically significant decrease in the risk (P for trend < 0.0001). Those individuals who gave up smoking for more than 25 years had relative risk of 1.9 (95% CI 1.1–3.1), while those who quit 0–2 years ago had relative risk of 4.2 (95% CI 2.8–6.4) (Lagergren et al. 2000). Similar trend was observed by Wu et al. (2001), both for cancer of gastric cardia (P for trend < 0.0002) and cancer of the distal stomach (P for trend < 0.002).

Significant association between smoking and risk persisted when relative risks were computed separately for intestinal and diffuse types of stomach cancer (Kato et al. 1990; Ye et al. 1999).

Number of cases of stomach cancer in women was generally small and the increases in risks associated with smoking were less than for men and statistically not significant

(Kato *et al.* 1990; Ji *et al.* 1996; Zaridze *et al.* 2000). However in the studies where sufficient number of cases of stomach cancer in women were included the size of relative risks were comparable with relative risk in men. For example in the study from Japan which included 995 cases of stomach cancer of which 344 were women showed statistically significant increase in relative risk among current smoking women (RR=1.74, 95% CI 1.28–2.36). Risk estimates were higher in women in the age of 60 years or more (RR=1.99, 95% CI 1.24–3.21) (Innoue *et al.* 1994). In the study of Kabat *et al.* (1993) current smoking women were at increased risk of adenocarcinoma of distal oesophagus and the gastric cardia (RR=4.8, 95% CI 1.7–5.4) and cancer of the distal stomach (RR=4.8, 95% CI 1.9–11.9). Highest relative risks were for those women who smoked for more than 21 years. Ever smoking Polish women were also at increased risk of stomach cancer (RR=1.8, 95% CI 1.1–3.0) (Chow *et al.* 1999). Risk was increased in current smokers (RR=1.8, 95% CI 1.0–3.3), as well as in former smokers (RR=1.8, 95% CI 0.9–3.7).

Of special interest is the mortality-based case–control study carried out in China (Liu *et al.* 1998). In this study 27 710 deaths (20 195 men and 7515 women) from stomach cancer were identified. The reference group included individuals who died from causes not related to smoking. Information on smoking habit was obtained from proxy interviews. It has been shown that in men smoking increases the risk of stomach cancer by 30%, while current smoking in women was associated with only 17% increase in the risk. According to this study 18% of death from stomach cancer in Chinese men and only 1.7% in women could be attributed to smoking. These figures reflect present not very high smoking rates in Chinese, specially in Chinese women, which unfortunately inevitably will rise. Similar trends will be seen in other countries, where smoking epidemics in women have not yet reached its maximum. Increase in smoking rates in women will be followed by rise of smoking-related relative risks of cancers, including stomach cancer and proportion of death attributable to smoking.

Diet and alcohol consumption, all associated with the risk of stomach cancer could be major confounding factors of the effect of smoking on the risk of cancer of this site (World Cancer Research Fund 1997; Zaridze *et al.* 2000). However, adjustment for alcohol drinking (De Stefani *et al.* 1990; You and Hsieh 1991; Kabat *et al.* 1993; Ji *et al.* 1996; Simieticky *et al.* 1996; Zhang *et al.* 1996; Gammon *et al.* 1997; De Stefani *et al.* 1998; Innoue *et al.* 1999; Ye *et al.* 1999; Lagergren *et al.* 2000; Zaridze *et al.* 2000), as well as for consumption of fresh fruits and vegetables (De Stefani *et al.* 1990; You and Hsieh 1991; Inoue *et al.* 1994; Semiaticki *et al.* 1995; Gajalakshmi and Shanta 1996; De Stefani *et al.* 1998; Innoue *et al.* 1999; Lagergren *et al.* 2000), did not materially effect the risk estimates associated with smoking.

Positive association between smoking and the risk of stomach cancer could be confounded by the effect of *H. pylori* infection status. A large body of evidence supports a causative role for *H. pylori* in stomach cancer. In 1994 IARC recognized *H. pylori* as a class 1 human carcinogen (IARC 1994).

Several surveys have shown that *H. pylori* infection status is not associated with the smoking habit. Limburg *et al.* (2001) examined association between seropositivity for *H. pylori* with different risk factors in Linxian prospective study. The proportion of seropositive individuals was similar in non-smokers (58%) and in smokers (61%). Moreover, the prevalence of CagA seropositive individuals was higher in non-smokers (32%), than in smokers (24%). Another study in China looked at association between prevalence of *H. pylori* infection and smoking, drinking, and diet. Prevalence of *H. pylori* positivity was higher among never smokers, relative risk for ever smoking being 0.9 (0.7–1.0). In highest category of smokers of more than 14 235 pack-years OR was 0.8 (0.6–1.1) (Brown *et al.* 2002). Similar evidence is observed in Europe. Prevalence of seropositive subjects is similar among never (50.9%), former (48.7%), and current smokers (45.1%). In fact, among never smokers proportion of *H. pylori* seropositives is somewhat higher than among current smokers (OR = 0.8, CI 0.7–0.9) (The EUROGAST study group 1993). In only one study conducted in north England smoking of more than 35 cigarettes/day turned to be associated with higher risk of *H. pylori* positivity. However, it should be noted that the proportion of subjects infected were identical in all lower smoking intensity categories. Overall there is no association between *H. pylori* infection status and smoking (Moaygedy *et al.* 2002).

Zaridze *et al.* (2000) computed the interaction between *H. pylori* seropositivity and smoking in relation to the risk of stomach cancer. *H. pylori* infection did not affect smoking-associated risk of stomach cancer. However, relative risk of stomach cancer was higher among *H. pylori* positive men. Similar results were obtained by Siman *et al.* (2001). The results of these analyses suggest that smoking potentiates the effect of *H. pylori* infection on the risk of stomach cancer.

The relative risk of gastric cancer associated with smoking is most probably underestimated in hospital-based case–control studies, due to substantial proportion of patient with smoking-related diseases in control groups. Of special concern are the studies in which prevalence of smoking was higher in controls than in cases and in which controls with smoking-associated diseases were recruited (Jedrichowski *et al.* 1986; Lee *et al.* 1990; Boeing *et al.* 1991; Agudo *et al.* 1992).

According to one widely accepted model of gastric carcinogenesis development of cancer in stomach is preceded by several stages, including chronic atrophic gastritis, intestinal metaplasia, and dysplasia. Relative risk of developing these lesions have been shown to be associated with smoking. Risk of both metaplasia ($P = 0.03$) and dysplasia ($P < 0.001$) increased significantly with increasing tobacco consumption, but the magnitude of association was much stronger for dysplasia. The odds ratio for dysplasia among heavy smokers (>20 cigarettes/day) compared with lifelong non-smokers exceeded 2 and was statistically significant (OR = 2.2, 95% CI 1.5–3.3). The risks of metaplasia and dysplasia also increased with increasing duration of smoking. *P* values for trend were 0.02 and < 0.001 for metaplasia and dysplasia, respectively. The risk of dysplasia also rose with increasing pack-years of smoking. (Kneller *et al.* 1993). You *et al.* (2000) assessed the effect of smoking on progression of gastric precursor lesions to dysplasia and cancer. Smoking duration for more than 25 years was associated with significant increase in the risk of progression to gastric cancer and dysplasia (OR = 1.6, 95% CI 1.0–2.1; *P* for trend = 0.04). The risk was also increased in those who smoked more than 20 cigarettes/day (OR = 1.4 95% CI 0.9–2.3).

Few studies have reported on cigar, pipe, or smokeless tobacco use in relation to stomach cancer. In most recent analyses of CPS II cohort, current smokers of exclusively cigars had significantly higher stomach cancer mortality than non-users of any tobacco (OR=2.29, CI 1.49–3.41) (Chao *et al.* 2002). In a cohort study of American men of German and Scandinavian origin regular pipe users were at very high risk (RR=4.4, CI 1.84–10.72). Relative risk remained marginally significant after stratification for pack-years of cigarette smoking (RR=2.3, CI 0.98–5.22). In case–control studies reported by Correa *et al.* (1985), Wu-Williams *et al.* (1990), and Lagergren *et al.* (2000) significant association between cigar and/or pipe smoking and risk of stomach cancer was observed. In case–control study conducted in India smoking of bidi (RR=3.3, CI 1.8–5.67) and chutta (RR=2.4, CI 1.18–4.93) was associated with statistically significant increase in the risk of gastric cancer, with dose–response relationship between intensity and duration of smoking and relative risk (Gajalakshmi and Shanta 1996). Chewing tobacco increased risk of stomach cancer in cohort study reported from America by Kneller *et al.* (1991). However after adjusting for cigarette smoking increase in the risk lost statistical significance. All Swedish studies reported no association between snus (snuff) dipping and stomach cancer incidence (Hansson *et al.* 1994; Ye *et al.* 1999; Lagergren *et al.* 2000).

Worldwide, it has been estimated that the smoking-attributable proportion of stomach cancer is 11% among men and 4% among women in developing countries, and 17% among men and 11% among women in developed countries (Tredaniel *et al.* 1997). According to Liu *et al.* (1998) 18% death from stomach cancer in men and 1.8% in women in China are caused by smoking. The proportion of incident cases of stomach cancer attributable to smoking has been estimated to be 20% in Poland (Chow *et al.* 1999) and 31% in India (Gajalakshmi and Shanta (1996). In US 28% of stomach cancer death in men and 14% in women are attributable to tobacco smoking (Chao *et al.* 2002). According to estimates of Siemieticky *et al.* (1995) smoking causes 35% of incidence cases of stomach cancer in US. Adding stomach cancer to the list of cancers caused by smoking would increase the total number of smoking-attributable death by at least 84 000 per year worldwide (Tredaniel *et al.* 1997) not accounting for recent increases in smoking prevalence or the expected rise in stomach cancer incidence due to ageing in the developing world.

In summary the existing scientific evidence suggest a causal association between smoking and stomach cancer.

References

Agudo, A., Gonzalez, C. A., Marcos, G., Sanz, M., Saigi, E., Verge, J., *et al.* (1992). Consumption of alcohol, coffee, and tobacco, and gastric cancer in Spain. *Cancer Causes Control*, 3, 137–43.

Akiba, S. and Hirayama, T. (1990). Cigarette smoking and cancer mortality risk in Japanese men and women—results from reanalysis of the six-prefecture cohort study data. *Environ. Health Perspect.*, 87, 19–26.

Armijo, R., Orellana, M., Medina, E., Coulson, A. H., Sayre, J. W., and Detels, R. (1981). Epidemiology of gastric cancer in Chile: Case-control study. *Int. J. Epidemiol.*, 10, 53–6.

Boeing, H., Frentzel-Beyme, R., Berger, M., Berdt, V., Gores, W., Korner, M., *et al.* (1991). Case-control study on stomach cancer in Germany. *Int. J. Cancer*, 47, 858–64.

Brown, L. M., Thomas, T. L., Ma, J., Chang, Y., You, W., Liu, W., *et al.* (2002). Helicobacter pylori infection in rural China: Demographic, lifestyle and environmental factors. *Int. J. Epidemiol.*, 31, 638–46.

Buiatti, E., Palli, D., Decarli, A., Amadori, D., Avellini, C., Bianchi, S., *et al.* (1989). A case-control study of gastric cancer and diet in Italy.
Int. J. Cancer, 44, 611–6.

Chao, A., Thun, M. J., Henley, S. J., Jacobs, E. J., McCullough, M. L., and Calle, E. E. (2002). Fatal stomach cancer in relation to cigarrete smoking and use of other forms of tobacco in Cancer Prevention Study II. *Int. J. Cancer* (in press).

Chen, Z. M., Xu, Z., Collins, R., Li, W. X., and Peto, R. (1997). Early health effects of the emerging tobacco epidemic in China: A 16-year prospective study. *J. Am. Med. Assoc.*, 278, 1500–4.

Chow, W. H., Swanson, C. A., Lissowska, J., Groves, F. D., Sobin, L. H., Nasierowska-Guttmejer, A., *et al.* (1999). Risk of stomach cancer in relation to consumption of cigarettes, alcohol, tea and coffee in Warsaw, Poland. *Int. J. Cancer*, 81, 871–6.

Correa, P., Fontham, E., Pickle, L. W., Chen, V., Lin, Y., and Haenszel, W. (1985). Dietary determinants of gastric cancer in South Louisiana. *J. Natl. Cancer Inst.*, 75, 645–54.

De Stefani, E., Boffetta, P., Carzoglio, J., Mendilaharsu, S., and Deneo-Pellegrini, H. (1998). Tobacco smoking and alcohol drinking as risk factors for stomach cancer: a case-control study in Uruguay. *Cancer Causes Control*, 9, 321–9.

De Stefani, E., Correa, P., Fierro, L., Carzoglio, J., Deneo-Pellegrini, H., and Zavala, D. (1990). Alcohol drinking and tobacco smoking in gastric cancer. A case-control study. *Rev. Epidemiol. Santé Publique*, 38, 297–307.

Devesa, S. S., Blot, W. J., and Fraumeni J. F. Jr. (1998). Changing patterns in the incidence of esophageal cancer and gastric carcinoma in the United States. *Cancer*, 83, 2049–53.

Dockerty, J. D., Marshall, S., Fraser, J., and Pearce, N. (1991). Stomach cancer in New Zealand: Time trends, ethnic group differences and a cancer registry-based case-control study. *Int. J. Epidemiol.*, 20, 45–53.

Doll, R., Peto, R., Wheatey, K., Gray, R., and Sutherland, E. (1994). Mortality in relation to smoking: 40 years' observation on male British doctors. *Br. Med. J.*, 309, 901–12.

Engeland, A., Andersen, A., Haldorsen, T., and Tretli, S. (1996). Smoking habits and risk of cancers other than lung cancer: 28 years' follow-up of 26, 000 Norwegian men and women. *Cancer Causes Control*, 7, 497–506.

Ferraroni, M., Negri, E., La Vecchia, C., D'Avanzo, X., and Franceschi, S. (1989). Socioeconomic indicators, tobacco and alcohol in the aetiology of digestive tract neoplasms. *Int. J. Epidemiol.*, 18, 556–62.

Gajalakshmi, C. K. and Shanta, V. (1996). Lifestyle and risk of stomach cancer: A hospital-based case-control study. *Int. J. Epidemiol.*, **25**, 1146–53.

Gammon, M. D., Schoenberg, J. B., Ahsan, H., Risch, H. A., Vaughan, T. L., Chow, W. H., *et al.* (1997). Tobacco, alcohol, and socioeconomic status and adenocarcinomas of the esophagus and gastric cardia. *J. Natl Cancer Inst.*, **89**, 1277–84.

Guo, W., Blot, W. J., Li, J. Y., Taylor, P. R., Liu, B. Q., Wang, W., *et al.* (1994). A nested case-control study of oesophageal and stomach cancers in the Linxian Nutrition Intervention Trial. *Int. J. Epidemiol.*, **23**, 444–50.

Haenszel, W., Kurihara, M., Segi, M., and Lee, R. K. C. (1972). Stomach cancer among Japanese in Hawaii. *J. Natl. Cancer Inst.*, **49**, 968–88.

Haenszel, W., Kurihara, M., Locke, F. B., Shimuzu, X., and Segi, M. (1976). Stomach cancer in Japan. *J. Natl. Cancer Inst.*, **56**, 265–78.

Hammond, E. C. (1966). Smoking in relation to the death rates of one million men and women. *Natl. Cancer Inst. Monogr.*, **19**, 127–204.

Hansson, L. E., Baron, J., Nyren, O., Bergstrom, R., Wolk, A., and Adami, H., pp. 2–8.O. (1994). Tobacco, alcohol and the risk of gastric cancer: A population-based case-control study in Sweden. *Int. J. Cancer*, **57**, 26–31.

Hirayma, T. (1982). Smoking and cancer in Japan. A prospective study on cancer epidemiology based on census population in Japan. Results of 13 years follow-up. In: *The UICC Smoking Control Workshop, Nagoya, Japan, August 24–25, 1981* (ed. S. Tominaga, and K. Aoki), The University of Nagoya Press, Nagoya.

Hoey, J., Montvernay, C., and Lambert, R. (1981). Wine and tobacco: Risk factors for gastric cancer in France. *Am. J. Epidemiol.*, **113**, 668–74.

Hoshiyama, Y., and Sasaba, T. (1992). A case-control study of stomach cancer and its relation to diet, cigarettes, and alcohol consumption in Saitama Prefecture, Japan. *Cancer Causes Control*, **3**, 441–8

Hu, J. F., Zang, S., Jia, E., Wang, Q., Liu, S., Liu, Y., *et al.* (1988). Diet and cancer of the stomach: Case-control study in China. *Int. J. Cancer*, **41**, 331–5.

IARC Monographs on the evaluation of carcinogenic risks to humans (1994). Schistosomes, liver flukes and Helicobacter pylori, Vol. 61, pp. 177–241, IARC, Lyon.

Inoue, M., Tajima, K., Hirose, K., Kuroishi, T., Gao, C. M., and Kitoh, T. (1994). Life-style and subsite of gastric cancer—Joint effect of smoking and drinking habits. *Int. J. Cancer*, **56**, 494–9.

Inoue, M., Tajima, K., Yamamura, Y., Hamajima, N., Hirose, K., Nakamura, S., *et al.* (1999). Influence of habitual smoking on gastric cancer by histologic subtype. *Int. J. Cancer*, **81**, 39–43.

Jedrychowski, W., Boeing, H., Wahrendorf, J., Popila, T., Tobiasz-Adamczyk, B., and Kulig, J. (1993). Vodka consumption, tobacco smoking and risk of gastric cancer in Poland. *Int. J. Epidemiol.*, **22**, 606–13.

Jedrychowski, W., Wahrendorf, J., Popila, T., and Rachtan, J. (1986). A case-control study of dietary factors and stomach cancer risk in Poland. *Int. J. Cancer*, **37**, 837–42.

Ji, B. T., Chow, W. H., Yang, G., McLaughlin, J. K., Gao, R. N., Zheng, W., *et al.* (1996). The influence of cigarette smoking, alcohol, and green tea consumption on the risk of carcinoma of the cardia and distal stomach in Shanghai, China. *Cancer.*, **77**, 2449–57.

Kabat, G. C., Ng, S. K., and Wynder, E. L. (1993). Tobacco, alcohol intake, and diet in relation to adenocarcinoma of the esophagus and gastric cardia. *Cancer Causes Control*, **4**, 123–32.

Kahn, H. A. (1966). The Dorn study of smoking and mortality among U.S. veterans: Report of eight and one-half years of observation. *Natl. Cancer Inst. Monogr.*, **19**, 1–125.

Kato, I., Tominaga, S., and Matsumoto, K. (1992a). A prospective study of stomach cancer among a rural Japanese population: A 6-year survey. *Jpn. J. Cancer Res.*, **83**, 568–75.

Kato, I., Tominaga, S., Ito, Y., Kobayashi, S., Yoshii, Y., Matsuura, A., *et al.* (1992b). A prospective study of atrophic gastritis and stomach cancer risk. *Jpn. J. Cancer Res.*, **83**, 1137–42.

Kato, I., Tominaga, S., Ito, Y., Kobayshi, S., Yoshii, Y., and Matsuura, A. (1990). A comparative case-control analysis of stomach cancer and atrophic gastritis. *Cancer Res.*, **50**, 6559–64.

Kneller, R. W., You, W. C., Chang, Y. S., Liu, W. D., Zhang, L., Zhao, L., *et al.* (1992). Cigarette smoking and other risk factors for progression of precancerous stomach lesions. *J. Natl Cancer Inst.*, **84**, 1261–6.

Kneller, R. W., McLaughlin, J. K., Bjelke, E., Schuman, L. M., Blot, W. J., Wacholder, S., *et al.* (1991). A cohort study of stomach cancer in a high-risk American population. *Cancer*, **68**, 672–8.

Kono, S., Ikeda, M., Tokudome, M., and Keratsune, M. (1987). Cigarette smoking, alcohol consumption and mortality: A cohort study of male Japanese physicians. *Jpn. J. Cancer Res.*, **78**, 1323–8.

Lagergren, J., Bergstrom, R., Lindgren, A., and Nyren, O. (2000). The role of tobacco, snuff and alcohol use in the aetiology of cancer of the oesophagus and gastric cardia. *Int. J. Cancer*, **85**, 340–6.

Lee, H. H., Wu, H. Y., Chuang, Y. C., Chang, A. S., Chao, H. H., Chen, K. Y., *et al.* (1990). Epidemiologic characteristics and multiple risk factors of stomach cancer in Taiwan. *Anticancer Res.*, **10**, 875–8.

Liaw, K. M. and Chen, C. J. (1998). Mortality attributable to cigarette smoking in Taiwan: A 12-year follow-up study. *Tob. Control*, **7**, 141–8.

Linburg, P. J., Qiao, Y., Mark, S. D., Wang, G., Perez-Perez, G. I., Blaser, M. J., *et al.* (2001). Helicobacter pylori seropositivity and subsite specific gastric cancer risks in Linxian, China. *J. Natl. Cancer Inst.*, **93**, 226–33.

Liu, B. Q., Peto, R., Chen, Z. M., Boreham, J., Wu, Y. P., Li, J. Y., Campbell, T. C., and Chen, J. S. (1998). Emerging tobacco hazards in China: 1 Retrospective proportional mortality study of one million death. *BMJ*, **317**, 1411–22.

Mathew, A., Gangadharan, P., Vargese, C., and Nair, M. K. (2000). Diet and stomach cancer: Case-control study in South India. *Eur. J. Cancer Prev.*, **9**, 89–97.

McLaughlin, J. K., Hrubec, Z., Blot, W. J., and Fraumeni, J. F. (1990). Stomach cancer and cigarette smoking among U.S. veterans, 1954–1980. *Cancer Res.*, **50**, 3804.

McLaughlin, J. K., Hrubec, Z., Blot, W. J., and Fraumeni, J. F. (1995). Smoking and cancer mortality among U.S. veterans: A 26-year follow-up. *Int. J. Cancer*, **60**, 190–3.

Moayyedi, P., Axon A. T. N., Feltbower, R., Duffet S., Crocombe, W., Braunholtz, D., *et al.* (2002). For the Leeds HELP Study Group. Relation of adult lifestyle and socioeconomic factors to the prevalence of Helicobacter pylori infection. *Int. J. Epidemiol.*, **31**, 624–31.

Nomura, A., Grove, J. S., Stemmermann, G. N., and Severson, R. K. (1990). A prospective study of stomach cancer and its relation to diet, cigarettes, and alcohol consumption. *Cancer Res.*, **50**, 627–31.

Nomura, A. M., Stemmermann, G. N., and Chyou, P. H. (1995). Gastric cancer among the Japanese in Hawaii. *Jpn. J. Cancer Res.*, **86**, 916–23.

Nordlund, L. A., Carstensen, J. M., and Pershagen, G. (1997). Cancer incidence in female smokers: A 26-year follow-up. *Int. J. Cancer*, **73**, 625–8.

Parkin, D. M. and Pisani, P. (1999). Estimates of the worldwide incidence of 25 major cancers in 1990. *Int. J. Cancer*, **80**, 827–41.

Pisani, P., Parkin, D. M., Bray, F., and Ferlay, J. (1999). Estimates of worldwide mortality from 25 cancers in 1990. *Int. J. Cancer*, **83**, 19–29.

Risch, H. A., Jain, M., Choi, N. W., Fodor, J. G., Pfeffer, C. L., Howe, G. R., *et al.* (1985). Dietary factors and incidence of cancer of the stomach. *Am. J. Epidemiol.*, **122**, 947–59.

Saha, S. K. (1991). Smoking habits and carcinoma of the stomach: A case-control study. *Jpn. J. Cancer Res.*, **82**, 497–502.

Siemiatycki, J., Krewski, D., Franco, E., and Kaiserman, M. (1995). Association between cigarette smoking and each of 21 types of cancer: A multi-site case-control study. *Int. J. Epidemiol.*, **24**, 504–14.

Siman, J. H., Forsgren, A., Berglund, G., and Floren, C. H. (2001). Tobacco smoking increases the risk for gastric adenocarcinoma among Helicobacter pylori-infected individuals. *Scand. J. Gastroenterol.*, **36**, 208–13.

Terry, P., Nyren, O., and Yuen, J. K. (1998). Protective effect of fruits and vegetables on stomach cancer in a cohort of Swedish twins. *Int. J. Cancer*, **76**, 35–7.

The Eurogast Study Group (1993). Epidemiology of, and risk factors for, Helicobacter pylori infection among 3 194 asymptomatic subjects in 17 populations. *Gut*, **34**, 1672–6.

Tredaniel, J., Boffetta, P., Buiatti, E., Saracci, R., and Hirsch, A. (1997). Tobacco smoking and gastric cancer: Review and meta-analysis. *Int. J. Cancer*, **72**, 565–73.

Tulinius, H., Sigfusson, N., Sigvaldason, H., Bjarnadottir, K., and Tryggvadottir, L. (1997). Risk factors for malignant diseases: A cohort study on a population of 22, 946 Icelanders. *Cancer Epidemiol. Biomarkers Prev.*, **6**, 863–73.

Tverdal, A., Thelle, D., Stensvold, I., Leren, P., and Bjartveit, K. (1993). Mortality in relation to smoking history: 13 years' follow-up of 68, 000 Norwegian men and women 35–49 years. *J. Clin. Epidemiol.*, **46**, 475–87.

World Cancer Research Fund/American Institute for Cancer Research (1997). *Food, nutrition and the prevention of cancer: A global perspective.* pp. 148-75, Washington, DC.

Wu, A., Wan, P., and Bernstein, L. (2001). A multicentric popoulation based case-control study of smoking, alcohol and body size and risk of adenocarcinoma of the stomach and esophagus (United States). *Cancer Causes Control*, **12**, 721–32.

Wu-Williams, A. H., Yu, M. C., and Mack, T. M. (1990). Life-style, work-place, and stomach cancer by subsite in young neb of Los Angeles County. *Cancer Res.*, **50**, 2569–76.

Ye, W., Ekstrom, A. M., Hansson, L. E., Bergstrom, R., and Nyren, O. (1999). Tobacco, alcohol and the risk of gastric cancer by sub-site and histologic type. *Int. J. Cancer*, **83**, 223–9.

You, W., Zhang, L., Gail, M. H., Chang, Y., Liu, W., Ma, J., *et al.* (2000). Gastric dysplasia and gastric cancer: Helicobacter pylori, serum vitamin C, and other risk factors. *J. Natl. Cancer Inst.*, **92**, 1607–12.

You, W. C., Blot, W., Chang, Y. S., Ershow, A. G., Yang, Z. T., An, Q., *et al.* (1988). Diet and high risk of stomach cancer in Shandong, China. *Cancer Res.*, **48**, 3518–23.

Yu, G. P., and Hsieh, C. C. (1991). Risk factors for stomach cancer: a population-based case-control study in Shanghai. *Cancer Causes Control*, **2**, 169–74.

Yu, G. P., Hsieh, C. C., Wang, L. Y., Yu, S. Z., Li, X. L., and Jin, T. H. (1995). Green-tea consumption and risk of stomach cancer: A population-based case-control study in Shanghai, China. *Cancer Causes Control*, **6**, 532–8.

Yuan, J. M., Ross, R. K., Wang, X. L., Gao, Y. T., Henderson, B. E., and Yu, M. C. (1996). Morbidity and mortality in relation to cigarette smoking in Shanghai, China: A prospective male cohort study. *J. Am. Med. Assoc.*, **275**, 1646–50.

Zaridze, D., Maximovitch, D., Yurchenko, V., Kozlovsky, O., and Chkhikvadze, V. (2002). Diet and stomach cancer. Results of case-control study from Russia. *Int. J. Cancer*, Supplement 13,

Abstract book, p. 90, 18th UICC International Cancer Congress, 30 June-5 July 2002, Oslo-Norway.

Zaridze, D., Borisova, E., Maximovitch, D., and Chkhikvadze, V. (2000). Alcohol consumption, smoking and risk of gastric cancer: Case-control study from Moscow, Russia. *Cancer Causes Control*, 11, 363–71.

Zhang, Z. F., Kurtz, R. C., Sun, M., Karpeh, M., Yu, G. P., Gargon, *et al.* (1996) Adenocarcinomas of the esophagus and gastric cardia: medical conditions, tobacco, alcohol, and socioeconomic factors. *Cancer Epidemiol. Biomarkers Prev.*, 5, 761–8.

Chapter 25

Cigarette smoking and colorectal cancer

Edward Giovannucci

Introduction

Our understanding of the potential association between tobacco and risk of colorectal cancer has had an interesting history. The landmark early studies, which covered the 1950s and 1960s, consistently did not support an association between tobacco and colorectal cancer risk (Hammond and Horn 1958, 1966; Higginson 1966; Kahn 1966; Staszewski 1969; Weir and Dunn 1970; Doll and Peto 1976; Williams and Horm 1977; Graham *et al.* 1978; Doll *et al.* 1980; Haenszel *et al.* 1980; Rogot and Murray 1980). Many of these studies had been instrumental in demonstrating important associations with other cancer sites. Generally, by the 1970s, tobacco was not considered an important risk factor for colorectal cancer. However, around this time colorectal adenomas had become established as cancer precursors through careful pathologic studies (Morson 1974; Lev 1990). Epidemiologists began studying risk factors for colorectal adenomas in studies conducted in the 1980s and 1990s, and smokers were consistently found to have an appreciably elevated risk. In 1994, a hypothesis, attempting to reconcile the apparent paradox findings between colorectal adenomas and cancers, stated that carcinogens from cigarette smoke cause irreversible genetic damage in colorectal epithelial cells, but several decades are required for completion of all the carcinogenic events following this initiating event (Giovannucci *et al.* 1994*a*, *b*). This hypothesis predicted that an association would be observed initially in adenomas, and then in cancers, after a certain period of time. Thus, the early studies may not have considered a sufficiently long time lag between smoking exposure and time of risk, and thus may have not yielded an association.

In recent years, the association between tobacco and colorectal cancer has been re-evaluated, including in studies that initially did not support an association but that had additional follow-up (Giovannucci 2001). In this chapter, the results for an association between tobacco and colorectal adenoma and cancer are summarized. Evidence addressing the likelihood of a causal association, and the implications of the findings, are then addressed.

Cigarette smoking and colorectal adenoma

Beginning in the 1980s, a number of studies have addressed the association between tobacco use and risk of colorectal adenoma. In almost every study, smokers had a higher risk of colorectal adenoma (Hoff *et al.* 1987; Demers *et al.* 1988; Kikendall *et al.* 1989; Cope *et al.* 1991; Monnet *et al.* 1991; Zahm *et al.* 1991; Honjo *et al.* 1992; Kune *et al.* 1992*b*; Lee *et al.* 1993; Olsen and Kronborg 1993; Giovannucci *et al.* 1994*a, b*; Jacobson *et al.* 1994; Boutron *et al.* 1995; Martinez *et al.* 1995; Longnecker *et al.* 1996; Terry and Neugut 1998; Nagata *et al.* 1999; Potter *et al.* 1999; Almendingen *et al.* 2000; Breuer-Katschinski *et al.* 2000). Typically, the studies have demonstrated dose–response relationships between adenoma risk with cigarettes per day among current smokers, and associations with duration of smoking, and with total cigarette pack-years. Generally, individuals who smoke one to two packs (20–40 cigarettes) daily, or who have accumulated 20–40 cigarette pack-years of smoking, have approximately a two- to threefold higher risk than non-smokers. The studies are remarkable in their consistency in both men and women; in stark contrast to these 21 studies, only two case–control studies found no or equivocal relationships. One of these studies, conducted in the US (Sandler *et al.* 1993), found a non-significant but suggestive twofold increased risk in women with higher numbers of pack-years, but no association was apparent in men. A Japanese study, based on only 86 cases, showed no association (Kono *et al.* 1990), but with 116 additional cases that occurred with continued follow-up, a strong positive association emerged (Honjo *et al.* 1992).

Several important observations are noteworthy. First, while smoking intensity is important, duration also appears to be critical. For example, a Japanese study (Nagata *et al.* 1999) found a higher risk among those who had smoked for 30+ years (relative risk (RR) = 1.60; 95% confidence interval (CI) = 1.02–2.62) but not less (RR = 1.10, 95% CI = 0.69–1.84). In two US studies of men (Giovannucci *et al.* 1994*b*) and women (Giovannucci *et al.* 1994*a*), elevated risks for large adenoma were observed only among individuals, who had smoked for at least 20 years. Other studies also tend to indicate that several decades of smoking may be required for a clear association to emerge for adenomas (Monnet *et al.* 1991; Zahm *et al.* 1991; Terry and Neugut 1998). This finding is noteworthy because adenomas typically arise a decade or more before malignancies; thus, this pattern would suggest at least several decades to elapse between smoking exposure and colorectal cancer risk. Second, the findings generally held for risk of large (>1 cm) adenoma (Zahm *et al.* 1991; Honjo *et al.* 1992; Kune *et al.* 1992*b*; Lee *et al.* 1993; Giovannucci *et al.* 1994*a, b*; Jacobson *et al.* 1994; Boutron *et al.* 1995; Longnecker *et al.* 1996; Terry and Neugut 1998; Nagata *et al.* 1999; Potter *et al.* 1999). Thirdly, an association has been observed relatively consistently among past smokers (Hoff *et al.* 1987; Monnet *et al.* 1991; Zahm *et al.* 1991; Honjo *et al.* 1992; Giovannucci *et al.* 1994*a, b*; Jacobson *et al.* 1994; Martinez *et al.* 1995; Longnecker *et al.* 1996). Finally, the association between tobacco and risk of colorectal adenoma persisted and was not appreciably attenuated in every study after controlling for potential confounders, including diet and alcohol in many of the studies.

The presence of an association is incontrovertible, suggesting that this association is causal, or represents a consistent bias or uncontrolled confounding. Arguing against confounding is the consistency of the findings in males and females in diverse populations, including the US, Norway, France, and Japan, the strength of the association, and the dose–response pattern for intensity and duration of smoking, and the similar results for age-adjusted and multivariate analyses (Hill 1965). A second possibility is that the results were due to some consistent bias. Of note, most studies were based on endoscopied individuals, it is plausible that smokers are more likely to undergo endoscopy for indications related to an underlying polyp as compared with non-smokers, creating a bias whereby smokers with adenomas would be preferentially entered into the study population. However, even in studies or sub-groups in which all in the defined population are screened regardless of symptoms (Hoff *et al.* 1987; Demers *et al.* 1988; Monnet *et al.* 1991; Zahm *et al.* 1991; Honjo *et al.* 1992; Giovannucci *et al.* 1994*a, b*), smokers are at higher risk. Another possibility is that adenomas might be more easily detectable during endoscopy for smokers, perhaps because of a relaxing effect of nicotine on the large bowel. However, this bias is more plausible for small adenomas but less so for large adenomas (Zahm *et al.* 1991; Honjo *et al.* 1992; Kune *et al.* 1992*b*; Lee *et al.* 1993; Giovannucci *et al.* 1994*a, b*; Jacobson *et al.* 1994; Boutron *et al.* 1995; Longnecker *et al.* 1996; Terry and Neugut 1998; Nagata *et al.* 1999; Potter *et al.* 1999); moreover, associations have been observed consistently in past smokers, where the putative relaxing influence of nicotine would no longer be present.

Smoking and colorectal cancer

Summary of studies in the United States

In general, the early studies on tobacco and colorectal cancer did not support an association (Hammond and Horn 1958, 1966; Higginson 1966; Kahn 1966; Staszewski 1969; Weir and Dunn 1970; Doll and Peto 1976; Williams and Horm 1977; Graham *et al.* 1978; Doll *et al.* 1980; Haenszel *et al.* 1980; Rogot and Murray 1980). For example, in the earliest report based on data from the Veterans Administration by Hammond and Horn, 187 783, men were followed from 1952 to 1955 and accrued 667 753 person-years (Hammond and Horn 1958). Compared to never smokers, cigarette smokers had a twofold excess risk of all cancers combined but not for cancers of the colon (84 cases observed, 108.4 expected) or rectum (55 observed, 58.8 expected). Following publication of data suggesting a 35 to 40-year induction period between smoking and risk for colorectal cancer (Giovannucci *et al.* 1994*a, b*), Heineman *et al.* (1994) further studied the Veterans Administration population for the period covering 1954–1980. In this new analysis, based on 3812 colon cancer deaths and 1100 rectal cancer deaths, risk increased with earlier age of initiating smoking (about a 40–50% increase for both colon and rectal cancers among those who began before the age of 15 years). This study offered strong support for the hypothesis that smoking primarily influences the early stages of colorectal cancers.

In contrast to the earlier published studies of US men, studies that have had follow-up time after 1970 have almost universally supported an association (Wu et al. 1987; Slattery et al. 1990, 1997; Giovannucci et al. 1994b; Heineman et al. 1994; Chyou et al. 1996; Le Marchand et al. 1997; Hsing et al. 1998; Chao et al. 2000; Stürmer et al. 2000). A study of male health professionals (Giovannucci et al. 1994b) demonstrated a twofold elevated risk in men who had accumulated at least 10 cigarette pack-years more than 35 years previously, even among those who had subsequently quit decades previously. In a cohort study of US males followed from 1980 to 1985, Wu et al. (1987) reported an elevated risk of colorectal cancer among current smokers (RR = 1.80), past smokers who stopped < 20 years (RR = 2.63) and ≥20 years (RR = 1.71). In a study of Hawaiian-Japanese men (Chyou et al. 1996), the results were not statistically significant up until 30 pack-years, but the RR = 1.48 (95% CI = 1.13–1.94) for colon cancer and RR = 1.92 (95% CI = 1.23–2.99) for rectal cancer for 30+ pack years. In the prospective Lutheran Brotherhood Study, a linear dose–response was observed between cigarettes/day in current smokers at baseline and colon cancer risk, although the number of cases was limited ($n = 120$) (Hsing et al. 1998). Relative to never smokers, the RR for past smokers was 1.45 (95% CI = 0.8–2.7); for current smokers (1–19 cigarettes per day), 1.1 (95% CI = 0.5–2.5); current smokers (20–29 cigarettes per day), 1.6 (95% CI = 0.7–3.4); current smokers (≥30 cigarettes per day), 2.3 (95% CI = 0.9–5.7).

Two recent cohorts have added further support. In the Physicians' Health Study, smoking status was examined in 1982 and men were followed for more than twelve years (Stürmer et al. 2000). In a multivariate model, the RR for colorectal cancer was elevated for current smokers (RR = 1.81; 95% CI = 1.28–2.55) and past smokers (RR = 1.49; 95% CI = 1.17–1.89). Smoking up to twenty years before baseline ($P = 0.05$) and smoking up to and including age 30 years ($P = 0.01$) were statistically significantly related to risk, even controlling for subsequent smoking history. The results indicated that smoking in the distant past is most critical, but recent past smoking may also be important. In the Cancer Prevention II Study (CPS II), a prospective study of mortality of 312 332 men and 469 019 women begun in 1982, smoking for ≥20 years after baseline increased risk of colorectal cancer in men (Chao et al. 2000). Dose–response relations were observed for cigarettes per day, pack-years smoked and earlier age started smoking for current and past smokers. In this study, risk was not elevated for those who quit smoking >20 years before baseline.

An association between smoking and risk of colorectal or colon cancer in men has also been observed in four case–control studies (Dales et al. 1979; Slattery et al. 1990; Le Marchand et al. 1997; Slattery et al. 1997). The study by Le Marchand et al. (1997) was notable in finding a positive association between smoking and colorectal cancer risk with a generally increasing risk with time since smoking. In the study by Slattery *et al.* (1997), the risk increased with number of cigarettes per day and remained elevated even in men who had quit for ≥15 years. A case-control study of US blacks conducted from 1973 to 76, which also included women, found an elevated risk of colorectal cancer with 20+ years of smoking (Dales *et al.* 1979).

Less relevant information is available for women, but the data also tend to suggest a long lag between smoking history and risk for colorectal cancer. Because women began smoking substantially in the US only during the late 1940s and 1950s (Pierce *et al.* 1989), a rise in the incidence of colorectal cancer would not have been expected until approximately the late 1980s assuming a 35–40-year induction period (Giovannucci *et al.* 1994*a, b*). In fact, up to around 1990, there do not appear to be studies that found a positive association between smoking and colorectal cancer risk among women in the US, but some supportive data have emerged recently. The first study to show a clear association was based on data from the Nurses' Health Study (Giovannucci *et al.* 1994*a*). This analysis found a twofold elevated RR among long-term smokers, including past smokers. Interestingly, an earlier analysis from this cohort, which included cases diagnosed from June of 1976 to May of 1984, found only a weak, statistically non-significant association between smoking and colon cancer, although past smoking was significantly associated with risk of rectal carcinoma (Chute *et al.* 1991). These results were confirmed for colorectal cancer mortality for women in the Cancer Prevention Study II (Chao *et al.* 2000). In that study, elevated risks of colorectal cancer mortality were observed after 20–30 years of smoking duration before baseline both in current smokers (RR = 1.41; 95% CI = 1.26–1.58) and past smokers (RR = 1.22; 95% CI = 1.09–1.37).

Three case–control studies supported an association between long-term tobacco use and colorectal cancer risk. Newcomb *et al.* (1995) found among women who smoked for at least 31 years, but not less, a dose–response relation with cigarettes per day. In addition, earlier age at smoking initiation was associated with an increased risk. Past smokers had a moderately increased risk. Slattery *et al.* (1997) found that >35 pack-years of smoking was associated with an elevated risk (RR = 1.38; 95% CI = 1.11–1.71) in women. Finally, Le Marchand *et al.* (1997) (1987–1991) also found an elevated risk of colorectal cancer for smokers; in this study, risk was particularly strong for women who had smoked for >30–40 years in the past.

Summary of recent studies in other countries

In recent years, a number of studies reporting on colorectal cancer risk and smoking have been conducted outside the United States. Almost all of these have been in European countries, except for a few studies in Japan. One of the landmark studies on tobacco and cancer is a long-term follow-up study of British male doctors (Doll *et al.* 1994). In recent analyses, smokers of 25+ cigarettes per day had a 4.4-fold higher rate of rectal cancer ($P < 0.001$), based on 168 cases. Colon cancer, based on 437 cases, exhibited only weak evidence of an increased risk (not statistically significant; RR = 1.44). This study had a follow-up of 40 years, but did not present time-lagged analyses. In a population-based case–control study of 174 colorectal cancer cases in Great Britain (Welfare *et al.* 1997), male and female smokers were at increased risk (OR = 1.77; 95% CI = 1.03–3.14).

A Norwegian cohort study of 68 825 men and women documented 51 fatal colon cancers and 40 fatal rectal cancers from 1972–88 (Tverdal *et al.* 1993). Males who had smoked in the past had a moderately increased risk for fatal colon cancer (RR = 1.2) and fatal rectal cancer (RR = 1.4), and male current smokers, but not female smokers, were at elevated risk from fatal colon cancer (RR = 1.5) and rectal cancer (RR = 1.8).

In a cohort study in Finland (Knekt *et al.* 1998), 56 973 men and women were followed from 1966–72 to 1994. A non-statistically significant overall association was observed, but for follow-up periods of between 11 and 20 years, a significant increased risk was observed for smokers (RR = 1.57; 95% CI = 1.09–2.24). At baseline, smokers had smoked for 20 years on average. This association was limited to men (RR = 1.94; 95% CI = 1.25–2.24), who smoked more than women. In a comparison of colorectal cancer risk for persons recorded as smokers in both of two baseline examinations, a significant increase in risk was observed in the consistent smokers (RR = 1.71; 95% CI = 1.09–2.68).

An Icelandic cohort study documented 145 colorectal cancers in 11 580 women and 193 cases in 11 366 men followed from 1968 to 1995 (Tulinius *et al.* 1997). In this cohort, the prevalence of current smoking at baseline was higher in women than in men (1–14 cigarettes/day: 11% of men, 20% of women; 15–24 cigarettes/day: 13% of men, 16% of women; 25+ cigarettes/day: 6% of men, 3% of women). Among women, risk of colorectal cancer increased with increasing level of cigarette smoking (multivariate RRs = 1.37, 1.53, 2.48). Results were not presented for men (Tulinius *et al.* 1997).

In a Yugoslavian hospital-based case–control study over 1984–86 (Jarebinski *et al.* 1988, 1989), risk of colorectal cancer was not elevated among men and women who had smoked for 1–30 years (RR = 1.0), but risk was elevated for total colorectal (RR = 2.0) and rectal cancer (RR = 2.7) among long-term smokers (30+ years).

The largest study non-supportive of a relationship between smoking and colorectal cancer risk was a hospital case–control study of 955 cases of colon cancer and 629 cases of rectal cancer in northern Italy (D'Avanzo *et al.* 1995). Cancers of the colon and rectum were not associated with number of cigarettes smoked, number of pack-years, duration, time since initiation, and time since quitting.

Several studies of smoking and colorectal cancer risk were conducted in Sweden, producing mixed results. A random sample of 26 000 Swedish women were asked about their smoking status in the early 1960s and then were followed for 26 years (Nordlund *et al.* 1997). No significant association was observed, except for a slight increase in smokers of 16+ cigarettes per day at baseline (RR = 1.42; 95% CI = 0.77–2.60). However, this study was conducted before 1990. A case–control study

(Baron *et al.* 1994) of 352 colon cancer cases and 217 rectal cancer cases found no association with tobacco, even among long-term smokers (40+) years. A cohort study of Swedish construction workers did not find any association among 713 men with colon cancer, and only a weak association with 505 rectal cancer cases (Nyrén *et al.* 1996). Among men with 30+ years of smoking at the start of follow-up, the RR was 1.03 (95% CI = 0.85–1.25) for colon cancer and 1.21 (95% CI = 0.96–1.53) for rectal cancer. However, in a prospective cohort study of 17 118 Swedish twins, long-term heavy tobacco use was associated with an increased risk of colorectal cancer (RR = 3.1, 95% CI = 1.4–7.1) (Terry *et al.* 2001).

The only non-US, non-European studies were conducted in Japan. A Japanese study of 59 male and 34 female colorectal cancer cases yielded null results (Tajima and Tominaga 1985), but smoking became prevalent in Japan only in the 1950s and this study was conducted from 1982 to 83. A hospital-based case–control study in Nagoya, Japan (Inoue *et al.* 1995), examined 'habitual' smoking (both past and current) and risk of colon cancer ($n=231$) and rectal cancer ($n=201$) over the years 1988–92. No relationship was observed for colon cancer, but 'habitual' smoking was associated with an increased risk of rectal cancer for both males (OR = 1.9; 95% CI = 1.1–3.2) and females (OR = 1.7; 95% CI = 1.0–3.1). A recent case–control study in Tokyo (Yamada *et al.* 1997) of 129 colorectal carcinoma-*in situ* cases, 66 colorectal cancers, and 390 controls from 1991 to 1993 found that cumulative exposure (pack years) to cigarette smoking within the prior 20 years was significantly associated with risk for colorectal carcinoma-*in situ* (RR = 3.7; 95% CI = 1.6–8.4 for ≥31 versus 0 pack-years; P(trend) = 0.0003), whereas smoking until 20 years before the diagnosis was associated with risk for colorectal cancer (RR = 5.0; 95% CI = 1.3–18.3; for ≥31 versus 0 pack-years; P(trend) = 0.005).

Assessment of evidence that smoking causally increases risk of colorectal cancer

The evidence summarized above strongly implicates long-term smoking as causally related to risk of cancers of the colon and rectum. Particularly if one examines the more recent studies, which can better study the impact of long-term smoking, the results are remarkably consistent with few exceptions. The following characteristics of the results support that this association is causal.

Firstly, in studies of US men with follow-up time exclusively after 1970, all 10 published studies report a positive association (Wu *et al.* 1987; Slattery *et al.* 1990, 1997; Giovannucci *et al.* 1994b; Heineman *et al.* 1994; Chyou *et al.* 1996; Le Marchand *et al.* 1997; Hsing *et al.* 1998; Chao *et al.* 2000; Stürmer *et al.* 2000). In addition, all 5 published studies for US women with follow-up time in the 1990s report statistically significant positive associations (Giovannucci *et al.* 1994a; Newcomb *et al.* 1995; Le Marchand *et al.* 1997; Slattery *et al.* 1997; Chao *et al.* 2000). In studies conducted outside of the US, although there have been several notable non-supportive studies (Baron *et al.* 1994; D'Avanzo *et al.* 1995; Nyrén *et al.* 1996; Nordlund *et al.* 1997), most recent studies (Jarebinski *et al.* 1988, 1989; Tverdal *et al.* 1993; Inoue *et al.* 1995; Tulinius *et al.* 1997; Welfare *et al.* 1997; Yamada *et al.* 1997; Knekt *et al.* 1998; Terry *et al.* 2001) found long-term smokers to be at elevated risk. Even accounting for possible publication bias, that these findings are all due to chance is implausible.

Secondly, the studies of cancers are complemented by studies of adenomas, for which almost all have supported an association with long-term smoking history. Perhaps, associations with small adenomas are less compelling, because only a small percentage progress to cancer and these are more prone to detection biases. However, all of 12 studies that examined large adenomas found a positive association with smoking history (Zahm *et al.* 1991; Honjo *et al.* 1992; Kune *et al.* 1992*b*; Lee *et al.* 1993; Giovannucci *et al.* 1994*a*, *b*; Jacobson *et al.* 1994; Boutron *et al.* 1995; Longnecker *et al.* 1996; Terry and Neugut 1998; Nagata *et al.* 1999; Potter *et al.* 1999). Large adenomas have acquired many genetic alterations observed in malignancies (Vogelstein *et al.* 1988), and the epidemiology for these lesions closely parallels that of cancers.

Thirdly, given the diversity of study designs for cancer, prospective, retrospective, and endoscopy-controlled studies for adenomas, for men and for women in different populations, it is unlikely that some consistent detection bias could account for all these observations. In addition, some of the theoretical biases should be opposing for adenomas and cancers. For example, if there is a stronger likelihood of smokers with adenomas being more likely to be diagnosed than non-smokers with adenomas, this should produce a positive detection bias for adenomas but a negative detection bias for cancers because their precursors would be removed preferentially for smokers. Also, while current smokers tend to have lower screening rates than the non-smokers, past smokers (especially in populations such as physicians, health professionals, and nurses) may have similar or even enhanced screening than never smokers, but both current and past smokers are at increased risk for colorectal cancer.

Fourthly, in every study of cancer or large adenoma that has adjusted for various potential confounders, results for smoking have not been appreciably attenuated. This pattern exists even in studies that adjusted for numerous potential lifestyle factors (e.g. physical activity, alcohol, diet) that could be plausibly related to tobacco use (Wu *et al.* 1987; Slattery *et al.* 1990, 1997; Giovannucci *et al.* 1994*b*; Newcomb *et al.* 1995; Chyou *et al.* 1996; Le Marchand *et al.* 1997; Chao *et al.* 2000; Stürmer *et al.* 2000). Moreover, past smokers, especially those who quit long in the past would tend to have different covariate patterns than continuing smokers, yet associations with tobacco use have been seen for both groups. Finally the relatively consistent findings for men and women in diverse populations from various countries argue against confounding.

Fifthly, the association has a high degree of biologic plausibility. Cigarette smoking is judged unequivocally to be causally related to at least eight different cancers, including those not directly related to smoke, such as the pancreas, kidney, and bladder

(U.S. Dept. of Health Education and Welfare *et al.* 1979). The burning of tobacco produces numerous genotoxic compounds, including polynuclear aromatic hydrocarbons, heterocyclic amines, nitrosamines, and aromatic amines (IARC Working Group on the Evaluation of the Carcinogenic Risk of Chemicals to Humans 1986; Manabe *et al.* 1991; Alexandrov *et al.* 1996; Hoffmann and Hoffman 1997). The large intestine is exposed to these compounds either through the circulatory (Yamasaki and Ames 1977) or digestive system (Kune *et al.* 1992*a*). DNA adducts to metabolites of benzo[*a*]pyrene, a carcinogenic polycyclic aromatic hydrocarbon, are detected more frequently in the colonic mucosa of smokers compared to non-smokers (Alexandrov *et al.* 1996). DNA adduct levels in the normal-appearing colonic epithelium of colorectal cancer patients occur at a higher frequency than in non-cancer patients (Pfohl-Leszkowicz *et al.* 1995). The apparently long induction period of at least 3 or 4 decades between the presumably genotoxic event and ultimately diagnosis of malignancy is consistent with the natural history of colorectal cancer (Giovannucci and Martínez 1996).

Unresolved issues and implications

The data just summarized strongly support an association between smoking and risk of colorectal cancer. Dose–response relations have been reported for pack-years, smoking duration, smoking intensity, smoking history in the distant past, and younger age at initiation of smoking. Relative risk comparing the high versus low categories of these factors have generally been in the range of 1.3–1.8. As most of these variables tend to be correlated, teasing out which are the most relevant factors is difficult, although clearly those who began early and smoked most intensely for many years are at highest risk. To what degree and how quickly risk drops after one ceases smoking remains somewhat in question, but most data suggest that part of the excess risk persists indefinitely in past smokers (Wu *et al.* 1987; Giovannucci *et al.* 1994*a, b*; Slattery *et al.* 1997; Stürmer *et al.* 2000). Only one study (Chao *et al.* 2000) found that the excess risk appears to approach zero after about 20 years since quitting. While smoking at any age has numerous health benefits, for colorectal cancer the avoidance of smoking at early ages appears particularly important.

Generally, associations have been observed for both colon and rectal cancers, although, in several studies (Doll and Peto 1976; Chute *et al.* 1991; Inoue *et al.* 1995; Nyrén *et al.* 1996), an association was observed or suggestive only with rectal cancer. However, in one of these studies (Chute *et al.* 1991), with additional follow-up (Giovannucci *et al.* 1994*a*), an association emerged for colon cancer. In most studies that have distinguished among colon and rectal cancer, the association has been stronger for rectal cancer (Tverdal *et al.* 1993; Doll *et al.* 1994; Giovannucci *et al.* 1994*a*; Heineman *et al.* 1994; Newcomb *et al.* 1995; Chyou 1996 #6191; Chao *et al.* 2000), though present for both. Overall, whether differences exist between the proximal and distal colon has not been adequately addressed.

Little is known whether smoking may preferentially increase risk of some molecular sub-types of colorectal cancer, though some early evidence is provocative. In one study, initiation of smoking at a young age and smoking for 35+ years was associated preferentially with colorectal cancer categorized by microsatellite instability (Slattery et al. 2000). An additional study found a higher risk of mismatch repair-deficient colorectal cancer in cigarette smokers (Yang et al. 2000). In another study (Freedman et al. 1996), current smoking and total pack-years of smoking were not associated with colorectal cancers that were positive for p53 mutations, but current and past smokers had a two-fold risk of developing cancers without p53 overexpression, and a dose–response relation was observed with increasing cigarette pack-years ($P=0.03$). These findings suggest that colorectal cancers related to smoking may proceed through a p53-independent pathway.

Most studies have focused on cigarette smoking, whereas relatively few have examined cigar or pipe smoking. In the large CPS II study, current smokers who had smoked exclusively cigars or pipes were at elevated risk of colorectal cancer mortality (multivariate RR = 1.34; 95% = 1.11–1.62) (Chao et al. 2000). Other studies have also indicated that cigar/pipe smoking may increase risk of colorectal cancer (Hammond and Horn 1966; Heineman et al. 1994; Slattery et al. 1997). As smoking of these products has increased in some segments of the population, further work in defining the association for pipe and cigar smoking is important.

Another area where further work would be of interest is determining whether specific individuals would be at higher risk because of their genetic background or other modifiable behavior. While there have been a number of studies of polymorphic genes encoding xenobiotic metabolizing enzymes in colorectal cancer, potential interactions with tobacco have been examined in a relatively small proportion of these (Brockton et al. 2000). This is a relatively untapped area. Only a few reports have considered whether there are smokers at relatively higher or lower risk of colorectal cancer based on behaviors or lifestyle characteristics.

In conclusion, the overall body of evidence indicates that colorectal cancer is a smoking-related malignancy. Two factors probably have contributed to the fact that this has not been appreciated until relatively recently. First, there appears to be a relatively long time lag between onset of smoking and period of risk, and second, colorectal cancers are common even in non-smokers so the population attributable risk has been moderate compared to other malignancies. In the United States, estimates of the population attributable risk due to smoking have been 21% of colorectal cancer in men (Giovannucci et al. 1994b), 16% of colon cancer and 22% of rectal cancer in men (Heineman et al. 1994); 12% of colorectal cancer mortality in men and women (Chao et al. 2000), and 11% of colon cancer and 17% of rectal cancer in women (Newcomb et al. 1995). From these estimates, approximately 7000–10 000 deaths from colorectal cancer per year would be attributable to cigarette smoking in the US (Chao et al. 2000). Because at least part of the excess risk appears to be permanent, the prevention of smoking in the young is especially important for this malignancy.

References

Alexandrov, K., Rojas, M., Kadlubar, F. F., Lang, N. P., and Bartsch, H. (1996). Evidence of *anti*-benzo[a]pyrene diolepoxide-DNA adduct formation in human colon mucosa. *Carcinogenesis* **17**, 2081–3.

Almendingen, K., Hofstad, B., Trygg, K., Hoff, G., Hussain, A., and Vatn, M. H. (2000). Smoking and colorectal adenomas: A case-control study. *Eur J Cancer Prev* **9**, 193–203.

Baron, J. A., Gerhardsson de, Verdier, M., and Ekbom, A. (1994). Coffee, tea, tobacco, and cancer of the large bowel. *Cancer Epidemiol Biomarkers Prev* **3**, 565–70.

Boutron, M. C., Faivre, J., Dop, M. C., Quipourt, V., and Senesse, P. (1995). Tobacco, alcohol, and colorectal tumors: A multistep process. *Am J Epidemiol* **141**, 1038–46.

Breuer-Katschinski, B., Nemes, K., Marr, A., Rump, B., Leiendecker, B., Breuer, N., *et al.* (2000). Alcohol and cigarette smoking and the risk of colorectal adenomas. *Dig Dis Sci* **45**, 487–93.

Brockton, N., Little, J., Sharp, L., and Cotton, S. C. (2000). N-acetyltransferase polymorphisms and colorectal cancer: A HuGE review. *Am J Epidemiol* **151**, 846–61.

Chao, A., Thun, M. J., Jacobs, E. J., Henley, S. H., Rodriguez, C., and Calle, E. E. (2000). Cigarette smoking and colorectal cancer mortality in the Cancer Prevention Study II. *JNCI* **92**, 1888–96.

Chute, C. G., Willett, W. C., Colditz, G. A., Stampfer, M. J., Baron, J. A., Rosner, B., *et al.* (1991). A prospective study of body mass, height, and smoking on the risk of colorectal cancer in women. *Cancer Causes Control* **2**, 117–24.

Chyou, P.-H., Nomura, A. M. Y., and Stemmermann, G. N. (1996). A prospective study of colon and rectal cancer among Hawaii Japanese men. *Ann Epidemiol* **6**, 276–82.

Cope, G. F., Wyatt, J. I., Pinder, I. F., Lee, P. N., Heatley, R. V., and Kelleher, J. (1991). Alcohol consumption in patients with colorectal adenomatous polyps. *Gut* **32**, 70–2.

Dales, L. G., Friedman, G. D., Ury, H. K., Grossman, S., Williams, S. R. (1979). A case-control study of relationships of diet and other traits to colorectal cancer in American blacks. *Am J Epidemiol* **109**, 132–44.

D'Avanzo, B., La Vecchia, C., Franceschi, S., Gallotti, L., and Talamini, R. (1995). Cigarette smoking and colorectal cancer: A study of 1,584 cases and 2,879 controls. *Prev Med* **24**, 571–9.

Demers, R. Y., Neale, A. V., Demers, P., Deighton, K., Scott, R. O., Dupuis, M. H., *et al.* (1988). Serum cholesterol and colorectal polyps. *J Clin Epidemiol* **41**, 9–13.

Doll, R., Gray, R., Hafner, B., and Peto, R. (1980). Mortality in relation to smoking: 22 years' observations on female British doctors. *British Journal of Medicine* **280**, 967–71.

Doll, R. and Peto, R. (1976). Mortality in relation to smoking: 20 years' observations on male British doctors. *British Medical Journal* **2**.

Doll, R., Peto, R., Wheatley, K., Gray, R., and Sutherland, I. (1994). Mortality in relation to smoking: 40 years' observations on male British doctors. *Br Med J* **309**, 901–11.

Freedman, A. N., Michalek, A. M., Marshall, J. R., Mettlin, C. J., Petrelli, N. J., Zhang, Z. F., *et al.* (1996). The relationship between smoking exposure and p53 overexpression in colorectal cancer. *Br J Cancer* **73**, 902–8.

Giovannucci, E. (2001). An updated review of the epidemiological evidence that cigarette smoking increases risk of colorectal cancer. *Cancer Epidemiol Biomarkers Prev* **10**, 725–31.

Giovannucci, E. and Martínez, M. E. (1996). Tobacco, colorectal cancer, and adenomas: A review of the evidence. *J Natl Cancer Inst* **88**, 1717–30.

Giovannucci, E., Colditz, G. A., Stampfer, M. J., Hunter, D., Rosner, B. A., Willett, W. C., *et al.* (1994a). A prospective study of cigarette smoking and risk of colorectal adenoma and colorectal cancer in U.S. women. *J Natl Cancer Inst* **86**, 192–9.

Giovannucci, E., Rimm, E. B., Stampfer, M. J., Colditz, G. A., Ascherio, A., Kearney, J., *et al*. (1994*b*). A prospective study of cigarette smoking and risk of colorectal adenoma and colorectal cancer in U.S. men. *J Natl Cancer Inst* **86**, 183–91.

Graham, S., Dayal, H., Swanson, M., Mittelman, A., and Wilkinson, G. (1978). Diet in the epidemiology of cancer of the colon and rectum. *J Natl Cancer Inst* **61**, 709–14.

Haenszel, W., Locke, F. B., and Segi, M. (1980). A case-control study of large bowel cancer in Japan. *J Natl Cancer Inst* **64**, 17–22.

Hammond, C. E. and Horn, D. (1966). Smoking in relation to the death rates of one million men and women. In: *National Cancer Institute Monograph 19* (ed. W. Haenszel), pp. 127–204, National Cancer Institute. Bethesda, MD.

Hammond, E. C. and Horn, D. (1958). Smoking and death rates: report on forty-four months of followup of 187,783 men. II. Death rates by causality. *JAMA* **166**, 1294–308.

Heineman, E. F., Zahm, S. H., McLaughlin, J. K., and Vaught, J. B. (1994). Increased risk of colorectal cancer among smokers: results of a 26-year follow-up of US veterans and a review. *Int J Cancer* **59**, 728–38.

Higginson, J. (1966). Etiological factors in gastrointestinal cancer in man. *J Natl Cancer Inst* **37**, 527–45.

Hill, A. B. (1965). The environment and disease: Association or causation? *Proc R Soc Med* **58**, 295–300.

Hoff, G., Vatn, M. H., and Larsen, S. (1987). Relationship between tobacco smoking and colorectal polyps. *Scand J Gastroenterol* **22**, 13–16.

Hoffmann, D. and Hoffman, I. (1997). The changing cigarette, 1950–1995. *J Toxicol Environ Health* **50**, 307–64.

Honjo, S., Kono, S., Shinchi, K., Imanishi, K., and Hirohata, T. (1992). Cigarette smoking, alcohol use and adenomatous polyps of the sigmoid colon. *Jpn J Cancer Res* **83**, 806–11.

Hsing, A. W., McLaughlin, J. K., Chow, W. H., Schuman, L. M., Co Chien, H. T., Gridley, G. *et al*. (1998). Risk factors for colorectal cancer in a prospective study among U.S. white men. *Int J Cancer* **77**, 549–53.

IARC Working Group on the Evaluation of the Carcinogenic Risk of Chemicals to Humans. (1986). Tobacco smoking.: World Health Organization, International Agency for Research on Cancer; 397 p. (IARC monographs on the evaluation of the carcinogenic risk of chemicals to humans). Lyon, France.

Inoue, M., Tajima, K., Hirose, K., Hamajima, N., Takezaki, T., Hirai, T., *et al*. (1995). Subsite-specific risk factors for colorectal cancer: A hospital-based case-control study in Japan. *Cancer Causes Control* **6**, 14–22.

Jacobson, J. S., Neugut, A. I., Murray, T., Garbowski, G. C., Forde, K. A., Treat, M. R., *et al*. (1994). Cigarette smoking and other behavioral risk factors for recurrence of colorectal adenomatous polyps (New York City, NY, USA). *Cancer Causes Control* **5**, 215–20.

Jarebinski, M., Adanja, B., and Vlajinac, H. (1989). Case-control study of relationship of some biosocial correlates to rectal cancer patients in Belgrade, Yugoslavia. *Neoplasma* **36**, 369–74.

Jarebinski, M., Vlajinac, H., and Adanja, B. (1988). Biosocial and other characteristics of the large bowel cancer patients in Belgrade (Yugoslavia). *Arch Geschwulstforsch* **58**, 411–17.

Kahn, H. A. (1966). The Dorn study of smoking and mortality among US Veterans on 8 years of observation. In: *National Cancer Institute Monograph 19* (ed. W. Haenszel). pp. 1–125. National Cancer Institute; Bethesda, MD.

Kikendall, J. W., Bowen, P. E., Burgess, M. B., Magnetti, C., Woodward, J., and Langenberg, P. (1989). Cigarettes and alcohol as independent risk factors for colonic adenomas. *Gastroenterology* **97**, 660–4.

Knekt, P., Hakama, M., Järvinen, R., Pukkala, E., and Heliövaara, M. (1998). Smoking and risk of colorectal cancer. *Br J Cancer* **78**, 136–9.

Kono, S., Ikeda, N., Yanai, F., Shinchi, K., and Imanishi, K. (1990). Alcoholic beverages and adenomatous polyps of the sigmoid colon: A study of male self-defence officials in Japan. *Int J Epidemiol* **19**, 848–52.

Kune, G. A., Kune, S., Vitetta, L., and Watson, L. F. (1992*a*). Smoking and colorectal cancer risk: Data from the Melbourne Colorectal Cancer Study and brief review of literature. *International Journal of Cancer* **50**, 369–72.

Kune, G. A., Kune, S., Watson, L. F., and Penfold, C. (1992*b*). Smoking and adenomatous colorectal polyps (letter). *Gastroenterology* **103**, 1370–1.

Le Marchand, L., Wilkens, L. R., Kolonel, L. N., Hankin, J. H., and Lyu, L.-C. (1997). Associations of sedentary lifestyle, obesity, smoking, alcohol use, and diabetes with the risk of colorectal cancer. *Cancer Res* **57**, 4787–94.

Lee, W. C., Neugut, A. I., Garbowski, G. C., Forde, K. A., Treat, M. R., Waye, J. D., *et al.* (1993). Cigarettes, alcohol, coffee, and caffeine as risk factors for colorectal adenomatous polyps. *Ann Epidemiol* **3**, 239–44.

Lev, R. (1990). *Adenomatous polyps of the colon*, p. 61. Springer-Verlag, New York.

Longnecker, M. P., Chen, M. J., Probst-Hensch, N. M., Harper, J. M., Lee, E. R., Frankl, H. D., *et al.* (1996). Alcohol and smoking in relation to the prevalence of adenomatous colorectal polyps detected at sigmoidoscopy. *Epidemiology* **7**, 275–80.

Manabe, S., Tohyama, K., Wada, O., and Aramaki, T. (1991). Detection of a carcinogen, 2-amino-1-methyl-6-phenylimidazo[4,5-b]pyridine (PhIP), in cigarette smoke condensate. *Carcinogenesis* **12**, 1945–7.

Martinez, M. E., McPherson, R. S., Annegers, J. F., and Levin, B. (1995). Cigarette smoking and alcohol consumption as risk factors for colorectal adenomatous polyps. *J Natl Cancer Inst* **87**, 274–9.

Monnet, E., Allemand, H., Farina, H., and Carayon, P. (1991). Cigarette smoking and the risk of colorectal adenoma in men. *Scand J Gastroenterol* **26**, 758–62.

Morson, B. C. (1974). Evolution of cancer of the colon and rectum. *Cancer* **34** (suppl), 845–9.

Nagata, C., Shimizu, H., Kametani, M., Takeyama, N., Ohnuma, T., and Matsushita, S. (1999). Cigarette smoking, alcohol use, and colorectal adenoma in Japanese men and women. *Dis Colon Rectum* **42**, 337–42.

Newcomb, P. A., Storer, B. E., and Marcus, P. M. (1995). Cigarette smoking in relation to risk of large bowel cancer in women. *Cancer Res* **55**, 4906–9.

Nordlund, L. A., Carstensen, J. M., and Pershagen, G. (1997). Cancer incidence in female smokers: A 26-year follow-up. *Int J Cancer* **73**, 625–8.

Nyrén, O., Bergström, R., Nyström, L., Engholm, G., Ekbom, A., Adami, H.-O., *et al.* (1996). Smoking and colorectal cancer: A 20-year follow-up study of Swedish construction workers. *J Natl Cancer Inst* **88**, 1302–7.

Olsen, J. and Kronborg, O. (1993). Coffee, tobacco and alcohol as risk factors for cancer and adenoma of the large intestine. *Int J Epidemiol* **22**, 398–402.

Pfohl-Leszkowicz, A., Grosse, Y., Carriere, V., Cugnenc, P. H., Berger, A., Carnot, F., *et al.* (1995). High levels of DNA adducts in human colon are associated with colorectal cancer. *Cancer Res* **55**, 5611–6.

Pierce, J. P., Fiore, M. C., Novotny, T. E., Hatziandreu, E. J., and Davis, R. M. (1989). Trends in cigarette smoking in the United States. Projections to the year 2000. *JAMA* **261**, 61–5.

Potter, J. D., Bigler, J., Fosdick, L., Bostick, R. M., Kampman, E., Chen, C., *et al.* (1999). Colorectal adenomatous and hyperplastic polyps: Smoking and N-acetyltransferase 2 polymorphisms. *Cancer Epidemiol Biomarkers Prev* **8**, 69–75.

Rogot, E. and Murray, J. L. (1980). Smoking and causes of death among US Veterans: 16 years of observation. *Public Health Reports* **95**, 213–22.

Sandler, R. S., Lyles, C. M., McAuliffe, C., Woosley, J. T., and Kupper, L. L. (1993). Cigarette smoking, alcohol, and the risk of colorectal adenomas. *Gastroenterology* **104**, 1445–51.

Slattery, M. L., Curtin, K., Anderson, K., Ma, K.-N., Ballard, L., Edwards, S., *et al.* (2000). Associations between cigarette smoking, lifestyle factors, and microsatellite instability in colon tumors. *JNCI* **92**, 1831–6.

Slattery, M. L., Potter, J. D., Friedman, G. D., Ma, K.-N., Edwards, S. (1997). Tobacco use and colon cancer. *Int J Cancer* **70**, 259–64.

Slattery, M. L., West, D. W., Robison, L. M., French, T. K., Ford, M. H., Schuman, K. L., *et al.* (1990). Tobacco, alcohol, coffee, and caffeine as risk factors for colon cancer in a low-risk population. *Epidemiology* **1**, 141–5.

Staszewski, J. (1969). Smoking and cancer of the alimentary tract in Poland. *Br J Cancer* **23**, 247–53.

Stürmer, T., Glynn, R. J., Lee, I. M., Christen, W. G., and Hennekens, C. H. (2000). Lifetime cigarette smoking and colorectal cancer incidence in the Physicians' Health Study I. *JNCI* **92**, 1178–81.

Tajima, K. and Tominaga, S. (1985). Dietary habits and gastro-intestinal cancer. A comparative case-control study of stomach and large intestinal cancers in Nagoya, Japan. *Jpn J Cancer Res* **76**, 705–16.

Terry, M. B. and Neugut, A. I. (1998). Cigarette smoking and the colorectal adenoma-carcinoma sequence: A hypothesis to explain the paradox. *Am J Epidemiol* **147**, 903–10.

Terry, P., Ekbom, A., Lichtenstein, P., Feychting, M., and Wolk, A. (2001). Long-term tobacco smoking and colorectal cancer in a prospective cohort study. *Int J Cancer* **91**, 585–7.

Tulinius, H., Sigfusson, N., Sigvaldason, H., Bjarnadottir, K., and Tryggvadottir, L. (1997). Risk factors for malignant diseases: A cohort study on a population of 22,946 Icelanders. *Cancer Epidemiol Biomarkers Prev* **6**, 863–73.

Tverdal, A., Thelle, D., Stensvold, I., Leren, P., and Bjartveit, K. (1993). Mortality in relation to smoking history: 13 years' follow-up of 68,000 Norwegian men and women 35–49 years. *J Clin Epidemiol* **46**, 475–87.

U.S. Dept. of Health Education and Welfare, Public Health Service, Office of the Assistant Secretary for Health, Office on Smoking and Health, (1997). Smoking and health: A report of the Surgeon General. U.S. Government Printing Office; 1979. (DHEW publication no. (PHS) 79-50066), Rockville, Md.

Vogelstein, B., Fearon, E. R., Hamilton, S. R., Kern, S. E., Preisinger, A. C., Leppert, M., *et al.* (1988). Genetic alterations during colorectal-tumor development. *N Engl J Med* **319**, 525–32.

Weir, J. M. and Dunn, J. E., Jr. (1970). Smoking and mortality: A prospective study. *Cancer* **25**, 105–12.

Welfare, M. R., Cooper, J., Bassendine, M. F., and Daly, A. K. (1997). Relationship between acetylator status, smoking, and diet and colorectal cancer risk in the north-east of England. *Carcinogenesis* **18**, 1351–4.

Williams, R. R. and Horm, J. W. (1977). Association of cancer sites with tobacco and alcohol consumption and socioeconomic status of patients: Interview study from the Third National Cancer Survey. *J Natl Cancer Inst* **58**, 525–47.

Wu, A. H., Paganini-Hill, A., Ross, R. K., and Henderson, B. E. (1987). Alcohol, physical activity and other risk factors for colorectal cancer: A prospective study. *British Journal of Cancer* **55**, 687–94.

Yamada, K., Araki, S., Tamura, M., Sakai, I., Takahashi, Y., Kashihara, H., *et al.* (1997). Case-control study of colorectal carcinoma *in situ* and cancer in relation to cigarette smoking and alcohol use (Japan). *Cancer Causes Control* **8**, 780–5.

Yamasaki, E. and Ames, B. N. (1977). Concentration of mutagens from urine by absorption with the nonpolar resin XAD-2: Cigarette smokers have mutagenic urine. *Proc Natl Acad Sci USA* **74**, 3555–9.

Yang, P., Cunningham, J. M., Halling, K. C., Lesnick, T. G., Burgart, L. J., Wiegert, E. M., *et al.* (2000). Higher risk of mismatch repair-deficient colorectal cancer in alpha1-antitrypsin deficiency carriers and cigarette smokers. *Mol Genet Metab* **71**, 639–45.

Zahm, S. H., Cocco, P., and Blair, A. (1991). Tobacco smoking as a risk factor for colon polyps. *Am J Public Health* **81**, 846–9.

Chapter 26

Smoking and cervical neoplasia

Anne Szarewski and Jack Cuzick

Squamous cell cervical cancer is primarily related to sexual activity (reviewed by Brinton 1992). Important risk factors are the number of sexual partners (of both the woman and her male partner) and early age at first intercourse. Use of barrier methods of contraception appears to be protective, whereas long-term use of the combined oral contraceptive pill appears to increase risk (Moreno *et al.* 2002; Skegg 2002). Overwhelming evidence now implicates the human papillomaviruses (HPVs), particularly certain so-called 'high-risk' types (e.g. 16, 18, 31, 33, 35, 39, 45, 51, 52, 56, 58, 59, and 68) as the causal sexually transmitted agents (Walboomers *et al.* 1999) although other sexually transmitted infections such as chlamydia, herpes simplex virus (HSV), and human immunodeficiency virus (HIV) may also have a role. The high frequency of infection with HPV and the relative rarity of cervical cancer suggest that other factors are needed to facilitate the carcinogenic process.

Winkelstein (1977) first drew attention to a possible role of cigarette smoking as a cofactor. Several studies had previously reported an association but it had been dismissed as a confounding factor for sexual variables, assumed to be either unmeasured or recorded inaccurately. Cigarette smoking and sexual behaviour are frequently related and the strong link between sexual behaviour and cervix cancer makes the evaluation of any relationship with smoking very difficult. However, as demonstrated below, the overall epidemiologic evidence supports the hypothesis that smoking is a cofactor or risk factor in its own right, even after controlling for sexual variables. In addition, there is now a substantial body of evidence from studies which have controlled for the effect of HPV, and which still show a significant effect of smoking. Three possible biological mechanisms have been proposed to explain the association, namely a direct carcinogenic effect on the cervix of cigarette smoke metabolites, an indirect effect mediated by an alteration of the host immune response, and an effect on antioxidants. These will be discussed later in this chapter.

We reviewed this topic extensively in the past (Szarewski and Cuzick 1998) and in this chapter propose to mainly update that review. Readers are therefore referred to the previous publication for details of studies not fully covered or referenced here. An additional feature provided here is a series of forest plots of the individual studies, which allow simple visualization of the data. We have focused on current smoking where the data were available, but if not, have used ever smoking as the exposure variable. No specific attempt has been made to summarize information on dose–response and duration.

Cohort studies

We are aware of 11 cohort studies in this field, with varying endpoints and mostly with limited information regarding smoking (Fig. 26.1). Ten of these show an increased risk in smokers and most also exhibit a dose–response relationship. In general, however, these studies did not adjust for sexual behaviour variables and this limits their value for assessing an independent effect of smoking. Only one cohort study included testing for HPV (Moscicki *et al.* 2001), but this study was small and concentrated on young women so that the endpoints were incidence of HPV and LSIL in the cohort.

Case–control studies

We have previously reviewed case–control studies in detail (Szarewski and Cuzick 1998). In the last 6 years, the majority of new studies published have included HPV testing and have therefore been of greater interest. Later in this chapter, we will therefore concentrate on those studies.

There are 32 case–control studies which have addressed the relationship between smoking and invasive cervical cancer (Eluf-Neto *et al.* 1994; Cuzick *et al.* 1996; Daling *et al.* 1996; Hirose *et al.* 1996, 1998; Kjaer *et al.* 1996; Chichareon *et al.* 1998; Ngelangel *et al.* 1998; Szarewski and Cuzick 1998; Atalah *et al.* 2001; Santos *et al.* 2001), summarized in Fig. 26.2. Of these, 29 make some adjustment for sexual behaviour variables and 21 show an increase in risk for current smokers, with relative risks for current smokers generally between 1.5 and 2.0 after adjustment for sexual variables. In addition, the majority also show a dose–response relationship.

Twenty case–control studies have specifically looked at carcinoma *in situ* or CIN 3 (Kjaer *et al.* 1996; Ho *et al.* 1998; Olsen *et al.* 1998; Roteli-Martins *et al.* 1998; Szarewski

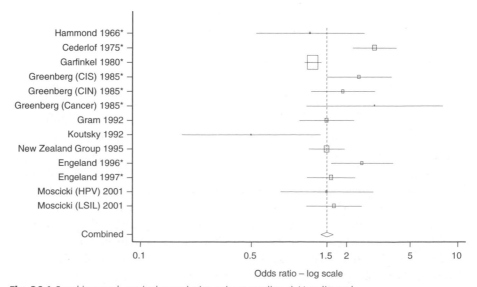

Fig. 26.1 Smoking and cervical neoplasia: cohort studies. * Unadjusted.

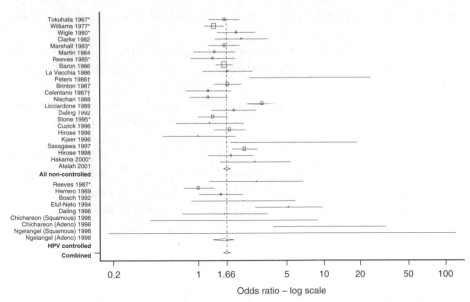

Fig. 26.2 Smoking and cervical neoplasia: case–control studies—cancer. *Unadjusted; †Heavy exposure group.

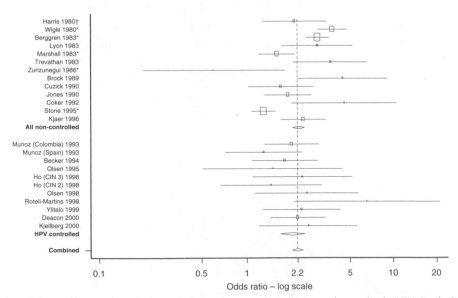

Fig. 26.3 Smoking and cervical neoplasia: case–control studies—carcinoma *in situ*/CIN Grade 3. *Unadjusted; †Heavy exposure group.

and Cuzick 1998; Ylitalo *et al.* 1999; Deacon *et al.* 2000; Kjellberg *et al.* 2000). All but one show a positive relationship with smoking and a dose–response relationship (Fig. 26.3). The adjusted odds ratios for current smokers are generally higher than those reported for invasive cancer, ranging between 1.7 and 6.6. The reasons for this are unclear, but could reflect a younger age group where current smoking is more prevalent.

Seven studies report data on both CIN (cervical intraepithelial neoplasia) and invasive cancer (Szarewski and Cuzick 1998; Hildesheim *et al.* 2001; Lacey *et al.* 2001; Zivaljevic *et al.* 2001). These studies generally encompass all grades of CIN and separate odds ratios for CIN and cancer are not given. All but one of these studies show a positive relationship with smoking, mostly with a dose–response, with adjusted odds ratios between 1.6 and 7.0 (Fig. 26.4).

Sixteen studies have looked at CIN only, of all grades (Kjaer *et al.* 1996; Sasagawa *et al.* 1997; Szarewski and Cuzick 1998; Derchain *et al.* 1999; Scholes *et al.* 1999). All but one of these show a positive relationship with smoking, with adjusted odds ratios between 1.4 and 5.8 for current versus never smokers (Fig. 26.5). Six studies show a dose–response, three studies do not, and seven do not have appropriate data for this analysis.

It is of interest that some studies which have looked separately at low and high grades of CIN have found that the relationship with smoking tends to be stronger for the higher grades. For example, in the study by Cuzick *et al.* (1990), the adjusted odds ratio for women with CIN 1 was 1.21 (NS), whereas for CIN 3 it was 1.72 ($p<0.05$). Schiffman *et al.* (1993) found a significant relationship of smoking with CIN 2/3 in HPV positive smokers (RR 2.7, 95% CI 1.1–6.5), but not in those with low- grade CIN. Similar results were reported by Vonka *et al.* (1984), Morrison *et al.* (1991), Brisson *et al.* (1994), Kjaer *et al.* (1996), and Derchain *et al.* (1999) in which the percentage of smokers increased steadily from controls to CIN 1, to high-grade CIN or cancer.

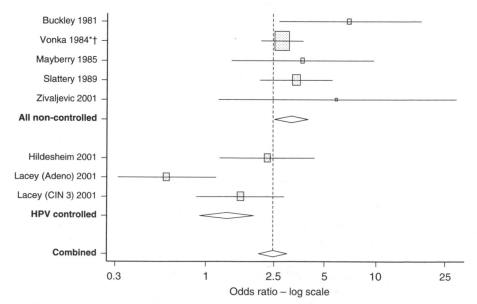

Fig. 26.4 Smoking and cervical neoplasia: case–control studies—both cancer and CIN. *Unadjusted; †Heavy exposure group.

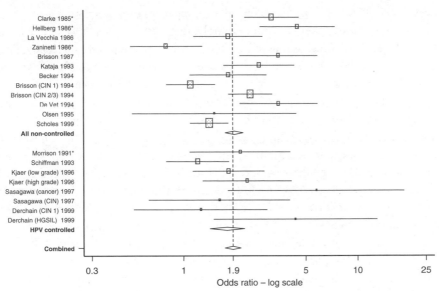

Fig. 26.5 Smoking and cervical neoplasia: case–control studies—CIN of all grades. *Unadjusted.

Luesley *et al.* (1994) studied 167 women referred to a colposcopy clinic with cervical smears showing mild dyskaryosis. Histological outcome was made on the basis of a large loop excision of the transformation zone (LLETZ). Current smoking was associated with an odds ratio of 4.6 (CI 2.29–9.37) for high-grade disease (CIN 2 or worse). In addition, lesion size was found to be significantly larger in smokers ($p=0.007$). Similar results were reported by Daly *et al.* (1998) who also reported a dose–response relationship between the number of cigarettes smoked and the risk of high-grade disease in women with mildly abnormal smears (OR 5.85, 95% CI 1.92–17.80 for women who smoked more than 20 cigarettes per day). Unfortunately, these studies did not include testing for HPV and did not adjust for sexual variables other than parity and contraceptive status.

Interaction with the human papillomavirus (HPV)

In 1982, Zur Hausen suggested that the HPV might be the primary cause of cervical cancer. Although it appears to be one of the few complete carcinogens (i.e. not necessarily requiring other cofactors) it is clear that carcinogenicity is greatly accelerated when cofactors are present. He postulated that, in the case of cervical cancer, both smoking and HSV were possible cocarcinogens. Since then, the evidence implicating HPV as the major causal agent has become overwhelming, with a number of high-risk types identified, in particular types 16 and 18 (Munoz *et al.* 1992; Walboomers *et al.* 1999).

The number of studies which have included information both on smoking and presence of HPV infection has increased considerably in recent years. Early studies used assays of limited accuracy, but more recent studies have mostly used a consensus PCR system or hybrid capture II. These studies will now be considered in greater detail (Figs. 26.1–26.5).

Reeves *et al.* (1987) were the first to use HPV typing in his case–control study of cervical cancer cases in Latin America. Unfortunately, the method chosen was filter *in situ* hybridization (FISH) which is now known to be of low sensitivity and specificity. There was no dose–response information from this study, but the unadjusted odds ratio for current smoking (number/day not specified) was 2.88 (95% CI 1.2–6.8). The results from this study are of limited value in view of the lack of a sexual behaviour adjusted odds ratio.

Herrero *et al.* (1989) reported another Latin American study of cancer cases, again using FISH for HPV detection. In this study, only 30 per cent of cases and controls had ever smoked for more than 6 months, and over half of these (in both groups) had smoked less than 10 cigarettes per day. This study did not show an overall effect of smoking (RR 1.7, 95% CI 0.8–3.6), but it is interesting that within the subgroup of women who were positive for HPV 16/18 there was some additional increased risk with smoking (RR 6.3, 95% CI 4.3–9.2), after adjustment for other sexual variables, and also a dose–response relationship (RR for >10/day 8.4, 95% CI 4.4–16.2).

Bosch *et al.* (1992) reported a Spanish/Latin American study of invasive cancer cases, using a consensus PCR technique to evaluate HPV status. The results were presented separately for Spain and Colombia, as there were some differences between the two countries. In Spain, only 26 per cent of the cases and 17 per cent of the controls had ever smoked, while in Colombia 50 per cent of the cases and 40 per cent of the controls had ever smoked. No information was available regarding the amount smoked. After adjusting for HPV and sexual variables, smoking was only marginally significant in this study (combined odds ratio 1.5 (95% CI 1.0–2.2)).

A study by Munoz *et al.* (1993) was carried out in parallel with the one by Bosch *et al.* (1992), this time looking specifically at cases with CIN 3/carcinoma *in situ* rather than invasive cancer. In Spain 59 per cent of cases and 34 per cent of controls were current smokers; in Colombia 38 per cent of cases and 14 per cent of controls were current smokers. However, in Spain 19 per cent of cases and 46 per cent of smoking controls had smoked for less than 5 pack-years and in Colombia the figures were 60 per cent of cases and 49 per cent of controls. Thus, even if the women smoked, they tended to be relatively light smokers. In Spanish women, although a significant overall association with current smoking was not found, there was a dose–response relationship ($p=0.003$), with an odds ratio of 3.1 (95% CI 2.0–4.7) for smokers of more than 5 pack-years. In Colombia, there was an association with current smoking, odds ratio 2.0 (95% CI 1.3–3.0), but no clear dose–response ($p=0.09$).

The International Agency for Research on Cancer (IARC) has carried out a series of studies in developing countries. These studies (Eluf-Neto *et al.* 1994; Chichareon *et al.* 1998; Ngalangel *et al.* 1998; Santos *et al.* 2001) have had a similar design and so will be discussed together. Women with invasive cancer were recruited, with controls from the same hospital. HPV testing was performed by the G5+/G6+ consensus PCR. A common problem in these studies is that relatively few women smoked, reducing their statistical power. In addition, smokers tended to smoke fewer than 10 cigarettes per day. Both squamous and adenocarcinoma were included, but not always reported separately (because of small numbers). The studies which looked at adenocarcinoma separately (Chichareon *et al.* 1998; Ngelangel *et al.* 1998) did not find a significant association with smoking. Three studies (Chichareon *et al.* 1998; Ngelangel *et al.* 1998; Santos *et al.* 2001) present results only from HPV positive cases and controls. However, this reduces the number of women still further and, although all show an elevated OR for smoking, none is statistically significant. IARC recognized that the individual studies lacked power and has recently published a meta-analysis (using only HPV positive cases and controls), which shows a significant association with smoking (OR 2.04, 95% CI 1.32–3.14) and a dose–response effect (Plummer *et al.* 2003).

Lacey *et al.* (2001) presented results for both adenocarcinoma and squamous cancer from a multi-centre study in the USA. Interestingly, there was a suggestion that current smoking was inversely related with adenocarcinoma, with an odds ratio of 0.6 (95% CI 0.3–1.1), though only 18 per cent of the 124 cases and 22 per cent of the 307 controls smoked. Numbers for the squamous cancer analysis were also small, with 91 invasive and 48 *in situ* cases, of whom 43 per cent smoked. There was a positive, though non-significant, association with current smoking (OR 1.6, 95% CI 0.9–2.9). HPV testing (by consensus PCR) was not carried out on all women and some only had post-treatment samples, which may have reduced the power of the study further.

Hildesheim *et al.* (2001) included both cancer and CIN in their Costa Rican study. The analysis was restricted to HPV positive cases and controls (using both hybrid capture II and PCR). Despite the fact that only 12 per cent of cases and 6 per cent of controls were smokers, a significant association was found with current smoking (OR, 2.3 95% CI 1.20–4.3) and there was a dose–response relationship for those smoking more than six cigarettes per day, having an odds ratio of 3.1 (95% CI 1.2–7.9).

Becker *et al.* (1994) compared Hispanic with non-Hispanic women in a university gynaecology clinic in New Mexico. HPV status was determined by a consensus PCR. Incident cases of CIN 2/3 were included, with the majority of both cases and controls (64%) being of Hispanic origin. The women were relatively young, with a median age of 26 and a range of 18–40 years. An increased risk of CIN 2/3 in current smokers persisted, even after adjustment for HPV (OR 1.8, 95% CI 1.1–3.0). Interestingly, a separate analysis by ethnic group showed that current smoking was significant only in non-Hispanic women, though the difference between the ethnic groups was not statistically significant.

Olsen *et al.* (1995) reported on women with CIN 2/3 in Norway, using PCR methods for HPV assessment. The women were relatively young (median age 31/32 years, range 20–44 years). They found a very strong association between HPV 16 and high-grade disease (adjusted OR 182.4, 95% CI 54.0–616.1). Information on smoking status was limited to ever versus never smokers; the crude OR of 4.1 (95% CI 2.1–8.1) was reduced to 1.5 (95% CI 0.5–4.3) after adjustment for HPV.

A further analysis of these data (Olsen *et al.* 1998) showed that HPV positive women who smoked were at greater risk of CIN 2/3 than HPV positive women who did not smoke (OR 2.54, 95% CI 1.13–5.72). In addition, statistical testing showed that 74 per cent of cases were attributable to the joint effect of smoking and HPV positivity.

Morrison *et al.* (1991) used a combination of Southern blotting and polymerase chain reaction (PCR) techniques to assess HPV status in his study, conducted in New York. This case–control study did not include cancer cases, restricting itself to CIN (of any grade). Once again, a high proportion of both cases (53%) and controls (44%) were of Hispanic origin and relatively few women (20% of cases and 9% of controls) smoked more than 10 cigarettes per day. The study showed an increased risk in smokers (OR 3.0, 95% CI 1.1–8.1) and a dose–response relationship, but the association was no longer significant after adjustment for HPV.

Schiffman *et al.* (1993) reported a case–control study from a health screening clinic in Oregon, using consensus PCR for determination of HPV status. Cases and controls were chosen on the basis of cytology results, which introduced misclassification problems in both case and control groups. Although not all cases had colposcopy and biopsy, of those who did, the majority were low-grade lesions. Based on cytology, there were 450 low-grade lesions and 50 of high grade. Thirty-five per cent of cases and 20 per cent of controls were current smokers; no data were presented regarding amount or duration of smoking. An increased risk in current smokers was observed (RR 1.7, $p < 0.05$), but this was no longer significant after adjustment for HPV (RR 1.2, 95% CI 0.8–1.8). However, an ancillary analysis showed that among HPV positive women, current smokers were almost three times as likely to have CIN 2/3 as non-smoking women (RR 2.7, 95% CI 1.1–6.5).

Kjaer *et al.* (1996) showed that even after adjustment for sexual behaviour and the presence of HPV (detected by consensus PCR), smoking remained an independent risk factor for both low- and high-grade cervical abnormalities (as measured by cytology). The adjusted relative risks (RR) were 1.8 (95% CI 1.1–2.8) for low-grade abnormalities and 2.3 (95% CI 1.3–4.2) for high-grade abnormalities. The study also showed that current smoking was a significant risk factor in both HPV positive (OR 1.9, 95% CI 1.2–3.2) and HPV negative women (OR 2.4, 95% CI 1.3–4.6).

Roteli-Martins *et al.* (1998) compared risk factors in women with biopsy-proven CIN 1 with those who had high-grade CIN, in their study in Brazil. HPV testing was performed by Hybrid Capture I. The 77 women were between 20 and 35 years of age. Smokers were significantly more likely to have high-grade CIN (35 per cent of women with CIN 1 smoked vs. 78 per cent of those with CIN 2/3, $p < 0.001$) and there was a trend towards an increasing risk with increasing duration of smoking ($p = 0.07$). In addition, smokers were significantly more likely to test positive for high-risk HPV types ($p = 0.046$).

Ho *et al.* (1998) also used women with CIN 1 as controls for those with high-grade CIN in their study from New York. In this larger study of 348 women, 90 per cent were Hispanic or Black. HPV testing was performed by PCR and Southern blotting. It was found that the risk of having CIN 3 was significantly greater in smokers (OR 2.37, 95% CI 1.09–5.15) and increased with the number of cigarettes smoked per day ($p = 0.03$) and duration of smoking ($p = 0.02$). This was not the case for CIN 2, however (OR for current smoking 1.46, 95% CI 0.67–3.19).

Ylitalo *et al.* (1999) in Sweden used all women without CIN 3 as controls for those with CIN 3 (thus the control group included even those with CIN 2). This was a case–control study nested in a screening cohort, so HPV testing for types 16 and 18 only was performed on archival smears by PCR. A doubling of risk for CIN 3 was found in current smokers (OR 1.94, 95% CI 1.32–2.85). The effect of smoking remained significant in women who were HPV positive (OR 2.34, 95% CI 1.28–4.27), but not in those who were HPV negative.

A similar nested case–control study was carried out by Deacon et al. (2000), and once again any women without CIN 3 were used as controls for those who had CIN 3. There were 199 HPV positive cases (by PCR), 181 HPV positive controls, and 203 HPV negative controls. The risk factors for HPV positivity and having CIN 3 were different, with smoking significant (with a dose–response) for CIN 3 (OR 2.57, 95% CI 1.49–4.45) but not for HPV infection. The authors suggest that this provides evidence for a synergism of smoking with HPV to cause cervical neoplasia.

Kjellberg et al. (2000) in Sweden looked at 137 women with high-grade CIN and 253 age-matched controls. HPV testing was performed by PCR. Smoking was significantly associated with high-grade CIN even after adjustment for the presence of HPV (OR 2.6, 95% CI 1.2–5.6). In addition, there was a dose–response for both duration and amount of smoking (adjusted OR for >15/day 6.0, 95% CI 2.7–13.3).

Sasagawa et al. (1997) in Japan found that smoking was a significant risk factor for invasive cancer after adjustment for HPV (OR 5.8, 95% CI 1.8–19.0), but not for CIN (OR 1.6, 95% CI 0.63–4.0). Smoking significantly elevated the risk of having an HPV infection (by PCR) in controls (OR 2.7, 95% CI 1.1–6.9) but not cases (OR 1.4, 95% CI 0.38–5.4), most of whom were in any case HPV positive.

Derchain et al. (1999) compared women with biopsy-proven CIN with those whose biopsies were normal (despite an abnormal colposcopy). After adjustment for the presence of HPV (by Hybrid Capture I), smoking was still associated with increased risk of high-grade CIN (OR 4.37, 95% CI 1.48–12.92).

Coker et al. (2002) have looked at both active and passive smoking as risk factors for CIN, using hybrid capture I as their HPV test. Current smoking was associated with a non-significant increase in risk of high-grade CIN (OR 1.81, 95% CI 0.71–4.6), with a similar, but again non-significant odds ratio for passive smoking exposure (OR 2.05, 95% CI 0.77–6.2).

The relationship between smoking and HPV infection

Ley et al. (1991) investigated HPV prevalence in a screening population, using PCR methods for HPV detection. The study consisted of a cross-sectional sample of 467 women attending a university health clinic in California for routine screening. The women were young (median age 22 years), mostly white (72%) and non-Hispanic (87%). On initial analysis, current smoking was correlated with presence of HPV (OR 2.3, 95% CI 1.1–5.2). The study did not investigate the women further and therefore no information is available regarding cervical abnormality in the two groups.

Rohan et al. (1991) conducted a similar cross-sectional university health clinic screening study, in Toronto. In this study, 105 women attending for routine cervical screening had samples taken for HPV typing (types 6, 11, 16, 18, and 33) by PCR. Once again, these women were young, with a mean age of 23 (range 20–27 years). Current smokers were more likely to have HPV infection of any type (OR 9.5, 95% CI 2.3–39.5). Ever-smokers were also more likely to be infected with HPV, of any type (OR 4.8, 95% CI 1.6–14.2) and of HPV 16 (OR 5.8, 95% CI 1.5–22.3). None of the women had an abnormal smear and no further investigations were performed.

Burger et al. (1993) in a study of 181 women with abnormal cervical smears found that the prevalence of HPV types 16, 18, and 33 (as measured by PCR) increased in accordance with the number of cigarettes smoked ($\chi^2_{trend}=10.75$, 1 df, $p=0.001$) even after adjustment for sexual variables.

In a separate, though overlapping study, Burger et al. (1996) found that the likelihood of women with CIN being HPV positive (by PCR) again increased significantly as their smoking intake increased (OR for >20/day 3.11, 95% CI 1.16–8.29).

Fairley et al. (1995) looked at the effect of stopping smoking in 49 women who originally tested positive for HPV. Based only on self-reports, no significant difference in HPV positivity (measured by PCR in material collected from tampons) at one year was found between the women who reported stopping smoking completely and the remaining women, some of whom were reported 'partial quitters'.

Chan et al. (2002) in a study of over 2000 women attending for routine screening found that current smoking was significantly associated with the presence of high-risk, but not low-risk HPV types (by PCR). The odds ratio for current smoking was 3.34 (95% CI 1.76–6.35).

Moscicki et al. (2001) carried out a longitudinal study in women aged 13–20 years in San Francisco. Women who were HPV negative at the beginning of the study were followed up for a median of 50 months. Smoking was not associated with development of incident HPV infection, but was a significant risk factor for development of low-grade CIN, in women who were HPV positive (OR 1.67, 95% CI 1.12–2.48), suggesting that HPV infections are more likely to lead to CIN in smokers.

Four studies (Hildesheim et al. 1994; Ho 1995; Liu et al. 1995; Remmink et al. 1995) have looked at factors affecting persistence of HPV infections. Of these, one showed no effect of smoking (Ho et al. 1995) and one did not collect enough information on smoking behaviour for analysis (Remmink et al. 1995). Liu et al. (1995) carried out a 6-month intervention trial of folate supplementation, in which they found that heavy smokers had a lower risk of progression of dysplasia (RR 0.79, 95% CI 0.66–0.94). Hildesheim et al. (1994) also found a lower risk of persistent HPV infection in current smokers compared to never smokers (OR 0.22, 95% CI 0.06–0.79). None of these studies was specifically designed to look at the effect of smoking and all had little information on smoking behaviour (indeed, too little for analysis in the case of Remmink et al. 1995). Several ongoing cohort studies should provide more definitive evidence on this important question.

Bosch and Munoz have published further analyses of the studies carried out in Spain (Bosch et al. 1996) and Colombia (Munoz et al. 1996). They have looked at the effect of male sexual behaviour and penile HPV carriage on the risk of cervical cancer and CIN 3 in the wives. In Spain, the presence of HPV DNA in the male (measured by PCR) conveyed a five-fold risk of cervical cancer for the wives (OR 4.9, 95% CI 1.9–12.6). However, even after controlling for the presence of HPV DNA, other infections, sexual behaviour, and the wife's smoking habit, smoking by the male partner was still a significant risk factor for cervical cancer (OR 2.8, 95% CI 1.8–4.4) and showed a dose–response relationship (OR for >26 pack years 3.3, 95% CI 2.0–5.5). In Colombia, by contrast, the presence of penile HPV DNA was not a significant factor (OR 1.2, 95% CI 0.6–2.3). However, after adjustment for the presence of HPV DNA and sexual behaviour, smoking was once again a significant factor, though less strongly than in the Spanish study (OR 1.7, 95% CI 1.1–2.5), with a suggestion of a dose–response relationship (OR for >26 pack-years 2.0, 95% CI 1.0–3.9).

Intervention studies

An intervention study (Szarewski *et al.* 1996) found a significant correlation between the extent of smoking reduction and reduction in the size of minor-grade lesions over a 6-month period. This study also looked at the effect of smoking reduction on immunological parameters (see below).

Possible mechanisms

Direct effects

During the last decade, evidence has accumulated to support a direct biological mechanism for the association of smoking with cervical neoplasia. It has been shown that nicotine and cotinine are both found in cervical mucus possibly at concentrations that are higher than in serum (Sasson *et al.* 1985; Hellberg *et al.* 1988). It has also been reported that the mucus concentrations correlate with reported cigarette consumption (Schiffman *et al.* 1987; McCann *et al.* 1992; Prokopczyk *et al.* 1997). Nicotine can be converted to nitrosamines, which are known to be carcinogenic (Hoffman *et al.* 1985), but polycyclic aromatic amines in cigarette smoke are thought to be more important for other sites. Studies have shown malignant transformation of HPV 16-immortalized human endocervical cells by cigarette smoke condensate (Nakao *et al.* 1996; Yang *et al.* 1996, 1997, 1998). In addition, DNA adducts (Simons *et al.* 1995; Mancini *et al.* 1999) and other evidence of genotoxic damage (Cerqueira *et al.* 1998) are detectable in cervical exfoliated cells. Winkelstein (1977) has pointed out that smoking is strongly associated with squamous cell carcinoma at other sites (lung, bladder) and that the vast majority of cervical carcinomas are of this type.

Immunologic effects

Immunosuppression is associated with an increased risk of cervical neoplasia and there is some evidence that smoking may induce immunological changes in the cervix. Women who are on immunosuppressive therapy are known to be at increased risk of developing condylomas, CIN, and cervical carcinoma (Porecco *et al.* 1975; Schneider *et al.* 1983; Sillman *et al.* 1984; Penn *et al.* 1986; Sillman *et al.* 1987; Alloub *et al.* 1989). In addition, a recent study (Alloub *et al.* 1989) has shown that these women are more likely to show positivity for HPV 16/18; in this study, 27 per cent of the immunosuppressed women versus 6 per cent of the controls were positive for HPV 16/18 ($p < 0.005$).

Women infected with the HIV have been shown to be at higher risk of developing both HPV infection and CIN (Byrne *et al.* 1989; Maiman *et al.* 1990; Johnson *et al.* 1991; Schafer *et al.* 1991; Vermund *et al.* 1991; Mandelblatt *et al.* 1992; Maggwa *et al.* 1993). Since these conditions share many of the same risk factors, confounding is always a possibility. However, it does appear that the degree of immunosuppression (as measured by CD4/CD8 ratio) in HIV positive women is related to the risk of CIN (Schafer *et al.* 1991; Conti *et al.* 1993) and also to the risk of recurrence of CIN after treatment (Maiman *et al.* 1993). It has been suggested that, by virtue of its immunosuppressive effects, HIV infection may facilitate infection with HPV and may also promote the effect of HPV in cervical carcinogenesis (Matorras *et al.* 1991; Vermund *et al.* 1991; Conti *et al.* 1993).

There is still controversy as to which immune parameters might be affected by smoking. In 1978 Rasp reported an impairment in adhesion of alveolar macrophages in smokers, which appeared to be reversible on cessation of smoking. Miller *et al.* (1982) found a reduced CD4/CD8 ratio in the blood of heavy smokers compared to non-smokers, and showed that the CD4/CD8 ratio returned to normal 6 weeks after cessation of smoking.

In recent years, attention has focused on the possible effect of smoking on Langerhans cells, epithelial dendritic cells which appear to have an important role in presenting antigen to T lymphocytes (Stingl *et al.* 1978; Hauser *et al.* 1992). It has been shown that application of a known skin carcinogen in mice results in a marked depletion of Langerhans cells (Muller *et al.* 1985). Smokers have been shown to have a reduced cutaneous inflammatory response to standard test irritants (Mills *et al.* 1993).

A number of studies have assessed the relationship between cervical neoplasia, HPV, and Langerhans cells. There is general agreement that Langerhans' cell density is reduced in the presence of HPV infection (Morris *et al.* 1983; Vayrynen *et al.* 1984; Caorsi *et al.* 1986; McArdle *et al.* 1986; Tay *et al.* 1987; Hawthorn *et al.* 1988; Morelli *et al.* 1993). However, some studies show that Langerhans' cell density is also reduced in CIN (Tay *et al.* 1987; Morelli *et al.* 1993; Szarewski *et al.* 2001), while others suggest that it is increased (Morris *et al.* 1983; Vayrynen *et al.* 1984; Caorsi *et al.* 1986; McArdle *et al.* 1986; Hawthorn *et al.* 1988). Interestingly, Morelli *et al.* (1993) compared Langerhans' cell density across the grades of CIN and found a decrease in CIN 1 (comparable to that seen with HPV infection) and an increase in the higher grades. A contrasting pattern was found by Spinillo *et al.* (1993), who showed a significant reduction in Langerhans' cell counts in HIV positive women who had CIN, compared with HIV negative controls. In this study, Langerhans' cell density was reduced in HIV positive women even after adjusting for the presence of HPV by *in situ* hybridization. In addition, significantly lower Langerhans' cell counts were found in high-grade compared with low-grade CIN. These studies are complicated by different techniques of measuring Langerhans' cell density, which may at least in part, account for the discrepancies observed.

Daniels *et al.* (1992) studied the effect of smokeless tobacco on Langerhans' cell density in oral mucosal premalignant lesions (leukoplakia) and found it to be significantly reduced. However, Cruchley *et al.* (1994) found no such reduction in the normal oral mucosa of smokers.

Barton *et al.* (1988) showed a reduction in Langerhans' cell counts in cervical biopsies from women with both CIN and HPV infection. In addition, current smokers had significantly reduced Langerhans' cell counts compared to non-smokers in both normal epithelium ($p=0.005$) and biopsies showing CIN and/or HPV ($p=0.03$). Poppe *et al.* (1995, 1996) confirmed these findings (in normal epithelium) and also showed a reduction of CD4 lymphocytes in the normal epithelium of smokers. However, Poppe *et al.* (1996) failed to show a correlation between the number of cigarettes smoked daily and the Langerhans' cell counts. Barton *et al.* (1988) did not distinguish between different smoking levels, differentiating only between current, ex-, and non-smokers.

By contrast, Szarewski *et al.* (2001) showed a significant increase in the number of Langerhans' cells with increasing levels of smoking, as measured by salivary cotinine levels. This study assessed changes in both Langerhans' cells and lymphocytes when women attempted to give up smoking: a significant trend towards a reduction in cell count with stopping smoking was found for Langerhans' cells ($p=0.05$), total lymphocytes ($p=0.02$), and CD8 lymphocytes ($p=0.05$). Heavy smoking was also significantly associated ($p=0.02$) with an increased chance of persistence of HPV in cervical biopsies.

Other immune parameters may also be involved in the aetiology of cervical HPV infection and CIN. A decrease in T cell counts, particularly of the CD4 component, has been reported, resulting in a reversed CD4/CD8 ratio (Tay *et al.* 1987). In the study of HIV positive women by Spinillo *et al.* (1993), both the reduction in Langerhans' cell count and increasing grade of CIN were correlated with a progressively greater reversal of the blood CD4/CD8 ratio. Several studies (Turner *et al.* 1988; Kesic *et al.* 1990; Soutter *et al.* 1994) have shown a lower CD4/CD8 ratio in the peripheral blood of women with CIN, compared to colposcopically normal controls. In the study by Soutter *et al.*, laser treatment of the CIN resulted in a rise in the CD4/CD8 ratio. The specific effects of smoking were not, however, evaluated in these studies.

Future studies need to take into account cytokine interactions, which recent studies suggest may be influenced by smoking (Eppel *et al.* 2000) and are significant in the immune response to HPV and CIN (Mota *et al.* 1999; Stanley *et al.* 1999).

Antioxidants

In recent years another aspect of the effect of smoking has come to light. It appears that smokers have a significantly different intake of many nutrients compared to non-smokers, and, in particular, a lower intake of foods providing antioxidants (Cade *et al.* 1991; Wichelow *et al.* 1991; Margetts *et al.* 1993). Smoking itself generates about 10^{15} free radicals with each puff, increasing the requirement for antioxidants which protect cells from damage by free radicals (Church *et al.* 1985). Smokers have been shown to have lower plasma levels of antioxidants compared with non-smokers (Palan *et al.* 1996). Not only do smokers have lower intakes of antioxidants such as β-carotene, α-tocopherol, and ascorbic acid, but, for a given intake, smokers have lower circulating blood levels of these vitamins compared to non-smokers (Stryker *et al.* 1988; Margetts *et al.* 1993). It has been suggested that the dietary intake of smokers and the metabolic effects of smoking on nutrient metabolism increase the risk of oxidative tissue damage in smokers above that which might be expected from the free radicals generated by smoking itself (Halliwell *et al.* 1993; Margetts *et al.* 1993). This may be of relevance to cervical neoplasia, where a number of studies have suggested a protective effect of antioxidant vitamins such as vitamin E (α-tocopherol), vitamin C (ascorbic acid) and β-carotene (Wassertheil-Smoller *et al.* 1981; Marshall *et al.* 1983; Romney *et al.* 1985; La Vecchia *et al.* 1988; Verreault *et al.* 1989; Cuzick *et al.* 1990; Slattery *et al.* 1990; Basu *et al.* 1991). Although the role of dietary factors in cervical neoplasia is still unclear, it, and the possible link with smoking, merits further investigation.

Adenocarcinoma

Adenocarcinoma of the cervix is relatively rare by comparison with the squamous cell type, accounting for approximately 5–10 per cent of all cervical cancer. However, the incidence appears to be increasing, particularly in young women (Kjaer *et al.* 1993). Studies in this field are limited by the rarity of the disease, which results in small numbers for comparison. This topic has been well reviewed by Kjaer *et al.* (1990); however, it is interesting to note that sexual behaviour, in particular, the number of sexual partners, and also HPV types 16 and especially 18, appear to be more strongly linked to adenocarcinoma than has previously been suspected. There are four studies (Parazzini *et al.* 1988; Brinton *et al.* 1990; Chichareon *et al.* 1998; Ngelangel *et al.* 1998) so far with sufficiently large numbers to present results for smoking in relation to adenocarcinoma, but even these have few cases. None has found a significant association. Larger studies are, however, needed before definite conclusions can be drawn.

Conclusion

Epidemiologic evidence strongly links smoking with squamous cell cervical cancer and high-grade CIN. However, some controversy still exists as to whether the link is causal or in some way reflects residual confounding with unmeasured aspects of sexual behaviour (Phillips *et al.* 1994). Attempts to adjust for sexual behaviour through variables such as age at first intercourse and number of sexual partners have generally reduced the strength of the relationship with smoking, but it has not disappeared: it remains at or above two-fold for current smokers and shows a dose–response relationship in many studies.

Recent studies which have collected data on HPV infection have further complicated the interpretation of the data. This is partly due to the much higher odds ratios found for HPV infection, which is clearly the major risk factor. In general, cases tend to be almost universally HPV positive whereas controls are primarily HPV negative, so that adjustment essentially results in a comparison of (HPV positive) cases to HPV positive controls. This situation leads to difficulties in obtaining an adequate number of HPV positive controls. Nevertheless, adjustment for HPV infection has not substantially reduced the odds ratios for smoking.

The current HPV-adjusted studies have two further major limitations. There is a concentration on women from developing countries, who generally smoke less and in whom other cofactors, such as other sexually transmitted diseases, may be more important. These studies have generally found positive odds ratios for smoking but have not been individually significant. European studies have had similar odds ratios (typically around two-fold), but because of the greater prevalence of smoking, these studies have more often been statistically significant.

More fundamental is the possibility that smoking leads to a weakened immune response which in turn increases the likelihood that an HPV infection will become persistent. If this were true, the persistent HPV infection becomes an intermediate endpoint, and adjusting for it would incorrectly indicate no effect of smoking on carcinogenesis. However, it is possible that smoking is in fact increasing the likelihood that an infection will become persistent.

To address these issues, further case–control studies are needed in non-Hispanic women with high-grade CIN and cancer. It is essential that detailed smoking histories are recorded and HPV assays by PCR techniques are performed. Controls can provide valuable information as to whether HPV positivity is increased in smokers in the absence of disease, which would shed light on its role in persistence of HPV infection in older women. Useful information about this should come from the current studies of HPV testing in primary screening (Clavel *et al.* 2001, Petry *et al.* 2003, Cuzick *et al.* 2003). Ideally, HPV positive controls should be tested again after one year to more accurately evaluate this hypothesis. In addition there is a need for cohort studies in young women which examine the factors leading to persistent HPV infections.

References

Alloub, M. I. (1989). Human papillomavirus infection and cervical intraepithelial neoplasia in women with renal allografts. *BMJ*, **298**, 153–6.

Atalah, E., *et al.* (2001). Diet, smoking and reproductive history as risk factors for cervical cancer. *Rev Med Chile*, **129**, 597–603.

Barton, S. E., *et al.* (1988). Effect of cigarette smoking on cervical epithelial immunity: a mechanism for neoplastic change? *Lancet*, **2**, 652–4.

Basu, J., *et al.* (1991). Plasma ascorbic acid and beta-carotene levels in women evaluated for HPV infection, smoking and cervix dysplasia. *Cancer Detect Prev*, **15**, 165–70.

Becker, T. M., *et al.* (1994). Sexually transmitted diseases and other risk factors for cervical cancer among southwestern Hispanic and non-Hispanic white women. *JAMA*, **271**, 1181–8.

Bosch, F. X., *et al.* (1992). Risk factors for cervical cancer in Colombia and Spain. *Int J Cancer*, **52**, 750–8.

Bosch, F. X., *et al.* (1996).Male sexual behaviour and human papillomavirus DNA: key risk factors for cervical cancer in Spain. *J Natl Cancer Inst*, **88**(15), 1060–7.

Brinton, L. A., *et al.* (1987). Epidemiology of cervical cancer by cell type. *Cancer Res*, **47**, 1706–11.

Burger, M. P. M., *et al.* (1993). Cigarette smoking and human papillomavirus in patients with reported cervical cytological abnormality. *BMJ*, **306**, 749–52.

Burger, M. P. M., *et al.* (1996). Epidemiological evidence of cervical intraepithelial neoplasia without the presence of human papillomavirus. *Br J Cancer*, **73**, 831–6.

Byrne, M. A., *et al.* (1989). The occurrence of human papillomavirus infection and intraepithelial neoplasia in women infected by HIV. *AIDS*, **3**, 379–82.

Cade, J. and Margetts, B. M. (1991). The relationship between diet and smoking: is the diet of smokers different? *J Epidemiol Community Health*, **45**, 270–2.

Caorsi, I. and Figueroa, C. D. (1986). Langerhan's cell density in the normal cervical epithelium and in cervical intraepithelial neoplasia. *Br J Obstet Gynaecol*, **93**, 993–8.

Cerqueira, E. M. *et al.*(1998). Genetic damage in exfoliated cells of the uterine cervix. Association and interaction between cigarette smoking and progression to malignant transformation? *Acta Cytol*, **42**, 639–49.

Chan, P. K. S., *et al.* (2002). Determinants of cervical human papillomavirus infection: differences between high and low-oncogenic risk types. *J Infect Dis*, **185**, 28–35.

Chichareon, S., *et al.* (1998). Risk factors for cervical cancer in Thailand: a case-control study. *J Natl Cancer Inst*, **90**, 50–7.

Church, D. F. and Pryor, W. A. (1985). Free-radical chemistry of cigarette smoke and its toxicological implications. *Environ Health Perspect*, **64**, 111–26.

Clavel, C., *et al.* (2001). Human papillomavirus testing in primary screening for the detection of high grade cervical lesions: a study of 7932 women. *Br J Cancer*, **89**(12), 1616–23.

Coker, A. L., *et al.* (2002). Active and passive smoking, high-risk papillomaviruses and cervical neoplasia. *Cancer Detection and Prevention*, **26**, 121–8.

Conti, M., *et al.* (1993). HPV, HIV infection and risk of cervical intraepithelial neoplasia in former intravenous drug abusers. *Gynecol Oncol*, **49**, 344–8.

Cruchley, A. T., *et al.* (1994). Langerhans' cell density in normal human oral mucosa and skin: relationship to age, smoking and alcohol consumption. *J Oral Pathol Med*, **23**, 55–9

Cuzick, J., *et al.* (2003).Management of women who test positive for high risk types of human papillomavirus: The HART study. *Lancet*, **362**, 1871–6.

Cuzick, J., *et al.* (1990).Vitamin A, vitamin E and the risk of cervical intraepithelial neoplasia. *Br J Cancer*, **62**, 651–2.

Cuzick, J., *et al.* (1996). Risk factors for invasive cervix cancer in young women. *Europ J Cancer*, **32A**(5), 836–41.

Daly, S. F., *et al.* (1998). Can the number of cigarettes smoked predict high-grade CIN among women with mildly abnormal cervical smears? *Am J Obstet Gynecol*, **179**, 399–402.

Daniels, T. E., *et al.* (1992). Reduction of Langerhans' cells in smokeless tobacco-associated oral mucosal lesions. *J Oral Pathol Med*, **21**, 100–4.

Deacon, J. M., *et al.* (2000). Sexual behaviour and smoking as determinants of cervical HPV infection and of CIN 3 among those infected: a case-control study nested within the Manchester cohort. *Br J Cancer*, **88**(11), 1565–72.

Derchain, S. F., *et al.* (1999). Association of oncogenic human papillomavirus DNA with high grade cervical intraepithelial neoplasia: the role of cigarette smoking. *Sex Transm Inf*, **75**, 406–8.

Eluf-Neto, J., *et al.* (1994). Human papillomavirus and invasive cervical cancer in Brazil. *Br J Cancer*, **69**, 114–19.

Engeland, A., *et al.* (1996). Smoking habits and risk of cancers other than lung cancer: 28 years' follow-up of 26,000 Norwegian men and women. *Cancer Causes and Control*, **7**, 497–506.

Engeland, A., *et al.* (1997). Use of multiple primary cancers to indicate associations between smoking and cancer incidence: an analysis of 500,000 cancer cases diagnosed in Norway during 1953–93. *Br J Cancer*, **70**, 401–7.

Eppel, W., *et al.* (2000). The influence of cotinine on interleukin 6 expression in smokers with cervical preneoplasia. *Acta Obstet Gynecol Scand*, **79**, 1105–11.

Fairley, C. K., *et al.* (1995). A cohort study comparing the detection of HPV DNA from women who stop and continue to smoke. *Aust NZ J Obstet Gynaecol*, **35**(2), 181–5.

Halliwell, B. (1993). Cigarette smoking and health: a radical view. *J R Soc Health*, **113**, 91–6.

Hauser, C. (1992). The interaction between Langerhans' cells and CD4+ T cells. *J Dermatol*, **19**, 722–5.

Hawthorn, R. J., *et al.* (1988). Langerhans' cells and subtypes of human papillomavirus in cervical intraepithelial neoplasia. *BMJ*, **297**, 643–6.

Hellberg, D., *et al.* (1988). Smoking and cervical intraepithelial neoplasia: nicotine and cotinine in serum and cervical mucus in smokers and nonsmokers. *Am J Obstet Gynecol*, **158**, 910–13.

Herrero, R., *et al.* (1989). Invasive cervical cancer and smoking in Latin America. *J Natl Cancer Inst*, **81**, 205–11.

Herrero, R., *et al.* (2000). Population-based study of human papillomavirus infection and cervical neoplasia in rural Costa Rica. *J Natl Cancer Inst*, 92, 464–74.

Hildesheim, A., *et al.* (1994). Persistence of type-specific human papillomavirus infection among cytologically normal women. *JID*, 169, 235–40.

Hildesheim, A., *et al.* (2001). HPV co-factors related to the development of cervical cancer: results from a population-based study in Costa Rica. *Br J Cancer*, 84(9), 1219–26.

Hirose, K., *et al.* (1996). Subsite (cervix/endometrium)-specific risk and protective factors in uterus cancer. *Jpn J Cancer Res*, 87, 1001–9.

Hirose, K., *et al.* (1998). Smoking and dietary risk factors for cervical cancer at different age group in Japan. *J Epidemiol*, 8, 6–14.

Ho, G. Y. F., *et al.* (1995). Persistent genital human papillomavirus infection as a risk factor for persistent cervical dysplasia. *J Natl Cancer Inst*, 87, 1365–71.

Ho, G. Y. F., *et al.* (1998). HPV 16 and cigarette smoking as risk factors for high-grade CIN. *Int J Cancer*, 78, 281–5.

Hoffmann, D. and Hecht, S. S. (1985). Nicotine-derived N-nitrosamines and tobacco-related cancer: current status and future directions. *Cancer Res*, 45, 935–44.

Johnson, J. C. *et al.* (1992). High frequency of latent and clinical human papillomavirus cervical infections in immune compromised human immunodeficiency virus infected women. *Obstet Gynecol*, 72, 321–7.

Kesic, V., *et al.* (1990). T lymphocytes in non-malignant, pre-malignant and malignant changes of the cervix. *Eur J Gynaecol Oncol*, 11, 191–4.

Kjaer, K. S. and Brinton, L. (1993). Adenocarcinomas of the uterine cervix: the epidemiology of an increasing problem. *Epidemiologic Reviews*, 15(2), 486–98.

Kjaer, S. K., *et al.* (1996). Case-control study of risk factors for cervical squamous cell neoplasia in Denmark. IV: role of smoking habits. *Europ J Cancer Prev*, 5, 359–65.

Kjaer, K. S., *et al.* (1996). Human papillomavirus – the most significant risk determinant of cervical intraepithelial neoplasia. *Int J Cancer*, 65, 601–6.

Kjellberg, L., *et al.* (2000). Smoking, diet, pregnancy and oral contraceptive use as risk factors for cervical intra-epithelial neoplasia in relation to human papillomavirus infection. *Br J Cancer*, 82(7), 1332–8.

Kvale, G., *et al.* (1988). Reproductive factors and risk of cervical cancer by cell type. A prospective study. *Br J Cancer*, 58, 820–4.

La Vecchia, C., *et al.* (1988). Dietary vitamin A and the risk of intraepithelial and invasive neoplasia. *Gynecol Oncol*, 30, 187–95.

Lacey, J.V., *et al.* (2001). Associations between smoking and adenocarcinomas and squamous cell _carcinomas of the uterine cervix (United States). *Cancer Causes and Control*, 12, 153–61.

Ley, C., *et al.* (1991). Determinants of genital human papillomavirus infection in young women. *J Natl Cancer Inst*, 83, 997–1003.

Liu, T., *et al.* (1995). A longitudinal analysis of human papillomavirus 16 infection, nutritional status and cervical dysplasia progression. *Cancer Epidemiology, Biomarkers & Prevention*, 4, 373–80.

Luesley, D., *et al.* (1994). Cigarette smoking and histological outcome in women with mildly dyskaryotic smears. *Br J Obstet Gynaecol*, 101, 49–52.

Maggwa, B. N., *et al.* (1993). The relationship between HIV infection and cervical intraepithelial neoplasia among women attending two family planning clinics in Nairobi, Kenya. *AIDS*, 7, 733–8.

Maiman, M., *et al.* (1990). Human immunodeficiency virus infection and cervical neoplasia. *Gynecol Oncol*, 38, 377–82.

Maiman, M., *et al.* (1993). Recurrent cervical intraepithelial neoplasia in human immunodeficiency virus seropositive women. *Obstet Gynecol*, 82, 170–4.

Mancini, R., et al. (1999). Polycyclic aromatic hydrocarbon-DNA adducts in cervical smears of smokers and non-smokers. Gynecol Oncol, 75, 68–71.

Mandelblatt, J. S., et al. (1992). Association between HIV infection and cervical neoplasia: implications for clinical care of women at risk for both conditions. AIDS, 6, 173–8.

Margetts, D. and Jackson, A. (1993). Interactions between people's diet and their smoking habits: the dietary and nutritional survey of British adults. BMJ, 307, 1381–4.

Matorras, R., et al. (1991). Human immunodeficiency virus-induced immunosuppression: a risk factor for human papillomavirus infection. Am J Obstet Gynecol, 164, 42–4.

McArdle, J. P. and Muller,H. K. (1986). Quantitative assessment of Langerhans' cells in human cervical intraepithelial neoplasia and wart virus infection. Am J Obstet Gynecol, 154, 509–15.

McCann, M. F., et al. (1992). Nicotine and cotinine in the cervical mucus of smokers, passive smokers and nonsmokers. Cancer Epidemiol, Biomarkers and Prev, 1, 125–9.

Miller, L.G., et al. (1982). Reversible alterations in immunoregulatory T cells in smoking. Chest, 5, 527–9.

Mills, C. M., et al. (1993). Altered inflammatory responses in smokers. BMJ, 307, 911.

Moreno, V., et al. (2002). Effect of oral contraceptives on risk of cervical cancer in women with human papillomavirus infection: the IARC multicentric case-control study. Lancet, 359, 1085–92.

Morelli, A. E., et al. (1992). Assessment by planimetry of Langerhans' cell density in penile epithelium with human papillomavirus infection. J Urol, 147, 1268–73.

Morelli, A. E., et al. (1993). Relationship between types of human papillomavirus and Langerhans' cells in cervical condyloma and intraepithelial neoplasia. Am J Clin Path, 99, 200–6.

Morris, H. H. B., et al. (1983). Langerhans' cells in human cervical epithelium: effects of wart virus infection and intraepithelial neoplasia. Br J Obstet Gynaecol, 90, 412–20.

Morrison, E. A. B., et al. (1991). Human papillomavirus infection and other risk factors for cervical neoplasia: A case-control study. Int J Cancer, 49, 6–13.

Moscicki, A. B., et al. (2001). Risks for incident human papillomavirus and low grade squamous intraepithelial lesion development in young females. JAMA, 285, 2995–3002.

Mota, F., et al. (1999). The antigen-presenting environment in normal and human papillomavirus (HPV)-related premalignant cervical epithelium. Clin Exp Immunol, 116, 33–40.

Munoz, N., et al. (1993). Risk factors for cervical intraepithelial neoplasia grade III/carcinoma in situ in Spain and Colombia. Cancer Epidemiol Biomarkers Prev, 2, 423–31.

Munoz, N., et al. (1996). Difficulty in elucidating the male role in cervical cancer in Colombia, a high risk area for the disease. J Natl Cancer Inst, 88, 1068–75.

Nakao, Y., et al. (1996).Malignant transformation of human ectocervical cells immortalized by HPV 18: in vitro model of carcinogenesis by cigarette smoke. Carcinogenesis, 17(3), 577–83.

Ngelangel, C., et al. (1998). Causes of cervical cancer in the Philippines: a case-control study. J Natl Cancer Inst, 90, 43–9.

Olsen, A. O., et al. (1995). Human papillomavirus and cervical intraepithelial neoplasia grads II-III: A population-based case-control study. Int J Cancer, 61, 312–15.

Olsen, A.O., et al. (1998). Combined effect of smoking and HPV 16 infection in cervical carcinogenesis. Epidemiology, 9, 346–9.

Palan, P., et al. (1996). Plasma levels of β-carotene, lycopene, canthaxanthin, retinol and α- and τ-tocopherol in cervical epithelial neoplasia and cancer. Clinical Cancer Research, 2, 181–5.

Parazzini, F., et al. (1988). Risk factors for adenocarcinoma of the cervix. Br J Cancer, 57, 201–4.

Penn, I. (1986). Cancers of the anogenital region in renal transplant recipients. Cancer, 58, 611.

Petry, K. U., et al. (2003). Inclusion of HPV testing in routine cervical cancer screening for women above 29 years in Germany: results for 8466 patients. Br J Cancer, 88, 1570–7.

Phillips, A. N. and Davey Smith, G. (1994). Cigarette smoking as a potential cause of cervical cancer: has confounding been controlled? Int J Epidemiol, 23, 42–9.

Plummer, M., *et al.* (2003). IARC Multi-center Cervical Cancer Study Group. Smoking and cervical cancer. *Cancer Causes Control*, 14, 805–14.

Poppe, W. A., *et al.* (1995). Tobacco smoking impairs the local immunosurveillance in the uterine cervix. An immunohistochemical study. *Gynecol Obstet Invest*, 39, 34–8.

Poppe, W. A. J., *et al.* (1996). Langerhans' cells and L1 antigen expression in normal and abnormal squamous epithelium of the cervical transformation zone. *Gynecol Obstet Invest*, 41, 207–13.

Porecco, R., *et al.* (1975). Gynaecological malignancies in immunosuppressed organ homograft recipients. *Obstet Gynecol*, 45, 359–64.

Prokopczyk, B., *et al.* (1997). Identification of tobacco-specific carcinogen in the cervical mucus of smokers and nonsmokers. *J Natl Cancer Inst*, 89, 868–73.

Reeves, W. C., *et al.* (1987). Case-control study of human papillomaviruses and cervical cancer in Latin America. *Int J Cancer*, 40, 450–4.

Remmink, A. J., *et al.* (1995). The presence of persistent high-risk HPV genotypes in dysplastic cervical lesions is associated with progressive disease. *Int J Cancer*, 61, 306–11.

Rohan, T., *et al.* (1991). PCR-detected genital papillomavirus infection: prevalence and association with risk factors for cervical cancer. *Int J Cancer*, 49, 856–60.

Romney, S. L., *et al.* (1985). Plasma vitamin C and uterine cervical dysplasia. *Am J Obstet Gynecol*, 151, 976–80.

Roteli-Martins, C. M., *et al.* (1998). Cigarette smoking and high risk HPV DNA as predisposing factors for high grade CIN in young Brazilian women. *Acta Obstet Gynecol Scand*, 77, 678–82.

Santos, C., *et al.* (2001). HPV types and cofactors causing cervical cancer in Peru. *Br J Cancer*, 85, 966–71.

Sasagawa, T., *et al.* (1997). Human papillomavirus infection and risk determinants for squamous intraepithelial lesion and cervical cancer in Japan. *Jpn J Cancer Res*, 88, 376–84.

Sasson, I. M., *et al.* (1985). Cigarette smoking and neoplasia of the uterine cervix: smoke constituents in cervical mucus. *N Eng J Med*, 312, 315–16.

Schafer, A., *et al.* (1991). The increased frequency of cervical dysplasia in women infected with the human immunodeficiency virus is related to the degree of immunosuppression. *Am J Obstet Gynecol*, 164, 593–9.

Schiffman, .M. H., *et al.* (1987). Biochemical epidemiology of cervical neoplasia. *Cancer Res*, 3886–8.

Schiffman, M. H., *et al.* (1993). Epidemiologic evidence showing that human papillomavirus infection causes most cervical intraepithelial neoplasia. *JNCI*, 85, 958–64.

Schlecht, N. F., *et al.* (2001). Persistant human papillomavirus infection as a predicator of cervical intraepithelial neoplasia. *JAMA*, 286, 3106–14.

Schneider, V., *et al.* (1983). Immunosuppression as a high risk factor in the development of condylomata acuminata and squamous neoplasia of the cervix. *Acta Cytol*, 27, 220–4.

Scholes, D., *et al.* (1999). The association between cigarette smoking and low-grade cervical abnormalities in reproductive-age women. *Cancer Causes and Control*, 10, 399–44.

Sillman, F., *et al.* (1984). The relationship between human papillomavirus and lower genital tract neoplasia in immunosuppressed women. *Am J Obstet Gynecol*, 150, 300–8.

Sillman, F. H. and Sedlis, A. (1987). Anogenital papillomavirus infection and neoplasia in immunodeficiant women. *Obstet Gynecol Clin North Am*, 14, 537–57.

Simons, A. M., *et al.* (1995). Demonstration of smoking-related DNA damage in cervical epithelium and correlation with human papillomavirus type 16, using exfoliated cervical cells. *Br J Cancer*, 71, 246–9.

Skegg, D. C. G. (2002). Oral contraceptives, parity and cervical cancer. *Lancet*, 359, 1080–1.

Slattery, M. L., *et al.* (1990). Dietary vitamins A, C and E and selenium as risk factors for cervical cancer. *Epidemiology*, 1, 8–15.

Soutter, W. P. and Kesic, V. (1994). Treatment of cervical intraepithelial neoplasia reverses CD4/CD8 lymphocyte abnormalities in peripheral venous blood. *Int J Gynecol Cancer*, 4, 279–82.

Spinillo, A., *et al.* (1993). Langerhans' cell counts and cervical intraepithelial neoplasia in women with Human Immunodeficiency Virus infections. *Gynaecol Oncol*, 48, 210–13.

Stanley, M. (1999).Mechanism of action of Imiquimod *Papillomavirus Report*, 10(2), 23–9.

Stingl, G., *et al.* (1978). Immunologic functions of 1a-bearing epidermal Langerhans cells. *J Immunol*, 121, 2005–13.

Stryker, W. S., *et al.* (1988). The relation of diet, cigarette smoking and alcohol consumption to plasma beta-carotene and alpha tocopherol levels. *Am J Epidemiol*, 127, 283–95.

Szarewski, A. and Cuzick, J. (1998). Smoking and cervical neoplasia: a review of the evidence. *J Epidemiol & Biostatistics*, 3, 229–56.

Szarewski, A., *et al.* (1996). The effect of smoking cessation on cervical lesion size. *Lancet*, 347, 941–3.

Szarewski, A., *et al.* (2001). The effect of stopping smoking on cervical Langerhans' cells and lymphocytes. *Br J Obstet Gynaecol*, 108, 295–303.

Tay, S. K., *et al.* (1987a). Subpopulations of Langerhans' cells in a cervical neoplasia. *Br J Obstet Gynaecol*, 94, 10–15.

Turner, M. J., *et al.* (1988). T lymphocytes and cervical intraepithelial neoplasia. *Irish J Med Science*, 81, 184.

Vayrynen, M., *et al.* (1984). Langerhans' cells in human papillomavirus (HPV) lesions of the uterine cervix identified by the monoclonal antibody OKT6. *Int J Gynaecol Obstet*, 22, 375–83.

Vermund, S. H., *et al.* (1991). High risk of human papillomavirus infection and cervical intraepithelial lesions among women with symptomatic human immunodeficiency syndrome. *Am J Obstet Gynecol*, 165, 392–400.

Verreault, R., *et al.* (1989). A case-control study of diet amd invasive cervical cancer. *Int J Cancer*, 48, 34–8.

Walboomers, J. M., *et al.* (1999). Human papillomavirus is a necessary cause of invasive cervical cancer worldwide. *J Pathol*, 189, 12–19.

Wassertheil-Smoller, S., *et al.* (1981). Dietary vitamin C and uterine cervical dysplasia. *Am J Epidemiol*, 114, 714–24.

Wichelow, M. J., *et al.* (1991). A comparison of the diets of non-smokers and smokers. *Br J Addict*, 86, 71–81.

Winkelstein, W. Jr. (1977). Smoking and cancer of the uterine cervix. *Am J Epidemiol*, 106, 257–9.

Yang, X., *et al.* (1996).Malignant transformation of HPV 16-immortalized human endocervical cells by cigarette smoke condensate and characterization of multistage carcinogenesis. *Int J Cancer*, 65, 338–44.

Yang, X., *et al.* (1997). Expression of cellular genes in HPV 16-immortalised and cigarette smoke condensate-transformed human endocervical cells. *J Cellular Biochem*, 66, 309–21.

Yang, X., *et al.* (1998). Enhanced expression of anti-apoptotic proteins in human papillomavirus-immortalized and cigarette smoke condensate-transformed human endocervical cells. *Molecular Carcinogenesis*, 22, 95–101.

Ylitalo, N., *et al.* (1999). Smoking and oral contraceptives as risk factors for cervical carcinoma in situ. *Int J Cancer*, 81, 357–65.

Zivaljevic, B., *et al.* (2001). Smoking as a risk factor for cervical cancer. *Neoplasma*, 48, 254–6.

zur Hausen, H. (1982). Human genital cancers: synergism between two virus infections or synergism between a virus infection and initiating events? *Lancet*, II, 1370–2.

Chapter 27

Tobacco and pancreas cancer

Patrick Maisonneuve

Introduction

In developed countries, pancreas cancer is the 10th most common form of cancer in men and the 9th most common form of cancer in women, but because of its very poor prognosis, it ranks as the fourth most common cause of cancer deaths in both sexes (Ferlay *et al.* 2000).

The risk of pancreatic cancer increases rapidly with age, with 80% of the cases being diagnosed after age 60. Pancreatic cancer has been predominantly a male disease, presumably because of past differences in smoking habits, but the sex ratio decreases with increasing age. Blacks are 50% more likely to contract pancreatic cancer than whites (Coughlin *et al.* 2000). The cause for this racial difference is poorly understood. There is little evidence to suggest that blacks smoke more than white, but suggestive evidence that there are racial differences in the ability to degrade carcinogens contained within tobacco smoke (Richie *et al.* 1997).

Risk factors for pancreas cancer comprise a diet rich in meat and fat, past medical history of pancreatitis or diabetes, exposure to certain chemicals, and hereditary factors, but tobacco smoking remains the major recognized risk factor for pancreatic cancer.

Prospective studies

The strongest evidence of the association between cigarette smoking and pancreatic cancer comes from a series of large prospective studies.

In 1966, Hammond and Horn investigated the relation between smoking and death rates in a large prospective study of one million US men and women (Hammond and Horn 1966). Between October 1959 and February 1960, 1 078 894 men and women were enrolled in the study and completed a detailed questionnaire including smoking habits. After 3 years of follow-up, the pancreatic cancer mortality ratio for men who ever smoked regularly compared to men who never smoked was 2.69 for subjects aged 45 to 64 and 2.17 for subjects over 65 years of age. For women aged 45 to 64, the mortality ratio was 1.81 for women who ever smoked regularly and 2.58 for women classified as "Heavier" cigarette smokers. (At that time, many female cigarette smokers smoked only a few cigarettes a day, did not inhale, and had been smoking for only few years.)

Similar results were found in a second similar prospective mortality study of 1.2 million American men and women enrolled in 1982 (Coughlin *et al.* 2000). Eighty percent of subjects were between the ages of 43 and 71. After 14 years of follow-up, cigarette smoking at baseline was associated with a two-fold risk of fatal pancreatic cancer in males. For former smokers, the risk decreased to levels similar to that of non-smokers 20 years after cessation.

Another large prospective study including 34 440 male British doctors recruited in 1951 provided strong evidence of the association between cigarette smoking and pancreatic cancer. After 20 years of observation, the annual age-standardized pancreatic cancer death rate per 100 000 men was 14 in non-smokers, 12 in ex-smokers, 14 in current smokers of less than 14 cigarettes/day, 18 in current smokers of 15–24 cigarettes/day, and 27 in current smokers of 25 or more cigarettes/day. No association was found for pipe or cigar smokers only (Doll and Peto 1976). After 40 years of observations, compared to never smokers, the mortality ratio was 1.4 for ex-smokers, 1.8 for current smokers of less than 25 cigarettes/day and 3.1 for current smokers of 25 or more cigarettes/day (Doll *et al.* 1994).

A combined analysis of two large ongoing prospective studies, the Nurses' Health Study and the Health Professionals Follow-up Study, including 118 339 women and 49 428 men again demonstrated a 2.5 fold increased risk of pancreatic cancer for current smokers (Fuchs *et al.* 1996). A significant positive trend in risk with increasing pack-years of smoking was observed ($p = 0.004$) however confined to cigarette consumption within the past 15 years. Former smokers had a 48% reduction in pancreatic cancer risk within 2 years of quitting and the risk of pancreas cancer among former smokers approached that for never smokers after less than 10 years of smoking cessation. It was also estimated from this study, that 25% of pancreatic cancers may be attributable to cigarette smoking.

Of interest, another large prospective cohort study was conducted in an elderly population consisting of 13 979 residents of a retirement community (Shibata *et al.* 1994). About 80% of the cohort members were between 65 and 85 years of age at entry in the study. After 9 years of follow-up, 65 pancreatic cancer cases had been identified and smoking was associated only with a modest non-significant elevation in risk indicating that, most likely, subjects susceptible to tobacco carcinogens would develop pancreatic cancer before reaching old age.

Case–control studies

In parallel to these large prospective studies, a large number of case-control studies have been conducted but, because pancreatic cancer is a very lethal disease, many of these studies were based on either retrospective data or on information gathered from proxy respondents, in which smoking habits may not be completely reliable. Still the vast majority of these studies identified cigarette smoking as a risk factor for pancreatic cancer, with similar effects than those described in the cohort studies.

Cigar, pipe, and chewing tobacco

While cigarette smoking remains the most common form of tobacco in westernized countries, alternative forms of tobacco are available. In particular, cigars became increasingly fashionable since mid-1990s in the United States and later in western Europe. The number of cigars consumed in the United States increased by approximately 50% between 1993 and 1998 (U.S. Department of Agriculture 1996, 1999). Still, little is known about the health hazard of cigar smoking, possibly because cigars were not required to carry a health warning from the Surgeon General until June 26, 2000 (U.S. Department of Health and Human Services 2000).

Most of the published case–control studies did not have sufficient statistical power to assess the association between either cigar, pipe, chewing tobacco, or oral snuff consumption and pancreatic cancer on their own. These forms of tobacco are less common and are often consumed in addition to cigarettes making difficult the evaluation of the effect of each single product. Still, in an hospital-based study of 484 male and female patients with pancreatic cancer and 954 control subjects, pipe or cigar smokers had a two-fold risk of developing pancreatic cancer (OR=2.1; 95% CI=1.2–3.8) while the risk was 3.6 (95% CI, 1.0–12.8) for tobacco chewers (Muscat, 1997). These results suggest that tobacco smoke causes pancreatic cancer when inhaled into the lungs and that tobacco juice may also cause pancreatic cancer when ingested or absorbed through the oral cavity. In a recent analysis of a large prospective mortality study in the United States, a significant association between cigar consumption and pancreas cancer was found but limited to current cigar smokers who reported that they inhaled the smoke (RR=2.7; 95% CI=1.3–9.9) (Shapiro *et al.* 2000).

Gene–environment interaction

Research in the area of gene–environment interaction is an important topic for various cancers because minimizing exposure to environmental risk factors could reduce the impact of inherited genetic susceptibility factors. A positive family history of pancreatic cancer and smoking are two independent risk factors, each of which approximately doubles the risk of pancreatic cancer but Schenk *et al.* found an interaction between these two risk factors (Schenk *et al.* 2001). Smokers who are related to a person who develops pancreatic cancer before the age 60 have 8 times the risk of pancreatic cancer as individuals lacking these two risk factors.

Another report focused on the impact of smoking in patients with hereditary pancreatitis, a rare pancreatic disorder associated with a 50- to 70-fold increased risk of pancreatic cancer (Lowenfels *et al.* 2001). In these patients, smoking doubled the risk of pancreatic cancer, as it does in the general population, but pancreatic cancer developed in average 20 years earlier in smokers than in non-smokers.

Histological and experimental studies

There is also strong evidence that smoking is associated with histologic alterations and molecular damages of the pancreas

In a large autopsy study based on 22 344 slides from 560 autopsied subjects, histological alterations in the ductal epithelium was strongly associated with smoking habits. Only 5.4% of the non-smokers had medium to high percentages of ductal cells with atypical nuclei. This rose to 50.7% in light smokers and to 74.9% in smokers of more than 40 cigarettes/day. Advanced findings (increased numbers) of cells with atypical nuclei were found in the acinar cells of the parenchyma in only 1.8% of non-smokers; 11.4% in smokers of less than 20 cigarettes/day; 29.2% in smokers of 20–39 cigarettes/day and 69.1% in smokers of more than 40 cigarettes/day. Moderate or advanced hyaline thickening of arterioles in 12.8% of the non-smokers increased to 74.4% in the heaviest smoking group. A similar relationship was observed for fibrous thickening in the arteries (Auerbach and Garfinkel 1986).

The nicotine-derived nitrosamine, nitrosamine 4-(methylnitrosamino)-1-(3-pyridyl)-1-butanone (NNK), is known to cause adenocarcinomas of the lung and pancreas in laboratory animals (Hoffmann *et al.* 1993, Schuller *et al.* 1993), and is thought to be largely responsible for the development of these cancers in smokers. In particular, NNK has genotoxic effects on cells, such as the formation of DNA adducts and mutations in the RAS gene. Experimental studies have demonstrated that aromatic amines and nitroaromatic hydrocarbons are metabolized by the pancreas and may be involved in the etiology of human pancreatic cancer (Anderson *et al.* 1997), and that DNA damage derived from carcinogen exposure is involved in pancreatic carcinogenesis and in particular that smoking was positively correlated to the level of total DNA adducts in pancreatic cancer tissue (Wang *et al.* 1998).

From these observations, it was hypothesized that polymorphisms in genes that encode carcinogen-metabolizing enzymes could also affect the risk of smoking-related pancreatic cancer. In particular, it has been shown that the glutathione S-transferase T1 (GSTT1) enzyme protects pancreatic cells from the damaging effects of tobacco smoking and that lacking this enzyme may increase the risk of smoking-related pancreatic cancer (Duell *et al.* 2002). Using biological material collected in a large case-control study in the San Francisco Bay Area, it was shown that the XRCC1 (X-ray repair cross-complementing group 1) 399Gln allele, which has been associated with elevated biomarkers of DNA damage in human cells, is also a potentially important determinant of susceptibility to smoking-induced pancreatic cancer (Duell *et al.* 2002). Still, previous smaller studies did not find significant associations between GSTM1, GSTT1, NAT1 or CYP1A1 polymorphisms and pancreatic cancer susceptibility (Bartsch *et al.* 1998; Liu *et al.* 2000).

Conclusion

Overall, tobacco smoking is associated with a two- to three-fold increased risk of pancreatic cancer and is responsible for approximately 25% of all pancreatic tumours. The risk is increasing with the amount of cigarette smoked and 10–15 years have to pass from quitting smoking until the risk fell to the level of a non-smoker. The risk seems to be higher for younger subjects and decreases to non-significant values among elderly people. Among individuals at high risk of pancreatic cancer such as patients with hereditary pancreatitis, smoking further advances the age at which cancer develops. Smoking has also been associated with histopathological alterations of the epithelial cells of the pancreas and the tobacco-related carcinogens. NNK induces adenocarcinoma of the pancreas in laboratory animals. Still, smoking remains the strongest risk factor amenable to preventive intervention.

References

Anderson, K. E., Hammons, G. J., Kadlubar, F. F., Potter, J. D., Kaderlik, K. R., Ilett, K. F., *et al.* (1997). Metabolic activation of aromatic amines by human pancreas. *Carcinogenesis*, **18**, 1085–92.

Auerbach, O. and Garfinkel, L. (1986). Histologic changes in pancreas in relation to smoking and coffee-drinking habits. *Dig Dis Sci*, **31**, 1014–20.

Bartsch, H., Malaveille, C., Lowenfels, A. B., Maisonneuve, P., Hautefeuille, A., and Boyle, P. (1998). Genetic polymorphism of N-acetyltransferases, glutathione S-transferase M1 and NAD(P)H:quinone oxidoreductase in relation to malignant and benign pancreatic disease risk. The International Pancreatic Disease Study Group. *Eur J Cancer Prev*, **7**, 215–23.

Coughlin, S. S., Calle, E. E., Patel, A. V., and Thun, M. J. (2000). Predictors of pancreatic cancer mortality among a large cohort of United States adults. *Cancer Causes Control*, **11**, 915–23.

Doll, R., Peto, R., Wheatley, K., Gray, R., and Sutherland, I. (1994). Mortality in relation to smoking: 40 years' observations on male British doctors. *Br Med J*, **309**, 901–11.

Duell, E. J., Holly, E. A., Bracci, P. M., Liu, M., Wiencke, J. K., and Kelsey, K. T. (2002). A population-based, case-control study of polymorphisms in carcinogen-metabolizing genes, smoking, and pancreatic adenocarcinoma risk. *J Natl Cancer Inst*, **94**, 297–306.

Duell, E. J., Holly, E. A., Bracci, P. M., Wiencke, J. K., and Kelsey, K. T. (2002). A population-based study of the Arg399Gln polymorphism in X-ray repair cross-complementing group 1 (XRCC1) and risk of pancreatic adenocarcinoma. *Cancer Res*, **62**, 4630–6.

Ferlay, J., Bray, F., Pisani, P., and Parkin, D. M. (2001). GLOBOCAN 2000: Cancer incidence, mortality and prevalence worldwide, Version 1.0. IARC CancerBase No. 5. IARC Press, Lyon.

Fuchs, C. S., Colditz, G. A., Stampfer, M. J., Giovannucci, E. L., Hunter, D. J., Rimm, E. B., *et al.* (1996). A prospective study of cigarette smoking and the risk of pancreatic cancer. *Arch Intern Med*, **156**, 2255–60.

Hammond, E.C. (1966). Smoking in relation to the death rates of one million men and women. *Natl Cancer Inst Monogr*, **19**, 127–204.

Hoffmann, D., Djordjevic, M. V., Rivenson, A., Zang, E., Desai, D., and Amin, S. (1993). A study of tobacco carcinogenesis. LI. Relative potencies of tobacco-specific N-nitrosamines as inducers of lung tumours in A/J mice. *Cancer Lett*, **71**, 25–30.

Liu, G., Ghadirian, P., Vesprini, D., Hamel, N., Paradis, A. J., Lal, G., *et al.* (2000). Polymorphisms in GSTM1, GSTT1 and CYP1A1 and risk of pancreatic adenocarcinoma. *Br J Cancer*, **82**, 1646–9.

Lowenfels, A. B., Maisonneuve, P., DiMagno, E. P., Elitsur, Y., Gates, L. K. Jr, Perrault, J., and Whitcomb, D. C. (1997). Hereditary pancreatitis and the risk of pancreatic cancer. International Hereditary Pancreatitis Study Group. *J Natl Cancer Inst*, **89**, 442–6

Lowenfels, A. B., Maisonneuve, P., Whitcomb, D. C., Lerch, M. M., and DiMagno, E. P. (2001). Cigarette smoking as a risk factor for pancreatic cancer in patients with hereditary pancreatitis. *JAMA*, **286**,169–70.

Muscat, J. E., Stellman, S. D., Hoffmann, D., and Wynder, E. L. (1997). Smoking and pancreatic cancer in men and women. *Cancer Epidemiol Biomarkers Prev*, **6**,15–9.

Richie, J. P., Jr, Carmella, S. G., Muscat, J. E., Scott, D. G., Akerkar, S. A., and Hecht, S. S. (1997). Differences in the urinary metabolites of the tobacco-specific lung carcinogen 4-(methylnitrosamino)-1-(3-pyridyl)-1-butanone in black and white smokers. *Cancer Epidemiol Biomarkers Prev*, **6**,783–90.

Schenk, M., Schwartz, A. G., O'Neal, E., Kinnard, M., Greenson, J. K., Fryzek, J. P., *et al.* (2001). Familial risk of pancreatic cancer. *J Natl Cancer Inst*, **93**,640–4.

Schuller, H. M., Jorquera, R., Reichert, A., and Castonguay, A. (1993). Transplacental induction of pancreas tumors in hamsters by ethanol and the tobacco-specific nitrosamine 4-(methylnitrosamino)-1-(3-pyridyl)-1-butanone. *Cancer Res*, **53**, 2498–2501.

Shapiro, J. A., Jacobs, E. J., and Thun, M. J. (2000). Cigar smoking in men and risk of death from tobacco-related cancers. *J Natl Cancer Inst*, **92**, 333–7.

Shibata, A., Mack, T. M., Paganini-Hill, A., Ross, R. K., and Henderson, B. E. (1994) A prospective study of pancreatic cancer in the elderly. *Int J Cancer*, **58**, 46–9.

U.S. Department of Agriculture (1996). Tobacco situation and outlook report. TBS-237. Washington (DC): U.S. Department of Agriculture, Commodity Economics Division, Economic Research Service.

U.S. Department of Agriculture (1999). Tobacco situation and outlook report. TBS-243. Washington (DC): U.S. Department of Agriculture, Commodity Economics Division, Economic Research Service.

U.S. Department of Health and Human Services (2000). Reducing tobacco use: A report of the Surgeon General. Atlanta, Georgia: U.S. Department of Health and Human Services, Centers for Disease Control and Prevention, National Center for Chronic Disease Prevention and Health Promotion, Office on Smoking and Health.

Wang, M., Abbruzzese, J. L., Friess, H., Hittelman, W. N., Evans, D. B., Abbruzzese, M. C., *et al.* (1998). DNA adducts in human pancreatic tissues and their potential role in carcinogenesis. *Cancer Res*, **58**, 38–41.

Wynder, E. L., Mabuchi, K., Maruchi, N., and Fortner, J. (1973) A case-control study of cancer of the pancreas. *Cancer*, **31**, 641–8.

Chapter 28

Smoking and lung cancer

Graham G. Giles and Peter Boyle

Summary

The establishment of the causal link between smoking and lung cancer was an epidemiological triumph won against considerable resistance marshalled by the tobacco industry. This chapter reviews how the evidence that smoking causes lung cancer was accumulated and weighed against criteria adopted to establish the causal significance of epidemiological associations between an exposure and disease. The history of elucidating the association between lung cancer and smoking is now fundamental to modern epidemiological thinking and practice but in the early to mid-twentieth century the science of epidemiology was new and in the making, and the research on smoking and lung cancer contributed to the development of epidemiology as a discipline (White 1990). In addition to the evaluation of epidemiological evidence, the case for causality was strengthened by evidence from human pathology and by evidence from experimental studies using animal models. Much of this material has been reviewed previously elsewhere (IARC 1986) to which the interested reader is referred for more detail than can be given here.

Introduction

The last century has witnessed a remarkable epidemic of lung cancer. The words of Adler (1912), today make salutatory reading. *'Is it worthwhile to write a monograph on the subject of primary malignant tumours of the lung? In the course of the last two centuries an ever-increasing literature has accumulated around this subject. But this literature is without correlation, much of it buried in dissertations and other out-of-the-way places, and, with but a few notable exceptions, no attempt has been made to study the subject as a whole, either the pathological or the clinical aspect having been emphasised at the expense of the other, according to the special predilection of the author. On one point, however, there is nearly complete consensus of opinion, and that is that primary malignant neoplasms of the lungs are among the rarest forms of the disease. This latter opinion of the extreme rarity of primary tumours has persisted for centuries.'*

The lung is the principal body organ susceptible to tobacco carcinogenesis and, apart from non-melanocytic skin cancer, in many populations it has been or remains the most commonly diagnosed cancer in men and an increasingly common cancer in women (Gilliland and Samet 1994). The smoking of tobacco is the principal cause of lung cancer. The IARC Monograph on Tobacco Smoking (IARC 1986) estimated the proportion of lung cancer deaths attributable to tobacco smoking in five developed countries (Canada, England and Wales, Japan, Sweden, and the United States) to range between 83 and 92 per cent for men and 57 and 80 per cent for women. Historically, the incidence of lung cancer has waxed and waned to a greater or lesser degree in different populations related to the timing, prevalence, and intensity of the smoking epidemic and the different local dose of carcinogens delivered per cigarette. In some countries, especially those in which the epidemic struck early and was supplied with high tar cigarettes, age-standardized annual incidence and mortality rates exceeded 100 per 100 000 men and subsequently declined with the falling prevalence of men smoking. In the same populations the uptake of smoking in women was delayed by one or two decades. This delay, and a contemporaneous marketing of the filter tipped and lower dose cigarettes, resulted in a slower rise in rates. Consistent with the historical rise and fall in the prevalence of smoking in men, in several populations lung cancer rates in men have now peaked or are falling. The prevalence of smoking in women has either continued to grow or has declined only slowly. There is evidence from some countries that lung cancer rates in women may be stabilizing but the scenario in most countries is one of continuing increases in incidence and mortality. In 2000 it was estimated globally that 1.2 million people were diagnosed with lung cancer (Parkin 2001). This number is expected to grow. Many countries of Europe, Asia, Africa, and South America have only recently achieved a high prevalence of smoking, especially in women. In terms of lung cancer alone, these populations will generate millions of additional deaths over the next few decades.

In men in all European countries, except Portugal, lung cancer is now the leading cause of cancer death. In the United States (and in all except a few Scandinavian countries) it is the commonest tumour in terms of incidence as well (although the recent inflation of prostate cancer incidence figures with very early cases is taking prostate cancer above lung cancer in terms of the incidence of the disease). The range of geographical variation in lung cancer mortality in Europe is three-fold in both sexes, the highest rates being observed in the United Kingdom, Belgium, the Netherlands, and Czechoslovakia, and lowest rates reported in southern Europe and also in Norway and Sweden (Levi et al. 1989). This overall pattern of age-standardized lung cancer mortality rates does not reveal the important and diverging cohort effects occurring in various countries: for instance, some of the countries in which there are now low rates such as those in southern Europe and parts of eastern Europe, experienced a later uptake and spread of tobacco use, and now appear among the most elevated rates in the younger age groups. This suggests that these same countries, including Italy, Greece, France, Spain, and several countries in eastern Europe, will have the highest lung cancer rates in men at the beginning of the next century in the absence of rapid intervention.

The importance of adequate intervention is shown by the low lung cancer rates in Scandinavian countries which have adopted, since the early 1970s, integrated central and local policies and programs against smoking (Bjartveit 1986; Della-Vorgia *et al.* 1990). These policies may have been enabled by the limited influence of the tobacco lobby in these countries. The experience in Finland provides convincing evidence of the favourable impact, after a relatively short delay, of well-targeted large-scale interventions on the most common cause of cancer death and of premature mortality in general.

With specific reference to women, current rates in most European countries (except the United Kingdom, Ireland, and Denmark) are still substantially lower than in the United States, where lung cancer is now the leading cause of cancer death in women. In several countries, including France, Switzerland, Germany, and Italy, where smoking is now becoming commoner in young and middle-aged women, overall national mortality rates are still relatively low, although appreciable upward trends have been registered over the last two decades. This is particularly worrisome in perspective, since smoking prevalence has continued to increase in subsequent generations of young women in these countries. Thus, the observation that lung cancer is still relatively rare in women, with smoking at present accounting only for approximately 40–60 per cent of all lung cancer deaths cannot constitute a reason for delaying efficacious interventions against smoking by women. The currently more favourable situation in Europe compared with the United States, together with the observation that smoking cessation reduces lung cancer risk after a delay of several years, should in the presence of adequate intervention, enable a major lung cancer epidemic in European women to be avoided.

A proportion of lung cancers, varying in various countries and geographical areas, may be due to exposures at work, and a small proportion to atmospheric pollution (Tomatis 1990). The effect of atmospheric pollution in increasing lung cancer risk appears to be chiefly confined to smokers. Lung cancer risk is elevated in atomic bomb survivors (Shimizu *et al.* 1987), patients treated for ankylosing spondylitis (Smith and Doll 1982), and in underground miners whose bronchial mucosa was exposed to radon gas and its decay products: this latter exposure was reviewed and it was concluded that there was 'sufficient evidence' that this occupational exposure caused lung cancer (IARC 1988). A greater risk of lung cancer is generally seen for individuals who are exposed at an older age. Investigation of the interaction with cigarette smoking among atomic bomb survivors suggests that it is additive (Kopecky *et al.* 1987) but the data from underground miners in Colorado are consistent with a multiplicative effect (Whittemore and McMillan 1983).

The overwhelming role of tobacco smoking in the causation of lung cancer has been repeatedly demonstrated over the past 50 years. Current lung cancer rates reflect cigarette smoking habits of men and women over past decades (Boyle and Robertson 1987; La Vecchia and Franceschi 1984; La Vecchia *et al.* 1988) but not necessarily current smoking patterns, since there is an interval of several decades between the change in smoking habits in a population and its consequences on lung cancer rates. Over 90 per cent of lung cancer may be avoidable simply through avoidance of cigarette smoking. Rates of lung cancer in central and eastern Europe at the present time are higher than those ever before recorded elsewhere; lung cancer has increased 10-fold in men and 8-fold in women in Japan since 1950; there is a worldwide epidemic of smoking among young women (Chollat-Traquet 1992) which will be translated in increasing rates of tobacco-related disease, including cancer, in the coming decades; there is another epidemic of lung cancer and tobacco-related deaths building up in China as the cohorts of men in whom tobacco smoking became popular reach ages where cancer is an important hazard (Boyle 1993) . Many solutions have been attempted to reduce cigarette smoking and increasingly many countries are enacting legislation to curb this habit (Roemer 1993).

The epidemiology of smoking and lung cancer

From the perspective of the early twenty-first century, a causal relationship between smoking and lung cancer is taken as self evident, but this was not always the case. An early observer of the then rare respiratory cancer (Rottman 1898) considered it an occupational hazard, possibly from exposure to tobacco dust. The association between tobacco smoking and the development of lung cancer appears to have been suggested in the United Kingdom in 1927 (Tylecote 1927). The first interview study on tobacco smoking and lung cancer seems to have been reported from Vienna (Fleckseder 1936) where lung cancer rates had risen dramatically. Fleckseder (1936) found 51 smokers among 54 patients he found with lung cancer. Thirty seven of these smoked between 20 and 90 cigarettes daily while excessive smoking of pipes, cigars, or both was rarer.

The same association was alluded to in a report from the United States (Ochsner and Debakey 1939) in a study primarily of a series of 79 patients treated by total pneumonectomy. A report from Cologne followed one year later (Muller 1940) based on the post-mortem records of 96 patients. The patient, or more usually the relatives of fatal cases, was interviewed as to their occupation, tobacco consumption, and exposure to specific 'inhalants'. Re-analysis of Muller's data provides relative risk of 3.1 among *moderate* smokers, 2.7 among *heavy* smokers, 16.8 among *very heavy* smokers and 29.2 among *excessive* smokers. Within the limitations of the study (e.g. small numbers, especially among non-smoking cases, possible inaccuracies in elucidation of precise smoking histories) these results were noticeably similar to results obtained from later case–control studies in the United States and, apart from a lack of increase among heavy smokers, there is the possible appearance of a dose–response relationship.

A study of smoking habits and occupation based on 195 post-mortem records of cases of lung cancer at the Pathology Institute at Jena for the years 1930–1941 was reported: useable replies were obtained from relatives of 93 men and 16 women. Of the women, 13 were non-smokers (Schairer and Schoniger 1943). The authors attempted to collect control information by interviewing 700 men in Jena between the ages of 53 and 54, the average age of the lung cancer patients at death (53.9 years). It was a study performed in Germany towards the end of the Second World War and only 270 men from Jena responded to the questionnaire. The authors showed great insight in concluding that wartime conditions (particularly the rationing system) may have favoured results from non-smokers. They reported a statistically significant difference in non-smokers and heavy smokers among lung cancer patients on the one hand and normal patients on the other. Realizing the possible errors in their material they concluded that there was a considerable probability that lung cancer was far more frequent among heavy smokers and far less frequent among non-smokers than expected. Their data is such that an approximate relative risk can be calculated and the risk relative to non-smokers was 1.9 among *light* smokers; 9.1 among *moderate* smokers, and 11.3 among *heavy/excessive* smokers. Again there appears to be a moderate dose–response relationship. A further study from the Netherlands (Wassink 1948) identified very similar associations between smoking and lung cancer.

Over the first few decades of the twentieth century, reports began not only to admit that the incidence of lung cancer was increasing (Clemmeson and Buck 1947) but also to associate the increase with smoking rather than better diagnosis or increased longevity of the population (Anon 1942). These findings were largely ignored until 1950, when five case–control studies of the topic were published (Doll and Hill 1950; Levin *et al.* 1950; Mills and Porter 1950; Schrek *et al.* 1950; Wynder and Graham 1950) that included altogether over 2000 cases, the two largest studies having over 600 cases each and an equivalent numbers of controls (Doll and Hill 1950; Wynder and Graham 1950). Their conclusions were virtually identical—that smoking, particularly cigarette smoking, was an important factor in the production of lung cancer. The evidence from these studies, however, failed to gain wide acceptance. Instead it attracted opposition, not only from the tobacco industry but also from some other scientists because, although an association between smoking and lung cancer had been demonstrated, few were willing to accept it as evidence of a causal relationship, as at this time the case–control design was considered by many to have too many defects for it to produce reliable, unbiased findings (Sadowsky *et al.* 1953; Hammond 1954).

The methodological problems of case–control studies were to be overcome by using another epidemiological design, and shortly after the publication of the first case–control studies, the results of two prospective cohort studies came to hand (Doll and Hill 1954; Hammond and Horn 1958). These two cohort studies essentially confirmed the strong associations that had been shown between cigarette smoking and lung cancer by the case–control studies, and gave additional information; e.g. with respect to the dose–response relationship between the amount smoked and the risk of lung cancer and the decrease in risk in those who were able to stop the habit.

The proof that smoking tobacco causes lung cancer

The evidence described above was not enough to satisfy powerful critics which, as well as tobacco Industry apologists such as Todd, included two other well-respected statisticians – Berkson and Fisher. Their criticisms of these epidemiological studies, however frustrating they might have been at the time, ultimately helped to refine the criteria used to assess whether epidemiological associations are causal. Causal reasoning in epidemiology had been developed from considerations of infectious diseases and, in hindsight, the application of Koch's postulates was unlikely to provide a comfortable fit with chronic disease causation. Although elaborated upon further by others, the criteria with which to assess causality were laid down by the mid-1960s (USPHS 1964; Hill 1966) as follows: the consistency, strength, specificity, temporal sequence and coherence of the association.

It is salutary to review the criticisms of the causal hypothesis made at the time. Todds's criticisms included the low correlation between national lung cancer mortality and tobacco consumption ($r=0.5$), the unreliability of smoking histories, and that the increase in mortality was more likely to be due to pollution (Anon 1991). Hill and Doll were able to dismiss the first criticism as, given the crudeness of the measures, a coefficient of this size strengthened their conclusions. In regard to the second criticism, if smoking histories were in fact unreliable, measurement error would have diluted the strength of the measured association. Furthermore, smoking histories were later found by Todd himself (White 1990) to be remarkably precise. In regard to pollution as a cause, there was simply no evidence to support the proposition.

Berkson's principal criticisms (Berkson 1958) were based on three observations; the first was the lack of specificity of action, the second was lack of biological evidence of a carcinogen and the third was the lower than expected death rates in the cohorts compared with their respective general populations. He was concerned that the studies found too many disease outcomes to be associated with smoking, rather than just with lung cancer that was the subject of investigation, and concluded that the findings were the result of many subtle and complicated biases. He supported his opinion with the failure of the attempts to produce cancer experimentally and to isolate the responsible carcinogen. The lower than expected rates experienced in the early years of the cohort he argued were also evidence of biased sampling.

The concept of specificity of action has limited utility when dealing with a complex mix of more than 4000 carcinogenic substances administered to the whole body rather than a single microorganism. In making this criticism Berkson also failed to take account of the extraordinary strength of the association between smoking and lung cancer and the wide range of relative risks associated with different diseases. Hill's rejoinder was that it was as if he said that milk could not be a cause of any disease because it spread tuberculosis, diptheria, scarlet fever, undulant fever, dysentery etc. (Hill 1966). On the other hand, his request to identify the active carcinogen was appropriate but it unfortunately hindered the widespread acceptance of the epidemiological evidence by some eminent authorities (Anon 1962). The 'healthy' cohort effect that gave rise to the early reduced risks compared with the general population was soon to disappear as the relative risk between smokers and non-smokers in the cohort increased.

Fisher, on the other hand, emphasized Doll and Hill's finding from their case–control study (Doll and Hill 1950), that smokers who developed lung cancer inhaled less often than smokers who remained free of the disease (Fisher 1958), to suggest that inhalation was protective against lung cancer. He also pointed to an apparent inconsistency in the secular trends by sex—that lung cancer rates were increasing more in men than women while the increase in smoking prevalence had recently been greatest in women (Fisher 1957). He did not comment on the cohort study findings. Because of his scientific interests, and possibly because of his smoking habit, he was interested in pursuing studies of genetic susceptibility but these plans were curtailed by his death in 1962.

The paradoxical findings with respect to inhalation patterns were a valid point of criticism that resisted clarification for some time. It is now known that the deposition of particulate matter in the bronchi differs by the depth of inhalation, deep inhalers depositing less in the bronchi and more particulates deep in the lungs (Wald *et al.* 1983). The concern about trends by gender was misplaced, as it failed to take into account the long latency period between exposure and the diagnosis of lung cancer and the strong cohort effects in the uptake of the smoking habit that differed between the sexes.

The consistency of the association

The consistency of the findings shown by the early case–control and cohort studies has been maintained in numerous additional studies since that time that have been conducted in many different populations (IARC 1986). The consistency of the evidence from these analytical studies has been reinforced further by ecological studies of lung cancer trends in populations that have shown a high correlation between smoking rates and lung cancer rates both within populations and internationally (Doll 1954; Doll and Peto 1981). Analysis of lung cancer mortality trends over time have shown pronounced cohort effects associated with the prevalence of smoking (USDHHS 1982), and in some populations where male smoking prevalence has fallen, so too is lung cancer mortality (Gilliland and Samet 1994).

The strength of the association

Strength of association is perhaps the single most important criterion in establishing causation. It is usually expressed as the ratio of the incidence of disease in those exposed to the causal agent (in this case smoking) to the incidence of the disease in the unexposed. In cohort studies this ratio is termed the relative risk, which is approximated in case–control studies by the odds ratio. In cohort studies, the estimates of relative risk of lung cancer comparing cigarette smokers with non-smokers range from 9 to 14-fold (Doll and Hill 1954; Hammond and Horn 1954; Hammond 1966; Cederlof *et al.* 1975; Doll and Peto 1976; Lund and Zeiner-Henriksen 1981).

Associations of this strength are likely to reflect a causal relationship and the likelihood is increased when a dose–response relationship can be demonstrated. Evidence of dose–response also supports the biological coherence of the association. In regard to lung cancer, several cohort studies have illustrated dose–response in several ways; in terms of the daily amount smoked, the duration of smoking, the age at onset of smoking, and the cumulative amount smoked. For example, in terms of number of cigarettes smoked, the mortality ratio compared with non-smokers for those who smoked 25 or more a day exceeded 25 for men and 29 for women in the British Physician's Study (Doll and Hill 1950). For age at onset less than 15 years the mortality ratio exceeded 16 for men in the ASC 25 state study (Hammond 1966) and 18 for men in the US Veteran's study (Rogot and Murray 1980).

The specificity of the association

As mentioned already, the specificity criterion for causality is a relict from Koch's postulates with respect to causal agents for infectious diseases. The specificity criterion, however, only reinforces a causal hypothesis and is not considered a necessary criterion (USPHS 1964; Hill 1966). Although tobacco smoke is measured epidemiologically as a single exposure, it is a complex mixture of carcinogenic chemicals that act together in a variety of ways to cause cancers in several organs and tissues. Of all the cancer types that can be at least partly attributed to smoking, the specificity for lung cancer is the greatest as evidenced by the strength of the association already noted above. The relative risks observed for smoking and lung cancer are much larger than those observed for cancers occurring in other organs, especially for cancers in tissues that are not directly exposed to tobacco smoke such as the kidney and the uterine cervix.

The temporal relationship of the association

Obviously, to be causally associated with the disease the suspect aetiological exposure has to antedate the diagnosis. One reason why the findings from major prospective cohort studies have been most useful in establishing a causal relationship between smoking and lung cancer is because the exposure to smoking was measured in advance of diagnosis in thousands of subjects who were free of disease at entry to the studies.

The coherence of the association

The coherence criterion links the epidemiological observations with other knowledge in regard to the biology and natural history of the disease. This takes into account other criteria, for example those of temporal sequence and dose–response relationship discussed above. Another piece of supportive evidence is the diminution of risk after smoking cessation, which shows a negative dose–response relationship with increasing time since quitting. In the British Physician's Study after quitting for 15 years or more the mortality ratio was 2 compared with 16 in those who had quit for less than 5 years (Doll and Peto 1976). This was similar to the mortality ratio for US Veterans who had quit for 20 years or more (Rogot and Murray 1980). Evidence from human pathology was also useful in establishing causality. Auerbach (Auerbach *et al.* 1979) examined pre-malignant changes in the bronchial epithelium from 402 male autopsies and discovered that atypical cells were more prevalent in the bronchial epithelium of smokers compared with non-smokers and that their prevalence increased in a dose–response fashion with the amount habitually smoked, the prevalence of atypical cells in non-smokers being very low.

Experimental evidence

A large amount of supportive evidence has been produced from experimental animal models of smoking carcinogenesis (IARC 1986). Some of this work faced difficulties especially in regard to the development of appropriate inhalation models. Unlike man, experimental animals avoid inhaling tobacco smoke and the delivery of carcinogenic doses of smoke to the lung can also be perturbed by anatomical differences in the animals' upper respiratory tracts compared with humans. It was also commonly observed that the loss of weight experienced by animals that were chronically exposed to smoke often extended their lives (Wynder and Hoffman 1967). Despite these inconsistencies, informative data were obtained on the carcinogenic effect of smoke in its gaseous phase. Further proof of carcinogenic potential was obtained by topical application of cigarette smoke condensate to mouse skin (Wynder and Hoffman 1967) and the injection of cigarette smoke condensate directly into rodents' lungs (Stanton *et al.* 1972).

Passive smoking and lung cancer risk

Having established a strong and consistent causal association between direct smoking and an increased risk of lung cancer, tobacco research turned recently to the association between exposure to environmental tobacco smoke (passive smoking) and a diversity of adverse health events, including lung cancer (Burns 1992; EPA 1992; Stockwell *et al.* 1992). On the basis of 30 epidemiological studies, the United States Environmental Protection Agency (EPA) concluded that environmental tobacco smoke (ETS) was a human lung carcinogen. It has been estimated that each year in the United States, 434 000 deaths are attributable to tobacco use, in particular cigarette smoking (CDC 1991), 112 000 of these smoking-related deaths from lung cancer (USDHHS 1989). There are an estimated 1500 deaths in non-smoking women due to passive smoking and 500 deaths in non-smoking men annually. The basis for these conclusions is a group of epidemiological studies that took spouse smoking as a measure of exposure to ETS (EPA 1992). The overall relative risk obtained from 11 studies conducted in the United States was 1.19; there was a tendency for a positive trend in risk to be found with increasing dose of smoking (EPA 1992). All the spousal smoking was assessed by questionnaire and the group of studies, with notable exceptions (Garfinkel *et al.* 1985; Fontham *et al.* 1991), is characterized by low statistical power and small increased relative risks with large confidence intervals frequently extending over unity.

Small increased risks such as this are below that which can be reliably detected by epidemiological methods and the exposure assessment in these studies is poor. The use of biomarkers for analysing and quantifying the role of ETS is much more complex for cancer than asthma, given the much longer interval between exposure and clinical manifestation of the disease. The critical reviewer could find shortcomings in the majority of the published studies of ETS and lung cancer. However, as was recognized by an IARC Working Party (IARC 1986) given current knowledge of the chemical constituents of both side stream and mainstream smoke, of the materials absorbed during passive smoking and of the quantitative relationships between dose and effect that are commonly observed from exposure to carcinogens, it could be concluded that passive smoking gives rise to some risk of lung cancer. The great deal that is known about the carcinogenic effects of active smoking (IARC 1986) has undoubtedly bolstered the interpretation of the epidemiological data on passive smoking.

Despite nearly half a century of careful epidemiological study and the scientific certainty that tobacco is carcinogenic there is still a need to quantify the risks of low level exposure.

Public health failure, 1960s onwards

It has been clear for the entire second half of the twentieth century that cigarette smoking causes lung cancer. Current low levels of smoking among physicians and research scientists, in many countries, have led many of them unconsciously to overlook tobacco smoking as an important cause of cancer (Boyle 1993b). There is, however, a very substantial body of evidence from many sources which indicates the carcinogenicity of tobacco smoking. Not only does cigarette smoking greatly increase the risk of lung cancer in smokers, but the risk of oral cavity cancer, larynx cancer, oesophageal cancer, bladder cancer, pancreas cancer, cervix cancer, stomach cancer, kidney cancer, and colorectal cancer are also increased (Boyle 1997).

There is at present a worldwide epidemic of tobacco-related diseases: not only does smoking cause increased levels of many different common forms of cancer, but it also increases the risk of cardiovascular disease. Deaths from lung cancer, the cancer site most strongly linked to cigarette smoking, have increased in Japan by a factor of 10 in men and 8 in women since 1950. In central and eastern Europe, more than 400 000 premature deaths are currently caused each year by tobacco smoking. In young men in all countries of central and eastern Europe, currently there are levels of lung cancer which are greater than anything seen before in the western countries and these rates are still rising. In Poland, a country severely hit by the tobacco epidemic, life-expectancy of a 45-year-old man has been falling for over a decade now due to the increasing premature death rates from tobacco-related cancers and cardiovascular disease (Zatonski and Boyle 1996). Tragically, cigarette smoking is still increasing in central and eastern Europe and also in China, where an epidemic of tobacco-related deaths is building up quickly. Tobacco smoking is also the most easily avoided risk factor for cancer.

The most important determinant of risk of lung cancer is the duration of smoking: long-term cigarette smokers have a one hundred-fold increased risk compared with never-smokers (Peto 1986). The content of cigarettes (low tar) produces only a three-fold variation in risks between the extremes (Low tar is frequently taken to include a number of features including filtered-tips as well as the active tar yield). Lung cancer is the major tobacco-related site and the leading cause of cancer death in men in almost all developed countries. Incidence rates are around 10–15 per 100 000 in non-smokers, between 80–100 per 100 000 in the highest-incidence population groups such as Afro-Americans and rates exceeding 200 per 100 000 have been reported in cities of central and eastern Europe. Lung cancer being frequently fatal, mortality rates are high and, consequently, the social costs are high.

The early concept that reducing tar and nicotine would reduce cancer risk was well founded on epidemiological studies, which showed a reduction in lung cancer risk, but not cardiovascular disease, of between twenty and fifty per cent in association with the move to filters which occurred over the fifties and sixties (Bross and Gibson 1968; Wynder et al. 1970; Dean et al. 1977; Hawthorne and Fry 1978; Wynder and Stellman 1979; Rimington 1981; Lubin 1984; Federal Trade Commission 1995). It was therefore logical that public health authorities should press for further reductions. However, the reductions which appeared in the yields as measured by the FTC system do not reflect, in a quantitative way, what passes into the lungs of smokers. That more intensive ('compensatory') smoking patterns are seen in smokers was demonstrated by Russell in 1980 and many others (Russell 1980; Herning et al. 1981; Kozlowski et al. 1982; United States Surgeon General 1986).

In the absence of systematic on-going analysis of what has been going into smokers lungs, we are left with biological outcomes as an index of what has been happening. There are three potentially important observations in this regard (Gray and Boyle 2000).

First of all, it is very difficult to imagine that the large fall in the tar content of cigarettes sold in the United Kingdom over the last fifty years (Wald et al. 1981) has not influenced the lung cancer death rate which has been falling for two decades in men in that country.

Secondly, and paradoxically, mortality from lung cancer in men increased between the first (CPS-I) and second (CPS-II) Cancer Prevention Studies of the American Cancer Society (Thun and Heath 1997; United States Surgeon General 1989): these studies recruited men from birth cohorts approximated 30 years apart. At first glance, the decrease in mortality promised by the yield reductions of the 1950s and 1960s has not been substantial over the 1970s and 1980s. However, this may be too simple an interpretation.

Information of the number of cigarettes smoked at time of enrolment to both studies may not mirror the lifelong patterns of smoking that cause lung cancer (Thun et al. 1977): data on smoking in early life, which critically determines duration of smoking, are sparse in both studies. Cigarette consumption during adolescence and early adult-hood was probably heavier among smokers in CPS-II for several reasons. Manufactured cigarettes were more readily available in the 1950s than in the 1930s, eras when smoking was likely to be initiated in the CPS-II and CPS-I cohort respectively.

Birth cohort analyses show that a prevalence of smoking among white men increased with each successive birth cohort born from 1900 to 1929 and decreased thereafter (Burns 1994). Age-specific lung cancer death rates have decreased in those born after 1930 (Devesa *et al.* 1989; Gilliland and Samet 1994).

The large increases in lung cancer death rates from CPS-I to CPS-II probably reflect unmeasured heavier smoking among CPS-II during the 1940s and 1950s as well as the measured increase in daily consumption and duration of smoking. In addition, CPS-II may include a more addicted 'hard-core' smokers, who find it virtually impossible to quit smoking, and CPS-II smokers, partly to compensate for lower nicotine content of modern cigarettes, may inhale more deeply, take more puffs per cigarette and retain smoke longer in the lungs than did smokers in the past. The impact of lower tar and nicotine cigarettes is difficult to elucidate with all these other changes in effect.

Thirdly, and what is clear, is that there has been a real swing towards higher rates of adenocarcinoma of the lung both in the United States and elsewhere (Cutler and Young 1975; Vincent *et al.* 1977; Cox and Resner 1979; Young *et al.* 1981; Beard *et al.* 1985; Wu *et al.* 1986; Johnson 1988; El-Torkey *et al.* 1990; Devesa *et al.* 1991; Wynder and Muscat 1995) which is consistent with the hypothesis that qualitative changes in cigarette smoke have led to a change in the observed pattern of lung cancer but not to a substantial decrease in mortality.

Women around the world have taken up cigarette smoking habit with gusto. For many years it appeared that their lung cancer rates were low and that tobacco was not having the same effect on men. This complacency, which crept in during the two decades from the mid-1960s especially, is now exposed as false: neither is there evidence that the effect of cigarette smoking on lung cancer risk is greater in women than in men. The dominance of the effect of duration of smoking means that a long period of time will pass between the exposure (large numbers of women smoking) until the effect (high levels of lung cancer). Lung cancer now exceeds breast cancer as the leading cancer cause of death in women in the United States, Canada, Scotland, and several other countries. In Canada, breast cancer mortality has remained at least constant for nearly four decades while lung cancer death rates have increased between 3 and 4-fold during the same period. While the higher case-fatality of lung cancer may be one factor in the mortality rates overtaking breast cancer, there is increasing evidence that there are regions of the world where the gap in the incidence rate is now closing. For example, in Glasgow, an area where lung cancer has been historically high, by 1990 the incidence rate for lung cancer (115 per 100 000) exceeded that for breast cancer (105 per 100 000) in 1990 (Gillis *et al.* 1992). In international Cancer Registries, there are some where the incidence of lung cancer now exceeds the incidence of breast cancer and others where there is still a gap. In the SEER (Surveillance Epidemiology and End Results) Programme of the US NCI, the incidence of lung cancer in both black and white women increased by over 90 per cent between 1973–1977 and 1988–1992: the increase in the incidence of breast cancer was around 25 per cent in both racial groups (comparison made between incidence rates age-adjusted using 1970 US population). Of great worry is that there does not appear to be any end in sight to this increase in lung cancer risk internationally: it is programmed to continue for several decades to come.

Part of the complacency over the effect on women was also due to the strong tendency for women to smoke brands of cigarettes which were lower in tar and nicotine content than men: it was assumed that this would have less of a risk on lung cancer than the higher tar cigarettes which men generally smoked. Now marked changes in the rates of the major histological cell types of lung cancer can be seen with particular increases in the risk of adenocarcinoma (Zheng *et al.* 1994; Levi *et al.* 1997). The changes seen are compatible with increased risk of adenocarcinoma due to increasing levels of smoking of light cigarettes ('low tar, low nicotine'). It appears that abandoning, high-tar cigarettes (15–45 mg tar) may have had some impact on reducing squam ous-cell carcinoma risk, there is now a 'balancing' by light cigarettes increasing risk of adenocarcinoma.

Cigarette smoking kills half of all those who adopt the habit with 50 per cent of these deaths occurring in middle age and each losing an average of 20 years of non-smokers life expectancy (Doll *et al.* 1994). It kills in over 24 different ways with lung cancer being the commonest cancer-site (Doll *et al.* 1994). Lung cancer rates have been declining in men and increasing in women: cigarette smoking in men has been declining while it has been increasing in women. These two are closely related. The move to 'light' cigarettes, which is increasingly common, now appears to be linked to increases in adenocarcinoma of the lung and shows no sign of being linked to a reduced risk overall. Clearly cigarettes are different but still seriously harmful after decades of self-regulation. There is no such thing as a safe cigarette. Smokers should be urged and helped to stop smoking, children and young adults should be convinced not to smoke. Tobacco can become an addictive drug: it should be left alone (Boyle *et al.* 1995).

Acknowledgements

It is a pleasure to acknowledge the support provided by the Cancer Council Victoria and the Italian Association of Cancer Research (*Associazione Italiana per la Ricerca sul Cancro*).

References

Adler, I. (1912). *Primary malignant growths of the lungs and bronchi: A pathological and clinical study.* London: Longmans, Green and Co.,

Anon, (1942). Cancer of the lung (editorial). *Br Med J*, **1**, 672–3.

Anon (1962). The cigarette as co-carcinogen (editorial). *Lancet*, 1, 85–6.

Anon (1991). Conversation with Sir Richard Doll (Journal interview 29). *Br J Addiction*, **86**, 365–77.

Auerbach, O., Hammond, E. C., and Garfinkel, L. (1979). Changes in bronchial epithelium in relation to cigarette smoking, 1955–1960 vs 1970–1977. *N Engl J Med*, **300**, 381–6.

Beard, M. C., Anneges, J. F., Woolner, L. B., and Kurland, L. T. (1985). Bronchiogenic carcinoma in Olmsted County, 1635–1979. *Cancer (Phila.)*, **55**, 2026–30.

Berkson, J. (1958). Smoking and lung cancer: some observations on two recent reports. *J Amer Stat Assoc*, **53**, 28–38.

Bjartveit, K. (1986). Legislation and political activity. In: *Tobacco: a major international health hazard* (ed. DG Zaridze and R Peto), pp. 285–98. IARC, Lyon.

Boyle, P. (1993). The hazards of passive and active smoking. *N Engl J Med*, **329**, 1581.

Boyle, P. (1993b). The hazards of passive and active smoking. *N Engl J Med*, 328, 1708–9

Boyle, P. (1997). Cancer, Cigarette smoking and premature death in Europe. A review including the Recommendations of European Cancer Experts Consensus Meeting. Helsinki, October 1996. *Lung Cancer*, **17**, 1–60.

Boyle, P. and Robertson, C. (1987). Statistical modelling of lung cancer and laryngeal cancer incidence data in Scotland, 1960–1979. *Am J Epidemiol*, **125**, 731–44.

Boyle, P., Veronesi, U., Tubiana, M., Alexander, F. E., Calais da Silva, F., Denis, L. J., *et al.* (1995). European School of Oncology Advisory Report to the European Commission for the "Europe Against Cancer Programme" European Code Against Cancer. *Eur J Cancer*, **9**, 1395–405.

Bross, I. D. J. and Gibson, R. (1968). Risks of lung cancer in smokers who switch to filter cigarettes. *Am J Publ Health*, **58**, 1396–403.

Burns, D. M. (1992). Environmental tobacco smoke: the price of scientific certainty. *J Natl Cancer Inst*, **84**, 1387–8.

Burns, D. M. (1994). *Tobacco Smoking*. In: *Epidemiology of Lung Cancer* (ed. J.M. Somet), pp 15–49. Marcel Dekker, New York.

Centres for Disease Control. (1991). Smoking-attributable mortality and years of potential life lost— United States, 1988. *MMWR*, **40**, 62–71.

Cederlof, R., Friberg, L., Hrubec, Z., and Lorich, U. (1975). *The relationship of smoking and some social covariates to mortality and cancer morbidity. A ten year follow-up in a probability sample of 55,000 Swedish subjects age 18–69, Part 1 and Part 2.* Stockholm: The Karolinska Institute.

Chollat-Traquet, C. (1992). *Women and Tobacco.* Geneva: World Health Organization.

Clemmesen, J. and Buck, T. (1947). On the apparent increase in the incidence of lung cancer in Denmark, 1931–1945. *Br J Cancer*, **1**, 253–9.

Cox, J. D. and Resner, R. A. (1979). Adenocarcinoma of the lung: recent results from the Veterans Administration lung group. *Am Rev Resp Dis*, **120**, 1025–9.

Cutler, S. J. and Young, J. L. (1975). Third National Cancer Survey: incidence data. *J Natl Cancer Inst Monogr*, **41**, 1–454.

Dean, G., Lee, P. N., Todd, G. F., and Wicken, A. J. (1977). Report on a second retrosepective study in Northeast England. Part 1. Factors related to mortality from lung cancer, bronchitis, heart disease, and stroke in cleveland county with particular emphasis on the relative risks associated with smoking filter and plain cigarettes. (Research Paper 14) London, Tobacco Research Council.

Della-Vorgia, P., Sasco, A. J., Skalkidis, Y., Katsouyani, K., and Trichopoulos, D. (1990). An evaluation of the effectiveness of tobacco-control legislative policies in European Community countries. *Scand J Soc Med*, **18**, 81–9.

Devesa, S. S., Blot, W. J., and Fraumeni, J. F. (1989). Declining lung cancer rates among young men and women in the United States: A cohort analysis. *J Natl Cancer Inst*, **81**, 1568–71.

Devesa, S. S., Shaw, G. L., and Blot, W. J. (1991). Changing patterns of cancer incidence by histologic type. *Cancer Epidemiol Biomarkers and Prev*, **1**, 29–34.

Doll, R. (1954). Review of: Cancer of the lung (Epidemiology). *Br Med J*, **2**, 1402.

Doll, R. and Hill, A. B. (1950). Smoking and carcinoma of the lung. *Br Med J*, **2**, 739–48.

Doll, R. and Hill, A. B. (1954). The mortality of doctors in relation to their smoking habits; a preliminary report. *Br Med J*, **1**, 1451–5.

Doll, R. and Peto, R. (1976). Mortality in relation to smoking: 20 years observations on male British doctors. *Br Med J*, **2**, 1525–36.

Doll, R. and Peto, R. (1981). The causes of cancer: quantitative estimates of avoidable risks of cancer in the United States today. *J Natl Cancer Inst*, **66**, 1191–308.

Doll, R., Peto, R., Wheatley, K., Gray, R., and Sutherland, I. (1994). Mortality in relation to smoking: 40 years' observations on male British doctors. *Br Med J*, **309**(6959), 901–11

El-Torkey, M., El-Zeky, F., and Hall, J. C. (1990). Significant changes in the distribution of histological types of lung cancer. A review of 4928 cases. *Cancer (Phila.)*, **65**, 2361–7,

EPA (United States Environment Protection Agency). (1992). *Respiratory health effects of passive smoking: lung cancer and other disorders.* US Environment Protection Agency, Washington, DC.

Federal Trade Commission. (1995). Tar, nicotine and carbon monoxide of the smoke of 1107 varieties of domestic cigarettes. Washington, DC, US Federal Trade Commission.

Fisher, R. A. (1957). Dangers of cigarette smoking. *Br Med J*, **2**, 43.

Fisher, R. A. (1958). Cancer and smoking. *Nature*, **182**, 596.

Fleckseder, R. (1936). Ueber den Bronchialkrebs und einge seiner Entstehungsbedingungen. *Munch Med Wochenschr Nr*, **36**, 1585–93.

Fontham, E. T.H., Correa, P., Wu-Williams, A., Reynolds, P., Greenberg, R. S., Buflier, P. A., *et al.* (1991). Lung cancer in non-smoking women: A multicentre case-control study. *Cancer Epidemiol Biomarkers Prev*, **1**, 35–43.

Garfinkel, L., Auerbach, O., and Hubert, L. (1985). Involuntary smoking and lung cancer: a case-control study. *J Natl Cancer Inst*, **75**, 465–9.

Gilliland, F. D. and Samet, J. M. (1994). Lung cancer. In: *Trends in Cancer Incidence and Mortality* (ed. R. Doll, J.F. Fraumeni, and C.S. Muir), pp. 175–95. Cold Spring Harbor Laboratory Press, Plainview, NY.

Gilliland, F. D. and Samet, J. M. (1994). Lung cancer. *Cancer Surveys*, **19**, 175–84.

Gillis, C. R., Hole, D. J., Lamont, D. W., Graham, A. C., and Ramage, S. (1992). The incidences of lung cancer and breast cancer in women in Glasgow. *Br Med J*, **305**, 1331.

Gray, N. and Boyle P. (2000). The regulation of tobacco and tobacco smoke. *Ann Oncol*, **11**, 909–14.

Hammond, E. C. (1954). Smoking in relation to lung cancer: A follow up study. *Conn State Med J*, **18**, 3–9.

Hammond, E. C. (1966). Smoking in relation to death rates of one million men and women. *Natl Cancer Inst Monogr*, **19**, 127–204.

Hammond, E. C., Garfinkel, L., Seidman, H., and Lew, E. A. (1976). 'Tar' and nicotine content of cigarette smoke in relation to death rates. *Environ Res*, **12**, 263–74.

Hammond, E. C. and Horn, D. (1954). The relationship between human smoking habits and death rates: A follow up study of 187,766 men. *J Amer Med Assoc*, **154**, 1316–28.

Hammond, E. C. and Horn, D. (1950). *Smoking in relation to death rates*, Manuscript distributed at the time of presentation at the meeting of the American Medical Association, New York, June 4, 1957 and subsequently published (Hammond and Horn, 1958).

Hawthorne, V. M. and Fry, J. S. (1978). Smoking and health. The association between smoking behaviour, total mortality and cardiorespiratory disease in West Scotland. *J Epidemiol Commun Health*, **32**, 260–6.

Herning, R. I., Jones, R. T., Bachman, J., and Mines, A. H. (1981). Puff volume increases when low nicotine cigarettes are smoked. *Br Med J Clin Res*, **283**, 187–9.

Hill, A. B. (1966). *Principles of Medical Statistics* (eighth edn), pp. 305–13. The Lancet, London.

IARC (International Agency for Research on Cancer). (1988). Man-made Mineral Fibers and Radon. Monogr Eval Carcinog Risk Hum; **43**, Lyon: IARC.

IARC (International Agency for Research on Cancer). (1986). *Tobacco Smoking*. Monogr Eval Carcinog Risk Hum; 38, Lyon: IARC

Johnson, W. W. (1988). Histologic and cytologic patterns of lung cancer in 2580 men and women over a 15-year period. *Acta Cytol*, **32**, 163–8.

Kopecky, K. J., Yamamoto, T., Fujikura, T., Tokuoka, S., Monzen, T., Nishimori, I., *et al.* (1987). *Lung cancer, radiation exposure and smoking among A-bomb survivors, Hiroshima and Nagasaki, 1950–1980.* Radiation Effects Research Foundation Technical Report 13-86. Hiroshima: Japan, Radiation Effects Research Foundation.

Kozlowski, L. T., Rickert, W. S., Pope, M. A., Robinson, J. C., and Frecker, R. C. (1982). Estimating the yields to smokers of tar, nicotine, and carbon monoxide from the lowest yield ventilated filter cigarettes. *Brit J Addict*, **77**, 159–165.

La Vecchia, C. and Franceschi, S. (1984). Italian lung cancer death rates in young males (Letter). *Lancet*, **I**, 406.

La Vecchia, C., Levi, F., Decarli, A., Wietlisbach, V., Negri, E., Gutzwiller, F. (1988). Trends in smoking and lung cancer mortality in Switzerland. *Prev Med*, **17**, 712–24.

Levi, F., Franceschi, S., La Vecchia, C., Randimbison, L., Van-Cong, T. (1997). Lung carcinoma trends by histologic type in Vaud and Neuchatel, Switzerland, 1974–1994. *Cancer*, **79**, 906–14.

Levin, M. L., Goldstein, H., and Gerhardt, P. R. (1950). Cancer and Tobacco Smoking. *J Am Med Assoc*, **143**, 336–8.

Levi, F., Maisonneuve, P., Filiberti, R., La Vecchia, C., Boyle, P. (1989). Cancer incidence and mortality in Europe. *Sozial und Praventivmedizin*, **34**(supp 2), 1–84.

Lubin, L. H. (1984). Modifying risk of developing lung cancer by changing habits of cigarette smoking. *Br Med J*, **289**, 1953–6.

Lund, E., Zeiner-Henriksen, T. (1981). Smoking as a risk factor for cancer among 26,000 Norwegian males and Females. *Tiddskv nor laegeforen*, **101**, 1937–40.

Mills, C. A. and Porter, M. M. (1950). Tobacco smoking habits and cancer of the mouth and respiratory system. *Cancer Res*, **10**, 539–42.

Muller, F. H. (1940). Tabaksmisbrauch und Lungenkarzinom. *Z f Krebsforsch*, **49**, 57–85.

Ochsner, A. and Debakey, M. (1939). Primary pulmonary malignancy. Treatment by total pneumonectomy. Analysis of 79 collected cases and presentation of 7 personal cases. *Surg Gynecol Obs*, **68**, 435–51.

Peto, R. (1986) Influence of dose and duration of smoking on lung cancer rates. *IARC Sci Publ*, **74**, 22–33.

Parkin, D. M. (2001). Global cancer statistics in the year 2000. *Lancet Oncol*, **2**, 533–43.

Rimington, J. (1981). The effects of filters on the incidence of lung cancer in cigarette smokers. *Environ Res*, **24**, 162–6.

Roemer, R. (1993). Legislative Action to combat the World Tobacco Epidemic. World Health Organisation, Geneva.

Rogot, E. and Murray J. L. (1980). Smoking and causes of death among US veterans: 16 years of observation. *Publ Health Rep*, **95**, 213–22.

Rottman H. (1898). Der primare lungencarcinoma. Inaugural-dissertation, Universitat Wurzburg.

Russell, M. A. H. (1980). The case for medium-nicotine, low tar, low carbon monoxide cigarettes. *Banbury Rep*, **3**, 297–310.

Sadowsksy, D. A., Gilliam, A. G., and Cornfield, G. (1953). Statistical association between smoking and cancer of the lung. *J Natl Cancer Inst*, **13**, 1237–58.

Schairer, E. and Schoniger E. (1943). Lungenkrebs und Tabaksverbrauch. *Z f Krebsforsch*, **54**, 261–9.

Schrek, R., Baker, L. A., Ballard, G. P., and Dolgoff, S. (1950). Tobacco smoking as an etiologic factor in disease. *Cancer Res*, **10**, 49–58.

Shimizu, Y., Kato, H., Schull, W. J., Preston, D. L., Fujita, S, and Pierce, D. A. (1987). *Life Span Study report 11, Part 1: comparison of risk coefficients for site specific cancer mortality based on the DS86 and T65DR shielded kerma and organ doses*. Radiation Effects Research Foundation Technical Report 12–87, Radiation Effects Research Foundation, Hiroshima, Japan.

Smith, P. G. and Doll, R. (1982). Mortality among patients with ankylosing spondylitis after a single treatment course with X-rays. *Br Med J*, **284**, 449–54.

Stanton, M. F., Miller, E., Wrench, C., and Blackwell, R. (1972). Experimental induction of epidermoid carcinoma in the lungs of rats by cigarette smoke condensate. *J Natl Cancer Inst*, **49**, 867–77.

Stockwell, H. G., Goldman, A. L., Lyman, G. H., Noss, C. I., Armstrong, A. W., Pinkham, P. A., *et al.* (1992). Environmental tobacco smoke and lung cancer risk in nonsmoking women. *J Natl Cancer Inst*, **84**, 1417–22.

Thun, M. J. and Heath, C. W. Jr. (1997). Changes in mortality from smoking in two American Cancer Society prospective studies since 1959. *Preventive Medicine*, **26**(4), 422–6.

Thun, M. J., Day-Lally, C., Myers, D. G., *et al. Trends in tobacco smoking and mortality from cigarette use in cancer prevention Studies I (1959 through 1965) and II (1982 through 1988).* In: *Changes in cigarette-related disease risks and their implication for prevention and control.* Bethesda, Maryland: National Cancer Institute, 1977: chapter 4. (NCI Monograph No 8).

Tomatis, L. (1990). *Air Pollution and Human cancer.* European School of Oncology Monographs, Springer-Verlag, Berlin.

Tylecote, F. E. (1927). Cancer of the Lung. *Lancet*, **2**, 256–7

United States Public Health Service. (1964). *Smoking and health.* Report of the Advisory Committee to the Surgeon General of the Public Health Service. U.S. Department of Health, Education and Welfare, Public Health Service, Centre for Disease Control, DHEW Publication no. 1103.

United States Department of Health, Education and Welfare, Public Health Service, Washington D C, DHEW Publication number (PHS) 79–50066, 1979.

USDHHS (United States Department of Health and Human Services). (1982). *The health consequences of smoking: Cancer.* A report of the Surgeon General. Washington, DC: US Public Health Service.

USDHHS (United States Department of Health and Human Services). (1989). *Reducing the health consequences of smoking: 25 years of progress.* A report of the Surgeon General. Washington, DC: US Government Printing Office.

United States Surgeon General. (1986). The Health Consequences of Smoking. NIH Pub.No. 86-7874, pp.1-639,Bethesda, MD· United States Department of Health and Human Services.

United States Surgeon General. United States Public Health Service. Reducing the Health Consequences of Smoking. (1989). A Report of the Surgeon Generale. U.S. Department of Health, and Human Services, Public Health Service, Centre for Disease Control, DHSS Publication no. (CDC) 89–8411, pp. 143.

Vincent, R. G., Pickren, J. W., Lane, W. W., Bross, I., Takita, H., Honten, L., *et al.* (1977). The changing histopathology of lung cancer. *Cancer (Phila.),* **39,** 1647–55.

Wald, N., Doll, R., and Copeland, G. (1981). Trends in tar, nicotine and carbon monoxide yields of UK cigarettes manufactured since 1934. *Br Med J Clin Res ed,* **282**(6266), 763–5

Wald, N. J., Idle, M., Boreham, J., and Bailey, A. (1983). Inhaling and lung cancer: an anomaly explained. *Br Med J,* **287,** 1273–75.

Wassink, W. F. (1948). Onstaansvoorwarden voor Longkanker. *Med Tijdschr Geneesk,* **92,** 3732–47.

White, C. (1990). Research on smoking and lung cancer: a landmark in the history of chronic disease epidemiology. *The Yale Journal of Biology and Medicine,* **63,** 29–46.

Whittemore, A. S. and McMillan, A. (1983). Lung cancer mortality among US uranium miners: a reapraisal. *J Natl Cancer Inst,* **71,** 489–99.

Wu, A. H., Henderson, B. E., Thomas, D. C., and Mack, T. M. (1986). Secular trends in histologic type of lung cancer. *J Nat Cancer Inst,* **77,** 53–6.

Wynder, E. L. and Graham, E. A. (1950). Tobacco smoking as a possible etiologic factor in bronchiogenic carcinoma. *J Am Med Assoc,* **143,** 329–36.

Wynder, E. L. and Hoffman, D. (1967). *Tobacco and tobacco smoke.* Studies in experimental carcinogenesis, Academic press, New York.

Wynder, E. L. and Stellman, S. D. (1979). The impact of long term filter usage on lung and larynx cancer risk: a case control study. *J Nat Cancer Inst,* **62,** 471–7.

Wynder, E. L. and Muscat, J. E. (1995). The changing epidemiology of smoking and lung cancer histology. *Environmental Health Perspectives,* **103** (8), 143–6.

Wynder, E. L., Mabuchi, K., and Beattie, E. J. Jr. (1970). The epidemiology of lung cancer. recent Trends. *J Am Med Assoc,* **213,** 2221–8.

Young, J. L., Percy, C. L., and Asire, A. J. (ed.) (1981). Cancer incidence and mortality in the United States, 1973–1977. *Nat Cancer Inst Monogr,* **57,** 1–1082.

Zatonski, W. A. and Boyle, P. (1996). Health transformations in Poland after 1988. *J Epi Bio,* **1**(4), 183–97.

Zheng, T., Holford, T., Boyle, P., Chen, Y., Ward, B. A., Flannery, J. *et al.* (1994). Time trend and age-period-cohort effect on the incidence of histologic types of lung cancer in Connecticut, 1960–1989. *Cancer,* **74,** 1556–1556.

Chapter 29

Tobacco smoking and cancer of the breast

Dimitrios Trichopoulos
and Areti Lagiou

Tobacco smoking is the most important human carcinogen, and breast cancer is, at least in the developed world, the type of cancer that causes more deaths among women (Lagiou and Adami 2002). If tobacco smoking were found to be a factor that increases the risk of breast cancer, the implications would extend beyond the potential prevention of a number of breast cancer cases, because of the emotional impact that this form of cancer has. The evidence, however, has been unusually puzzling.

Biologic considerations

It has been reported that active smoking may increase (Lash and Aschengrau 1999; Johnson *et al.* 2000), reduce (Vessey *et al.* 1983), or be unrelated to (MacMahon 1990; Egan *et al.* 2002) the risk of breast cancer. More recently, it has been indicated that passive smoking may increase the risk of this disease (Morabia *et al.* 1996). Various biological plausibility arguments have been invoked in support of each of the various possibilities:

- *Tobacco smoking may reduce the risk of breast cancer.* Tobacco smoking has established anti-estrogenic effects (MacMahon *et al.* 1982; Baron 1984; Michnovicz *et al.* 1986) and estrogens are important determinants of breast cancer risk (Hankinson and Hunter 2002). The anti-estrogenicity of tobacco smoking is manifested in several associations with estrogen-dependent diseases or conditions, including associations with earlier menopause (Cooper *et al.* 1999), osteoporosis (Hopper and Seeman 1994), and endometrial cancer (Terry *et al.* 2002). An inverse association between tobacco smoking and breast cancer has been reported for men (Casagrande *et al.* 1988; Petridou *et al.* 2000) among whom tobacco smoking also has anti-estrogenic effects (Michnovicz and Fishman 1990).

- *Tobacco smoking may increase the risk of breast cancer.* Tobacco smoke is an established human carcinogen (IARC Monographs 1986) and causes cancer in several non-respiratory sites, including pancreas (Lowenfels and Maisonneuve 2002) and liver (Kuper *et al.* 2000). It contains several fat-soluble compounds with carcinogenic potential that can be activated into electrophilic substances by enzymes in the human mammary cells (Phillips *et al.* 2001; Morabia 2002). Nipple aspirates of smokers contain metabolites of compounds of cigarette smoke, which can be geno-toxic (Petrakis *et al.* 1980; Morabia, 2002). As it is true for other breast carcinogens, notably ionizing radiation (Hoel and Dinse 1990, Land IIa 1995; Hankinson and Hunter 2002), tobacco smoking could exert its carcinogenic potential particularly among young women or among women who have never been pregnant and whose mammary epithelium has not been terminally differentiated (Russo *et al.* 2001).

◆ *Tobacco smoking is unrelated to breast cancer risk.* Tobacco smoking may be unrelated to breast cancer risk or may have dual effects that incorporate a detrimental effect during the early life initiation stage and a beneficial anti-estrogenic effect during the late life tumour progression stage. Dual effects on breast cancer risk are well established with respect to obesity, which acts in a beneficial way before menopause and in a detrimental way after it (Hankinson and Hunter 2002).

◆ *Passive smoking may increase the risk of breast cancer.* At source, environmental tobacco smoke contains high concentrations of most tobacco carcinogens. Although nicotine inhalation (and cotinine excretion) through passive smoking is two orders of magnitude lower than that through active smoking, this may not apply to other agents, including carcinogenic agents. Exposure to environmental tobacco smoke may start shortly after birth and the carcinogenic effects of tobacco smoke depend exponentially on total duration of exposure (Dockery and Trichopoulos 1997). Early life exposures, before terminal mammary differentiation induced by a full-term pregnancy, are thought to have higher carcinogenic potential on the breast (Adami *et al.* 1998).

◆ *Passive smoking is unrelated to breast cancer risk.* In every instance in which passive smoking has been implicated in disease causation, active smoking has been an established cause of the corresponding disease with a considerably higher relative risk. Paradigms are lung cancer (Dockery and Trichopoulos 1997) and chronic obstructive lung disease (Kalandidi *et al.* 1987). Even if there is a weak positive association between breast cancer and active smoking, an association of the disease with passive smoking would be extremely weak and empirically undetectable.

Epidemiological evidence on active smoking and breast cancer

Until the late 1980s, tobacco smoking had not been explicitly studied in relation to breast cancer and whatever evidence was available was a side-product of investigations with different primary objectives. MacMahon was the first to critically evaluate this evidence (MacMahon 1990). He noted that hospital-based case–control studies had indicated an inverse association, which was probably due to the fact that many diseases represented among hospital controls are positively associated with tobacco smoking.

He further noted that case–control studies relying on population controls, or on controls with diseases unrelated to smoking, pointed to a weak positive association, as did cohort studies in which selection bias is unlikely.

An additional refinement in epidemiological studies was introduced when the possibility was raised that passive smoking may increase the risk of breast cancer (Morabia *et al.* 1996). Non-smokers were subdivided into those genuinely non-exposed to tobacco smoking (that is non-smokers that have not been passively exposed to tobacco smoke) and those passively exposed to environmental tobacco smoke. In an exhaustive and thoughtful review, Morabia (2002) identified 11 case–control studies that evaluated active smoking in relation to breast cancer using as referent women who were not exposed to either active or passive smoking. In all of these studies, the point estimate of the adjusted odds ratio for breast cancer among active smokers was higher than the null value of 1 and in six of them the relative risk elevation was statistically significant. However, the results of a recent large cohort study, in which passive smokers were excluded from the non-smoking referent group, were less clearcut (Egan *et al.* 2002); the relative risk (and 95 per cent confidence interval (CI)) for breast cancer was 1.04 (0.94–1.15) among current active smokers and 1.09 (1.00–1.18) among past active smokers.

The results of case–control studies may have been biased because exposure histories were collected after disease onset, and health conscious women, who are generally non-smokers, may have been over-represented among controls. Indeed, there is some evidence, discussed later on, that points to information bias in case–control studies. On the other hand, the fact that smokers have, as a rule, an earlier age at menopause (Cooper *et al.* 1999) which is associated with lower breast cancer risk (Hankinson and Hunter 2002), tends to introduce negative confounding that has not always been accounted for. It should also be noted that in perhaps the most powerful epidemiological study (Egan *et al.* 2002), a significant increase in breast cancer risk was found, as predicted, among women who begun smoking before the age of 17 years (RR = 1.19, 95 per cent CI 1.03–1.37). The results of another study have pointed to the same direction (Innes and Byers 2001). In addition, findings indicating that cigarette smoking may modify the prevalence and spectrum of p53 mutations in breast tumours (Conway *et al.* 2002), evidence that smoking may selectively increase breast cancer risk in high-risk families (Couch *et al.* 2001), and reports that smoking is associated with an increased occurrence of hormone receptor negative tumours (Morabia *et al.* 1998; Manjer *et al.* 2001) cannot be explained on the basis of simple forms of information and selection bias.

Epidemiological evidence on passive smoking and breast cancer

The fact that passive smoking was found to be a significant predictor of coronary heart disease among non-smoking women in the Nurses' Health Study (Kawachi *et al.* 1997), even though the relative risk linking active smoking to this disease is rarely more than three-fold, imparts an element of credibility to the hypothesis that passive smoking may increase the risk of breast cancer. At least 11 case–control studies reviewed by Morabia (2002) have evaluated passive smoking in relation to breast cancer risk. In all these studies, the odds ratio estimates were higher than 1, and in five of them the excess breast cancer risk among passive smokers was statistically significant. Thus, the evidence from case–control studies is strongly supportive of a weak positive association between passive smoking and breast cancer risk.

The evidence from two cohort studies, however, points to no association between passive smoking and breast cancer risk. In the Jee *et al.* study (Jee *et al.* 1999) the relative risk was 1.3 with 95 per cent CI from 0.9 to 1.8, whereas in the Egan et al. study (2002), the corresponding relative risk was 0.9 with 95 per cent CI from 0.7 to 1.2.

In a mechanistic meta-analysis of all epidemiological studies, the empirical evidence would support a positive association between passive smoking and breast cancer risk, but the inherently higher validity of cohort investigations forces a re-examination of the results of the case–control studies. As has been pointed out by Egan *et al.* (2002), information bias is a major concern in case–control studies, because exposure histories are generally collected after disease onset. This is particularly true for an emotionally charged disease with largely unknown aetiology, studied in relation to an exposure (passive smoking) which is subject to misclassification and which can be viewed with hostility. In situations like these, women with breast cancer, who are not themselves smokers (an exposure which is not likely to be misclassified), may tend to allocate themselves to the category of passive smokers, thus removing themselves from the category of genuinely non-exposed to either active or passive smoking.

Logical as this argument may be, it is still hypothetical. However, there is an indirect way to evaluate it. All case–control studies that have examined passive smoking in relation to breast cancer risk have also evaluated active smoking in relation to this risk, using as referent women who were genuinely non-exposed to either active or passive smoking. These studies have been termed 'second generation', because they have used a more appropriate referent in comparison to earlier studies of active smoking, in which passive smokers were not excluded from the referent group of non-smoking women (Morabia 2002). Table 29.1 abstracts information presented by Morabia (Morabia 2002). If some non-smoking women with breast cancer were inclined to incorrectly designate themselves as passive smokers, the odds ratio for breast cancer in relation to passive smoking would be inflated because of an increase at the numerator of the odds ratio formula. Moreover, the odds ratio for breast cancer in relation to active smoking would also be inflated because of a decrease in the denominator of the formula. Under the hypothesis of information bias, the predicted net result would be a positive correlation of the breast cancer odds ratio estimates among active and passive smokers from each of the 11 studies. The Pearson and Spearman correlation

Table 29.1 Odds ratios (and 95 per cent confidence intervals) for breast cancer among passive smokers and among active smokers in comparison to neither-active-nor-passive smokers. Results of 11 case–control studies*

Case–control studies	Adjusted OR (95 per cent CI)	
	Passive smoking	Active smoking
Wells 1992 (Sandler)	1.6 (0.8–3.4)	1.2 (0.6–2.5)
Morabia et al. 1996	2.3 (1.5–3.7)	2.5 (1.6–3.8)**
van Leeuwen et al. 1997 (Rookus)	1.2 (0.8–1.7)	1.2 (0.8–1.6)
Wells 1998 (Smith)	1.6 (0.8–3.1)	2.0 (0.98–4.1)
Lash and Aschengrau 1999	2.0 (1.1–3.7)	2.0 (1.1–3.6)
Zhao et al. 1999	2.5 (1.7–3.8)	3.5 (1.3–9.3)
Millikan et al. 1998; Marcus et al. 2000	1.3 (0.9–1.9)	1.1 (0.8–1.6)**
Delfino et al. 2000	1.9 (0.8–4.3)	1.4 (0.8–2.7)**
Johnson et al. 2000—pre-menopausal	2.3 (1.2–4.6)	2.3 (1.2–4.5)
Johnson et al. 2000—post-menopausal	1.2 (0.8–1.8)	1.5 (1.0–2.3)
Chang-Claude et al. 2001	1.5 (1.0–2.3)	1.4 (0.9–2.2)

*Modified from: Morabia 2002.
**Crude OR.

coefficients from the data in Table 29.1 are $+0.85$ ($p<0.001$) and $+0.81$ ($p<0.05$), respectively. Compatibility of the empirical evidence with the working hypothesis of information bias does not, of course, establish the validity of this hypothesis, but it lends credibility to it.

Conclusion

There is little evidence that passive smoking increases the risk of breast cancer, although one cannot reject this possibility. The problem is the more general one of distinguishing between a null association from a weakly positive one, or, indeed, a weakly negative one, on the basis of epidemiological evidence alone.

With respect to active smoking, the overall epidemiological evidence is also weak. There are findings, however, suggestive of interaction of this exposure with the differentiation status of the mammary gland, as reflected by age at exposure and parity, and these findings cannot be explained by simple forms of information bias. There are also reports that active smoking affects selectively hormone receptor negative tumours, and that it modifies the spectrum of p53 mutations in breast tumours. These results may reflect chance or selective reporting, but, if they were to be replicated and further supported by epidemiological results, they could mean that active smoking affects breast cancer risk. At this stage, and if one were to adopt the International Agency for Research on Cancer terminology concerning the evaluation of carcinogenicity, the likely verdict on active smoking in relation to breast cancer risk would be that it is a 'possible' carcinogen.

References

Adami, H. -O., Signorello, L. B., and Trichopoulos, D. (1998). Towards an understanding of breast cancer etiology. In: *Progress and enigmas in cancer epidemiology* (ed. H.-O. Adami and D. Trichopoulos) *Seminars in Cancer Biology*, **8**, 255–62.

Baron, J. A. (1984). Smoking and estrogen-related disease. *Am. J. Epidemiol.*, **119**, 9–22.

Casagrande, J. T., Hanisch, R., Pike, M. C., Ross, R. K., Brown, J. B., and Henderson, B. E. (1988). A case-control study of male breast cancer. *Cancer Res.*, **48**, 1326–30.

Chang-Claude, J., Kropp, S., Bartsch, H., and Risch, A. (2001). Active and passive smoking, N-acetyltransferase 2 genotype and breast cancer risk [abstract]. AACR Annual Meeting.

Conway, K., Edmiston, S. N., Cui, L., Drouin, S. S., Pang, J., He, M., *et al.* (2002). Prevalence and spectrum of p53 mutations associated with smoking in breast cancer. *Cancer Res.*, **62**, 1987–95.

Cooper, G. S., Sandler, D. P., and Bohlig, M. (1999). Active and passive smoking and the occurrence of natural menopause. *Epidemiology*, **10**, 771–3.

Couch, F. J., Cerhan, J. R., Vierkant, R. A., Grabrick, D. M., Therneau, T. M., Pankratz, V. S., *et al.* (2001). Cigarette smoking increases risk for breast cancer in high-risk breast cancer families. *Cancer Epidemiol. Biomarkers Prev.*, **10**, 327–32.

Delfino, R. J., Smith, C., West, J. G., Lin, H. J., White, E., Liao, S. Y., Gim, J. S., Ma, H. L., Butler, J., Anton-Culuer, H. (2000). Breast cancer, passive and active cigarette smoking and N-acetyltransferase 2 genotype. *Pharmacogenetics*, **10**, 461–9.

Dockery, D. W. and Trichopoulos, D. (1997). Risk of lung cancer from environmental exposures to tobacco smoke. *Cancer Causes and Control*, **8**, 333–45.

Egan, K. M., Stampfer, M. J., Hunter, D., Hankinson, S., Rosner, B. A., Holmes, M., *et al.* (2002). Active and passive smoking in breast cancer: prospective results from the Nurses' Health Study. *Epidemiology*, **13**, 138–45.

Hankinson, S. and Hunter, D. (2002). Breast cancer. In: *Textbook of cancer epidemiology* (eds. Adami, Hunter, and Trichopoulos). Oxford University Press, New York, pp. 301–339.

Hoel, D. G. and Dinse, G. E. (1990). Using mortality data to estimate radiation effects on breast cancer incidence. *Environ. Health Perspect.*, **87**, 123–9.

Hopper, J. L. and Seeman, E. (1994). The bone density of female twins discordant for tobacco use. *N. Engl. J. Med.*, **330**, 387–92.

IARC Monographs on the Evaluation of Carcinogenic Risks (1986). *Tobacco smoking*, Vol. 38. Lyon, pp. 421.

Innes, K. E. and Byers, T. E. (2001). Smoking during pregnancy and breast cancer risk in very young women (United States). *Cancer Causes Control*, **12**, 179–85.

Jee, S. H., Ohrr, H., and Kim, I. S. (1999). Effects of husbands' smoking on the incidence of lung cancer in Korean women. *Int. J. Epidemiol.*, **28**, 824–8.

Johnson, K. C., Hu, J., and Mao, Y. (2000). Passive and active smoking and breast cancer risk in Canada, 1994–97. The Canadian Cancer Registries Epidemiology Research Group. *Cancer Causes Control*, **11**, 211–21.

Kalandidi, A., Trichopoulos, D., Hatzakis, A., Tzannes, S., and Saracci, R. (1987). Passive smoking and chronic obstructive lung disease. *Lancet*, **2**, 1325–6.

Kawachi, I., Colditz, G. A., Speizer, F. E., Manson, J. E., Stampfer, M. J., Willett, W. C., *et al.* (1997). A prospective study of passive smoking and coronary heart disease. *Circulation*, **95**, 2374–9.

Kuper, H., Tzonou, A., Kaklamani, E., Hsieh, C. C., Lagiou, P., Adami, H. O., *et al.* (2000). Tobacco smoking, alcohol consumption and their interaction in the causation of hepatocellular carcinoma. *Int. J. Cancer*, **85**, 498–502.

Lagiou, P. and Adami, H. O. (2002). Burden of cancer. In: *Textbook of cancer epidemiology* (ed. Adai, Hunter,and Trichopoulos). Oxford University Press, New York, pp. 3–28.

Land, C. E. (1995). Studies of cancer and radiation dose among atomic bomb survivors. The example of breast cancer. *JAMA*, **274**, 402–7.

Lash, T. L. and Aschengrau, A. (1999). Active and passive cigarette smoking and the occurrence of breast cancer. *Am. J. Epidemiol.*, **149**, 5–12.

Lowenfels, A. B. and Maisonneuve, P. (2002). Epidemiologic and etiologic factors of pancreatic cancer. *Hematol. Oncol. Clin. North Am.*, **16**, 1–16.

MacMahon, B. (1990). Cigarette smoking and cancer of the breast. In: *Smoking and hormone-related disorders* (eds. Wald and Baron). Oxford University Press, Oxford, pp. 154–66.

MacMahon, B., Trichopoulos, D., Cole, P., and Brown, J. (1982). Cigarette smoking and urinary estrogens. *N. Engl. J. Med.*, **307**, 1062–5.

Manjer, J., Malina, J., Berglund, G., Bondeson, L., Garne, J. P., and Janzon, L. (2001). Smoking associated with hormone receptor negative breast cancer. *Int. J. Cancer*, **91**, 580–4.

Marcus, P. M., Newman, B., Millikan, R. C., Moorman, P. G., Baird, D. D., and Qaqish, B. (2000). The associations of adolescent cigarette smoking, alcoholic beverage consumption, environmental tobacco smoke, and ionizing radiation with subsequent breast cancer risk (United States). *Cancer Causes Control*, **11**, 271–8.

Michnovicz, J. J. and Fishman, J. (1990). Increased oxidative metabolism of oestrogens in male and female smokers. In: *Smoking and hormone-related disorders* (eds. Wald and Baron). Oxford University Press, Oxford, pp. 197–208.

Michnovicz, J. J., Hershcopf, R. J., Naganuma, H., Bradlow, H. L., and Fishman, J. (1986). Increased 2-hydroxylation of estradiol as a possible mechanism for the anti-estrogenic effect of cigarette smoking. *N. Engl. J. Med.*, **315**, 1305–9.

Millikan, R. C., Pittman, G. S., Newman, B., Tse, C. K., Selmin, O., Rockhill, B., *et al.* (1998). Cigarette smoking, N-acetyltransferases 1 and 2, and breast cancer risk. *Cancer Epidemiol. Biomarkers Prev.*, **7**, 371–8.

Morabia, A. (2002). Smoking (active and passive) and breast cancer: epidemiologic evidence up to June 2001. *Environ. Mol. Mutagen.*, **39**, 89–95.

Morabia, A., Bernstein, M., Heritier, S., and Khatchatrian, N. (1996). Relation of breast cancer with passive and active exposure to tobacco smoke. *Am. J. Epidemiol.*, **143**, 918–28.

Morabia, A., Bernstein, M., Ruiz, J., Heritier, S., Diebold Berger, S., Borisch, B. (1998). Relation of smoking to breast cancer by estrogen receptor status. *Int. J. Cancer*, **75**, 339–42.

Petrakis, N. L., Maack, C. A., Lee, R. E., and Lyon, M. (1980). Mutagenic activity in nipple aspirates of human breast fluid. *Cancer Res.*, **40**, 188–9.

Petridou, E., Giokas, G., Kuper, H., Mucci, L. A., and Trichopoulos, D. (2000). Endocrine correlates of male breast cancer risk: a case-control study in Athens, Greece. *Br. J. Cancer*, **83**, 1234–37.

Phillips, D. H., Martin, F. L., Grover, P. L., and Williams, J. A. (2001). Toxicological basis for a possible association of breast cancer with smoking and other sources of environmental carcinogens. *J. Women's Cancer*, **3**, 9–16.

Russo, J., Hu, Y. F., Silva, I. D., and Russo, I. H. (2001). Cancer risk related to mammary gland structure and development. *Microsc. Res. Tech.*, **52**, 204–23.

Terry, P. D., Miller, A. B., and Rohan, T. E. (2002). A prospective cohort study of cigarette smoking and the risk of endometrial cancer. *Br. J. Cancer*, **86**, 1430–5.

Van Leeuwen, F. E., de Vries, F., van der Kooy, K., and Rookus, M. (1997). Smoking and breast cancer risk [abstract]. *Am. J. Epidemiol.*, **145**, S29.

Vessey, M., Baron, J., Doll R., McPherson, K, and Yeates, D. (1983). Oral contraceptives and breast cancer: final report of an epidemiological study. *Br. J. Cancer*, **47**, 455–62.

Wells, A. J. (1992). Re: 'Breast cancer, cigarette smoking, and passive smoking' [reply]. *Am. J. Epidemiol.*, **135**, 710–12.

Wells, A. J. (1998). Re: 'Breast cancer, cigarette smoking, and passive smoking'. *Am. J. Epidemiol.*, **147**, 991–2.

Zhao, Y., Shi, Z., and Liu, L. (1999). [Matched case-control study for detecting risk factors of breast cancer in women living in Chengdu] (in Chinese). *J. Epidemiol.*, **20**, 91–4.

Chapter 30

Smoking and ovarian cancer

Crystal N. Holick and Harvey A. Risch

Epidemiology

Ovarian cancer causes more deaths than any other cancer of the female reproductive system and ranks second in incidence among gynecologic cancers, accounting for 4 per cent of all cancers, with 23 300 new cases estimated among women in the United States in 2002 (American Cancer Society 2002). Risk of ovarian cancer increases with age and peaks in the late 70s. Mutations in the genes *BRCA1* or *BRCA2* account for about 10 per cent of all epithelial ovarian cancers (Risch *et al.* 2001). Pregnancies and use of oral contraceptives are known to reduce the risk of developing ovarian cancer, and nulliparous women are more likely to develop it (Daly and Obrams 1998). In addition to female reproductive factors, personal and environmental exposures including diet practices (Cramer *et al.* 1984; Risch *et al.* 1994), coffee consumption (La Vecchia *et al.* 1984), alcohol intake (Polychronopoulou *et al.* 1993), and smoking history (Doll *et al.* 1980) may also modify the risk of ovarian cancer. Recently, evidence has emerged that risk factors for ovarian cancer—including tobacco smoking (Kuper *et al.* 2000; Marchbanks *et al.* 2000; Green *et al.* 2001), parity (Kvale *et al.* 1988; Risch *et al.* 1996), and oral contraceptive use (The WHO Collaborative Study of Neoplasia and Steroid Contraceptives 1989; Risch *et al.* 1996)—may vary by histologic type.

Hypotheses of ovarian carcinogenesis

The carcinogenic process of epithelial ovarian cancer is not fully understood. Several mechanisms of ovarian pathogenesis have been hypothesized, each of which could have involvement by tobacco smoking.

Incessant ovulation

Increased cell division, stimulated by internal and external factors, increases the accumulation of genetic errors and is thought to enhance the risk of neoplastic transformation (Preston-Martin *et al.* 1990). Fathalla, in 1971, theorized that regularly repeated ovulation in women may increase the likelihood of ovarian malignancy (Fathalla 1971). According to this hypothesis, repeated ovulation-induced disruption and repair of the ovarian epithelium increases epithelial proliferation and risk of DNA damage, leading to neoplastic transformation and thus to ovarian cancer.

Casagrande *et al.* (1979) extended this concept by suggesting that anovulation, resulting from oral contraceptive use, reduces the risk of ovarian cancer. Epithelial clefts and inclusion cysts frequently form within the ovarian stroma as part of ovulatory repair. Cells lining the clefts or inclusion cysts may undergo metaplasia to resemble serous, mucinous, or endometrioid epithelium, as well as neoplastic transformation to produce tumors of serous, mucinous, or endometrioid histologic varieties.

The incessant-ovulation hypothesis is supported by inferences from epidemiologic studies of ovarian cancer (Risch *et al.* 1983; The Cancer and Steroid Hormone Study 1987; Whittemore *et al.* 1992; Schildkraut *et al.* 1997). Hormonal, reproductive, and environmental factors, such as oral contraceptive use, pregnancy, and tobacco smoking, may modify risk of ovarian cancer via an impact on ovulation. A dose–response decrease in risk with increasing parity (Hankinson *et al.* 1995) and with increasing duration of oral contraceptive use (Gross and Schlesselman 1994) is consistently observed in most studies. Evidence also suggests that tobacco smoking may impair ovulation in women, since smoking is observed to be associated with delayed conception (Baird and Wilcox 1985) and with reduced ovulatory response to gonadotropin stimulation (Van Voorhis *et al.* 1992). Furthermore, ovarian atresia, caused by exposure to polycyclic aromatic hydrocarbons contained in cigarette smoke, has been shown in other species (e.g. rodents) (Mattison and Thorgeirsson 1978). Cigarette smoking also results in earlier age at natural menopause (Cooper *et al.* 1999; Hardy *et al.* 2000). With cigarette smokers having fewer lifetime ovulations than nonsmokers, the repeated ovulation model predicts a lower risk of ovarian cancer among smokers.

Although the incessant ovulation hypothesis is supported by the above evidence as well as by animal studies showing the proliferative behavior of the ovarian epithelium following ovulation (Godwin *et al.* 1992), it is unable to explain appreciable discrepancies between the amount of anovulation and the magnitude of effect on risk for several ovulation-related factors (Risch 1998). Tobacco smoking may therefore influence the risk of ovarian cancer through additional biologic mechanisms, unrelated to ovulation, for example involving hormonal factors.

Gonadotropin–estrogen theory

Stimulation of the ovary by steroid hormones may play a causative role in the pathogenesis of ovarian cancer. Under the gonadotropin–estrogen (hormonal) theory, the initial stage in the development of epithelial ovarian cancer, as in the incessant-ovulation hypothesis, involves repeated proliferation and invagination of the ovarian surface epithelium to form clefts and inclusion cysts within the ovarian stroma. Subsequent events including differentiation, further proliferation, and eventual malignant transformation are mediated through hormonal stimulation (Cramer and Welch 1983). Specifically, increased pituitary gonadotropin [follicle-stimulating hormone (FSH) or luteinizing hormone (LH)] action and the resulting excessive estrogen (or estrogen precursor) stimulation of ovarian epithelial cells is responsible for the increased risk of ovarian cancer development. Factors that affect estrogen regulation would influence gonadotropin stimulation and risk indirectly (Cramer and Welch 1983).

The gonadotropin–estrogen hypothesis predicts that higher concentrations of FSH and LH, leading to greater ovarian estrogen synthesis, would increase the risk of developing ovarian cancer. This observation is consistent with reports showing increased risk associated with exogenous menopausal estrogen use (Hoover et al. 1977; Parazzini et al. 1994; Rodriguez et al. 1995; Purdie et al. 1996; Risch 1996;). A number of common chemicals or drugs are believed to enhance hepatic estrogen degradation or metabolism (Helzlsouer et al. 1995). It is possible therefore that tobacco smoking may influence the risk of epithelial ovarian cancer through hormonal mechanisms by altering the levels of circulating estrogens. Women who smoke appear to have lower levels of urinary estrogens, and other evidence of endogenous estrogen-deficiency (Wynder et al. 1969; Van Voorhis et al. 1992). The reduced circulating estrogens in smokers could thus result in a decreased risk of ovarian cancer.

There is very little direct evidence bearing on the gonadotropin–estrogen hypothesis. The site distribution of ovarian epithelial tumors shows a larger fraction arising within epithelial inclusion cysts, compared with the epithelial cells on the ovarian surface, and the smallest fraction in the peritoneal mesothelium which has the greatest surface area (Godwin et al. 1992; Resta et al. 1993). This suggests a hormonal influence on neoplastic transformation. Studies evaluating the presence of ovarian epithelial cell steroid–hormone receptors show at least low levels of estrogen receptors (al-Timimi et al. 1985). Ovarian cancers mostly arise in the postmenopausal years, after the large perimenopausal rise in gonadotropin levels. On the other hand, a nested case–control study of prediagnostic serum gonadotropin and steroid hormone levels showed that women with lower FSH levels were at increased risk of subsequently developing ovarian cancer; there was no association with estrogen levels (Helzlsouer et al. 1995).

Beyond estrogens: progesterone and androgens

The presence of progesterone and androgen receptors within ovarian epithelial cells (al-Timimi et al. 1985; Zeimet et al. 1994) suggests that the epithelial cells are exposed to and respond to both these hormones, and this has led to speculation on the involvement of these hormones in the etiology of ovarian carcinogenesis (Risch 1998). It has been suggested that the progestin exposure in oral contraceptive use (and in pregnancy, for that matter) may be responsible for the protective effect, independent of or in addition to anovulation (Risch 1998). One mechanism underlying the progestin hypothesis may involve enhanced apoptosis of the ovarian epithelium (Rodriguez et al. 1998). The degree of protection associated with oral-contraceptive use may be related to the progestin potency of the formulation (Schildkraut et al. 2002).

Various epidemiologic and other studies support a role for androgens in the etiology of ovarian cancer (reviewed in Risch 1998). In postmenopausal women, smoking appears to be related to increased levels of adrenal androgens. In premenopausal women, smoking increases the androgen–estrogen ratio of follicular fluid (Van Voorhis *et al.* 1992), to which the ovarian epithelium is exposed. It seems reasonable that smoking could thus act on the ovarian epithelium through hormonal effects, but more studies are needed.

Tobacco smoking and risk of ovarian cancer

Several mechanisms support the biologic plausibility of an association between tobacco smoking and ovarian cancer, however given the above discussion, it is uncertain in which direction, to increase or decrease risk, the association should be. Results from early studies evaluating the association between cigarette smoking and risk of ovarian cancer lead IARC in 1987 to report that ovarian cancer was not considered to be a tobacco-related cancer (IARC 1987). With the exception of a British cohort study (Doll *et al.* 1980), no association has been found between tobacco smoking and risk of ovarian cancer in subsequent prospective studies (Engeland *et al.* 1996), and additional case–control studies have found null or inconsistent results (Trichopoulos *et al.* 1981; Smith *et al.* 1984; Tzonou *et al.* 1984; Baron *et al.* 1986; Franks *et al.* 1987; Hartge *et al.* 1989; Franceschi *et al.* 1991; Polychronopoulou *et al.* 1993). Some studies have observed nonsignificant reductions in risk among smokers (Byers *et al.* 1983; La Vecchia *et al.* 1984). In a Japanese case–control study of alcohol consumption and risk of breast, corpus uteri, and ovarian cancer, Kato *et al.* (1989) found a nonsignificant relative risk of 0.78 (95% CI: 0.56–1.08) for ever smokers versus never smokers. Evaluating several reproductive, dietary, genetic, or environmental factors on the development of ovarian cancer, studies by Whittemore *et al.* (1988), Mori *et al.* (1988), and Slattery *et al.* (1989) reported no significant differences in tobacco use between cases and controls, though no details were given. An increase in ovarian cancer risk associated with tobacco smoking has also been observed (Cramer *et al.* 1984; Stockwell and Lyman 1987). Cramer *et al.* (1984) conducted a population-based case–control study of dietary factors and ovarian cancer that found a nonsignificant increased relative risk of 1.8 (95% CI: 0.54–5.97) for smokers versus nonsmokers. Those authors found no significant trends in risk in relation to lifetime pack-years of cigarette smoking (Cramer *et al.* 1984). Several of the studies (Cramer *et al.* 1984; Mori *et al.* 1988; Slattery *et al.* 1989; Polychronopoulou *et al.* 1993) did not control for all of the most potentially important confounding factors including age, parity, and oral contraceptive use, and this is a limitation in considering their results.

Risk differences according to histologic subtype

There is evidence that various risk factors involved in the development of epithelial ovarian cancer—including parity and oral contraceptive use—might vary by the histologic type of the tumor (Risch *et al.* 1996). Germline *BRCA1* or *BRCA2* mutations do not occur in women with mucinous tumors (Risch *et al.* 2001). A follow-up study of more than 60 000 females in Norway found a protective effect of increasing parity among serous, endometrioid, and other epithelial tumors but not for mucinous tumors (Kvale *et al.* 1988). In The WHO Collaborative Study of Neoplasia and Steroid Contraceptives, oral contraceptive use was significantly inversely associated with epithelial ovarian cancer risk for all the principal histologic types except for mucinous tumors (The WHO Collaborative Study of Neoplasia and Steroid Contraceptives 1989). Similarly, Risch *et al.* (1996) reported a population-based study of dietary and reproductive factors and epithelial ovarian cancer, which found decreasing oral contraceptive- and parity-related trends in risk for all of the particular histologic varieties of ovarian tumors except mucinous tumors. These case–control studies, as well as one other (Cramer *et al.* 1982), consistently found odds ratios closer to (or even above) unity associated with ever use of oral contraceptives in mucinous tumors compared to serous, endometrioid, clear cell, or other (nonmucinous) epithelial tumors.

Few studies have evaluated relationships between tobacco smoking and risks of the different histologic subtypes of ovarian cancer. There is however some evidence for an increase in risk of mucinous ovarian cancer with tobacco smoking. An early report by Franks *et al.* (1987), using data from The Cancer and Steroid Hormone Study, found no association between epithelial ovarian cancer overall and smoking dose or duration, age started smoking, time since started smoking, or latency of smoking. A recent re-examination of the association in that study according to histologic subtype found current cigarette smoking to be a risk factor for mucinous epithelial ovarian cancer (odds ratio (OR) = 2.9; 95% CI: 1.7–4.9), but not for the other histologic types (Marchbanks *et al.* 2000). This association remained significantly elevated regardless of age started smoking and number of years since first use of cigarettes (Marchbanks *et al.* 2000). Risk of mucinous epithelial ovarian cancer for current smokers increased slightly with increasing cumulative pack-years of smoking; this same pattern was not observed for serous, endometrioid, or other histologic types (Marchbanks *et al.* 2000). Moreover, another recent study provided support for Marchbanks *et al.*'s findings, reporting some evidence for an association between mucinous ovarian tumors and heavy daily tobacco smoking (Kuper *et al.* 2000). Investigating the association between cigarette smoking and risk of ovarian cancer in a large case–control study, Green *et al.* (2001) concluded that current cigarette smoking was a risk factor for ovarian cancer, but especially for mucinous borderline and invasive types. Significantly elevated risks for mucinous epithelial tumors were seen among both current smokers (OR=3.2; 95% CI: 1.8–5.7) and past smokers (OR=2.3; 95% CI: 1.3–3.9) compared to never smokers (Green *et al.* 2001).

If steroid hormones are involved in the etiology of ovarian cancer, variation in hormone metabolism and degradation could affect disease risk, and exposures such as tobacco smoking may modify these associations through induction effects on enzymes that activate or detoxify both polycyclic hydrocarbons and other (pro)carcinogens found in tobacco smoke, as well as steroid hormones. Thus, it has been suggested that tobacco smoking may affect the relationships between several genetic polymorphic variants and risk of ovarian cancer (Goodman *et al.* 2001). A common high-activity variant in the gene for microsomal epoxide hydrolase (EPHX1), which detoxifies endogenous steroids and exogenous xenobiotics, was observed in one study to be associated with increased risk of ovarian cancer (Lancaster *et al.* 1996). Spurdle *et al.* (2001) evaluated the effect of both this variant and smoking and risk of ovarian cancer, taking into account histologic classification. They found smoking to be associated with increased risk of mucinous tumors, regardless of EPHX1 genotype, and that the heterozygote and fast variants of this polymorphism were associated with decreased risk of mucinous tumors among nonsmokers (Spurdle *et al.* 2001). These results appear to suggest that smoking may be associated with risk of mucinous ovarian tumors, that this risk may not be mediated through effects on induction of microsomal epoxide hydrolase, but that this enzyme might still be involved in the metabolism of other substances that could be associated with risk.

Histology: mucinous ovarian tumors

The various findings above are consistent with our suggestion that mucinous ovarian tumors comprise a distinct etiologic entity, separate from the other types of epithelial ovarian neoplasms (Risch *et al.* 1996). Differing from most types of ovarian cancer, mucinous tumors are thought to reflect a neoplastic morphologic continuum, from mucinous cystadenomas, through low-malignant potential (borderline) tumors, to invasive cancers, and many cases show the coexistence of these features within a single neoplasm (Rodriguez and Prat 2002). It has been speculated that the major effect of smoking may occur in the early stages of the mucinous cystadenoma-to-carcinoma sequence (Green *et al.* 2001). Mucinous tumors of the ovary, as well as serous and endometrioid ones, all share a common histogenetic ancestry with other structures of the reproductive tract, and show morphologic similarities to endocervical (or intestinal), endosalpingeal, and endometrial tumors, respectively (Parmley and Woodruff 1974). The resemblance of mucinous ovarian tumor cells to tumor cells of the endocervix or colon, or even pancreas, leads to two possibilities, that (a) risk factors for these tumor types might be shared, or (b) that mucinous ovarian tumors are frequently improperly diagnosed as such but are metastatic from unrecognized intestinal primaries. The latter issue is a recognized problem in diagnosing mucinous ovarian primaries (Lash and Hart 1987; Young and Hart 1989), and it is unclear to what degree the various epidemiologic studies showing positive associations with mucinous neoplasms were able to resolve the true origin of these tumors. Nicotine, benzo[*a*]pyrene, and other metabolites of cigarette smoke have been found in the cervical mucus of smokers (Feyerabend *et al.* 1982; Sasson *et al.* 1985) and it is possible that these substances are also present in the local environment of the ovary. Though cigarette smoking does not appear to be associated with risk of cervical adenocarcinoma (Lacey *et al.* 2001), it is related to risk of both colon cancer (Giovannucci 2001) and pancreas cancer (Muscat *et al.* 1997), and at least the enteric variety of mucinous ovarian tumors might reflect the same association.

Summary

Several possible mechanisms by which various factors may affect the risk of developing epithelial ovarian cancer have been hypothesized. It is possible that incessant ovulation and gonadotropin–estrogen hypotheses may work together in the etiology of this disease. However, evidence points to additional hormonal influences on the behavior of ovarian epithelial cells. The harmful effects of tobacco smoking may not be limited to these proposed mechanisms of ovarian carcinogenesis. Cigarette smoke contains polycyclic aromatic hydrocarbons, N-nitrosamines, and other carcinogenic substances, and it is unknown if these constituents of the smoke reach the epithelium of the ovary to exert a local effect, as has been suggested elsewhere (Mattison and Thorgeirsson 1978; Hellberg and Nilsson 1988). Early studies reported no association between tobacco smoking and risk of epithelial ovarian cancer, but more recent studies looking at the particular histologic varieties of ovarian cancer appear to show associations between tobacco smoking and increased risk of mucinous ovarian tumors. Ovarian cancer may very well be a heterogeneous disease with several distinct etiologic pathways. Analysing the associations between smoking and ovarian cancer, while taking into account histologic heterogeneity, may provide clues to the different underlying etiologies that comprise ovarian cancer pathogenesis.

References

al-Timimi, A., Buckley, C. H., and Fox, H. (1985). An immunohistochemical study of the incidence and significance of sex steroid hormone binding sites in normal and neoplastic human ovarian tissue. *Int. J. Gynecol. Pathol.* **4**, 24–41.

American Cancer Society. (2002). *Cancer facts and figures.* American Cancer Society, Inc., Atlanta.

Baird, D. D. and Wilcox, A. J. (1985). Cigarette smoking associated with delayed conception. *JAMA*, **253**, 2979–83.

Baron, J. A., Byers, T., Greenberg, E. R., Cummings, K. M., and Swanson, M. (1986). Cigarette smoking in women with cancers of the breast and reproductive organs. *J. Natl. Cancer Inst.*, **77**, 677–80.

Byers, T., Marshall, J., Graham, S., Mettlin, C., and Swanson, M. (1983). A case–control study of dietary and nondietary factors in ovarian cancer. *J. Natl. Cancer Inst.*, **71**, 681–6.

Casagrande, J. T., Louie, E. W., Pike, M. C., Roy, S., Ross, R. K., and Henderson, B. E. (1979). 'Incessant ovulation' and ovarian cancer. *Lancet*, **2**, 170–3.

Cooper, G. S., Sandler, D. P., and Bohlig, M. (1999). Active and passive smoking and the occurrence of natural menopause. *Epidemiology*, **10**, 771–3.

Cramer, D. W. and Welch, W. R. (1983). Determinants of ovarian cancer risk. II. Inferences regarding pathogenesis. *J. Natl. Cancer Inst.*, **71**, 717–21.

Cramer, D. W., Hutchison, G. B., Welch, W. R., Scully, R. E., and Knapp, R. C. (1982). Factors affecting the association of oral contraceptives and ovarian cancer. *N. Engl. J Med.*, **307**, 1047–51.

Cramer, D. W., Welch, W. R., Hutchison, G. B., Willett, W., and Scully, R. E. (1984). Dietary animal fat in relation to ovarian cancer risk. *Obstet. Gynecol., 63*, 833–8.

Daly, M. and Obrams, G. I. (1998). Epidemiology and risk assessment for ovarian cancer. *Semin. Oncol.* **25**, 255–64.

Doll, R., Gray, R., Hafner, B., and Peto R. (1980), Mortality in relation to smoking: 22 years' observations on female British doctors. *Br. Med. J., 280*, 967–71.

Engeland, A., Andersen, A., Haldorsen, T., and Tretli, S. (1996). Smoking habits and risk of cancers other than lung cancer: 28 years' follow-up of 26,000 Norwegian men and women. *Cancer Causes Control*, **7**, 497–506.

Fathalla, M. F. (1971). Incessant ovulation—a factor in ovarian neoplasia? *Lancet*, **2**, 163.

Feyerabend, C., Higenbottam, T., and Russell, M. A. (1982). Nicotine concentrations in urine and saliva of smokers and non-smokers. *Br. Med. J. (Clin. Res. Ed.)*, **284**, 1002–4.

Franceschi, S., La Vecchia, C., Booth, M., Tzonou, A., Negri, E., Parazzini, F., *et al.* (1991). Pooled analysis of 3 European case–control studies of ovarian cancer: II. Age at menarche and at menopause. *Int. J. Cancer*, **49**, 57–60.

Franks, A. L., Lee, N. C., Kendrick, J. S., Rubin, G. L., and Layde, P. M. (1987). Cigarette smoking and the risk of epithelial ovarian cancer. *Am. J. Epidemiol.*, **126**, 112–7.

Giovannucci, E. (2001). An updated review of the epidemiological evidence that cigarette smoking increases risk of colorectal cancer. *Cancer Epidemiol. Biomarkers Prev.*, **10**, 725–31.

Godwin, A. K., Perez, R. P., Johnson, S. W., Hamaguchi, K., and Hamilton, T. C. (1992). Growth regulation of ovarian cancer. *Hematol. Oncol. Clin. North Am.*, **6**, 829–41.

Godwin, A. K., Testa, J. R., Handel, L. M., Liu, Z., Vanderveer, L. A., Tracey, P. A., *et al.* (1992). Spontaneous transformation of rat ovarian surface epithelial cells: association with cytogenetic changes and implications of repeated ovulation in the etiology of ovarian cancer. *J. Natl. Cancer Inst.*, **84**, 592–601.

Goodman, M. T., McDuffie, K., Kolonel, L. N., Terada, K., Donlon, T. A., Wilkens, L. R., *et al.* (2001). Case–control study of ovarian cancer and polymorphisms in genes involved in catecholestrogen formation and metabolism. *Cancer Epidemiol. Biomarkers Prev.*, **10**, 209–16.

Green, A., Purdie, D., Bain, C., Siskind, V., and Webb, P. M. (2001). Cigarette smoking and risk of epithelial ovarian cancer (Australia). *Cancer Causes Control*, **12**, 713–9.

Gross, T. P. and Schlesselman, J. J. (1994). The estimated effect of oral contraceptive use on the cumulative risk of epithelial ovarian cancer. *Obstet. Gynecol.*, **83**, 419–24.

Hankinson, S. E., Colditz, G. A., Hunter, D. J., Willett, W. C., Stampfer, M. J., Rosner, B., *et al.* (1995). A prospective study of reproductive factors and risk of epithelial ovarian cancer. *Cancer*, **76**, 284–90.

Hardy, R., Kuh, D., and Wadsworth, M. (2000). Smoking, body mass index, socioeconomic status and the menopausal transition in a British national cohort. *Int. J. Epidemiol.*, **29**, 845–51.

Hartge, P., Schiffman, M. H., Hoover, R., McGowan, L., Lesher, L., and Norris, H. J. (1989). A case–control study of epithelial ovarian cancer. *Am. J. Obstet. Gynecol.*, **161**, 10–6.

Hellberg, D. and Nilsson, S. (1988). Smoking and cancer of the ovary. *N. Engl. J. Med.*, **318**, 782–3.

Helzlsouer, K. J., Alberg, A. J., Gordon, G. B., Longcope, C., Bush, T. L., Hoffman, S. C., *et al.* (1995). Serum gonadotropins and steroid hormones and the development of ovarian cancer. *JAMA*, **274**, 1926–30.

Hoover, R., Gray, L. A., Sr., and Fraumeni, J. F., Jr. (1977). Stilboestrol (diethylstilbestrol) and the risk of ovarian cancer. *Lancet*, **2**, 533–4.

IARC (1987). Overall evaluations of carcinogenicity: an updating of IARC Monographs volumes 1 to 42. *IARC Monogr. Eval. Carcinog. Risks. Hum. Suppl.*, **7**, 1–440.

Kato, I., Tominaga, S., and Terao, C. (1989). Alcohol consumption and cancers of hormone-related organs in females. *Jpn. J. Clin. Oncol.*, **19**, 202–7.

Kuper, H., Titus-Ernstoff, L., Harlow, B. L., and Cramer, D. W. (2000). Population based study of coffee, alcohol and tobacco use and risk of ovarian cancer. *Int. J. Cancer*, **88**, 313–8.

Kvale, G., Heuch, I., Nilssen, S., and Beral, V. (1988). Reproductive factors and risk of ovarian cancer: a prospective study. *Int. J. Cancer*, **42**, 246–51.

Lacey, J. V., Jr., Frisch, M., Brinton, L. A., Abbas, F. M., Barnes, W. A., Gravitt, P. E., *et al.* (2001). Associations between smoking and adenocarcinomas and squamous cell carcinomas of the uterine cervix (United States). *Cancer Causes Control*, **12**, 153–61.

Lancaster, J. M., Brownlee, H. A., Bell, D. A., Futreal, P. A., Marks, J. R., Berchuck, A., *et al.* (1996). Microsomal epoxide hydrolase polymorphism as a risk factor for ovarian cancer. *Mol. Carcinog.*, **17**, 160–2.

Lash, R. H. and Hart, W. R. (1987). Intestinal adenocarcinomas metastatic to the ovaries. A clinicopathologic evaluation of 22 cases. *Am. J. Surg. Pathol.*, **11**, 114–21.

La Vecchia, C., Franceschi, S., Decarli, A., Gentile, A., Liati, P., Regallo, M., *et al.* (1984). Coffee drinking and the risk of epithelial ovarian cancer. *Int. J. Cancer*, **33**, 559–62.

Marchbanks, P. A., Wilson, H., Bastos, E., Cramer, D. W., Schildkraut, J. M., and Peterson, H. B. (2000). Cigarette smoking and epithelial ovarian cancer by histologic type. *Obstet. Gynecol.*, **95**, 255–60.

Mattison, D. R. and Thorgeirsson, S. S. (1978). Smoking and industrial pollution, and their effects on menopause and ovarian cancer. *Lancet*, **1**, 187–8.

Mori, M., Harabuchi, I., Miyake, H., Casagrande, J. T., Henderson, B. E., and Ross, R. K. (1988). Reproductive, genetic, and dietary risk factors for ovarian cancer. *Am. J. Epidemiol.*, **128**, 771–7.

Muscat, J. E., Stellman, S. D., Hoffmann, D., and Wynder, E. L. (1997). Smoking and pancreatic cancer in men and women. *Cancer Epidemiol. Biomarkers Prev.*, **6**, 15–9.

Parazzini, F., La Vecchia, C., Negri, E., and Villa, A. (1994). Estrogen replacement therapy and ovarian cancer risk. *Int. J. Cancer*, **57**, 135–6.

Parmley, T. H. and Woodruff, J. D. (1974). The ovarian mesothelioma. *Am. J. Obstet. Gynecol.*, **120**, 234–41.

Polychronopoulou, A., Tzonou, A., Hsieh, C. C., Kaprinis, G., Rebelakos, A., Toupadaki, N., *et al.* (1993). Reproductive variables, tobacco, ethanol, coffee and somatometry as risk factors for ovarian cancer. *Int. J. Cancer*, **55**, 402–7.

Preston-Martin, S., Pike, M. C., Ross, R. K., Jones, P. A., and Henderson, B. E. (1990). Increased cell division as a cause of human cancer. *Cancer Res.*, **50**, 7415–21.

Purdie, D., Green, A., Bain, C., Siskind, V., Ward, B., Hacker, N., *et al.* (1996). Estrogen replacement therapy and risk of epithelial ovarian cancer [abstract]. *Am. J. Epidemiol.*, **143**, S43.

Resta, L., Russo, S., Colucci, G. A., and Prat, J. (1993). Morphologic precursors of ovarian epithelial tumors. *Obstet. Gynecol.*, **82**, 181–6.

Risch, H. A. (1996). Estrogen replacement therapy and risk of epithelial ovarian cancer. *Gynecol. Oncol.*, **63**, 254–7.

Risch, H. A. (1998). Hormonal etiology of epithelial ovarian cancer, with a hypothesis concerning the role of androgens and progesterone. *J. Natl. Cancer Inst.*, **90**, 1774–86.

Risch, H. A., Jain, M., Marrett, L. D., and Howe, G. R. (1994). Dietary fat intake and risk of epithelial ovarian cancer. *J. Natl. Cancer Inst.*, **86**, 1409–15.

Risch, H. A., Marrett, L. D., Jain, M., and Howe, G. R. (1996). Differences in risk factors for epithelial ovarian cancer by histologic type. Results of a case–control study. *Am. J. Epidemiol.*, **144**, 363–72.

Risch, H. A., McLaughlin, J. R., Cole, D. E., Rosen, B., Bradley, L., Kwan, E., *et al.* (2001). Prevalence and penetrance of germline BRCA1 and BRCA2 mutations in a population series of 649 women with ovarian cancer. *Am. J. Hum. Genet.*, **68**, 700–10.

Risch, H. A., Weiss, N. S., Lyon, J. L., Daling, J. R., and Liff, J. M. (1983). Events of reproductive life and the incidence of epithelial ovarian cancer. *Am. J. Epidemiol.*, **117**, 128–39.

Rodriguez, I. M. and Prat, J. (2002). Mucinous tumors of the ovary: a clinicopathologic analysis of 75 borderline tumors (of intestinal type) and carcinomas. *Am. J. Surg. Pathol.*, **26**, 139–52.

Rodriguez, C., Calle, E. E., Coates, R. J., Miracle-McMahill, H. L., Thun, M. J., and Heath, C. W., Jr. (1995). Estrogen replacement therapy and fatal ovarian cancer. *Am. J. Epidemiol.*, **141**, 828–35.

Rodriguez, G. C., Walmer, D. K., Cline, M., Krigman, H., Lessey, B. A., Whitaker, R. S., *et al.* (1998). Effect of progestin on the ovarian epithelium of macaques: cancer prevention through apoptosis? *J. Soc. Gynecol. Investig.*, **5**, 271–6.

Sasson, I. M., Haley, N. J., Hoffmann, D., Wynder, E. L., Hellberg, D., and Nilsson, S. (1985). Cigarette smoking and neoplasia of the uterine cervix: smoke constituents in cervical mucus. *N. Engl. J. Med.*, **312**, 315–6.

Schildkraut, J. M., Bastos, E., and Berchuck, A. (1997). Relationship between lifetime ovulatory cycles and overexpression of mutant p53 in epithelial ovarian cancer. *J. Natl. Cancer Inst.*, **89**, 932–8.

Schildkraut, J. M., Calingaert, B., Marchbanks, P. A., Moorman, P. G., and Rodriguez, G. C. (2002). Impact of progestin and estrogen potency in oral contraceptives on ovarian cancer risk. *J. Natl. Cancer Inst.*, **94**, 32–8.

Slattery, M. L., Schuman, K. L., West, D. W., French, T. K., and Robison, L. M. (1989). Nutrient intake and ovarian cancer. *Am. J. Epidemiol.*, **130**, 497–502.

Smith, E. M., Sowers, M. F., and Burns, T. L. (1984). Effects of smoking on the development of female reproductive cancers. *J. Natl. Cancer Inst.*, **73**, 371–6.

Spurdle, A. B., Purdie, D. M., Webb, P. M., Chen, X., Green, A., and Chenevix-Trench, G. (2001). The microsomal epoxide hydrolase Tyr113His polymorphism: association with risk of ovarian cancer. *Mol. Carcinog.*, **30**, 71–8.

Stockwell, H. G. and Lyman, G. H. (1987). Cigarette smoking and the risk of female reproductive cancer. *Am. J. Obstet. Gynecol.*, **157**, 35–40.

The Cancer and Steroid Hormone Study of the Centers for Disease Control and the National Institute of Child Health and Human Development (1987). The reduction in risk of ovarian cancer associated with oral-contraceptive use. *N. Engl. J. Med.*, **316**, 650–5.

The WHO Collaborative Study of Neoplasia and Steroid Contraceptives (1989). Epithelial ovarian cancer and combined oral contraceptives. *Int. J. Epidemiol.*, **18**, 538–45.

Trichopoulos, D., Papapostolou, M., and Polychronopoulou, A. (1981). Coffee and ovarian cancer. *Int. J. Cancer*, **28**, 691–3.

Tzonou, A., Day, N. E., Trichopoulos, D., Walker, A., Saliaraki, M., Papapostolou, M., *et al.* (1984). The epidemiology of ovarian cancer in Greece: a case–control study. *Eur. J. Cancer Clin. Oncol.*, **20**, 1045–52.

Van Voorhis, B. J., Syrop, C. H., Hammitt, D. G., Dunn, M. S., and Snyder, G. D. (1992). Effects of smoking on ovulation induction for assisted reproductive techniques. *Fertil. Steril.*, **58**, 981–5.

Whittemore, A. S., Harris, R., and Itnyre, J. (1992). Characteristics relating to ovarian cancer risk: collaborative analysis of 12 US case–control studies. II. Invasive epithelial ovarian cancers in white women. Collaborative Ovarian Cancer Group. *Am. J. Epidemiol.*, **136**, 1184–203.

Whittemore, A. S., Wu, M. L., Paffenbarger, R. S., Jr., Sarles, D. L., Kampert, J. B., Grosser, S., *et al.* (1988). Personal and environmental characteristics related to epithelial ovarian cancer. II. Exposures to talcum powder, tobacco, alcohol, and coffee. *Am. J. Epidemiol.*, **128**, 1228–40.

Wynder, E. L., Dodo, H., and Barber, H. R. (1969). Epidemiology of cancer of the ovary. *Cancer*, **23**, 352–70.

Young, R. H. and Hart, W. R. (1989). Metastases from carcinomas of the pancreas simulating primary mucinous tumors of the ovary. A report of seven cases. *Am. J. Surg. Pathol.*, **13**, 748–56.

Zeimet, A. G., Muller-Holzner, E., Marth, C., and Daxenbichler, G. (1994). Immunocytochemical versus biochemical receptor determination in normal and tumorous tissues of the female reproductive tract and the breast. *J. Steroid. Biochem. Mol. Biol.*, **49**, 365–72.

Chapter 31

Endometrial cancer

Paul D. Terry, Thomas E. Rohan, Silvia Franceschi
and Elisabete Weiderpass

Endometrial adenocarinoma accounts for approximately one of every 10 cancers diagnosed among women worldwide, with incidence rates varying at least 10-fold between
areas of low incidence (such as North Africa and China) and high incidence (such as
North America) (Parker *et al.* 1997; Parkin *et al.* 1999). The use of exogenous estrogens, and of estrogen replacement therapy in particular, has been strongly related to
increased risk in epidemiological studies (IARC 1999; Akhmedkhanov *et al.* 2001).
Exogenous estrogens unopposed by progesterone have been hypothesized to increase
the risk of this malignancy through increased mitotic activity of endometrial cells,
increased number of DNA replication errors, and somatic mutations resulting in the
malignant phenotype (Akhmedkhanov *et al.* 2001). Hence, factors associated with
estrogen absorption or metabolism may alter the risk of this malignancy. In this
regard, it has been hypothesized that cigarette smoking might be associated with anti-
estrogenic effects, and through this mechanism reduce the risk of endometrial cancer
(Baron 1984; Baron *et al.* 1990). Our aim here is to review the current literature on
cigarette smoking and endometrial cancer risk. We review published studies identified
through searches of the Medline and Cancerlit databases and cross-matching the references of relevant articles. Virtually all published reports are in the English language,
and we have restricted our review to those.

Studies of cigarette smoking and endometrial cancer risk

To date, at least 26 epidemiological studies have examined the association between
smoking and endometrial cancer risk (Williams and Horm 1977; Weiss *et al.* 1980;
Kelsey *et al.* 1982; Smith *et al.* 1984; Lesko *et al.* 1985; Tyler *et al.* 1985; Baron *et al.*
1986; Franks *et al.* 1987; Lawrence *et al.* 1987, 1989; Levi *et al.* 1987; Stockwell
and Lyman 1987; Koumantaki *et al.* 1989; Elliott *et al.* 1990; Rubin *et al.* 1990; Austin
et al. 1993; Brinton *et al.* 1993; Engeland *et al.* 1996; Goodman *et al.* 1997; Shields *et al.*
1999; Terry *et al.* 1999, 2002*a*, *b*; Jain *et al.* 2000; McCann *et al.* 2000; Newcomer *et al.*
2001; Weiderpass and Baron 2001). These studies have been categorized according
to their basic design (case–control or cohort) and the type of smoking measures used
(qualitative or quantitative). Studies that have used both qualitative (e.g. 'ever', 'current',

or 'former' smoker) and quantitative measures (e.g. number of cigarettes per day or years of smoking duration) are reviewed in both sections.

Current, former, ever, and never smokers

Cohort studies

Cohort studies are those in which exposure assessment precedes the quantification of disease occurrence in exposed and unexposed individuals. To date, there have been three prospective cohort studies (Engeland *et al.* 1996; Terry *et al.* 1999, 2002*a*) of the association between cigarette smoking and endometrial cancer risk (Table 31.1). These studies do not support clearly a reduction in endometrial cancer risk among current or former smokers compared with never smokers. However, the results of two of these studies (Engeland *et al.* 1996; Terry *et al.* 1999) were based on a small number of cases and a limited number of women with long-term or intense cigarette smoking.

Case–control studies

The results of 12 population-based case–control studies (Smith *et al.* 1984; Tyler *et al.* 1985; Franks *et al.* 1987; Elliott *et al.* 1990; Rubin *et al.* 1990; Brinton *et al.* 1993; Goodman *et al.* 1997; Shields *et al.* 1999; Jain *et al.* 2000; McCann *et al.* 2000; Newcomer *et al.* 2001; Weiderpass and Baron 2001), that have included between 46 and 740 endometrial cancer cases, generally have shown small to moderate reduced risks among current smokers compared to never smokers, but have shown no association with risk among former smokers compared to never smokers (Tables 31.1 and 31.3). The results of six hospital-based case–control studies (Kelsey *et al.* 1982; Lesko *et al.* 1985; Levi *et al.* 1987; Stockwell and Lyman 1987; Koumantaki *et al.* 1989; Austin *et al.* 1993), that have included between 83 and 1374 endometrial cancer cases, are consistent with those of population-based studies in showing moderate (e.g. 30–40%) lower risks among current compared with never smokers, but do not show altered risks (or perhaps small 10–20% reduced risks) in former compared to never smokers (Table 31.1). The largest of the hospital-based studies (Stockwell and Lyman 1987), with 1374 cases and 3921 controls, found both former and current smokers to be at moderately (approximately 30%) reduced risk of endometrial cancer.

Quantitative measures of smoking

Cohort studies

Two (Terry *et al.* 1999, 2002*a*) of the three (Engeland *et al.* 1996; Terry *et al.* 1999, 2002*a*) prospective cohort studies mentioned in the previous section have examined quantitative smoking measures in relation to endometrial cancer risk. The results of these studies were consistent with the inverse associations with current smoking (but not former smoking) observed in the case–control studies (Table 31.2). Of these two

Table 31.1 Epidemiological studies of cigarette smoking and endometrial cancer risk: current, former, and never smokers

First author, study year	Study design	Cases/ controls (# in Cohort)	Age range at recruitment	Ever smoking vs. never OR (95% CI)	Former smoking vs. never OR (95% CI)	Current smoking vs. never OR (95% CI)	Adjustment for:*
Engeland et al. 1996	Prospective cohort	140/26 000	32–72	–	1.2 (0.6–2.2)	1.1 (0.7–1.6)	Not specified
Terry 1999	Prospective cohort	123/11 659	42–82	–	0.7 (0.3–2.0)	0.9 (NO CI)†	Age, weight, parity
Terry 2002	Prospective cohort	403/70 591	40–59	–	1.0 (0.8–1.3)	0.8 (0.6–1.1)	Age, BMI, HRT, parity
Brinton et al. 1993	Population case–control	405/297	20–74	0.8 (0.5–1.1)	1.1 (0.7–1.6)	0.4 (0.2–0.7)	Age, weight, HRT, parity, diabetes, age at menopause
Elliot et al. 1990	Population case–control	46/138	–	–	1.4 (0.6–3.5)	0.2 (0.1–0.6)	Age, BMI, HRT, parity, diabetes
Franks et al. 1987	Population case–control	79/416	20–55	0.5 (0.3–0.8)	–	–	Age, BMI, HRT, parity, diabetes, age at menopause
Goodman et al. 1997	Population case–control	332/511	18–84	0.8 (0.6–1.2)	–	–	Age, BMI, HRT, parity, diabetes
Jain et al. 2000	Population case–control	220/223	30–79	1.0 (0.8–1.3)	–	–	None
McCann et al. 2000	Population case–control	236/639	40–85	0.6 (0.4–0.8)	–	–	Age
Newcomer et al. 2001	Population case–control	740/2372	40–79	0.8 (0.7–0.9)	0.8 (0.7–1.0)	0.8 (0.6–1.0)	Age, BMI, HRT, parity, diabetes
Rubin et al. 1990	Population case–control	196/986	20–54	–	0.8 (0.5–1.2)	0.7 (0.5–1.0)	Age, BMI, treatment for diabetes
Shields et al. 1999	Population case–control	553/752	45–64	–	0.8 (0.6–1.2)‡	0.6 (0.4–0.8)‡	Age, BMI

Table 31.1 (continued) Epidemiological studies of cigarette smoking and endometrial cancer risk: current, former, and never smokers

First author, study year	Study design	Cases/controls (# in Cohort)	Age range at recruitment	Ever smoking vs. never OR (95% CI)	Former smoking vs. never OR (95% CI)	Current smoking vs. never OR (95% CI)	Adjustment for:*
Smith et al. 1984	Population case–control	70/612	20–54	0.8 (0.4–1.5)	–	–	Age, BMI, HRT, parity, age at menopause
Tyler et al. 1985	Population case–control	437/3200	20–54	0.9 (0.7–1.1)	1.0 (0.7–1.4)	0.8 (0.7–1.1)	Age, Weight, HRT, age at menopause
Weiderpass and Baron, 2001	Population case–control	709/3368	50–74	–	0.9 (0.7–1.1)	0.6 (0.5–0.8)	Age, BMI, HRT, parity, diabetes, age at menopause
Austin et al. 1993	Hospital case–control	168/334	40–82	–	0.8 (0.5–1.5)	0.7 (0.4–1.2)	Age, BMI, HRT, parity, diabetes
Kelsey et al. 1982§	Hospital case–control	167/903	45–74	0.8 (NO CI)	–	–	Age, HRT, age at menopause
Koumantaki et al. 1989	Hospital case–control	83/164	40–79	–	–	0.5 (0.2–1.3)¶	Age, height, weigh, HRT, parity, age at menopause
Lesko et al. 1985	Hospital case–control	510/727	18–69	–	0.9 (0.6–1.2)	0.8 (NO CI)†	Age, BMI, HRT, age at menopause, parity, diabetes
Levi et al. 1987	Hospital case–control	357/1122	31–74	–	0.9 (0.5–1.5)	0.5 (0.3–0.7)	Age, BMI, HRT, parity, age at menopause
Stockwell and Lyman 1987	Hospital case–control	1374/3921	–	–	0.6 (0.5–0.8)	0.7 (NO CI)†	Age

*Covariates considered here are: age, body mass index (BMI), hormone replacement therapy (HRT), age at menopause, parity, diabetes.

†Crude measures of association were calculated from the data provided.

‡Results shown are for women not taking unopposed estrogens. Among estrogen users, smokers were also at higher risk than nonsmokers.

§Results reported in Baron (1984).

¶Former smokers were combined with never smokers in this analysis.

Note: The table was originally published in Lancet Oncology 2002;3:470–80 and has been reproduced with permission.

studies (Terry *et al.* 1999, 2002*a*), one (Terry *et al.* 1999) found a 50 per cent reduced risk among current smokers in the highest level of intensity (11 cigarettes per day or more) compared to nonsmokers, but the number of cases was low and the confidence intervals correspondingly wide. The more recent and larger of the two cohort studies (Terry *et al.* 2002*a*) found a statistically significant 40 per cent reduced risk among current smokers of more than 20 cigarettes per day, but showed somewhat weaker and statistically nonsignificant reductions in risk with smoking of long duration or high consumption of pack-years. In contrast, the risk among former smokers was similar to that among never smokers.

Case–control studies

To date, six population-based case–control studies (Lawrence *et al.* 1987, 1989; Tyler *et al.* 1985; Brinton *et al.* 1993; Newcomer *et al.* 2001; Weiderpass and Baron 2001) have examined quantitative measures of smoking in relation to endometrial cancer risk, generally showing inverse associations to be strongest among current smokers of high intensity or long duration (Tables 31.2 and 31.3). However, one population-based study of late-stage endometrial cancer (Lawrence *et al.* 1989) did not show an association with any measure of smoking (although the number of cases in that study was relatively small); in another small study (Lawrence *et al.* 1987), the same investigators found that smoking more than 20 cigarettes per day was associated with a reduced risk of early-stage endometrial cancer among both current and former smokers. While the majority of these studies adjusted their relative risk estimates for potentially confounding variables, such as body mass index (BMI) (weight (kg)/height (m)^2), hormone replacement therapy (HRT), parity, diabetes, and age at menopause (Table 31.1), studies that did not adjust for these variables tended to show similar inverse associations. Within individual studies, statistical adjustment for the effects of BMI and other covariates often made little difference, although some attenuation of relative-risk estimates have been noted (Weiderpass and Baron 2001; Terry *et al.* 2002*a*).

Six hospital-based case–control studies of endometrial cancer that examined quantitative measures of smoking have mostly shown statistically significant 30–60 per cent reduced risks with current or recent smoking of high intensity (Lesko *et al.* 1985; Levi *et al.* 1987; Stockwell and Lyman 1987), with smoking of long duration (Koumantaki *et al.* 1989), or with a relatively large number of pack-years (Table 31.2) (Williams and Horm 1977; Baron *et al.* 1986). However, the fact that the various smoking measures are correlated with each other complicates the differentiation of their independent effects. For example, smokers of high intensity also tend to be smokers of long duration (Terry *et al.* 2002*a*), and the latter also tend to have commenced smoking at an early age.

Effect modification

A number of studies have examined the association between smoking and endometrial cancer risk according to factors that are known determinants of endogenous hormone

Table 31.2 Epidemiological studies of cigarette smoking and endometrial cancer risk: smoking frequency, duration, and pack-years

First author, study year	Study design	# Cases/controls (# in cohort)	Age range	Smoking intensity (cigarettes/day)		Smoking duration (years)		Pack-years (packs/day*years)	
				Comparison	OR (95% CI)	Comparison	OR (95% CI)	Comparison	OR (95% CI)
Terry 1999	Prospective cohort	123/11 659	42–82	Current 11+ vs. never	0.5 (0.1–2.0)	–	–	–	–
Terry 2002	Prospective cohort	403/70 591	40–59	Former >20 vs. never	0.9 (0.6–1.3)	Former >20 vs. never	1.1 (0.8–1.6)	Former >20 vs. never	1.0 (0.7–1.5)
				Current >20 vs. never	0.6 (0.4–0.9)*	Current >20 vs. never	0.8 (0.6–1.1)	Current >20 vs. never	0.7 (0.5–1.1)
Brinton 1993	Population case-control	405/297	20–74	Ever 30+ vs. never	0.7 (0.4–1.4)	Ever 40+ vs. never	0.5 (0.3–0.9)*	–	–
				Former 30+ vs. never	1.4 (NO CI)	Former 40+ vs. never	0.5 (NO CI)		
				Current 30+ vs. never	0.3 (NO CI)	Current 40+ vs. never	0.5 (NO CI)		
Lawrence 1987	Population case-control	301/289	40–69	Former >20 vs. never	0.6 (NO CI)	–	–	–	–
				Current >20 vs. never	0.5 (NO CI)				
Lawrence 1989	Population case-control	84/168	40–69	Former > 20 vs. never	1.0 (NO CI)	–	–	–	–
				Current >20 vs. never	1.0 (NO CI)				

Study	Design	Cases/controls	Age	Exposure	OR (95% CI)	Exposure	OR (95% CI)	Exposure	OR (95% CI)
Newcomer 2001	Population case-control	740/2372	40–79	–	–	–	–	Ever 80+ vs. never	0.9 (0.5–1.4)
Tyler, 1985	Population case-control	437/3200	20–54	–	–	–	–	Ever 15+ vs. never	1.0 (0.7–1.2)
Weiderpass 2001	Population case-control	709/3368	50–74	Maximum 20+ vs. never	0.7 (0.4–1.3)	Lifelong 45+ vs. never	0.6 (0.3–0.9)	–	–
Baron 1986	Hospital case-control	476/2128	40–89	–	–	–	–	Ever 15+ vs. never	0.6 (0.4–0.9)*
Koumantaki 1989	Hospital case-control	83/164	40–79	–	–	20+ (continuous variable)	0.5 (0.3–0.9)*	–	–
Lesko 1985	Hospital case-control	510/727	18–69	Current 25+ vs. never	0.5 (0.3–0.8)	–	–	–	–
Levi 1987	Hospital case-control	357/1122	31–74	Current 15+ vs. never	0.4 (0.2–0.9)*	–	–	–	–
Stockwell and Lyman 1987	Hospital case-control	1374/3921	–	Current >40 vs. never	0.5 (0.3–0.9)	–	–	–	–
Williams and Horm 1977	Hospital case-control	358/3189	25–76	–	–	–	–	Ever 40+ vs. never	0.7 (NS)

*Statistically significant test of trend reported.

Note: The table was originally published in Lancet Oncology 2002;3:470–80 and has been reproduced with permission.

Table 31.3 Epidemiological studies of cigarette smoking and endometrial cancer risk according to menopausal status

First author, study year	Study design	# Cases/controls (# in cohort)	Comparison	Premenopausal OR (95% CI)	Postmenopausal OF (95% CI)
Terry 2002	Prospective Cohort	403/70,591	Current >20 cigarettes/day vs. never	0.7 (0.4–1.3)	0.5 (0.3–1.1)
Brinton 1993	Population case–control	405/297	Former vs. never smokers	3.0 (1.2–7.4)	0.8 (0.4–1.2)
			Current vs. never smokers	0.5 (0.1–1.7)	C.4 (0.2–0.7)
			Ever 30+ years vs. never	6.2 (0.9–42.3)	0.6 (0.4–1.0)*
			Ever 30+ cigarettes/day vs. never	1.3 (0.2–7.1)	0.6 (0.3–1.3)*
Franks 1987	Population case–control	79/416	Ever vs. never smokers	–	0.5 (0.3–0.8)
Lawrence 1987	Population case–control	301/289	Current vs. never smokers	0.6 (NO CI)	0.6 (NO CI)
Smith 1984	Population case–control	70/612	Ever vs. never smokers	1.3 (0.7–2.5)	0.4 (0.2–1.0)
Weiderpass and Baron2001	Population case–control	709/3368	Current (highest level of duration)	0.9 (0.4–2.0)	0.4 (0.2–0.8)
Koumantaki 1989	Hospital case–control	83/164	Current vs. former+nonsmokers	2.3 (NO CI)	0.2 (NO CI)
Lesko 1985	Hospital case–control	510/727	Current 25+vs. never smokers	0.9 (0.4–2.2)	0.5 (0.2–0.9)
Levi 1987	Hospital case–control	357/1122	Current vs. never smokers	0.5 (0.2–0.9)	0.4 (0.3–0.7)
Stockwell 1987†	Hospital case–control	1374/3921	Current >40 vs. never smokers	1.9 (0.5–7.8)	0.4 (0.2–0.8)

*Statistically significant test of trend reported

†In this study the stratification categories were <50 vs. 50 + years

Note: The table was originally published in Lancet Oncology 2002;3:470–80 and has been reproduced with permission.

levels, and which may counteract or augment possible tobacco-related hormonal changes. These factors include menopausal status, HRT, and BMI. Effect modification can reflect true underlying differences in the association across strata, for example, if cigarette smoking acted to reduce or modify estrogen levels differently in one group compared to another, but can also reflect methodological factors, such as differences that occur by chance or through the varying prevalence of confounding variables.

Menopausal status

Although endometrial cancer is rare among premenopausal women, several studies have examined the association between cigarette smoking and endometrial cancer risk according to menopausal status, including one prospective cohort study (Terry *et al.* 2002*a*), five population-based case–control studies (Smith *et al.* 1984; Franks *et al.* 1987; Lawrence *et al.* 1987; Brinton *et al.* 1993; Weiderpass and Baron 2001), and four hospital-based case–control studies (Lesko *et al.* 1985; Levi *et al.* 1987; Stockwell and Lyman 1987; Koumantaki *et al.* 1989) (Table 31.3). In all but one of these studies, a study of early stage endometrial cancer (Lawrence *et al.* 1987), the inverse association was (to varying degrees) stronger among postmenopausal than premenopausal women. Among premenopausal women, the relative risk estimates for cigarette smoking have been inconsistent, sometimes showing increased risks with certain measures of cigarette smoking (Smith *et al.* 1984; Stockwell and Lyman 1987; Koumantaki *et al.* 1989; Brinton *et al.* 1993), sometimes showing decreased risks (Lawrence *et al.* 1987; Levi *et al.* 1987; Brinton *et al.* 1993; Terry *et al.* 2002*a*), and sometimes showing practically no association (Lesko *et al.* 1985; Weiderpass and Baron 2001). In analyses limited to postmenopausal women, on the other hand, all showed between 20 and 80 per cent reduced risks of endometrial cancer with the various smoking measures.

Hormone replacement therapy (HRT)

Given the possibility that cigarette smoking is associated with blood hormone levels mostly among women who are taking HRT (Jensen *et al.* 1985; Jensen and Christiansen, 1988; Cassidenti *et al.* 1990), one might speculate that an inverse association between smoking and endometrial cancer risk would be stronger among HRT users than among nonusers. However, the results of studies that have examined the association between smoking and endometrial cancer risk according to HRT use (Weiss *et al.* 1980; Franks *et al.* 1987; Lawrence *et al.* 1987; Levi *et al.* 1987; Terry *et al* 2002*a*) are equivocal in showing such a pattern (Table 31.4). While two studies (Franks *et al.* 1987; Levi *et al.* 1987) observed a larger reduction in risk among smokers taking HRT than among smokers not taking HRT, two other studies (Lawrence *et al.* 1987; Terry *et al.* 2002*a*) found no difference in the association according to HRT status, including a large prospective cohort study (Terry *et al.* 2002*a*). Thus, although effect modification by HRT status is biologically plausible, the available epidemiological evidence is equivocal.

Table 31.4 Epidemiological studies of cigarette smoking and endometrial cancer risk according to hormone replacement therapy (HRT) use

First author, study year	Study design	# Cases/controls (# in cohort)	Comparison	No HRT OR (95% CI)	HRT OR (95% CI)
Terry et al. 2002	Prospective cohort	403/70,591	Current > 20 cigarettes/day vs. never	0.6 (0.4–1.0)*	0.6 (0.3–1.3)
Franks et al. 1987	Population case–control	79/416	Ever vs. never smokers	0.5 (0.3–0.9)	0.3 (0.1–0.8)
Lawrence et al. 1987	Population case–control	301/289	Current vs. never smokers	0.6 (NO CI)	0.6 (NO CI)
Weiss et al. 1980	Population case–control	322/289	Ever vs. never smokers	0.4 (0.2–0.7)	–
Levi et al. 1987	Hospital case–control	357/1122	Current vs. never smokers	0.5 (0.3–0.7)	0.2 (0.1–0.7)

*Statistically significant test of trend reported.

Note: The table was originally published in Lancet Oncology 2002;3:470–80 and has been reproduced with permission.

Relative body weight

Obesity is an established risk factor for endometrial cancer (IARC 2002). Given the fact that smokers tend to have lower BMI than nonsmokers (although former smokers tend to have a higher BMI than current or never smokers) (Baron *et al.* 1990), two case–control studies have examined the association between cigarette smoking and endometrial cancer risk according to BMI (Levi *et al.* 1987; Elliott *et al.* 1990). Neither of these studies, one hospital-based (Levi *et al.* 1987) and one population-based (Elliott *et al.* 1990), found any clear differences in the association between smoking and endometrial cancer risk according to BMI. Another study (Lawrence *et al.* 1987), a population-based case–control study of early stage endometrial cancer, observed the inverse association with cigarette smoking to become stronger with increasing absolute rather than relative body weight.

Studies of cigarette smoking and blood hormone levels

Whether mediated through changes in the amount of adipose tissue, altered age at menopause, or anti-estrogenic effects, blood hormone levels might be an important link between smoking and the reduced risk of endometrial cancer observed in most of the studies discussed above. The estrogens that have typically been studied in relation to cigarette smoking include estrone, sex-hormone binding globulin (SHBG)-bound estradiol, and estriol. Blood levels of androgens, typically androstenedione and dehydroepiandrosterone (DHEAS), have also been studied, since these are biological precursors of estrone. Studies that have examined blood levels of SHBG are less common, and studies of unbound (free) estradiol are scarce.

Smoking and blood estrogen levels

Studies of cigarette smoking and blood hormone levels have been conducted mostly among postmenopausal women who were not taking HRT (Table 31.5). Of these studies, nine examined serum (Friedman *et al.* 1987; Cauley *et al.* 1989; Slemenda *et al.* 1989; Schlemmer *et al.* 1990; Cassidenti *et al.* 1992; Austin *et al.* 1993; Law *et al.* 1997) or plasma (Khaw *et al.* 1988; Longcope and Johnston 1988) estrone, ten examined serum (Friedman *et al.* 1987; Cauley *et al.* 1989; Slemenda *et al.* 1989; Schlemmer *et al.* 1990; Key *et al.* 1991; Cassidenti *et al.* 1992; Austin *et al.* 1993; Law *et al.* 1997) or plasma (Khaw *et al.* 1988; Longcope and Johnston 1988) estradiol, and two examined serum (Cassidenti *et al.* 1992) or plasma-free (Longcope and Johnston 1988) estradiol. As shown in Table 31.5, these studies have been consistent in showing little or no association between smoking and blood estrogen levels among postmenopausal women who were not taking hormone replacement therapy. Among premenopausal women, three studies (Longcope and Johnston 1988; Key *et al.* 1991; Berta *et al.* 1992) found no clear association between cigarette smoking and estrogen levels. Studies that adjusted hormone measurements for the effects of BMI (and other covariates) showed similar

Table 31.5 Studies of cigarette smoking and blood hormone levels

First author, study year	Study population	Sex hormones examined	Major differences in blood hormone levels between smokers and nonsmokers	Additional adjustment for BMI
Austin et al. 1993	209 postmenopausal women not taking HRT	Serum E1, E2, Δ^4A	No major differences	Yes
Berta et al. 1992	694 premenopausal women with BMI < 25	Plasma E1, E2	No major differences	No
Cassidenti et al. 1990	25 postmenopausal women randomized to take 1 or 2 mg micronized E2	Serum E1, E2, unbound E2, SHBG	Unbound E2 (lower) and SHBG-binding capacity (higher) in smokers	Randomization
Cassidenti et al. 1992	38 postmenopausal women not taking HRT	Serum E1, E2, SHBG, non-SHBG-bound E2, Δ^4A, DHEAS	Δ^4A (higher) and DHEAS (higher) in smokers	Yes
Cauley et al. 1989	143 postmenopausal women not taking HRT	Serum E1, E2, Δ^4A	Δ^4A (higher) in smokers	Yes
Friedman et al. 1987	25 postmenopausal women not taking HRT	Serum E1, E2, Δ^4A, DHEAS	Δ^4A (higher) and DHEAS (higher) in smokers	Yes
Jensen et al. 1985	136 postmenopausal women randomized to 4, 2, or 1 mg E2, or placebo	Serum E1, E2	E1 (lower) and E2 (lower) in smokers	Randomization
Jensen and Christiansen 1988	110 postmenopausal women randomized to oral or percutaneous E2 or placebo	Serum E1, E2	E1 (lower) and E2 (lower) in smokers after oral E2	Randomization

Study	Population	Measurements	Findings	
Key et al. 1991	147 pre- and postmenopausal women not taking HRT	Serum E2, DHEAS	No major differences	Yes
Khaw et al. 1988	233 postmenopausal women not taking HRT	Plasma DHEAS, Δ^4A, E1, E2, SHBG	Δ^4A (higher) and DHEAS (higher) in smokers	Yes
Lapidus et al. 1986	253 postmenopausal women not taking HRT	Serum SHBG	No major differences	Yes
Law et al. 1997	1219 pre- and postmenopausal women not taking HRT	Serum E1, E2, Δ^4A, DHEAS, SHBG	No major differences	Yes
Longcope and Johnston 1988	88 pre- and postmenopausal women not taking HRT	Plasma Δ^4A, E1, E2, free E2, SHBG	Δ^4A (higher) in smokers	Yes
Michnovicz et al. 1986	27 premenopausal women not taking HRT, BMI<25	2-Hydroxylation of injected radiolabeled E2	2-Hydroxylation of E2 (higher) in smokers	No
Schlemmer et al. 1990	267 women in the early postmenopause	Serum E1, E2, Δ^4A	Δ^4A (higher) in smokers	No
Slemenda et al. 1989	84 peri- and postmenopausal women	Serum E1, E2, Δ^4A	Δ^4A (higher) in smokers	No

Abbreviations: E1 (estrone), E2 (estradiol), Δ^4A (androstenedione), DHEAS (dehydroepiandrosterone), SHBG (sex-hormone binding globulin), HRT (hormone replacement therapy), BMI (body mass index).

Note: The table was originally published in Lancet Oncology 2002;3:470–80 and has been reproduced with permission.

results to those that did not, suggesting that BMI is not a strong confounding variable in this association.

Two studies examined the association between cigarette smoking and blood estrogen levels after randomization of women to groups receiving either estradiol or placebo (Table 31.5) (Jensen and Christiansen 1988; Cassidenti *et al.* 1990). In a small study of 25 postmenopausal women (Cassidenti *et al.* 1990), unbound estradiol was significantly lower among smokers than nonsmokers both at baseline and shortly after taking micronized estradiol orally. No important differences were observed between smokers and nonsmokers in serum levels of either estrone or bound estradiol. In contrast, a study in which 110 postmenopausal women were randomized to take hormones (either orally or percutaneously) or a placebo (Jensen and Christiansen 1988) found that smokers had lower levels of both estrone and bound estradiol than nonsmokers after oral (but not percutaneous) hormone treatment for at least one year (levels of free estrogens were not examined). These results indicate that smoking might affect the absorption or metabolism of hormones used in replacement therapy.

Smoking and blood sex-hormone binding globulin (SHBG) levels

Of the five studies that have examined the association between cigarette smoking and serum (Lapidus *et al.* 1986; Cassidenti *et al.* 1992; Law *et al.* 1997) or plasma (Khaw *et al.* 1988; Longcope and Johnston 1988) SHBG, none found any clear association. However, one of these studies (Khaw *et al.* 1988) found an inverse association between smoking and the ratio of bound estradiol to SHBG, a measure of estrogen activity. In this context, it is interesting to note that Cassidenti *et al.* (1990) found unbound (but not SHBG-bound) estradiol significantly lower among smokers than nonsmokers both at baseline and after taking oral estradiol, suggesting an increased SHBG-binding capacity in the women who smoked.

Smoking and blood androgen levels

In postmenopausal women, androgens are the major source of estrone, converted through an aromatization process in fat deposits. Thus, adiposity is positively correlated with estrogen levels in postmenopausal women. Of the nine studies that examined blood levels of androstenedione in smokers (Friedman *et al.* 1987; Khaw *et al.* 1988; Longcope and Johnston 1988; Cauley *et al.* 1989; Slemenda *et al.* 1989; Schlemmer *et al.* 1990; Cassidenti *et al.* 1992; Austin *et al.* 1993; Law *et al.* 1997), all found higher circulating levels among current than never or former smokers (Table 31.5). However, these same studies did not show clear variation in blood estrone levels by smoking status, perhaps suggesting a reduced conversion of androstenedione to estrone among smokers. Of the five studies that have examined cigarette smoking and DHEAS levels, three (Friedman *et al.* 1987; Khaw *et al.* 1988; Cassidenti *et al.* 1992) found increased blood levels among current smokers, while the other two (Key *et al.* 1991; Law *et al.* 1997) found no clear differences according to smoking status.

Studies of cigarette smoking and urinary hormone levels

Seven studies have examined cigarette smoking and urinary estrogen levels (MacMahon *et al.* 1982; Michnovicz *et al.* 1986, 1988; Trichopoulos *et al.* 1987; Berta *et al.* 1992; Key *et al.* 1996; Berstein *et al.* 2000) (Table 31.6), and of these, three found no major differences according to smoking status (Trichopoulos *et al.* 1987; Michnovicz *et al.* 1988; Berta *et al.* 1992). The remaining four studies each showed lower urinary estriol levels among smokers than nonsmokers, but mixed results for urinary estrone and estradiol (MacMahon *et al.* 1982; Michnovicz *et al.* 1986; Key *et al.* 1996; Berstein *et al.* 2000). The results of two of these studies (Michnovicz *et al.* 1988; Berstein *et al.* 2000) showed lower levels of 2-hydroxyestrone among smokers than nonsmokers.

Studies of cigarette smoking and age at menopause

Age at natural menopause varies substantially under the influence of genetic and environmental factors (McKinlay 1996). A relatively early age at menopause has been associated with reduced risk of endometrial cancer (Kelsey *et al.* 1982; Baron 1984; Baron *et al.* 1990; Akhmedkhanov *et al.* 2001). For example, a one year decrease in age at menopause has been associated approximately with a 7 per cent decrease in risk (Kelsey *et al.* 1982). In this regard, it has been proposed that cigarette smoking decreases the age at natural menopause (Baron *et al.* 1990), and might reduce endometrial cancer risk through reduced exposure to endogenous estrogens. At least 19 studies have examined the association between cigarette smoking and age at natural menopause (Hammond 1961; Daniell 1976, 1978; Bailey *et al.* 1977; Jick and Porter 1977; McNamara *et al.* 1978; Lindquist and Bengtsson 1979; van Keep *et al.* 1979; Kaufman *et al.* 1980; Adena and Gallagher 1982; Andersen *et al.* 1982; Willett *et al.* 1983; McKinlay *et al.* 1985; Brinton *et al.* 1986; Hiatt and Fireman 1986; Stanford *et al.* 1987; Brownson *et al.* 1988; Chu *et al.* 1990; Field *et al.* 1992) (Table 31.7). In these studies, differences in age at menopause between smokers and nonsmokers were measured in terms of differences in means (Daniell 1976, 1978; McNamara 1978; Kaufman *et al.* 1980; Adena and Gallagher 1982; Hiatt and Fireman 1986; Field *et al.* 1992; Weiderpass *et al.* 1999), medians (McKinlay *et al.* 1985; Brinton *et al.* 1986; Stanford *et al.* 1987; Brownson *et al.* 1988; Chu *et al.* 1990), or the percentage of women who reached menopause by a certain age (Hammond 1961; Bailey *et al.* 1977; Jick and Porter 1977; Lindquist and Bengtsson 1979; van Keep *et al.* 1979; Andersen *et al.* 1982; Willett *et al.* 1983) (these latter studies are not shown in Table 31.7). These studies have shown that, on average, smokers have menopause 1–1.5 years earlier than nonsmokers. There are no clear differences in the results of studies that adjusted estimates for obesity (and other covariates) compared to those that did not.

Table 31.6 Studies of cigarette smoking and urinary hormone levels

First author, study year	Study population	Sex hormones examined	Differences in urinary hormone excretion levels between smokers and nonsmokers	Additional adjustment for BMI
Bernstein et al. 2000	16 postmenopausal women before and after taking 2 mg per os/d E2	Urinary E1, E2, E3, 16αOHE$_1$, 2OHE$_1$	E1 and E3 (lower), E2 and 2OHE$_1$ (higher) in smokers after treatment	No
Berta et al. 1992	694 premenopausal women, BMI<25	Urinary E1, E2, E3	No major differences	No
Key et al. 1996	367 pre- and postmenopausal women	Urinary E1, E2, E3	E3 (lower) in postmenopausal smokers	Yes
MacMahon et al. 1982	106 premenopausal women not taking HRT	Urinary E1, E2, E3	E1, E2, E3 (lower) in smokers in the luteal phase of the menstrual cycle	No
Michnovicz et al. 1988	29 premenopausal women not taking HRT, BMI<25	Urinary E1, E2, E3, 16αOHE$_1$, 2OHE$_1$	E3 (lower) and 2OHE$_1$ (higher) in smokers	No
Michnovicz et al. 1986	27 premenopausal women not taking HRT, BMI<25	Urinary E1, E3	E3 (lower) and the ratio of E3 to E1 (lower) in smokers	No
Trichopoulos et al. 1987	220 postmenopausal women not taking HRT	Urinary E1, E2, E3	No major differences	Height and weight

Abbreviations: E1 (estrone), E2 (estradiol), E3 (estriol), 16α-OEH1 (16-alpha-hydroxyestrone), 2-OEH1 (2-hydroxyestrone), HRT (hormone replacement therapy), BMI (body mass index).

Note: The table was originally published in Lancet Oncology 2002;3:470–80 and has been reproduced with permission.

Table 31.7 Studies of cigarette smoking and age at menopause (median or mean age at menopause (in years))

First author, study year	Study sample size	Nonsmokers	Ever smokers	Former smokers	Current smokers	Difference in years (current–nonsmokers)	Adjustment for BMI
Adena and Gallagher 1982	15 464	50.9	–	50.5	49.9	1.0	No
Brinton et al. 1986	1930	50.6	50.5	–	–	–	No
Brownson et al. 1988	2149	50.3	49.9	50.1	49.6	0.7	No
Chu et al. 1990	9402	Cases: 50.5 Controls: 49.9	–	Cases: 50.6 Controls: 49.6	Cases: 49.3 Controls: 48.7	1.2 1.2	No
Daniell et al. 1976	1279	49.1	47.6	–	–	–	Yes
Daniell et al. 1978	236	49.4	47.4	–	–	–	Yes
Field et al. 1992	3234	Cases: 50.3 Controls: 49.3	Cases: 49.3 Controls: 48.8	–	–	–	No
Hiat and Fireman 1986	84 172	48.9	–	48.4	48.0*	0.9	Yes
Kaufman et al. 1980	656	49.4	–	49.2	47.7*	1.7	Yes
McKinlay et al. 1985	7828	52.0	–	–	50.3	1.7	No
McNamara et al. 1978	1405	50.1	–	–	49.3	0.8	No
Stanford et al. 1987	3497	51	50	–	–	–	No
Weiderpass et al. 1999	3368	Cases: 52 Controls: 50	–	–	Cases: 51 Controls: 50	1 0	No

*Crude values were calculated from the data provided.

BMI, body mass index.

Note: The table was originally published in Lancet Oncology 2002;3:470–80 and has been reproduced with permission.

Comments

The results of at least 26 epidemiological studies to date suggest that current or recent smoking is associated with a small to moderate decreased risk of endometrial cancer, particularly among postmenopausal women who smoked for many years at high intensity. Associations between cigarette smoking and increased risk of osteoporosis (Baron 1984; Jensen et al. 1985; Jensen and Christiansen 1988; Baron et al. 1990), and attenuated effects of HRT among smokers (Jensen and Christiansen 1988), suggest an 'antiestrogenic' effect of smoking (Baron 1984; Baron et al. 1990). However, circulating levels of estrogen generally do not differ according to categories of cigarette smoking. A positive association between smoking and blood androgen levels has been observed consistently, especially with androstenedione, although its relevance to the association between smoking and endometrial cancer risk remains unclear.

Regarding the effects of smoking on estrogenic profiles, the type, rather than the absolute levels, of circulating estrogens may be important. In particular, smoking may increase estradiol 2-hydroxylation, which has been observed to decrease mammary epithelial proliferation rates in experimental studies (Bradlow et al. 1996). Although active smokers and nonsmokers may have the same concentrations of estrogens overall, smokers might have a lower concentration of more biologically active estrogens (primarily 16-alpha-hydroxyestrone). However, only one study (Michnovicz et al. 1986) has directly examined 2-hydroxylation in relation to cigarette smoking, finding a 50 per cent increased estradiol 2-hydroxylation in premenopausal women who smoked at least 15 cigarettes per day compared to nonsmokers. Although based on relatively small sample sizes, the findings of lowered levels of urinary estriol, and increased urinary 2-OEH1, among smokers observed in two studies (Michnovicz et al. 1988; Berstein et al. 2000) may support the hypothesis that smoking decreases the formation of active estrogen metabolites along the 16-alpha-hydroxylation pathway.

Since adipose tissue is the main determinant of estrogen levels among postmenopausal women, and is inversely associated with smoking, BMI may partly mediate the inverse association between cigarette smoking and estrogen. Most studies have adjusted for current BMI, although more relevant measures may include changes in body weight over time, waist-to-hip ratio, or duration of obesity. In addition, smoking appears to lower the age at which women reach menopause by an average of about 1–1.5 years, an association that seems to weaken with time since smoking cessation. Statistical adjustment for the effects of age at menopause generally has not altered the inverse associations between smoking and endometrial cancer risk. While a lower average body weight and earlier age at menopause among current smokers compared to nonsmokers certainly mediates some of the inverse association between smoking and endometrial cancer risk, the extent of this mediation remains unclear.

Effect-modification may provide clues to the mechanisms underlying associations observed in epidemiological studies. However, the data regarding effect modification of the association between cigarette smoking and endometrial cancer risk by other factors remain equivocal. On the one hand, 10 studies have shown a reduced endometrial cancer risk with current smoking that is stronger among, or limited to, postmenopausal women (Smith *et al.* 1984; Lesko *et al.* 1985; Brinton *et al.* 1993; Weiderpass and Baron 2001), women using HRT (Franks *et al.* 1987; Levi *et al.* 1987; Weiss *et al.* 1980), parous women (Terry *et al.* 2002*a*), and women who are obese (Lawrence *et al.* 1987; Brinton *et al.* 1993). On the other hand, nine studies have failed to demonstrate important differences in the association according to menopausal status (Lawrence *et al.* 1987; Levi *et al.* 1987; Terry *et al.* 2002*a*), obesity (Levi *et al.* 1987; Terry *et al.* 2002*a*), or HRT use (Lawrence *et al.* 1987; Brinton *et al.* 1993; Weiderpass and Baron 2001; Terry *et al.* 2002*a*). However, the validity of a single estrogen measurement as an indicator of a woman's usual levels is unclear, and none of the published reports has had sufficient statistical power to address meaningfully the issue of effect modification.

In summary, the available data suggest that cigarette smoking is associated with reduced risk of endometrial cancer among current smokers, mainly among postmenopausal women, and that the association weakens with time since quitting. Studies that examined quantitative measures of exposure to cigarette smoke have shown greater reductions in risk among women who were current smokers and smoked either more intensely or for a longer duration than women who smoked relatively less. The mechanisms by which this association may be driven remain unclear.

References

Adena, M. A. and Gallagher, H. G. (1982). Cigarette smoking and the age at menopause. *Ann. Hum. Biol.*, **9**, 121–30.

Akhmedkhanov, A., Zeleniuch-Jacquotte, A., and Toniolo, P. (2001). Role of exogenous and endogenous hormones in endometrial cancer: review of the evidence and research perspectives. *Ann. N. Y. Acad. Sci.*, **943**, 296–315.

Andersen, F. S., Transbol, I., and Christiansen, C. (1982). Is cigarette smoking a promotor of the menopause? *Acta Med Scand*, **212**, 137–9.

Austin, H., Drews, C., and Partridge, E. E. (1993). A case-control study of endometrial cancer in relation to cigarette smoking, serum estrogen levels, and alcohol use. *Am. J. Obstet. Gynecol.*, **169**, 1086–91.

Bailey, A., Robinson, D., and Vessey, M. (1977). Smoking and age of natural menopause. *Lancet*, **2**, 722.

Baron, J. A. (1984). Smoking and estrogen-related disease. *Am. J. Epidemiol.*, **119**, 9–22.

Baron, J. A., Byers, T., Greenberg, E. R., Cummings, K. M., and Swanson, M. (1986). Cigarette smoking in women with cancers of the breast and reproductive organs. *J. Natl. Cancer. Inst.*, **77**, 677–80.

Baron, J. A., La Vecchia, C., and Levi, F. (1990). The antiestrogenic effect of cigarette smoking in women. *Am. J. Obstet. Gynecol.*, **162**, 502–14.

Berstein, L. M., Tsyrlina, E. V., Kolesnik, O. S., Gamajunova, V. B., and Adlercreutz, H. (2000). Catecholestrogens excretion in smoking and non-smoking postmenopausal women receiving estrogen replacement therapy. *J. Steroid. Biochem. Mol. Biol.*, **72**, 143–7.

Berta, L., Frairia, R., Fortunati, N., Fazzari, A., and Gaidano, G. (1992). Smoking effects on the hormonal balance of fertile women. *Horm. Res.*, **37**, 45–8.

Bradlow, H. L., Telang, N. T., Sepkovic, D. W., and Osborne, M. P. (1996). 2-Hydroxyestrone: the 'good' estrogen. *J. Endocrinol.*, **150 Suppl**, S259–65.

Brinton, L. A., Schairer, C., Stanford, J. L., and Hoover, R. N. (1986). Cigarette smoking and breast cancer. *Am J Epidemiol*, **123**, 614–22.

Brinton, L. A., Barrett, R. J. Berman, M. L., Mortel, R., Twiggs, L. B., and Wilbanks, G. D. (1993). Cigarette smoking and the risk of endometrial cancer. *Am. J. Epidemiol.*, **137**, 281 91

Brownson, R. C., Blackwell, C. W., Pearson, D. K., Reynolds, R. D., Richens, J. W., Jr. and Papermaster, B. W. (1988). Risk of breast cancer in relation to cigarette smoking. *Arch. Intern. Med.*, **148**, 140–4.

Cassidenti, D. L., Vijod, A. G., Vijod, M. A., Stanczyk, F. Z., and Lobo, R. A. (1990). Short-term effects of smoking on the pharmacokinetic profiles of micronized estradiol in postmenopausal women. *Am. J. Obstet. Gynecol.*, **163**, 1953–60.

Cassidenti, D. L., Pike, M. C., Vijod, A. G., Stanczyk, F. Z., and Lobo, R. A. (1992). A reevaluation of estrogen status in postmenopausal women who smoke. *Am. J. Obstet. Gynecol.*, **166**, 1444–8.

Cauley, J. A., Gutai, J. P., Kuller, L. H., LeDonne, D., and Powell, J. G. (1989). The epidemiology of serum sex hormones in postmenopausal women. *Am. J. Epidemiol.*, **129**, 1120–31.

Chu, S. Y., Stroup, N. E., Wingo, P. A., Lee, N. C., Peterson, H. B., and Gwinn, M. L. (1990). Cigarette smoking and the risk of breast cancer. *Am J Epidemiol*, **131**, 244–53.

Daniell, H. W. (1976). Osteoporosis of the slender smoker. Vertebral compression fractures and loss of metacarpal cortex in relation to postmenopausal cigarette smoking and lack of obesity. *Arch. Intern. Med.*, **136**, 298–304.

Daniell, H. W. (1978). Smoking, obesity, and the menopause. *Lancet*, **2**, 373.

Elliott, E. A., Matanoski, G. M., Rosenshein, N. B., Grumbine, F. C., and Diamond, E. L. (1990). Body fat patterning in women with endometrial cancer. *Gynecol. Oncol.*, **39**, 253–8.

Engeland, A., Andersen, A., Haldorsen, T., and Tretli, S. (1996). Smoking habits and risk of cancers other than lung cancer: 28 years' follow-up of 26,000 Norwegian men and women. *Cancer Causes Control*, **7**, 497–506.

Field, N. A., Baptiste, M. S., Nasca, P. C., and Metzger, B. B. (1992). Cigarette smoking and breast cancer. *Int. J. Epidemiol.*, **21**, 842–8.

Franks, A. L., Kendrick, J. S., and Tyler, C. W., Jr. (1987). Postmenopausal smoking, estrogen replacement therapy, and the risk of endometrial cancer. *Am. J. Obstet. Gynecol.*, **156**, 20–3.

Friedman, A. J., Ravnikar, V. A., and Barbieri, R. L. (1987). Serum steroid hormone profiles in postmenopausal smokers and nonsmokers. *Fertil Steril*, **47**, 398–401.

Goodman, M. T., Hankin, J. H., Wilkens, L. R., Lyu, L. C., McDuffie, K., Liu, L. Q., and Kolonel, L. N. (1997). Diet, body size, physical activity, and the risk of endometrial cancer. *Cancer Res.*, **57**, 5077–85.

Hammond, E. C. (1961). Smoking in relation to physical complaints. *Arch Environ Health*, **3**, 28–164.

Hiatt, R. A. and Fireman, B. H. (1986). Smoking, menopause, and breast cancer. *J. Natl. Cancer. Inst.*, **76**, 833–8.

IARC (1999). *IARC monograph on the evaluation of carcinogenic risks to humans, vol. 72. Hormonal contraception and postmenopausal hormonal therapy.* IARC, Lyon.

IARC (2002). *IARC handbook of cancer prevention, vol. 6. Weight control and physical activity.* IARC Press, International Agency for Research on Cancer, Lyon.

Jain, M. G., Howe, G. R., and Rohan, T. E. (2000). Nutritional factors and endometrial cancer in Ontario, Canada. *Cancer Control*, **7**, 288–96.

Jensen, J. and Christiansen, C. (1988). Effects of smoking on serum lipoproteins and bone mineral content during postmenopausal hormone replacement therapy. *Am. J. Obstet .Gynecol.*, **159**, 820–5.

Jensen, J., Christiansen, C., and Rodbro, P. (1985). Cigarette smoking, serum estrogens, and bone loss during hormone-replacement therapy early after menopause. *N. Engl. J. Med.*, **313**, 973–5.

Jick, H. and Porter, J. (1977). Relation between smoking and age of natural menopause. Report from the Boston Collaborative Drug Surveillance Program, Boston University Medical Center. *Lancet*, **1**, 1354–5.

Kaufman, D. W., Slone, D., Rosenberg, L., Miettinen, O. S., and Shapiro, S. (1980). Cigarette smoking and age at natural menopause. *Am. J. Public Health*, **70**, 420–2.

Kelsey, J. L., LiVolsi, V. A., Holford, T. R., Fischer, D. B., Mostow, E. D., Schwartz, P. E., *et al.* (1982). A case-control study of cancer of the endometrium. *Am. J. Epidemiol.*, **116**, 333–42.

Key, T. J., Pike, M. C., Baron, J. A., Moore, J. W., Wang, D. Y., Thomas, B. S., and Bulbrook, R. D. (1991). Cigarette smoking and steroid hormones in women. *J. Steroid. Biochem. Mol. Biol.*, **39**, 529–34.

Key, T. J., Pike, M. C., Brown, J. B., Hermon, C., Allen, D. S., and Wang, D. Y. (1996). Cigarette smoking and urinary oestrogen excretion in premenopausal and post-menopausal women. *Br. J. Cancer*, **74**, 1313–6.

Khaw, K. T., Tazuke, S., and Barrett-Connor, E. (1988). Cigarette smoking and levels of adrenal androgens in postmenopausal women. *N. Engl. J. Med.*, **318**, 1705–9.

Koumantaki, Y., Tzonou, A., Koumantakis, E., Kaklamani, E., Aravantinos, D., and Trichopoulos, D. (1989). A case-control study of cancer of endometrium in Athens. *Int. J. Cancer*, **43**, 795–9.

Lapidus, L., Lindstedt, G., Lundberg, P. A., Bengtsson, C., and Gredmark, T. (1986). Concentrations of sex-hormone binding globulin and corticosteroid binding globulin in serum in relation to cardiovascular risk factors and to 12-year incidence of cardiovascular disease and overall mortality in postmenopausal women. *Clin. Chem.*, **32**, 146–52.

Law, M. R., Cheng, R., Hackshaw, A. K., Allaway, S., and Hale, A. K. (1997). Cigarette smoking, sex hormones and bone density in women. *Eur. J. Epidemiol.*, **13**, 553–8.

Lawrence, C., Tessaro, I., Durgerian, S., Caputo, T., Richart, R., Jacobson, H., and Greenwald, P. (1987). Smoking, body weight, and early-stage endometrial cancer. *Cancer*, **59**, 1665–9.

Lawrence, C., Tessaro, I., Durgerian, S., Caputo, T., Richart, R. M., and Greenwald, P. (1989). Advanced-stage endometrial cancer: contributions of estrogen use, smoking, and other risk factors. *Gynecol. Oncol.*, **32**, 41–5.

Lesko, S. M., Rosenberg, L., Kaufman, D. W., Helmrich, S. P., Miller, D. R., Strom, B., *et al.* (1985). Cigarette smoking and the risk of endometrial cancer. *N. Engl. J. Med.*, **313**, 593–6.

Levi, F., la Vecchia, C., and Decarli, A. (1987). Cigarette smoking and the risk of endometrial cancer. *Eur. J. Cancer Clin. Oncol.*, **23**, 1025–9.

Lindquist, O. and Bengtsson, C. (1979). Menopausal age in relation to smoking. *Acta. Med. Scand.*, **205**, 73–7.

Longcope, C. and Johnston, C. C., Jr. (1988). Androgen and estrogen dynamics in pre- and postmenopausal women: a comparison between smokers and nonsmokers. *J. Clin. Endocrinol. Metab.*, **67**, 379–83.

MacMahon, B., Trichopoulos, D., Cole, P., and Brown, J. (1982). Cigarette smoking and urinary estrogens. *N. Engl. J. Med.*, **307**, 1062–5.

McCann, S. E., Freudenheim, J. L., Marshall, J. R., Brasure, J. R., Swanson, M. K., and Graham, S. (2000). Diet in the epidemiology of endometrial cancer in western New York (United States). *Cancer. Causes. Control.*, **11**, 965–74.

McKinlay, S. M. (1996). The normal menopause transition: an overview. *Maturitas*, **23**, 137–45.

McKinlay, S. M., Bifano, N. L., and McKinlay, J. B. (1985). Smoking and age at menopause in women. *Ann. Intern. Med.*, **103**, 350–6.

McNamara, P. M., Hjortland, M. C., Gordon, T., and Kannel, W. B. (1978). Natural history of menopause: the Framingham Study. *J. Cont. Ed. Obstet Gynecol*, **20**, 27–35.

Michnovicz, J. J., Hershcopf, R. J., Naganuma, H., Bradlow, H. L., and Fishman, J. (1986). Increased 2-hydroxylation of estradiol as a possible mechanism for the anti-estrogenic effect of cigarette smoking. *N. Engl. J. Med.*, **315**, 1305–9.

Michnovicz, J. J., Naganuma, H., Hershcopf, R. J., Bradlow, H. L., and Fishman, J. (1988). Increased urinary catechol estrogen excretion in female smokers. *Steroids*, **52**, 69–83.

Newcomer, L. M., Newcomb, P. A., Trentham-Dietz, A., and Storer, B. E. (2001). Hormonal risk factors for endometrial cancer: modification by cigarette smoking (United States). *Cancer Causes Control*, **12**, 829–35.

Parker, S. L., Tong, T., Bolden, S., and Wingo, P. A. (1997). Cancer statistics, 1997. *CA Cancer J. Clin.*, **47**, 5–27.

Parkin, D. M., Pisani, P., and Ferlay, J. (1999). Estimates of the worldwide incidence of 25 major cancers in 1990. *Int. J. Cancer.*, **80**, 827–41.

Rubin, G. L., Peterson, H. B., Lee, N. C., Maes, E. F., Wingo, P. A., and Becker, S. (1990). Estrogen replacement therapy and the risk of endometrial cancer: remaining controversies. *Am. J. Obstet. Gynecol.*, **162**, 148–54.

Schlemmer, A., Jensen, J., Riis, B. J., and Christiansen, C. (1990). Smoking induces increased androgen levels in early post-menopausal women. *Maturitas*, **12**, 99–104.

Shields, T. S., Weiss, N. S., Voigt, L. F., and Beresford, S. A. (1999). The additional risk of endometrial cancer associated with unopposed estrogen use in women with other risk factors. *Epidemiology*, **10**, 733–8.

Slemenda, C. W., Hui, S. L., Longcope, C., and Johnston, C. C., Jr. (1989). Cigarette smoking, obesity, and bone mass. *J. Bone. Miner. Res.*, **4**, 737–41.

Smith, E. M., Sowers, M. F., and Burns, T. L. (1984). Effects of smoking on the development of female reproductive cancers. *J. Natl. Cancer. Inst.*, **73**, 371–6.

Stanford, J. L., Hartge, P., Brinton, L. A., Hoover, R. N., and Brookmeyer, R. (1987). Factors influencing the age at natural menopause. *J. Chronic Dis.*, **40**, 995–1002.

Stockwell, H. G. and Lyman, G. H. (1987). Cigarette smoking and the risk of female reproductive cancer. *Am. J. Obstet. Gynecol.*, **157**, 35–40.

Terry, P., Baron, J. A., Weiderpass, E., Yuen, J., Lichtenstein, P., and Nyren, O. (1999). Lifestyle and endometrial cancer risk: a cohort study from the Swedish Twin Registry. *Int. J. Cancer*, **82**, 38–42.

Terry, P., Miller, A. B., and Rohan, T. E. (2002a). A prospective cohort study of cigarette smoking and the risk of endometrial cancer. *Br. J. Cancer*, **86**, 1430–5.

Terry, P. D., Rohan, T. E., Franceschi, S., and Weiderpass, E. (2002b). Cigarette smoking and the risk of endometrial cancer. *Lancet. Oncol*, **3**, 470–80.

Trichopoulos, D., Brown, J., and MacMahon, B. (1987). Urine estrogens and breast cancer risk factors among post-menopausal women. *Int. J. Cancer*, **40**, 721–5.

Tyler, C. W., Jr., Webster, L. A., Ory, H. W., and Rubin, G. L. (1985). Endometrial cancer: how does cigarette smoking influence the risk of women under age 55 years having this tumor? *Am. J. Obstet. Gynecol.*, **151**, 899–905.

van Keep, P. A., Brand, P. C., and Lehert, P. (1979). Factors affecting the age at menopause. *J. Biosoc. Sci. Suppl.*, 37–55.

Weiderpass, E., and Baron, J. A. (2001). Cigarette smoking, alcohol consumption, and endometrial cancer risk: a population-based study in Sweden. *Cancer Causes Control*, **12**, 239–47.

Weiderpass, E., Adami, H. O., Baron, J. A., Magnusson, C., Bergstrom, R., Lindgren, A., *et al.* (1999). Risk of endometrial cancer following estrogen replacement with and without progestins. *J. Natl. Cancer. Inst.*, **91**, 1131–7.

Weiss, N. S., Farewall, V. T., Szekely, D. R., English, D. R., and Kiviat, N. (1980). Oestrogens and endometrial cancer: effect of other risk factors on the association. *Maturitas*, **2**, 185–90.

Willett, W., Stampfer, M. J., Bain, C., Lipnick, R., Speizer, F. E., Rosner, B., Cramer, D., and Hennekens, C. H. (1983). Cigarette smoking, relative weight, and menopause. *Am. J. Epidemiol.*, **117**, 651–8.

Williams, R. R. and Horm, J. W. (1977). Association of cancer sites with tobacco and alcohol consumption and socioeconomic status of patients: interview study from the Third National Cancer Survey. *J. Natl. Cancer. Inst.*, **58**, 525–47.

Part 7

Tobacco and heart disease

Chapter 32

Tobacco and cardiovascular disease

Konrad Jamrozik

Introduction

At the level of the whole population, tobacco causes far more harm via its contribution to cardiovascular disease (CVD) than it does through its effects on either the risk of lung cancer or of chronic obstructive pulmonary disease (COPD). This occurs because, in the absence of smoking, lung cancer and COPD are both very rare conditions. CVD, by contrast, is now the commonest cause of death of *Homo sapiens* (World Health Organization 1999). Thus, for a given prevalence of smoking in a population, the small increase in risk of CVD, in relative terms, that is associated with smoking generates many additional cases of CVD. By contrast, the much larger relative risks for lung cancer and COPD associated with smoking generate fewer additional cases of these conditions because these risks are applied to 'background' incidence rates that are much lower than the lifetime risk of CVD in non-smokers (Wald 1978).

Nevertheless, and despite some relationship between smoking and heart disease having been described for at least a century (Bruce 1901), more than twenty years elapsed between publication of the original report on the effects of smoking and health by the Royal College of Physicians of London (1962), which concentrated on lung cancer, and the appearance of a report from the Surgeon-General of the United States dedicated to the adverse effects of smoking on the cardiovascular system (United States Department of Health and Human Services 1983). Even the latter report is remarkable for the number of aspects of CVD about which information on the impact of smoking was either entirely lacking or inadequate to draw firm conclusions. This emphasizes how much more was learnt about active smoking and CVD in the last two decades of the twentieth century. That picture is now very close to complete, although, as this chapter will show, some significant questions remain unanswered and, arguably, we have yet to distil all of the lessons that might be taught by the knowledge that we have available.

To some extent, history has repeated itself in relation to passive smoking. The first reports of an increased incidence of major respiratory illness in infants and children who were passive smokers appeared in the English-language literature in 1974 (Colley *et al.* 1974; Harlap and Davies 1974), and data implicating passive smoking as a cause of lung cancer in adults were first published in 1981 (Hiryama 1981; Trichopoulos *et al.* 1981). However, another four years elapsed before equivalent studies of CVD appeared (Garland *et al.* 1985), even though a literature on the short-term consequences of passive smoking for cardiovascular function had been amassing since at least 1969 (Ayres *et al.* 1969). This chapter will demonstrate that after more than three decades of research, the epidemiological picture of passive smoking and CVD is still far from complete.

Scope of this chapter

Although the cardiovascular system has both arterial and venous sides, the emphasis here is on arterial disease related to smoking, and on the similarities and differences of the effects of smoking on disease in the four principal arterial 'territories'—those in the head (cerebrovascular tree), heart (coronary arterial tree), abdomen (principally the aorta, but also the mesenteric arteries supplying the gut), and legs (peripheral arterial tree). The corresponding conditions of principal interest are: cerebrovascular disease (CeVD), including stroke and transient cerebral ischaemic attack (TIA); ischaemic heart disease (IHD), including acute myocardial infarction (AMI); abdominal aortic aneurysm (AAA); and peripheral arterial disease (PAD).

The coronary equivalent of TIA is angina pectoris, transient chest pain that is classically brought on by exercise and relieved by rest before permanent damage is done to the muscle of the heart (which is what does occur in AMI, commonly known as 'heart attack'). The peripheral arterial equivalent of TIA and angina is intermittent claudication (IC), cramping pain in the muscles of the calf, thigh, or buttock that also is brought on by exercise, and specifically walking, and is relieved by rest. In contrast to angina and IC, the precipitants of TIA are not well understood, but the syndrome is analogous insofar as there is a temporary disruption of neurological function that is ascribed to a short-term inadequacy in the supply of blood to part of the brain, relative to its needs, and the symptoms resolve before obvious permanent damage is done to the underlying tissue.

One approach to this chapter would be to consider smoking and disease in each of the four principal arterial territories in turn. However, the material has instead been organized according to the criteria proposed by Sir Austin Bradford Hill for assessing whether statistical associations are likely to reflect underlying causal relationships (Hill 1965). As will become apparent, this allows us to see quickly not only areas of research where the volume of knowledge is such that we can safely regard a particular question as definitively answered, but also where unanswered questions remain or where persisting inconsistencies should cause us to think again about what we hold to be the underlying biological mechanisms. In addition, the Bradford Hill criteria have proved very useful as a framework for evaluating the emerging evidence regarding passive smoking and disease where, in general, the effects of exposure on risk are much smaller than for active smoking (National Health and Medical Research Council 1997) but the policy response throws into sharp focus issues surrounding the right of society to curtail the 'private' behaviour of individuals in public places and workplaces.

With the literature on smoking and health now running to tens of thousands of scientific papers, any review, even one restricted to a particular subset of diseases, is necessarily selective. In the case of active smoking, the references cited here are a mixture of citations of some of the best-known studies and of work conducted by the author in Perth, Western Australia. At first sight, the latter might seem an obscure choice, but it has been made for two reasons. First, Perth is one of few communities worldwide where the same methods have been used to assess the impact of active smoking on disease in each of the four principal arterial territories identified above, ascertainment of all of the cases and selection of control subjects have both been population-based, and internationally agreed criteria have been used to define cases. Framingham, Massachusetts, is another such community (Dawber 1980), but after more than fifty years of study, the numbers of events of the more uncommon arterial syndromes experienced by an inception cohort of just 5209 individuals is still too small to be statistically meaningful. Application of the same methods of enquiry to mathematically informative numbers of events in the different arterial territories in members of the same population provides a firmer basis on which to judge similarities and differences in relationships than does drawing together information from different communities that are widely dispersed in space and time.

The second reason for giving prominence to work from Western Australia is that the context of the investigations, in terms of prevailing patterns and trends in smoking, is well documented. Many of the 'classical' studies of health and smoking were begun, if not also completed, in settings where unfiltered cigarettes dominated the local market and the prevalence of smoking was very high in men and still rising sharply in women. This might beg the question as to how relevant are the findings now when, internationally, filtered cigarettes are completing their takeover of virtually all markets for tobacco products. Set against a background of stable or rising prevalences of smoking, the 'classical' studies probably are relevant to many developing countries now, where the uptake of smoking by both sexes still continues. However, for some time the prevalence of smoking has been falling significantly in many developed countries, especially in the English-speaking world and Scandinavia (Molarius et al. 2001). Perth is representative of such settings (Macfarlane and Jamrozik 1993), and therefore potentially much more informative as to the risks associated with modern patterns of smoking of modern cigarettes.

After examining the evidence regarding active and passive smoking and arterial disease, this chapter briefly considers effects of smoking on the venous system before closing with a section identifying a relatively small number of areas where further research on smoking and CVD might be worthwhile.

The Bradford Hill criteria

The decision having been taken to organize the information on smoking and arterial disease according to the Bradford Hill criteria, it becomes necessary to introduce those criteria in their own right.

Sir Austin Bradford Hill was an eminent statistician whose long list of accomplishments includes involvement in the original Medical Research Council trial of streptomycin for tuberculosis (Medical Research Council 1948), publication, with Sir Richard Doll, of the first English case–control studies of smoking and lung cancer (Doll and

Hill 1950, 1952), and establishment, again with Doll, of the long-running cohort study of smoking in British doctors (Doll *et al.* 1980, 1994). His criteria for assisting judgements about the likelihood of causal relationships explaining associations seen in observational data were published in 1965, with the original paper emphasizing that, as a true experiment, a randomized controlled trial involving human subjects should always provide the best evidence for answering such questions (Hill 1965). The criteria are listed and briefly explained in Table 32.1. Various other individuals and groups have proposed extensions and embellishments to the list of criteria, but Hill's formulation has the claim of simplicity as well as precedence, and therefore has been adopted here.

In relation to diseases purportedly caused by tobacco, the weight of evidence available by at least the early 1960s had made such experiments unethical, even if they were practical, while experimental studies conducted in laboratory animals could contribute only to Hill's criterion of biological plausibility because the potential for between-species differences limited their applicability to humans. Nevertheless, so-called 'natural experiments', in which the incidence of cardiovascular and other diseases are tracked as the smoking habits of a given population change, have contributed important information bearing on the criteria of temporal sequence and reversibility. These observations fall into a category known to epidemiologists as 'ecological studies'

Table 32.1 The Bradford Hill criteria for judgements about causation

Criterion	Test and its interpretation
Strength	Is the statistical relationship strong? Does it show a dose–response relationship—is a higher level of exposure to the putative cause associated with a greater risk of the disease?
Consistency	Is the relationship seen consistently in studies conducted at different historical periods, in different places, in different people (for example, in men as well as in women, in young people as well as in older ones, in different ethnic groups), and using different epidemiological methods (such as case–control and cohort studies)?
Temporal sequence	Do at least some of the studies provide incontrovertible evidence that exposure to the putative cause *preceded* development of the alleged effect?
Reversibility	Is a reduction in exposure followed by a reduced risk of the disease of interest? This question is best answered in data from individuals, but indicative information may also be derived from studies of whole populations
Specificity	Is exposure to the putative causal factor associated with development of an outcome that is unique to that exposure?
Biological plausibility	Is there supportive evidence from experimental studies in other species and from laboratory work on relevant organs, tissues, and other physiological systems? A systematic search for, and failure to find, evidence that would *not* support a conclusion of biological plausibility can be very useful here in demonstrating that the overall body of evidence is 'coherent'.

because the data on both exposure and disease are collected at the level of an entire community rather than for individuals, and care must be taken that some other factor that influences the pattern of the disease of interest more directly, quickly, or profoundly has not also changed during the period under study. In the case of Australia, for example, the evidence suggests that smoking among men peaked either during or soon after World War II (Hyndman *et al.* 1991) (see Fig. 32.1), which might

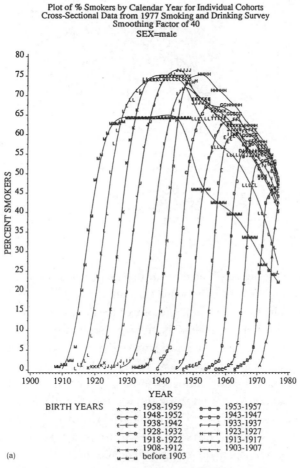

Fig. 32.1 Retrospective cohort analyses of smoking habits of Australian (a) men and (b) women

Footnote, Each line on a graph plots the evolution of smoking habits in the set of men or women born in a particular five-year period. The peak prevalence occurred among men in their twenties at the time of World War II, and far preceded and exceeded that among women, as did the rate of decline once the peak was passed. Overall, Australian women have been slower to stop starting and to start stopping than their male counterparts.

Source: Hyndman *et al.* (1991)

Copyright: Health Department of Western Australia

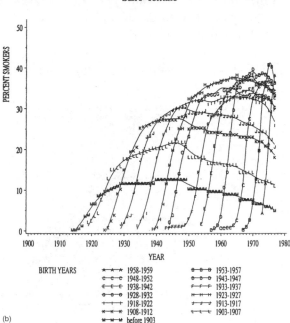

Plot of % Smokers by Calendar Year for Individual Cohorts
Cross-Sectional Data from 1977 Smoking and Drinking Survey
SEX=female

(b)

Fig. 32.1 (continued).

have contributed to the unprecedented downturn in mortality from IHD that occurred in the late 1960s and has continued since (Dwyer and Hetzel 1980) (see Fig. 32.2). However, the same change in the epidemiology of the disease also 'fits' with the major shift from plain to filter cigarettes that occurred from the late 1950s onwards. On the other hand, neither the change in level of smoking nor the type of cigarette smoked would explain why mortality from stroke, the more lethal manifestation of CeVD, began falling in the early 1950s (Jamrozik 1997), unless the time-trend for reduction of risk, specifically after cessation of smoking, was significantly faster for CeVD than for IHD. Development of effective pharmacological treatments for high blood pressure might conceivably have triggered the downturn in mortality from CeVD, even though hypertension is also a major independent and modifiable risk factor for IHD. Data on other potentially important factors, such as changes in dietary patterns consequent on the arrival of significant numbers of migrants from continental Europe and on developments in kitchen appliances, are extremely scant (Jamrozik *et al.* 1992), and those on levels of blood lipids and patterns of physical activity virtually non-existent.

The example of secular trends in mortality from arterial disease in Australia serves to illustrate several important points. While application of the Bradford Hill criteria to observational data on individuals itself requires considerable judgement, interpretation

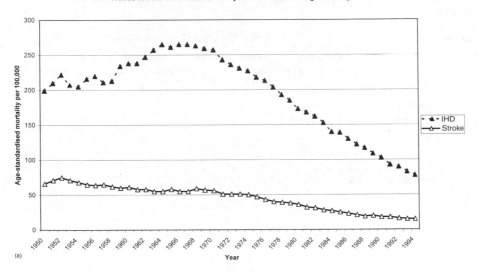

(a)

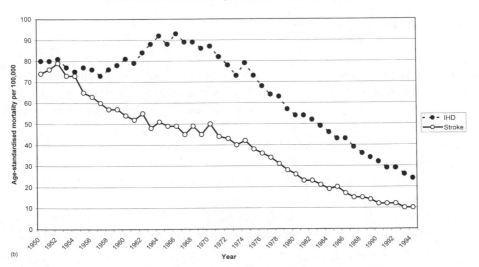

(b)

Fig. 32.2 Trends in mortality from IHD and stroke in Australian (a) men and (b) women
Footnote: In both sexes, mortality from stroke began falling early in the 1950s, while that
from IHD continued to increase until the late 1960s before beginning to fall sharply and contin-
uously. Taken together, the two patterns are not entirely consistent with the graphs shown in
Fig. 32.1, suggesting that factors other than changes in smoking habits are also at play.
Source: National Heart Foundation of Australia (1996)
Copyright: National Heart Foundation of Australia

Table 32.2 Application of Bradford Hill criteria to the evidence on ACTIVE smoking and arterial disease

Criterion	Manifestation of arterial disease			
	Ischaemic heart disease	Cerebrovascular disease	Abdominal aortic aneurysm	Peripheral arterial disease
Strength	✓	✓	✓	✓
dose–response	✓	✓	✓	✓
Consistency				
time	✓	✓	✓	✓
place	✓	✓	✓	✓
person	✓	✓	✓	✓
epidemiological method	✓	✓	?	✓
Temporal sequence	✓	✓	?	✓
Reversibility				
individual	✓	✓	✗	✗
population	✓	?	?	?
Specificity	✗	✗	✗	✗
Biological plausibility	✓	✓	✓	✓

✓ = Evidence available and supports criterion.

✗ = Available evidence does not support criterion.

? = Evidence either not available or inconclusive.

of secular trends in these diseases in whole communities, and the role that changes in smoking habits play in initiating and maintaining those trends, is even more difficult. Secondly, as the foregoing discussion makes clear, smoking is just one of several major, independent, and potentially modifiable risk factors for development of CVD, which has direct implications for Bradford Hill's criterion of specificity. Thirdly, if both cigarettes and patterns of their use change simultaneously, it may be close to impossible to discern, at least retrospectively, how much, if any, each change contributed to a population's experience of CVD.

But all of this is to run before we can walk. Let us first consider the individual criteria proposed by Bradford Hill and how they apply to the data on active smoking. Table 32.2 summarizes such a survey.

Strength and dose–response

As may be seen from Table 32.2, active smoking of cigarettes is a strong risk factor for disease in each of the four principal arterial territories, and shows an obvious dose–response in each. The dose–response relationships shown in Tables 32.3 and 32.4 are representative of those seen internationally, and those for IHD in Perth are further supported by data from cohort studies conducted in the same population (see Table 32.5). Unexpectedly, follow-up of healthy subjects recruited to the earlier case–control study

Table 32.3 Case–control studies of active smoking and ischaemic heart disease in Perth, Western Australia

Type of arterial disease (Period of study) [Reference] Sex and age-groups	Definition and source of cases	Daily consumption of cigarettes	Cases	Controls	Odds ratio	95% Confidence limits	Adjusted for:
Ischaemic heart disease (1989) (Liew 1989) Men only; 25–64 years	AMI: Perth MONICA Register	Never smoked	n = 174	n = 843	1.0	–	age, history of hypertension, maternal history of IHD, vigorous exercise
		Ex-smoker					
		1–24			1.71	0.87, 3.37	
		25+			2.37	1.14, 4.96	
		Current smoker					
		1–24			2.07	1.06, 4.05	
		25+			6.65	3.27, 13.5	
Ischaemic heart disease (1994) (Spencer et al. 1999) Men only; 25–64 years	AMI: Perth MONICA Register	Never smoked	n = 336	n = 735	1.0	–	age, dietary salt, fat, meat, alcohol, exercise, obesity, diabetes, history of hypertension, angina, low cholesterol diet
		Ex-smoker			2.0	1.25, 3.33	
		Current smoker			2.5	1.67, 3.33	
Ischaemic heart disease (1990–1993) (Lambert 2000) Women only; 25–64 years	AMI: Perth MONICA Register	Never smoked	n = 416	n = 935	1.0	–	age, marital status, source of income, alcohol, exercise, dietary fat, diabetes
		Ex-smoker			1.34	0.94, 1.91	
		Current smoker			3.87	2.67, 5.61	

Table 32.4 Case–control studies of active smoking and other arterial disease in Perth, Western Australia

Type of arterial disease (Period of study) [Reference] Sex and age-groups	Definition and source of case	Daily consumption of cigarettes	Cases	Controls	Odds ratio	95% Confidence limits	Adjusted for:
Cerebrovascular disease (1989–1990) (Jamrozik et al. 1994) Both sexes; ages ≥18 years	Stroke: Perth Community Stroke Study	Never smoked	n=295	n=553	1.0	–	history of hypertension, alcohol, claudication, previous CeVD, dietary milk, meat, salt, fish; matched for age and sex
		Ex-smoker			0.75	0.46, 1.24	
		1–20			1.99	1.04, 3.79	
		21+			3.52	1.35, 9.14	
Abdominal aortic aneurysm (1996–1998) (Jamrozik et al. 2000a) Men only: 65–83 years	AAA ≥ 30mm WA* AAA Program	Never smoked	n=875	n=11 328	1.0	–	age, place of birth, height, family history of AAA, dietary salt, exercise, waist: hip ratio
		Ex-smoker			2.5	2.0, 3.1	
		1–24			4.5	3.5, 5.8	
		25+			6.0	4.0, 9.0	
Peripheral arterial disease (1996–1998) (Fowler et al. 2002) Men only: 65–83 years	IC or ABI ≤ 0.9 WA AAA Program	Never smoked	n=744	n=3726	1.0	–	age, diabetes, exercise, history of hyperlipidaemia
		Ex-smoker			2.1	1.6, 2.6	
		1–14			3.9	2.7, 5.6	
		15–24			6.6	4.2, 10.5	
		25+			7.3	4.2, 12.8	

*WA=Western Australia; AAA=abdominal aortic aneurysm; IC=intermittent claudication; ABI=ankle:brachial index of systolic blood pressure.

Table 32.5 Cohort studies of active smoking and arterial disease in Perth, Western Australia

Type of arterial disease (Period of study) [Reference] Sex and age-groups	Definition and source of data	Daily consumption of cigarettes	Events	Size of cohort	Odds ratio	95% confidence limits	Adjusted for:
Ischaemic heart disease (1978–1994) [unpublished data] Men only, ages ≥18 years Five years of follow-up	First AMI*: Perth Cohort Study	Never smoked	n=72	n=4805	1.0	–	age, diastolic blood pressure, cholesterol, diabetes (men with CVD excluded)
		Ex-smoker			0.99	0.53, 1.88	
		1–14			1.42	0.61, 3.33	
		15–24			1.68	0.67, 4.12	
		25–34			4.10	1.98, 8.49	
		35+			2.83	0.79, 10.1	
Cerebrovascular disease (1989–1994) (Jamrozik et al. 2000b) Both sexes; ages ≥18 years Five years of follow-up	Major CVD*: Perth Community Stroke Study	Never smoked	n=141	n=931	1.0	–	age, sex, history of AMI, diabetes, intake of meat, use of full fat milk
		Current smoker			0.43	0.19, 0.995	

*AMI = acute myocardial infarction; 'major CVD' = death from IHD, CeVD, AAA, PAD or mesenteric thrombosis, plus non-fatal AMI or stroke.

of stroke (Jamrozik *et al.* 1994) revealed an inverse relationship between current smoking and major cardiovascular events (Jamrozik *et al.* 2000*b*).

Apart from the long-running studies in Framingham (Dawber 1980) and of British doctors (Doll *et al.* 1980, 1994) that have already been mentioned, new cohorts continue to be established in a wide variety of countries. Individual studies take some time to 'mature', although much useful information has already been obtained from the very large cohorts under follow-up in the Nurses Health Studies (Hu *et al.* 2000) and Health Professionals Study (Verhoef 1998) and from men screened for participation in the Multiple Risk Factor Intervention Trial (MRFIT) (Stamler *et al.* 1986). In addition, patients with AMI who participated in the ISIS-2 trial of aspirin and streptokinase have now been included in one of the largest case–control comparisons ever conducted for a non-communicable disease (Parish *et al.* 1995). Once again, the results show a strong and dose-related increase in risk of major coronary events associated with active smoking.

A recent, large case–control study of stroke in New Zealand (Bonita *et al.* 1999) stands out from all of these studies for two reasons apart from its focus on events in the cerebral rather than the coronary arteries. The first is that ascertainment of cases was population-based and therefore less subject to bias related to either the selected nature of the participants or the fact that, to be included, those suffering an event had to survive to reach hospital alive. Secondly, it has been one of the first studies deliberately to exclude passive smokers from the control group, a problem that may have affected many of the 'classical' studies and that, as Bonita *et al.* demonstrate, serves to underestimate the effects of active smoking on risk of disease (1999). The difference between their two sets of estimates, seen in Table 32.6, is sufficiently large to support a recommendation that exclusion of passive smokers should now be the 'gold standard' in such studies, especially since the spread of smoke-free policies has reached a point where large proportions of many communities are now able to live, travel, work, and relax in smoke-free environments if they so choose.

Smoking has long been accepted as a risk factor for both AAA and particularly PAD, but, as we shall see later, the relative lack of systematic study of these conditions appears to have contributed to a delay in our learning some important lessons about them.

Consistency

As has already been intimated, that active smoking is an important risk factor for the development of IHD is now supported by close to fifty years of research that includes both men and women, both case–control and cohort investigations, and evidence from a wide variety of geographical settings. Much the same is true of stroke, with one important proviso to which we will return. The more limited data on PAD and AAA demonstrate the same features, although both of these tend to be disproportionately diseases of men, the former possibly because men took up smoking much sooner than women, the latter at least partly because of a genetic component.

Table 32.6 Effect of exclusion of passive smokers from the control group on the apparent risk of stroke associated with active smoking

Smoking status	With passive smokers INCLUDED				With passive smokers EXCLUDED			
	Cases $n=521$ (%)	Controls $n=1851$ (%)	Odds ratio*	95% CLs	Cases $n=521$ (%)	Controls $n=1851$ (%)	Odds ratio*	95% CLs
Never smoked	31.1	48.7	1.0**	–	21.1 / 29.8	35.7 / 36.5	1.0§ / 1.82¶	– / 1.34, 2.49
Current smoker	31.5	13.8	4.14	3.04, 5.63	31.5	13.8	6.33	4.50, 8.91
1–4 per day	5.2	2.1	2.56	1.35, 4.88	5.2	2.1	3.89	2.03, 7.47
5–14 per day	8.1	3.4	4.37	2.61, 7.32	8.1	3.4	6.63	3.89, 11.3
15+ per day	18.2	8.3	4.59	3.17, 6.63	18.2	8.3	7.06	4.75, 10.5
Ex-smoker	33.4	36.2	1.0	0.75, 1.32	13.6	12.7	2.21	1.50, 3.27
<2 years	4.2	2.4	2.30	1.24, 4.27	4.2	2.4	3.45	1.84, 6.46
2–10 years	9.4	10.3	1.23	0.80, 1.88	9.4	10.3	1.89	1.21, 2.93
>10 years	19.8	23.5	0.79	0.57, 2.51				

Source: Adapted from Bonita et al. (1999).

*Adjusted for age, sex, diabetes, hypertension, and history of heart disease.

**Includes never smokers who were passively exposed.

§Unexposed never smokers and unexposed ex-smokers of more than 10 years' standing.

¶Passively exposed never smokers and ex-smokers of more than 10 years' standing.

The outstanding issue with regard to stroke is that it consists of three different pathological syndromes: subarachnoid haemorrhage (SAH), accounting for about 4% of all strokes and due in 85% of cases to rupture of a saccular aneurysm of an artery at the base of the brain external to the brain tissue (van Gijn and Rinkel 2001); primary intracerebral haemorrhage (PICH), responsible for about 11% of strokes in popula tions of European origin (Jamrozik *et al.* 1999) and due to haemorrhage from a small blood vessel within the brain tissue; and occlusive stroke, accounting for most of the remaining cases and due to thrombosis or to an embolus from the heart or neck, blocking a blood vessel in the brain. That the risk factors for these in general, and the role of smoking in particular, are not necessarily the same has received only limited attention, at least partly because routine CT examination to establish the pathological basis of stroke has become available only relatively recently. In fact, a case–control study conducted as part of the Perth Community Stroke Study (PCSS) was one of the first to provide evidence that active smoking is a risk factor for both occlusive stroke and PICH, although it did point to intriguing differences between these syndromes in regard to their associations with certain other risk factors (Jamrozik *et al.* 1994).

The PCSS alone included too few cases of SAH to permit separate analysis of risk factors for this form of stroke, but a large population-based series amassed retrospectively in the southwest of England suggests that smokers are more likely to survive an episode of SAH than are non-smokers (Pobereskin 2001*a*). As an editorial accompanying this report noted, such a finding is unexpected and potentially controversial (Juvela 2001). Of itself, it provides no clues as to the role of smoking in the *aetiology* of SAH, and Pobereskin concedes that it has not been consistently reported from other series. Most of those have not examined either question or not published the results if they have done so, and few are individually large enough to have a reasonable chance of seeing the effect on survival if it exists. Pobereskin is also open in acknowledging that data on smoking habits are most difficult to collect for patients who do not survive to reach hospital or who die soon after being admitted. Potentially this could lead to a bias in which smoking was apparently associated with better survival, but Pobereskin is confident that this problem has not affected his data (Pobereskin 2001*b*). If his original observation is correct, it may be one of several hints that the relationship between smoking and aneurysmal disease differs fundamentally from that with occlusive, atherosclerotic arterial disease.

Temporal sequence

In practice, the question of temporal sequence—exposure to the putative cause (smoking) preceding development of the alleged outcome (arterial disease)—is rarely a problem in relation to major non-communicable diseases related to tobacco because most smokers acquire the habit in their teens and the consequent diseases usually do not manifest themselves before later middle age. Nevertheless, the issue of temporal sequence is readily addressed by cohort studies to which recruitment is limited to subjects with no evidence of the relevant disease at baseline. With the proviso that any screening test almost certainly generates some false negatives, such cohort studies are certainly available for IHD and CeVD. This is of critical importance as 'temporal sequence' is the only one of the criteria proposed by Bradford Hill that *must* be fulfilled if one is to conclude that a causal relationship does explain the statistical associations observed between an exposure of interest and its putative effect.

Very large studies would be required in the case of AAA, where the prevalence of surgically significant lesions is still less than 1% in men in early old age (Jamrozik *et al.* 2000*a*). The prevalence of PAD, diagnosed either by symptoms (IC) or a reduced ankle:brachial index of systolic blood pressure, is at least six times higher in the same age–sex group (Fowler *et al.* 2002), making cohort studies more feasible. For example, Bowlin *et al.* found that current smokers of more than 20 cigarettes daily doubled their risk of developing IC within five years relative to never smokers (1994).

Reversibility

Good evidence was already available at the time of the 1983 report from the Surgeon-General (United States Department of Health and Human Services 1983) that after an individual stops smoking his or her excess risk of IHD associated with active smoking dissipates rapidly, compared with the equivalent pattern for lung cancer, and probably has disappeared entirely within seven to ten years. While much of the research available at that time was dominated by studies of men whose careers as smokers spanned the change from plain to filter cigarettes, more recent confirmatory evidence of the same pattern is available from the Nurses' Health Study for women (Kawachi *et al.* 1994) and from two of the Australasian centres in the World Health Organization MONICA Project for men (McElduff 1998*a*). The Nurses' Health Study has demonstrated a very similar pattern of reduction of excess risk of stroke after cessation of smoking (Kawachi *et al.* 1993), and the same findings are evident for both the coronary and cerebral arterial territories in studies conducted in Western Australia (Liew 1989; Jamrozik *et al.* 1994; Spencer *et al.* 1999; Lambert 2000) (see Tables 32.3 and 32.4).

In the case of AAA and PAD, however, there is evidence from Western Australia of long persistence of residual excess risk after a man gives up smoking. The sets of data for these conditions displayed in Table 32.4 both come from cross-sectional case–control comparisons based on a large randomized controlled trial of screening for AAA involving men aged 65–83 years selected at random from electoral rolls, enrolment to vote being compulsory for all adult Australian citizens (Jamrozik *et al.* 2000). Information on smoking habits was collected via a self-completed questionnaire that was answered by the men before the screening examinations for AAA and PAD were undertaken. However, claims to have stopped smoking were not verified biochemically, although many men were accompanied to the screening examination by a wife or partner who was all too willing to act as their 'conscience'.

Table 32.7 Long-term persistence of excess risk of PAD in ex-smokers (Fowler *et al.* 2002)

Smoking status	Odds ratio	95% CLs
Never smoked	1.0	–
Ex-smoker	2.1	1.6, 2.6
20+ years	1.3	1.0, 1.7
10–19 years	2.7	2.0, 3.6
5–9 years	3.7	2.5, 5.3
1–4 years	3.8	2.5, 5.7
<1 year	5.4	2.4, 11.9
Current smoker		
1–14 / day	3.9	2.7, 5.6
15–24 per day	6.6	4.2, 10.5
25+ per day	7.3	4.2, 12.8

CLs = confidence limits; odds ratios adjusted for age, physical activity, diabetes, and history of high triglyceride and cholesterol levels.

Table 32.7 shows that stratification of ex-smokers, who constituted some 60% of all men screened, by reported time since cessation of smoking did reveal an inverse relationship with apparent risk of PAD, but the excess risk of each condition was still statistically significant among men who claimed to have stopped smoking more than twenty years previously. Misclassification of continuing smokers as ex-smokers could conceivably contribute to these findings, despite the overall pattern of responses regarding smoking status being consistent with the retrospective cohort analysis mentioned previously (Hyndman *et al.* 1991). At the same time, calculations showed that if the apparent excess risk in those who had ever smoked was correct and causal, some 40% of cases of PAD in this population were attributable to previous smoking and a further 32% to current smoking (Fowler *et al.* 2002). Thus, while there is no uncertainty surrounding the reversibility of the excess risk of IHD and stroke if a smoker gives up the habit before overt disease develops in these arterial territories, the same may not be true of the aorta and arteries of the lower limb. Since AAA is, by definition, aneurysmal disease, while PAD is occlusive disease, the explanation for the contradiction cannot lie in a different pathological process affecting arteries below the diaphragm compared with that above it. In any case, the puzzle is compounded further when one considers that atherosclerosis plays a role in all four arterial syndromes.

Fewer analyses are available of the relationships between population-wide trends in smoking and those for the incidence or mortality from arterial disease, but, as discussed earlier, the interpretation of such data is fraught with hazard because all of the cigarettes themselves, patterns of smoking, the medical management of cardiovascular risk factors and events, and the epidemiology of the diseases changed rapidly and significantly over the last five decades of the twentieth century.

Specificity

The entries in Table 32.2 for 'specificity', meaning exposure to the putative causal factor being associated with development of an outcome that is unique to that exposure, stand out as the one row for which the evidence on smoking and CVD currently available does not support the criterion proposed by Bradford Hill. The explanation for this lies in the fact that many factors increase the risk of atherosclerotic CVD and, with a final pathological process that is common to all of them, it is very difficult to discern epidemiologically whether any given risk factor makes a contribution that is unique to itself. As is discussed further below, the apparent lack of specificity for smoking in the genesis of CVD has been a matter of scientific note for at least twenty years (Anonymous 1980), and the whole issue has been re-examined very thoroughly more recently in the context of evidence that, relative to active smoking, passive smoking seems to carry a risk for IHD that is disproportionately high compared with its contribution to the development of lung cancer in non-smokers.

Biological plausibility

Randomized, blinded controlled trials have provided incontrovertible evidence that smoking, exposure to tobacco smoke, or exposure to components of tobacco smoke such as carbon monoxide, produce clinically observable effects on various parts of the cardiovascular system including the electrical system of the heart (Sheps *et al.* 1987), the coronary circulation (Ayres *et al.* 1969; Aronow and Rokaw 1971; Sumida *et al.* 1998; Otsuka *et al.* 2001), and the peripheral arteries (Celermajer *et al.* 1996). This evidence is supported by cross-sectional studies demonstrating increased asymptomatic thickening of the lining 'intima' layer of the carotid arteries in both active and passive smokers (Howard *et al.* 1994), with follow-up of the same individuals showing greater rates of evolution of these 'plaques' in smokers (Diez-Roux *et al.* 1995; Howard *et al.* 1998). Since the carotid arteries are the main blood vessels supplying the brain, greater degrees of occlusion at the anatomical sites examined in these studies are associated with neurological symptoms, and surgical clearance of such obstructions reduces the risk of stroke, these findings clearly are of direct relevance to the role purportedly played by smoking in the aetiology of CeVD.

These studies in intact humans are complemented by a wealth of laboratory research on other species (Penn and Snyder 1996; Penn *et al.* 1996, 2001) and on human tissues (Davis *et al.* 1989; Kritz *et al.* 1995). Glantz and Parmley (1995) provide a wide-ranging review of the evidence that passive smoking, in particular, could plausibly cause an increase in risk of CVD in non-smokers and point to a number of mechanisms through which this could occur. It is true that there are differences in chemical and other characteristics between the smoke inhaled directly from cigarettes by smokers and that inhaled from ambient air by non-smokers. However, the overall exposure of the latter to particular constituents of the smoke is so obviously lower that, taken with the evidence of direct, potentially harmful effects of active smoking on parts of the cardiovascular system, the convincing argument regarding the biological plausibility of passive smoking as a cause of CVD means that the case in regard to active smoking must be even more compelling. Significantly, the identification of a number of different mechanisms via which tobacco smoke could harm the arterial tree makes it very difficult to modify cigarettes to make them 'safer' in regard to the risk of CVD in smokers.

Passive smoking and arterial disease

The evidence that passive smoking increased the incidence of severe respiratory infections in infants and young children (Colley *et al.* 1974; Harlap and Davies 1974) was not seriously challenged when it emerged. This is probably because it was known by the 1970s that active smoking caused COPD (Fletcher and Peto 1976) and was associated with increased mortality from pneumonia in adults (Doll and Peto 1976), it was obvious that children of this age could be heavily exposed if their parents smoked around them, and the implications for policy were limited because the majority of that exposure occurred in private homes, a domain that most communities are loathe to regulate. However, the tobacco industry having been alerted in 1978 to the threat to its well-being posed by the issue of passive smoking (Roper Organization 1978), the publication, in 1981, of evidence (Hirayama 1981; Trichopoulos *et al.* 1981) that passive smoking was associated with lung cancer in adults was accompanied by very considerable controversy. The possible contribution of passive smoking to IHD, first identified epidemiologically in 1985 (Garland *et al.* 1985), has proved even more contentious because it appears to be similar in magnitude to the effect of passive smoking on the risk of lung cancer, whereas the multiplying effect of active smoking on the risk of lung cancer is at least five times its effect on IHD.

The National Heart Foundation of Australia was one of the first health organizations to react to the paper from Garland *et al.* (1985), publishing a pamphlet on passive smoking and heart disease entitled, "So you think you're a non-smoker" (National Heart Foundation of Australia 1985) in the same year. More systematic reviews of the scientific evidence on passive smoking generally were published by the Surgeon-General in the United States in 1986 (United States Department of Health and Human Services 1986) and the National Health and Medical Research Council (NHMRC) in Australia in 1987 (National Health and Medical Research Council 1987), but neither body was persuaded at that time that passive smoking caused CVD. When the NHMRC visited the question of passive smoking again (1997), many more epidemiological and laboratory reports on the issue of CVD had been published, leading that body to a conclusion that the evidence for a causal relationship was 'strongly suggestive'. In Britain, the Scientific Committee on Tobacco and Health was unambiguous in its report published in 1998 that passive smoking is a cause of IHD (Department of Health 1998), and Law *et al.*, working in the same country, had been persuaded by the evidence available in the preceding year (1997), as had the California Environmental Protection Agency (Office of Environmental Health Hazard Assessment 1997).

Table 32.8 Application of Bradford Hill criteria to the evidence on passive smoking and arterial disease

Criterion	Manifestation of arterial disease			
	Ischaemic heart disease	Cerebrovascular disease	Abdominal aortic aneurysm	Peripheral arterial disease
Strength	✗	✗	?	?
dose–response	✓	✓	?	?
Consistency				
time	✓	✓	?	?
place	✓	✓	?	?
person	✓	?	?	?
epidemiological method	✓	?	?	?
Temporal sequence	✓	✗	?	?
Reversibility				
individual	?	?	?	?
population	?	?	?	?
Specificity	✗	✗	?	?
Biological plausibility	✓	✓	✓	✓

✓ = Evidence available and supports criterion.

✗ = Available evidence does not support criterion.

? = Evidence either not available or inconclusive.

The epidemiological evidence implicating passive smoking as a cause of IHD continues to mount (Ciruzzi *et al.* 1998; McElduff *et al.* 1998*b*; Thun *et al.* 1999; Irabarren *et al.* 2001; Rosenlund *et al.* 2001), with new meta-analyses appearing at frequent intervals (He *et al.* 1999), and the data on stroke are also growing (Bonita *et al.* 1999). However, as may be seen from Table 32.8, little attention has been afforded to the role of passive smoking in the genesis of AAA and PAD, and the question of whether the risk of any of the arterial diseases falls when a non-smoking individual stops being passively exposed to tobacco smoke has not been studied systematically.

Although the elevation in risk of IHD associated with passive smoking is modest, both coronary disease and exposure to tobacco smoke are so common among non-smokers that the aggregate number of additional cases of heart attack potentially attributable to passive smoking is very large indeed (Wells 1994). The sceptics, some of whom openly acknowledge support from the tobacco industry, regularly advance arguments about misclassification of continuing smokers as ex-smokers, publication bias (LeVois and Layard 1995)—the tendency for studies showing no association not to be submitted or accepted for publication—and confounding—systematic differences in the lifestyles of non-smokers who are and are not passive smokers that render the former more prone to development of IHD—as possible explanations for pattern of positive findings in the available literature. These objections are theoretical and largely speculative, but each has been examined systematically and discounted (Steenland *et al.* 1998; Wells *et al.* 1998).

Two further papers, both including authors who are associated with the tobacco industry, proffer elaborate but slightly different arguments about the overall dose–response relationship between tobacco smoke and CVD. Gori (1995) calculates that a pooled estimate of the epidemiological data on the excess risk of IHD associated with active smoking of five cigarettes daily is not statistically significant and therefore that there is a threshold of exposure to tobacco smoke, whether through active or passive smoking, below which individuals suffer no adverse cardiovascular consequences. Smith *et al.* (2000) argue that combining the epidemiological data for active and passive smoking produces a non-linear dose–response curve that is biologically implausible. The best counter to both these observations is a simple experiment that showed that exposure to tobacco smoke in the corridor of a hospital for just 20 minutes resulted in significant 'activation' of the platelets of non-smokers but not those of smokers, platelets being small cells in the bloodstream that play a critical role in thrombosis, including coronary thrombosis and occlusive stroke (Kritz *et al.* 1995).

In summary, the epidemiological association between passive smoking and at least IHD is definitely real, and the available evidence points to it being both based on a causal relationship and of considerable public health significance, even though the excess risk in individual passive smokers is small.

Active smoking and venous disease

Smokers have significantly increased mortality from the most lethal form of venous disease, pulmonary embolism (PE) secondary to deep vein thrombosis (DVT) (Doll *et al.* 1994), which is perhaps a consequence of the higher levels of fibrinogen and activation of platelets in smokers, as well as their increased risk of cancer. Beyond the known interaction with use of the oral contraceptive pill (Farmer *et al.* 2000), it is uncommon to see smoking cited as increasing the risk of DVT and PE. Nevertheless, smoking does appear to be an independent risk factor for these conditions (Hansson *et al.* 1999). Interest in this association may be increased following publication of evidence that cessation of smoking before major elective surgery reduces post-operative complications, of which DVT and PE are among the most serious (Moller *et al.* 2002).

One might also predict a relationship between smoking and varicose veins, perhaps mediated through the 'smoker's cough', but this is evident in some (Brand *et al.* 1988) but not all (Fowkes *et al.* 2001) of the studies that have sought such an association.

Unanswered questions

The case against active smoking as an avoidable cause of major diseases in each of the four principal arterial territories is overwhelming. However, as well as the issue of passive smoking and the somewhat limited investigation of the role of smoking in diseases of the venous system mentioned above, a number of questions surrounding smoking and arterial CVD remain unanswered. Some of these are of considerable significance in terms of public health, others suggest novel lines of enquiry into the biology of vascular disease, and yet others potentially have ramifications in both these spheres.

Type of tobacco product

The great bulk of the evidence concerning the impact of smoking on CVD is derived from studies of users of manufactured cigarettes. When pipes and cigars receded from the tobacco markets in most developed countries in the 1970s and 1980s, epidemiological interest in these products also waned, but it has been rekindled by a recent resurgence in the smoking of cigars. There is little doubt that use of such products is associated with significant hazard (Hein *et al.* 1992; Jacobs *et al.* 1999). Much less information is available concerning hazards potentially associated with traditional forms of smoking in other communities.

Changes over time in manufactured cigarettes raise a related set of questions, especially as it is not clear which component or components of tobacco smoke are responsible for the increased risk of arterial disease in smokers. In practice, with the epidemiology at least of IHD also changing rapidly, it would be very difficult to detect whether changes in the source and blend of tobacco, other additives, cigarette papers or filters affected the risk of vascular events in smokers. Nevertheless, because manufacturers attempt to tailor their products to particular markets, divergences between the patterns of vascular disease in otherwise similar countries might potentially provide clues as to which aspects of tobacco products or their use are particularly relevant to the development of atherosclerosis.

On the other hand, there is little uncertainty regarding one question relating to type of tobacco product and risk of CVD. The evidence already cited suggests that smokers of cigarettes should not be encouraged to change to other tobacco products in an attempt to reduce their risk of CVD. Direct support for this inference is available from a long-term prospective study of 'switching'. Former smokers of cigarettes who changed to pipes and cigars experienced a significant reduction in risk compared with men who continued smoking cigarettes but also a 57% excess risk of dying from one of IHD, lung cancer, and COPD compared with those who stopped smoking entirely (Wald and Watt 1997). The explanation almost certainly lies in the fact that former smokers of cigarettes continue to inhale the smoke when they change to other forms of tobacco product (Goldman 1977).

Lack of reversibility in AAA and PAD

As already noted, case–control studies from Western Australia suggest that the elevation in risk of AAA and PAD persists long after the individual stops smoking, in contrast to the rapid declines in excess risk of IHD and CeVD. Wilmink *et al.* (1999) reported a relative risk for AAA of 3.0 (95% CL 1.4–6.4) in ex-smokers, but Blanchard *et al.* (2000), who summarized a history of smoking in terms of pack-years, did not draw attention to this phenomenon. A major review of the literature by English *et al.* (1995) considered all non-coronary and non-cerebral arterial disease as a single category and therefore does not permit examination of the question. Whether arterial disease related to smoking behaves differently in different anatomical territories bears further investigation as this may provide new insights into the basic biology of atherosclerosis. Any new studies should include independent verification of claims by affected individuals to have stopped smoking before development of their symptoms.

Aneurysmal disease

There is growing evidence that smoking has a protective effect in regard to development of retinopathy in patients with diabetes mellitus (Janghorbani *et al.* 2001; Keen *et al.* 2001; Stratton *et al.* 2001). As the key lesion in this condition is an arterial micro-aneurysm, there is a sharp contrast with the elevated risk in smokers of macro-aneurysmal disease in the cerebral (Shinton and Beevers 1989) and aortic circulations (Jamrozik *et al.* 2000). Again, further investigation of this paradox might reveal new lessons about the pathogenesis of arterial disease.

Smoking and survival from major vascular events

While smoking has a strong influence on the incidence of major arterial disease events, its relationship to survival after such events is less clear. One Australian population-based study of middle-aged patients with AMI who reached hospital alive suggested that case fatality at 28 days was significantly lower in current smokers (Nidorf *et al.* 1990), while another, which included all major coronary events in a defined population, found no significant association in either direction between smoking and short-term survival (McElduff and Dobson 2001). Apparently protective effects of current smoking have also been observed in major trials of acute coronary care (Barbash *et al.* 1995), but careful work in New Zealand suggests that the reduced case-fatality of smokers after they are admitted to hospitals with an AMI is balanced by worse out-of-hospital survival, with no significant relationship apparent overall (Sonke *et al.* 1997). This does not appear to be the explanation for the observation, cited earlier (Pobereskin 2001*a*), that smokers fare better, in terms of survival, after subarachnoid haemorrhage. However, it does underline the importance of taking a population-wide view of rapidly fatal phenomena, lest artefacts related to differential survival to reach hospital alive be accepted at face value.

In the overall picture, sorting out the details of the relationships between smoking and the outcome of major vascular events is not a high priority compared with the need to reduce the contribution of smoking to the incidence of such episodes. Nevertheless, the availability of clear answers would permit unambiguous advice to be given to patients and their families.

Conclusion

The smoking of tobacco is a major independent risk factor for life-threatening diseases in all four principal arterial territories. The totality of the evidence indicates that this relationship goes beyond statistical association to one of cause-and-effect. Most importantly, compared with other factors such as hypertension, hypercholesterolaemia, and lack of physical activity, cessation of smoking requires a once-only change on the part of the individual, and a change to non-smoking is followed by a rapid and complete disappearance of the excess risk of IHD and stroke, the two most common fatal manifestations of arterial disease. *How* smoking harms the arterial tree is not completely clear, but several plausible candidate mechanisms have been identified. A number of other scientifically intriguing questions about smoking and both arterial and venous diseases also remain open. But it is beyond any doubt that smoking does most of its harm in terms of deaths, not through cancer or COPD, but through vascular disease.

Acknowledgements

The author's interest in tobacco was originally kindled by Godfrey Fowler and fostered by Nicholas Wald, Sir Richard Peto, and Sir Richard Doll. Michael Hobbs and Bruce Armstrong designed the Perth MONICA Project, which formed the framework for the Western Australian studies of ischaemic heart disease cited in this chapter, while Ted Stewart-Wynne, Craig Anderson, Sue Forbes, and Graeme Hankey have been pillars of the Perth Community Stroke Study. Robyn Broadhurst has not only managed most of the data for that project, but also is prime mover for the Perth Cohort Study, also cited here. Paul Norman, Michael Lawrence-Brown, Raywin Tuohy, Carole Spencer, and Jim Dickinson have played vital roles in the Western Australian Abdominal Aortic Aneurysm Program, and Bess Fowler made a memorable contribution to the work on peripheral arterial disease. Financial support for these projects has been provided, in various combinations, by the National Health and Medical Research Council, the National Heart Foundation of Australia, Healthway—the Western Australian Health Promotion Foundation, and State and Federal Governments in Australia.

References

Anonymous (1980). How does smoking harm the heart? *Br Med J*, **281**, 573–4.

Aronow, W. S., and Rokaw, S. N. (1971). Carboxyhaemoglobin caused by smoking non-nicotine cigarettes. *Circulation* **44**, 782–8.

Ayres, S. M., Mueller, H. S., Gregory, J. J., Gianelli, S., and Penny, J. L. (1969). Systemic and myocardial haemodynamic response to relatively small concentrations of carboxyhaemoglobin (COHb). *Arch Environ Health* **18**, 699–709.

Barbash, G. I., Reiner, J., White, H. D., Wilcox, R. G., Armstrong, P. W., Sadowski, Z., *et al.* (1995). Evaluation of paradoxic beneficial effects of smoking in patients receiving thrombolytic therapy for acute myocardial infarction: mechanism of the "smoker's paradox" from the GUSTO-I trial, with angiographic insights. *J Am College Cardiol* **26**, 1222–9.

Blanchard, J. F., Armenian, H. K., and Friesen, P. P. (2000). Risk factors for abdominal aortic aneurysm: results of a case-control study. *Am J Epidemiol* **151**, 575–83.

Bonita, R., Duncan, J., Truelsen, T., Jackson, R. T., and Beaglehole, R. (1999). Passive smoking as well as active smoking increases the risk of acute stroke. *Tob Control* **8**, 156–60.

Bowlin, S. J., Medalie, J. H., Flocke, S. A., Zyzanski, S. J., and Goldbourt, U. (1994). Epidemiology of intermittent claudication in middle-aged men. *Am J Epidemiol* **140**, 418–30.

Brand, F. N., Dannenberg, A. L., Abbott, R. D., and Kannel, W. B. (1988). The epidemiology of varicose veins: the Framingham Study. *Am J Prev Med* **4**, 96–101.

Bruce, J. M. (1901). Diseases and disorders of the heart and arteries in middle life and advanced age. *Lancet* **i**, 844–8.

Celermajer, D. S., Adams, M. R., Clarkson, P., *et al.* (1996). Passive smoking and impaired endothelium-dependent arterial dilatation in healthy young adults. *N Eng J Med* **334**, 150–4.

Ciruzzi, M., Pramparo, P., Esteban, O., *et al.* (1998). Case-control study of passive smoking at home and risk of acute myocardial infarction. *J Am Coll Cardiol* **31**, 797–803.

Colley, J. R. T., Holland, W. W., and Corkhill, R. T. (1974). Influence of passive smoking and parental phlegm on pneumonia and bronchitis in early childhood. *Lancet* **ii**, 1031–4.

Davis, J., Shelton, L., Watanabe, I. S., and Arnold, J. (1989). Passive smoking affects endothelium and platelets. *Arch Intern Med* **149**, 386–9.

Dawber, T. R. (1980). The Framingham Study: The epidemiology of atherosclerotic disease. Cambridge, Mass.: Harvard University Press.

Department of Health. (1998). Report of the Scientific Committee on Tobacco and Health. London: Stationery Office.

Diez-Roux, A. V., Nieto, F. J., Comstock, G. W., Howard, G., and Szklo, M. (1995). The relationship of active and passive smoking to carotid atherosclerosis 12–14 years later. *Prev Med* **24**, 48–55.

Doll, R. and Hill, A. B. (1950). Smoking and carcinoma of the lung: preliminary report. *Br Med J* **ii**, 739–48.

Doll, R. and Hill, A. B. (1952). A study of the aetiology of carcinoma of the lung. *Br Med J* **ii**, 1271–86.

Doll, R. and Peto, R. (1976). Mortality in relation to smoking: 20 years' of observations in male British doctors. *Br Med J* **ii**,

Doll, R., Gray, R., Hafner, B., and Peto, R. (1980). Mortality in relation to smoking: 22 years' observations on female British doctors. *Br Med J* **280**, 967–71.

Doll, R., Peto, R., Wheatley, K., Gray, R., and Sutherland, I. (1994). Mortality in relation to smoking: 40 years' observations on male British doctors. *Br Med J* **309**, 901–11.

Dwyer, T. and Hetzel, B. S. (1980). A comparison of coronary heart disease mortality in Australia, USA and England and Wales with reference to three major risk factors—hypertension, cigarette smoking and diet. *Intl J Epidemiol* **9**, 65–71.

English, D. R., Holman, C. D. J., Milne, E., *et al.* (1995). The quantification of drug caused morbidity and mortality in Australia 1995 edition. Canberra: Commonwealth Department of Human Services and Health.

Farmer, R. D., Lawrenson, R. A., Todd, J. C., Williams, T. J., MacRae, K. D., Tyrer, F., and Leydon, G. M. (2000). A comparison of the risks of venous thromboembolic disease in association with different combined oral contraceptives. *Br J Clin Pharmacol* **49**, 580–90.

Fletcher, C. M. and Peto, R. (1977). The natural history of chronic airflow obstruction. *Br Med J* **i**, 1654–8.

Fowkes, F. G., Lee, A. J., Evans, C. J., Allan, P. L., Bradbury, A. W., and Ruckley, C. V. (2001). Lifestyle risk factors for lower limb venous reflux in the general population: Edinburgh Vein Study. *Int J Epidemiol* **30**, 846–52.

Fowler, B. V., Jamrozik, K., Allen, Y., and Norman, P. E. (2002). Prevalence of peripheral arterial disease: Persistence of excess risk in former smokers. *ANZ J Public Health* **26**, 219–24.

Garland, C., Barrett-Connor, E., Suarez, L., *et al.* (1985). Effects of passive smoking on ischaemic heart disease mortality of nonsmokers. *Am J Epidemiol* **121**, 645–9.

Glantz, S. A. and Parmley, W. W. (1995). Passive smoking and heart disease. Mechanisms and risk. *JAMA* **273**, 1047–53.

Goldman, A. L. (1977). Carboxyhemoglobin levels in primary and secondary cigar and pipe smokers. *Chest* **72**, 33–5.

Gori, G. B. (1995). Environmental tobacco smoke and coronary heart syndromes: Absence of an association. *Regul Toxicol Pharmacol* **21**, 281–95.

Hansson, P. O., Eriksson, H., Welin, L., Svardsudd, K., and Wilhelmsen, L. (1999). Smoking and abdominal obesity: risk factors for venous thromboembolism among middle-aged men: "the study of men born in 1913". *Arch Intern Med* **159**, 1886–90.

Harlap, S. and Davies, A. M. (1974). Infant admissions to hospital and maternal smoking. *Lancet* **i**, 529–32.

He, J., Vupputuri, S., Allen, K., Prerost, M. R., Hughes, J., and Whelton, P. K. (1999). Passive smoking and the risk of coronary heart disease – a meta-analysis of epidemiologic studies. *N Eng J Med* **340**, 920–6.

Hein, H. O., Suadicani, P., and Gyntelberg, F. (1992). Ischaemic heart disease incidence by social class and form of smoking: the Copenhagen Male Study—17 years' follow-up. *J Intern Med* **231**, 477–83.

Hill, A. B. (1965). The environment and disease: association or causation. *Proc Roy Soc Med* **58**, 295–300.

Hirayama, T. (1981). Non-smoking wives of heavy smokers have a higher risk of lung cancer: a study from Japan. *Br Med J* **282**, 183–5.

Howard, G., Burke, G. L., Szklo, M., Tell, G. S., Eckfeldt, J., Evans, G., and Heiss, G. (1994). Active and passive smoking are associated with increased carotid wall thickness. The Atherosclerosis Risk in Communities (ARIC) Study. *Arch Intern Med* **154**, 1277–82.

Howard, G., Wagenknecht, L. E., Burke, G. L., *et al.* (1998). Cigarette smoking and progression of atherosclerosis: The Atherosclerosis Risk in Communities (ARIC) Study. *JAMA* **279**, 119–24.

Hu, F. B., Stampfer, M. J., Manson, J. E., Grodstein, F., Colditz, G. A., Speizer, F. E., and Willett, W. C. (2000). Trends in the incidence of coronary heart disease and changes in diet and lifestyle in women. *N Engl J Med* **343**, 530–7.

Hyndman, J., Hobbs, M., Jamrozik, K., Hockey, R., and Parsons, R. (1991). A retrospective cohort study of smoking habits in Australia. In: (ed. B. Durston, and K. Jamrozik). Proceedings of the 7th World Conference on Tobacco and Health. Perth: Health Department of Western Australia, 264–7.

Irabarren, C., Friedman, G. D., Klatsky, A. L., and Eisner, M. D. (2001). Exposure to environmental tobacco smoke: association with personal characteristics and self reported health conditions. *J Epidemiol Community Health* **55**, 721–8.

Jacobs, E. J., Thun, M. J., and Apicella, L. F. (1999). Cigar smoking and death from coronary heart disease in a prospective study of US men. *Arch Intern Med* **159**, 2413–8.

Jamrozik, K., Jamieson, R., and Fitzgerald, C. (1992). An oral history of changes in the Australian diet. *Med J Aust* **157**, 759–61.

Jamrozik, K., Broadhurst, R. J., Anderson, C. S., and Stewart-Wynne, E. G. (1994). The role of lifestyle factors in the aetiology of stroke: A population-based case-control study in Perth, Western Australia. *Stroke* **25**, 51–9.

Jamrozik, K. (1997). Stroke—a looming epidemic? *Aust Fam Physician* **26**, 1137–43.

Jamrozik, K., Broadhurst, R. J., Lai, N., Hankey, G. J., Burvill, P. W., and Anderson, C. S. (1999). Trends in the incidence, severity and outcome of stroke in Perth, Western Australia. *Stroke* **30**, 2105–11.

Jamrozik, K., Norman, P., Spencer, C. A., Parsons, R. W., Tuohy, R., Lawrence-Brown, M. M., and Dickinson, J. A. (2000a). Screening for abdominal aortic aneurysm: lessons from a population-based study. *Med J Aust* **173**, 345–50.

Jamrozik, K., Broadhurst, R. J., Forbes, S., Hankey, G. J., and Anderson, C. S. (2000b). Predictors of death and vascular events in the elderly: The Perth Community Stroke Study. *Stroke* **31**, 863–8.

Janghorbani, M., Jones, R. B., Murray, K. J., and Allison, S. P. (2001). Incidence of and risk factors for diabetic retinopathy in diabetic clinic attenders. *Ophthalmic Epidemiol* **8**, 309–25.

Juvela, S. (2001). Cigarette smoking and death following subarachnoid haemorrhage. *J Neurosurg* **95**, 551–4.

Kawachi, I., Colditz, G. A., Stampfer, M. J., *et al.* (1993). Smoking cessation and decreased risk of stroke in women. *JAMA* **269**, 232–6.

Kawachi, I., Colditz, G. A., Stampfer, M. J., *et al.* (1994). Smoking cessation and time course of decreased risks of coronary heart disease in middle-aged women. *Arch Intern Med* **154**, 169–75.

Keen, H., Lee, E. T., Russell, D., Miki, E., Bennett, P. H., and Lu, M. (2001). The appearance of retinopathy and progression to proliferative retinopathy: the WHO Multinational Study of Vascular Disease in Diabetes. *Diabetologia* **44 Suppl 2**, S22–30.

Kritz, H., Schmid, P., and Sinzinger, H. (1995). Passive smoking and cardiovascular risk. *Arch Intern Med* **155**, 1942–8.

Lambert L. J. (2000). Hysterectomy, hormones and coronary heart disease. Doctor of Philosophy thesis. University of Western Australia, Perth.

Law, M. R., Morris, J. K., and Wald, N. J. (1997). Environmental tobacco smoke exposure and ischaemic heart disease: an evaluation of the evidence. *Br Med J* **315**, 973–80.

LeVois, M. E. and Layard, M. W. (1995). Publication bias in the environmental tobacco smoke/coronary heart disease epidemiologic literature. *Regul Toxicol Pharmacol* **21**, 184–91.

Liew, D. (1989). Bachelor of Medical Science Honours thesis. Melbourne: Monash University.

McElduff, P., Dobson, A., Beaglehole, R., and Jackson, R. (1998a). Rapid reduction in coronary risk for those who quit cigarette smoking. *Aust NZ J Public Health* **22**, 787–91.

McElduff, P., Dobson, A. J., Jackson, R., Beaglehole, R., Heller, R. F., and Lay-Yee, R. (1998b). Coronary events and exposure to environmental tobacco smoke: a case-control study from Australia and New Zealand. *Tob Control* **7**, 41–6.

McElduff, P. and Dobson, A. J. (2001). Case fatality after an acute cardiac event: the effect of smoking and alcohol consumption. *J Clin Epidemiol* **54**, 58–67.

Macfarlane, J. E. and Jamrozik, K. (1993). Tobacco in Western Australia: an examination of patterns of tobacco smoking among adults in Western Australia from 1974 to 1991. *Aust J Public Health* **17**, 350–8.

Medical Research Council (1948). Streptomycin treatment of pulmonary tuberculosis. *Br Med J* **ii**, 769–82.

Molarius, A., Parsons, R. W., Dobson, A. J., Evans, A., Fortmann, S. P., Jamrozik, K., *et al.* (2001). for the WHO MONICA Project. Trends in cigarette smoking in 36 populations from the early 1980s to the mid 1990s: Findings from the WHO MONICA Project. *Am J Pub Health* **91**, 206–12.

Moller, A. M., Villebro, N., Pedersen, T., and Tonnesen, H. (2002). Effect of preoperative smoking intervention on postoperative complications: a randomised clinical trial. *Lancet* **359**, 114–7.

National Health and Medical Research Council (1987). Effects of passive smoking on health – Report of the NHMRC Working Party on the Effects of Passive smoking on Health. Canberra: Australian Government Publishing Service.

National Health and Medical Research Council (1997). The health effects of passive smoking: A scientific information paper. Canberra: Australian Government Publishing Service.

National Heart Foundation of Australia (1985). So you think you're a non-smoker. Canberra: National Heart Foundation.

National Heart Foundation of Australia (2000). Heart Facts Report – 1996. Canberra: National Heart Foundation of Australia.

Nidorf, S. M., Parsons, R. W., Thompson, P. L., Jamrozik, K., and Hobbs, M. S. T. (1990). Reduced risk of death at 28 days in patients taking a beta-blocker before admission to hospital with myocardial infarction. *Br Med J* **300**, 71–4.

Office of Environmental Health Hazard Assessment. (1997). Health effects of exposure to environmental tobacco smoke. Sacramento: California Environmental Protection Agency.

Otsuka, R., Watanabe, H., Hirata, K., *et al.* (2001). Acute effects of passive smoking on the coronary circulation in healthy young adults. *JAMA* **286**, 436–41.

Parish, S., Collins, R., Peto, R., *et al.* (1995). Cigarette smoking, tar yields, and non-fatal myocardial infarction: 14,000 cases and 32,000 controls in the United Kingdom. The International Studies of Infarct Survival (ISIS) Collaborators. *Br Med J* **311**, 471–7.

Penn, A., Keller, K., Snyder, C., Nadas, A., and Chen, L. C. (1996). The tar fraction of cigarette smoke does not promote arteriosclerotic plaque development. *Environ Health Perspect* **104**, 1108–13.

Penn, A., and Snyder, C. A. (1996). Butadiene inhalation accelerates atherosclerotic plaque development in cockerels. *Toxicology* **113**, 351–4.

Penn, A., Nath, R., Pan, J., Chen, L., Widmer, K., Henk, W., and Chung, F. L. (2001). 1,N(2)-propanodeoxyguanosine adduct formation in aortic DNA following inhalation of acrolein. *Environ Health Perspect* **109**, 219–24.

Pobereskin, L. H. (2001a). Influence of premorbid factors on survival following subarachnoid haemorrhage. *J Neurosurg* **95**, 555–9.

Pobereskin, L. H. (2001b). Incidence and outcome of subarachnoid haemorrhage, a retrospective population-based study. *J Neurol Neurosurg Psychiatry* **70**, 340–3.

Roper Organization. (1978). A study of public attitudes toward cigarette smoking and the tobacco industry. (Vol 1) Roper Organization Inc.

Rosenlund, M., Berglind, N., Gustaavsson, A., *et al.* (2001). Environmental tobacco smoke and myocardial infarction among never-smokers in the Stockholm Heart Epidemiology Program (SHEEP). *Epidemiology* **12**, 558–64.

Royal College of Physicians of London (1962). Smoking and health: a report of the Royal College of Physicians of London on smoking in relation to cancer of the lung and other diseases. London: Pitman Medical.

Sheps, D. S., Adams, K. S., Bromberg, P. A., *et al.* (1987). Lack of effect of low levels of carboxyhaemoglobin on cardiovascular function in patients with ischaemic heart disease. *Arch Environ Health* **42**, 108–16.

Shinton, R., and Beevers, G. (1989). Meta-analysis of relation between cigarette smoking and stroke. *Br Med J* **298**, 789–94.

Smith, C. J., Fischer, T. H., and Sears, S. B. (2000). Environmental tobacco smoke, cardiovascular disease, and the non-linear dose-response hypothesis. *Toxicol Sci* **54**, 462–72.

Sonke, G. S., Stewart, A. W., Beaglehole, R., Jackson, R., and White, H. D. (1997). Comparison of case fatality in smokers and non-smokers after acute cardiac event. *Br Med J* **315**, 992–3.

Spencer, C. A., Jamrozik, K., Lambert, L. J. (1999). Do simple prudent health behaviours protect men from myocardial infarction? *Intl J Epidemiol* **28**, 846–52.

Stamler, J., Wentworth, D., and Neaton, J. D. (1986). Is relationship between serum cholesterol and risk of premature death from coronary heart disease continuous and graded? Findings in 356,222 primary screenees of the Multiple Risk Factor Intervention Trial (MRFIT). *JAMA* **256**, 2823–8.

Stratton, I. M., Kolmei, D. M., Aldington, S. J. Turner, R, C., Holman, R. R., Manley, S. E., and Matthews, D. R. (2001). UKPDS 50: risk factors for incidence and progression of retinopathy in Type II diabetes over 6 years from diagnosis. *Diabetologia* **44**, 156–63.

Steenland, K., Sieber, K., Etzel, R. A., Pechacek, T., and Maurer, K. (1998). Exposure to environmental tobacco smoke and risk factors for heart disease among never smokers in the Third National Health and Nutrition Examination Survey. *Am J Epidemiol* **147**, 932–9.

Sumida, H., Watanabe, H., Kugiyama, K., Ohgushi, M., Matsumura, T., and Yasue, H. (1998). Does passive smoking impair endothelium-dependent coronary artery dilation in women? *J Am Coll Cardiol* **31**, 811–5.

Thun, M., Henley, J., and Apicella, L. (1999). Epidemiologic studies of fatal and nonfatal cardiovascular disease and ETS exposure from spousal smoking. *Environ Health Perspect* **107** Suppl 6, 841–6.

Trichopoulos, D., Kalandidi, A., Sparros, L., and MacMahon, B. (1981). Lung cancer and passive smoking. *Intl J Cancer* **27**, 1–4.

United States Department of Health and Human Services (1986). The health consequences of involuntary smoking. Washington DC: US Government Printing Office.

United States Department of Health and Human Services (1983). The health consequences of smoking: cardiovascular disease. Washington DC: US Government Printing Office.

van Gijn, J., and Rinkel, G. J. E. (2001). Subarachnoid haemorrhage: diagnosis, causes and management. Brain **124**, 249–78.

Verhoef, P., Rimm, E. B., Hunter, D. J., Chen, J., Willett, W. C., Kelsey, K., and Stampfer, M. J. (1998). A common mutation in the methylenetetrahydrofolate reductase gene and risk of coronary heart disease: results among U.S. men. *J Am Coll Cardiol* **32**, 353–9.

Wald N. J. (1978). Smoking in relation to lung cancer and coronary heart disease. *Bull Intl Union Against TB* **53**, 325–33.

Wald, N. J. and Watt, H. C. (1997). Prospective study of effect of switching from cigarettes to pipes or cigars on mortality from three smoking related diseases. *Br Med J* **314**, 1860–3.

Wells, A. J. (1994). Passive smoking as a cause of heart disease. *J Am Coll Cardiol* **24**, 546–54.

Wells, A. J., English, P. B., Posner, S. F., Wagenknecht, L. E., and Perez-Stable, E. J. (1998). Misclassification rates for current smokers misclassified as nonsmokers. *Am J Public Health* **88**, 1503–9.

Wilmink, T. B., Quick, C. R., and Day, N. E. (1999). The association between cigarette smoking and abdominal aortic aneurysms. *J Vasc Surg* **30**, 1099–105.

World Health Organization (1999). The world health report 1999: Making a difference. WHO, Geneva.

Part 8

Tobacco and respiratory disease

Chapter 33

Chronic obstructive pulmonary disease

David M. Burns

Introduction

Tobacco use antedates the arrival of Columbus in the Americas, and tobacco leaf became a mainstay of trade between America and Europe over the next several centuries. However, use of tobacco as cigarettes is a behavior largely confined to the twentieth and now the twenty-first century (USDHHS 2001). Milder blends of flue-cured tobaccos are used for most cigarettes, and they produce a more acid smoke than the tobacco used for pipes and cigars (IARC 1986). Nicotine, the addictive agent sought by the smoker, is less readily absorbed across the oral mucosa from this more acid smoke; and, to satisfy the smokers need for this drug, smoke must be inhaled into much larger surface area of the lung to allow sufficient absorption. This obligatory inhalation of cigarette smoke by the addicted smoker makes cigarette smoking the most hazardous form of tobacco use, and the deposition and retention of tobacco smoke in the lung causes chronic obstructive pulmonary disease (COPD). An extensive body of literature has examined the relationship of tobacco smoke inhalation to chronic lung disease, and that literature is reviewed elsewhere (USDHHS 1984, 1990, 2001, in press). This chapter presents a synthesis of the available information, but it does not attempt to provide an exhaustive set of references to this substantial body of literature.

Lung damage from tobacco smoke inhalation is described using a variety of terms including chronic bronchitis, emphysema, chronic obstructive lung disease (COLD), COPD, and chronic airflow obstruction. The pathophysiological pattern of this injury is often separated into three overlapping pictures which are each present to a variable extent in most long-term cigarette smokers. The first pattern consists of inflammatory changes in the larger airways with hypertrophy of the airway lining and an increased number of mucus-secreting glands, and it commonly presents with the clinical symptom of a chronic cough productive of small amounts of sputum. This set of clinical symptoms is technically defined as chronic bronchitis when it is present for three or more months in two or more years. However, in common medical usage, the diagnosis of chronic bronchitis sometimes also includes individuals with emphysema and airflow limitation rather than just chronic cough. This overlapping usage of terms, which have specific scientific definitions but are commonly used in medical and scientific discourse to include all forms of tobacco-induced chronic lung injury, occurs for all of the common names for smoking-induced lung disease; and it causes confusion in the medical and lay literature. In this chapter we will use the term COPD to encompass all of the patterns of lung injury produced by cigarette smoking.

A second pathophysiological pattern is that of inflammatory changes in the smaller and more distal airways of the lung which narrows these airways and increases their resistance to airflow. These changes can progress to produce the decreased expiratory airflow characteristic of clinically significant COPD.

Inflammatory cells present in the peribronchiolar spaces release digestive enzymes that ultimately damage and disrupt the alveolar walls producing emphysema, the third pathophysiological pattern of injury. As the alveolar walls rupture, the lung becomes composed of a smaller number of much larger airspaces with a reduced surface area and decreased elastic recoil. When examined at autopsy, this digested lung appears full of holes of various sizes. During life, it functions poorly for gas exchange and ventilation. The decreased elastic recoil of an emphysematous lung reduces the pressure available to drive expiratory airflow and allows the airways to collapse during expiration, further worsening the rate of expiratory airflow produced by the inflammatory changes in the small airways described above.

Composition of tobacco smoke

Tobacco smoke is a complex aerosol with particles largely within the range of 0.1–1.0 microns in diameter (Stratton *et al.* 2001). These particles are small enough that they are not removed in the upper airway and deposit largely on the alveolar and airway surfaces of the lung. The pattern of lung deposition is consistent with particles of a somewhat larger size since there is more deposition in the airways and on the alveolar surfaces than would be expected from extrapolations based on particle size alone (Stratton *et al.* 2001). The difference in deposition location is likely due to aggregation of particles in the very dense aerosol of mainstream smoke or because the particles may grow in size as they are humidified in the airway.

Tobacco smoke contains over 4800 individual constituents and the composition of the smoke is undergoing rapid chemical change as it is inhaled (IARC 1986). Biologically active free radicals are generated as tobacco is burned, and they persist long enough to interact with lung tissue following inhalation. The constituents of smoke have at least three toxicities important for causing injury to the lung in COPD. Tobacco smoke as whole smoke, and several of its constituents, are potent irritants to the airways capable of creating an inflammatory response in the airways even with initial use. This acute irritant response, manifest as a reflex cough in many adolescents with their first inhalation of cigarette smoke, disappears as the airway adapts to repetitive exposure to smoke. It is replaced by a chronic low-grade inflammation of the airways.

Many of the constituents in both the gas phase and the particulate phase of smoke paralyse the cilia lining the airways. Cilia are the hair-like structures on the surface of airway cells that rhythmically beat to move mucus up and out of the lung aiding in the removal of particles deposited on the surface of the airways. Paralysis interferes with the clearance process of the lung and results in a longer residence time in the airway for toxic smoke constituents. Lastly, smoke can oxidatively inactivate some of the protective proteins in the blood, most notably the antiproteases that prevent lung digestion.

Early responses of the lung to cigarette smoking

Acute cough and bronchoconstriction are common reactions to the first inhalation of cigarette smoke. When this protective warning of the airways is ignored and regular smoking is begun, inflammatory changes appear in the small (>2 mm) airways of the lung. These changes are evident in some smokers within the first few years of smoking; and, after smoking for 10–15 years, the majority of smokers have evidence of abnormal function in these small airways. Much of the functional limitation of expiratory airflow in COPD results from increased resistance to expiratory airflow in these same small airways (Hogg et al. 1968). However, development of inflammatory changes in the small airways early in the smoking experience is not a useful predictor of the likelihood of subsequently developing clinically significant COPD. These early changes are likely a nearly universal response to the inhaled irritants in the smoke, and it is other biologic or genetic determinants of how the lung responds to chronic irritation that define which smokers will go on to develop COPD.

Even during adolescence and early adulthood, cigarette smoking is associated with a lower level of lung function and an increased frequency of respiratory symptoms, particularly cough (USDHHS 1994). Adolescent smokers have a lower rate of increase in lung function as they grow into adulthood when compared to nonsmoking adolescents, and there is evidence that they reach a lower level of peak lung function (Tager et al. 1988). There is also concern that their decline in lung function may begin at an earlier age. Changes in lung development documented in actively smoking adolescents are likely superimposed on similar changes produced by exposure to environmental tobacco smoke during infancy and early childhood.

Changes in lung function in smokers and nonsmokers

The most widely used measure of lung function abnormality in COPD is the volume of air that can be expired during the first second with a maximal effort (FEV_1). Among populations of heavy smokers, an excess decline in the FEV_1 is first seen at age 25–34 for both males and females in comparison with never smokers. An excess decline in FEV_1 is seen among both light and heavy smokers by age 35–44 (Beck et al. 1981).

This excess decline in lung function is greater among those who smoke more cigarettes per day and worsens with increasing duration of smoking (Burrows *et al.* 1977; USDHHS 1984).

The relationship between smoking and lung function as measured by FEV_1 at various ages is presented in Fig. 33.1. When more than 70 per cent of lung function is lost, it is common for smokers to have symptoms from their ventilatory limitation, most notably shortness of breath on exertion. Once 90 per cent of lung function has been lost ventilatory limitation can compromise survival and death from ventilatory failure becomes an increasingly likely and unavoidable outcome. Among normal individuals who do not smoke, and who do not have substantive exposure to environmental tobacco smoke, lung function increases as a child grows and the FEV_1 reaches a peak between ages 20 and 25 years. Thereafter, it slowly declines. This experience is presented as a thick solid line in Fig. 33.1. Children who are exposed to environmental tobacco smoke have a lower rate of lung growth. That effect of environmental tobacco smoke exposure is portrayed by the dotted line prior to age 20 in the figure. This lower

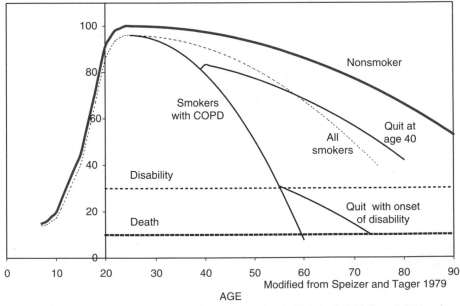

Fig. 33.1 FEV_1 as a per cent of the value at age 25 for smokers, nonsmokers, and those who quit. The values presented are the FEV_1 as a percentage of the value for an individual at age 25 years. The heavy solid line represents those who have never smoked, the dashed line represents the entire population of smokers including those exposed to environmental tobacco smoke as children, the thin solid line represents those smokers who are going to develop COPD, thin solid lines also represent those who quit at age 40 years and when symptoms develop. See text for description.

rate of growth in lung function may be worsened, and the age of peak lung growth may be reached earlier, if the adolescent begins to actively smoke cigarettes. There is considerable concern that these changes in the developing lung may predispose the adult lung to a more rapid decline in function with increasing age, particularly with continued smoking during adulthood.

When the entire population of adult smokers is examined, their rate of lung function decline with age is substantially steeper than that for nonsmokers, reflecting progressive damage to the airways and alveoli of the their lungs. This change with advancing age and duration of smoking is presented in Fig. 33.1 as a dashed line labeled 'all smokers'. However, the rate of decline is not sufficient to cause respiratory disability for the majority of smokers, in part because of the large ventilatory reserve of the lung. When an abnormal FEV_1 is used as the criteria for diagnosis of COPD, approximately one-third of smokers over age 55 (Sherrill et al. 1994) have COPD, and that percentage increases to over 45 per cent when smokers over age 65 are examined (Higgins et al. 1993). These high prevalences of abnormal lung function are supported by autopsy studies which show evidence of at least some emphysema in the lungs of approximately 90 per cent of long-term cigarette smokers (Auerbach et al. 1972; Sutinen et al. 1978).

Many smokers with abnormal lung function may be unaware of the presence of lung injury and may have no symptoms related to their lung damage. A minority of cigarette smokers, in the range of 15 per cent, will have a more rapid decline in lung function and will develop clinically significant COPD. These smokers are more likely to have smoked more cigarettes per day and to have smoked for a longer duration, but known characteristics of smoking behavior do not fully explain why some smokers will develop COPD and others with similar smoking patterns do not. Differences in genetic susceptibility or differences in response to inflammation have been postulated as reasons for the differences in the rate of progression to clinically significant disease.

The thin solid line in Fig. 33.1 represents those smokers who go on to develop COPD. They have a more rapid decline in lung function with time, as must be expected since they have developed more extensive disease. Having an abnormal FEV_1 by early middle age (age 45) is a strong predictor of developing COPD, but it is less clear that the rate of decline over one period of time is a good predictor of the future rate of decline or of the likelihood of developing COPD. Identification of smokers with abnormal lung function in early middle age offers the opportunity to intervene with smoking cessation assistance before clinically significant ventilatory limitation develops. Those who quit smoking are likely to have a small improvement in lung function during the first year of abstinence, and their rate of decline in lung function slows to that of the never smoker (Anthonisen et al. 1994; Scanlon et al. 2000). This pattern of change is depicted by the thin solid line in Fig. 33.1 labeled 'quit at age 40'. If smokers quit before there is extensive lung damage and remain abstinent, it is likely that most of them will never develop clinically significant COPD.

In contrast to interventions early in the course of lung injury from smoking, getting smokers to quit once they have developed disease extensive enough to be disabling has more limited benefits. Even for this group with extensive damage, there is a slowing in the rate of decline in lung function with cessation of smoking; but the individuals usually remain symptomatic. The effect is simply to prolong the interval between the onset of symptoms and death rather than to eliminate the disability. This effect is depicted by the thin solid line in Fig. 33.1 labeled 'Quit with onset of disability'.

Chronic cough is a less disabling but far more common result of cigarette smoking than is ventilatory limitation. Increased prevalence of chronic cough is evident even among adolescent and young adult smokers. The prevalence increases with increasing duration of smoking and is present in the majority of moderate to heavy smokers over age 60 years (Lebowitz and Burrows 1977). This cough begins as a dry cough but progresses with longer duration of smoking to become productive of small amounts of mucus.

Mechanisms of lung injury

Airway inflammation and enzymatic digestion of lung structural proteins (elastin and collagen) are mechanisms that define the injury to the lung in COPD. Early in the smoking exposure, the changes are edema and inflammatory cell (cytotoxic T lympho-cytes and macrophages) infiltration in the walls of the small airways of the lung. Inflammation is due to epithelial cell injury that increases permeability and releases proinflammatory mediators. These mediators draw in neutrophils, and the result is a pathological picture typical of chronic inflammation. The vast majority of smokers develop these changes, and many develop them within the first year or two of smoking. These early changes can reverse within one year following cessation among smokers with a short smoking duration (Buist et al. 1976, 1979). With longer duration of smok-ing, epithelial hyperplasia, smooth muscle hypertrophy, and peribronchiolar fibrosis are commonly found in most smokers (Cosio et al. 1978, 1980). At least modest degree of emphysema is found in most continuing smokers over the age of 60 years (Auerbach et al. 1972; Sutinen et al. 1978), and the severity of the emphysematous change increases with the number of cigarettes smoked per day.

The neutrophils and macrophages that characterize the inflammatory response to cigarette smoke in the lung release enzymes capable of digesting the elastin and colla-gen that make up the structural elements of the lung. Antiproteases, released from macrophages and found in the blood, block the action of these enzymes (Barnes 2000). The result is a balance that preserves the integrity of normal lung while allowing the lung to respond to external infectious agents by releasing digestive enzymes. Oxidants in cigarette smoke inactivate the antiproteases unbalancing this relationship and lead-ing to digestion of lung tissue, rupture of alveolar walls, and emphysematous dilation of the alveolar spaces (Barnes 2000).

In contrast to the inflammatory changes in the small airways, emphysema is usually manifested later in life (over age 50) and is not reversible.

Death rates from COPD in smokers and nonsmokers

Death from infection, respiratory failure, or other complications of COPD is an end result of the slowly accumulating lung damage produced by smoking. Because symptoms and disability may be present for a decade or more before death from COPD, and because individuals may die with COPD without it being the cause of death, death rates from COPD underestimate both the extent of cigarette-induced lung injury among smokers and the prevalence of COPD for the general population. Comparisons of mortality rates between smokers and nonsmokers (e.g. relative risks) yield very high values at most ages, since the occurrence of COPD is largely limited to smokers and very low rates of disease or death from COPD occur among never smokers. Mortality-based relative risks increase with increasing number of cigarettes smoked per day and increasing duration of smoking (USDHHS 1984).

The effect of smoking on rates of death from COPD can also be examined using the excess death rate in smokers. An excess death rate is simply the age and disease-specific death rates in never smokers subtracted from the same age and disease-specific death rates in smokers, and it offers a different perspective on the absolute risks of the diseases due to smoking at different ages.

Figure 33.2 presents excess death rates for lung cancer, coronary heart diseases, and COPD for male smokers examined in the American Cancer Society Cancer Prevention Study II (Thun *et al.* 1997). It is evident that coronary heart disease results in substantial excess mortality among smokers by age 40 years, and excess death rates from lung cancer increases rapidly after age 50. However, death from COPD is largely confined to ages over 60–65 years. This later onset of excess death rates from COPD is due to the slowly progressive nature of the disease process and the large ventilatory reserve of the lung, but it is also the reason why morbidity and health care costs from COPD are much larger than one might expect from comparisons based solely on numbers of deaths from different causes.

The late rise in smoking attributable death rate from COPD also helps to explain why national death rates from heart disease and lung cancer rise more rapidly than do death rates from COPD as cigarette smoking is first adopted by the population of a country, and correspondingly why death rates from COPD decline more slowly than those of heart disease and cancer as the prevalence of smoking declines.

Changes with cessation of smoking

The risk of dying from COPD declines following cessation of cigarette smoking when compared to that of continuing smokers (USDHHS 1990). The decline in risk is slower than that for heart disease and lung cancer, and there remains a small increase in risk even after prolonged abstinence (NCI 1997). The fraction of the excess risk of dying of COPD, lung cancer, and coronary heart disease that remains after abstinence of various durations is presented in Fig. 33.3. It takes longer for the excess risk of death from

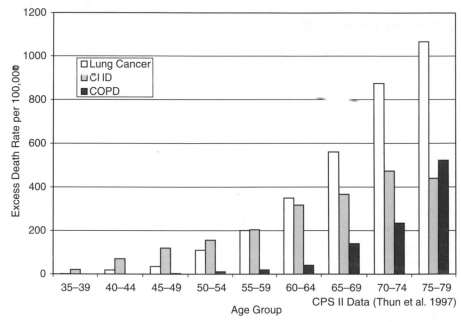

Fig. 33.2 Male excess death rates* from smoking-caused diseases (*rates in smokers minus the rate in never smokers). Excess rates are calculated by subtracting the age-specific death rate for a given disease experienced by smokers from that for never smokers in the American Cancer Society Cancer Prevention Study II as published by Thun *et al.* (1997). Rates are presented for male smokers.

COPD to decline following cessation, and the death rate remains substantially elevated in former smokers even after 20 years of abstinence.

As described above, lung function may improve slightly following cessation probably due to a decrease in airway inflammation once the exposure to the irritants in tobacco smoke ceases. The rate of lung function decline with advancing age also slows following cessation and returns to that of the never smoker (Anthonisen *et al.* 1994; Scanlon *et al.* 2000). However, the emphysema present in the lung at the time of cessation does not repair, and lung function rarely returns to normal among smokers with substantial lung injury at the time of cessation.

Respiratory symptoms, most notably a chronic productive cough, often improve following cessation and may disappear altogether.

Pipe and cigar smoking

Cigarette smokers are much more likely to inhale tobacco smoke than are those who have only smoked pipes and cigars, and this distinction is evident in the pattern of disease risks found among smokers of different forms of tobacco. Pipe and cigar smokers have risks similar to those of cigarette smokers for cancers of the oral cavity where

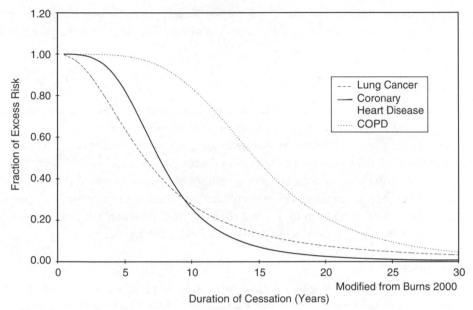

Fig. 33.3 Fraction of excess risk remaining with increasing duration of cessation. The data presented are the fraction of the excess death rate (rate in smokers minus the rate in never smokers of the same age) that remains after different numbers of years following successful smoking cessation. Data are modeled from the American Cancer Society Cancer Prevention Study I as described in Burns (2000).

exposure to smoke is similar whether the smoker inhales or not; but cancer of the lung and COPD are much less common among pipe and cigar smokers than among cigarette smokers (Shanks *et al.* 1998). These distinctions in disease risks disappear if pipe and cigar smokers inhale more deeply, an observation of considerable concern since cigarette smokers who have switched to pipes or cigars are much more likely to report that they inhale the smoke than are smokers who have only used these forms of tobacco.

Cigarettes with lower machine-measured yields of tar and nicotine

The yield of tar and nicotine as measured by machine has declined substantially for commercial cigarettes sold over the past 50 years, and these newer and filtered cigarettes have been presented to the public as safer alternatives to unfiltered and higher tar cigarettes (Pollay and Dewhirst 2002). Smokers of these types of cigarettes report them as being 'smoother on the throat and lighter on their chest' (Shiffman *et al.* 2001), and there is some evidence to suggest that smokers of these products may have a lower prevalence of chronic cough (Higenbottam *et al.* 1980). However, the evidence does not suggest a difference in the extent of lung function impairment or mortality from

COPD with use of these cigarettes (NCI 2001). Whatever symptomatic benefits may occur, they are clearly dwarfed by the increases in disease risk that accrue with continued smoking.

Summary

Cigarette smoking is the dominant cause of chronic obstructive pulmonary disease for both men and women. Changes in the lungs of smokers can be demonstrated within a few years of beginning to smoke. By the age 25–34 years, evidence of functional loss is evident in populations of smokers. The risks of developing ventilatory impairment and of dying of COPD increase with increasing number of cigarettes smoked per day and increased duration of smoking. Cessation of smoking alters the rate of lung function decline and risk of dying from COPD, but the benefits of cessation are greatest when cessation can be achieved early before substantial lung injury has occurred.

References

Anthonisen, N. R., Connett, J. E., Kiley, J. P., Altose, M. D., Bailey, W. C., Buist, A. S., *et al.* (1994). Effects of smoking intervention and the use of inhaled anticholinergic bronchodilator on the rate of decline in FEV_1: the Lung Health Study. *Journal of the American Medical Association*, **272**, 1497–505.

Auerbach, O., Hammond, E. C., Garfinkel, L., and Benante, C. (1972). Relation of smoking and age to emphysema. Whole-lung section study. *New England Journal of Medicine*, **286**, 853–7.

Barnes, P. J. (2000). Chronic obstructive pulmonary disease. *New England Journal of Medicine*, **343**, 269–80.

Beck, G. J., Doyle, C. A., and Schachter, E. N. (1981). Smoking and lung function. *American Review of Respiratory Disease*, **123**, 149–55.

Buist, A. S., Sexton, G. J., Nagy, J. M., and Ross, B. B. (1976). The effect of smoking cessation and modification on lung function. *American Review of Respiratory Disease*, **114**, 115–22.

Buist, A. S., Nagy, J. M., and Sexton, G. J. (1979). The effect of smoking cessation on pulmonary function: a 30-month follow-up of two smoking cessation clinics. *American Review of Respiratory Disease*, **120**, 953–7.

Burns, D. M. (2000). Primary prevention, smoking, and smoking cessation—implications for future trends in lung cancer prevention. *Cancer*, **89**, No. 11 (Suppl), 2506–9.

Burrows, B., Knudson, R. J., Cline, M. G., and Lebowitz, M. D. (1977). Quantitative relationships between cigarette smoking and ventilatory function. *American Review of Respiratory Disease*, **115**, 195–205.

Cosio, M. G., Chezzo, H., Hogg, J. C., Corbin, R., Lovelnd, M., Dosman, J., and Macklem, P. T. (1978). The relations between structural changes in the small airways and pulmonary function tests. *New England Journal of Medicine*, **298**, 1277–81.

Cosio, M. G., Hale, K. A., and Niewoehner, D. E. (1980). Morphologic and morphometric effects of prolonged cigarette smoking on the small airways. *American Review of Respiratory Disease*, **122**, 265–71.

Higenbottam, T., Clark, T. J. H., Shipley, M. J., and Rose, G. (1980). Lung function and symptoms of cigarette smokers related to tar yield and number of cigarettes smoked. *Lancet*, **1**(8165), 409–11.

Higgins, M. W., Enright, P. L., Kronmal, R. A., Schenker, M. B., Anton-Culver, H., and Lyles, M. (1993). Smoking and lung function in elderly men and women: the Cardiovascular Health Study. *Journal of the American Medical Association*, **269**, 2741–8.

Hogg, J. C., Macklem, P. T., and Thurlbeck, W. M. (1968). Site and nature of airway obstruction in chronic lung disease. *New England Journal of Medicine*, **278**, 1355–60.

International Agency for Research on Cancer (1986). *IARC Monographs on the carcinogenic risk of chemicals to humans: tobacco smoking*. Vol. 38. IARC, Lyon, France.

Lebowitz, M. D. and Burrows, B. (1977). Quantitative relationships between cigarette smoking and chronic productive cough. *International Journal of Epidemiology*, **6**, 107–13.

National Cancer Institute. *Smoking and Tobacco Control Monograph # 8: Changes in cigarette-related disease risks and their implications for prevention and control* (ed. D. Burns, L. Garfinkel, and J Samet), U.S. Department of Health and Human Services, Public Health Service, National Institutes of Health, National Cancer Institute. NIH Publication No. 97-4213, 1997.

National Cancer Institute. *Smoking and Tobacco Control Monograph No.13. Risks associated with smoking cigarettes with low machine yields of tar and nicotine*. U.S. Department of Health and Human Services, Bethesda. NCI, October 2001.

Pollay, R. W. and Dewhirst, T. (2002). The dark side of marketing seemingly 'light' cigarettes: successful images and failed fact. *Tobacco Control*, **11**(Suppl 1), I18–31.

Scanlon, P. D., Connett, J. E., Waller, L. A., Altose, M. D., Bailey, W. C., Buist, A. S., and Tashkin, D. P. (2000). Smoking cessation and lung function in mild-to-moderate chronic obstructive pulmonary disease: the Lung Health Study. *American Journal of Respiratory and Critical Care Medicine*, **161**, 381–90.

Shanks, T. and Burns, D. (1998). Disease consequences of cigar smoking. In: *Cigar smoking in the United States: Health effects and trends. Smoking and Tobacco Control Monograph No. 9* (ed. D. Burns, K.M. Cummings, and D. Hoffman), USDHHS NIH NCI, Chapter 4.

Sherrill, D. L., Holberg, C. J., Enright, P. L., Lebowitz, M. D., and Burrows, B. (1994). Longitudinal analysis of the effects of smoking onset and cessation on pulmonary function. *American Journal of Respiratory and Critical Care Medicine*, **149**, 591–7.

Shiffman, S., Pillitteri, J. L., Burton, S. L., Rohay, J. M., and Gitchell, J. G. (2001). Smokers beliefs about 'light' and 'ultra light' cigarettes. *Tobacco Control*, **10**(Suppl I), i17–i23.

Speizer, F. E. and Tager, I. B. (1979). Epidemiology of chronic mucus hypersecretion and obstructive airways disease. *Epidemiology Reviews*, **1**, 124–42.

Stratton, K., Shetty, P., Wallace, R., and Bondurant, S., eds. (2001). *Clearing the smoke. Assessing the science base for tobacco harm reduction*. National Academy Press, Washington DC.

Sutinen, S., Vaajalahti, P., and Paakko, P. (1978). Prevalence, severity, and types of pulmonary emphysema in a population of deaths in a Finnish city. Correlation with age, sex and smoking. *Scandinavian Journal of Respiratory Disease*, **59**, 101–15.

Tager, I. B., Segal, M. R., Speizer, F. E., and Weiss, S. T. (1988). The natural history of forced expiratory volumes: effect of cigarette smoking and respiratory symptoms. *American Review of Respiratory Disease*, **138**, 837–49.

Thun, M., Myers, D., Day-Lally, C., Namboodiri, M., Calle, E., Flanders, W. D., *et al*. (1997). Age and the exposure-response relationships between cigarette smoking and premature death in Cancer Prevention study II, Chapter 5. In: *Changes in cigarette-related disease risks and their implications for prevention and control: smoking and tobacco control monograph # 8*. (ed. D. Burns, L. Garfinkel, and J. Samet). U.S. Department of Health and Human Services, Public Health Service, National Institutes of Health, National Cancer Institute, NIH Publication No. 97-4213, pp. 383–476.

U.S. Department of Health and Human Services (1984). *The health consequences of smoking: chronic obstructive lung disease. A report of the surgeon general*. U.S. Department of Health and Human Services, Public Health Service, Office on Smoking and Health, DHHS Publication No. (PHS) 84-50205.

U.S. Department of Health and Human Services (1990). *The health benefits of smoking cessation*. U.S. Dept of Health and Human Services, Public Health Service, Centers for Disease Control, National Center for Chronic Disease Prevention and Health Promotion, Office on Smoking and Health, DHHS Publication No. (CDC) 90-8416.

U.S. Department of Health and Human Services (1994). *Preventing tobacco use among young people: A report of the surgeon general*. U.S. DHHS, Public Health Service, Centers for Disease Control and Prevention, National Center for Chronic Disease Prevention and Health Promotion, Office on Smoking and Health, Atlanta G.

U.S. Department of Health and Human Services (2001). *Women and smoking: a report of the surgeon general*. Atlanta, U.S. Department of Health and Human Services, Public Health Service, Centers for Disease Control and Prevention, National Center for Chronic Disease Prevention and Health Promotion, Office on Smoking and Health, Georgia.

U.S. Department of Health and Human Services (in press) *The health consequences of tobacco use: A report of the surgeon general*. U.S. Department of Health and Human Services, Public Health Service, Centers for Disease Control and Prevention, National Center for Chronic Disease Prevention and Health Promotion, Office on Smoking and Health, Atlanta, Georgia.

Part 9

Tobacco and other diseases

Chapter 34

Smoking and other disorders

Allan Hackshaw

Introduction

Given that smoking consists of several thousand chemicals and toxins it is no wonder that it is associated with a wide range of diseases. Since the first epidemiological studies linking smoking with lung cancer, there has been an abundance of studies (epidemiological and biological) that have shown smokers to be at a higher (or in a few cases, lower) risk of developing certain disorders. Smoking is an established cause of several cancers, respiratory disease, and cardiovascular disease; these are described elsewhere in this book. Here, I describe disorders other than those just mentioned and provide an overview of published reviews and the results of published meta-analyses where available. I also present the results from cohort studies that are based on incident cases (where possible), thus aiming to ensure that smoking has preceded the disorder and avoiding some of the possible biases associated with case–control studies. The studies referenced here may not be all that are available. The disorders reviewed here are by no means all those that are or may be associated with smoking. They represent ones that are relatively common in the population and in which smoking has, in the past, been regarded as a risk factor.

Gastrointestinal system

Smoking is associated with several disorders of the gastrointestinal tract. Table 34.1 shows pooled relative risks of some of the main disorders obtained from meta-analyses.

Peptic ulcer

Peptic ulcers (gastric or duodenal) are relatively common amongst adults. Many epidemiological studies have shown that smokers are about twice as likely to develop peptic ulcers than non-smokers, including several large cohort studies that looked at incidence of the disease (Table 34.2). Risk increases with increasing cigarette consumption (Paffenberger *et al.* 1974; Anda *et al.* 1990) and it is lower in ex-smokers (Anda *et al.* 1990; Vessey *et al.* 1992; Doll *et al.* 1994). Studies have also showed that smoking can delay the healing process once ulcers have developed and it can increase the risk of recurrence. The evidence is consistent with that from biological studies from which

Table 34.1 Published pooled relative risks associated with smoking and gastrointestinal disease

Disorder	Author	Number of epidemiological studies in analysis	Gender	Relative risk (95% CI) in smokers compared to non-smokers
Peptic ulcer	Kurata and Nogawa 1997	20	Men and women	2.2 (2.0–2.3)
Crohn's disease	Logan 1990	7	Men and Women	2.4 (2.0–2.9)
	English et al. 1995	7	Men	2.24 (1.45–3.46)
		7	Women	4.76 (3.10–7.31)
Ulcerative colitis	Logan 1990	8	Men and women	0.47 (0.39–0.56)
Gallstone disease	English et al. 1995	4	Men and women	1.24 (1.16–1.32)

Table 34.2 Cohort studies that reported results on peptic ulcer and smoking

Study	Country	Number of subjects	Total number of ulcers diagnosed	Gender	Relative risk in current smokers compared to never-smokers (95% CI)
Paffenberger et al. 1974	USA	26 954	487	Men	1.30 (1.07–1.58)
Stemmermann et al. 1989	USA (Hawaii)	5933	326	Men	2.12 (1.60–2.80)
Anda et al. 1990	USA	2851	140	Women	1.8 (1.2–2.6)
Kurata et al. 1992	USA	34 198	154	Men	1.50 (0.47–4.81)
				Women	1.48 (0.35–6.24)
Vessey et al. 1992	UK	17 032	175	Women	1.74 (not reported)
Doll et al. 1994	UK	34 439	134*	Men	3.00 (not reported)
Johnsen et al. 1994	Norway	6864	165	Men	2.66 (1.88–3.77)
		6907	78	Women	2.28 (1.42–3.67)

*Deaths from peptic ulcer.

several mechanisms have been proposed. Smoking affects factors that can promote the development of ulcers, for example by increasing gastric secretions such as pepsin and causing the reflux of contents in the duodenum back into the stomach. It also has a detrimental effect on the defensive mechanisms in the gastroduodenal mucosa, which in the absence of smoking would aid ulcer healing. There have been several reviews on this topic, for example, see Ashley (1997), Eastwood (1997), Parasher and Eastwood (2000).

However, with the recent discovery of the micro-organism *Helicobacter pylori* as an important cause of peptic ulcer, it is possible that the effect of smoking as an independent risk factor is less than originally thought. It is proposed that smokers are only more susceptible to *H. pylori* infection and that smoking enhances the adverse effects of the infection (Parasher and Eastwood 2000). Furthermore, there is evidence that once the infection has been eradicated, smoking has little or no effect on ulcer development or recurrence (Marshall *et al.* 1988; Borody *et al.* 1992; O'Connor *et al.* 1995; Chan *et al.* 1997; Kadayifci *et al.* 1997). Whatever the true mechanism may be, smoking is an important risk factor, either by causing some ulcers directly or indirectly by leading to *H. pylori* infection.

Inflammatory bowel disease

It is well documented that smoking increases the risk of Crohn's disease but decreases the risk of ulcerative colitis, and this has been consistent between studies, most of which have been case–control studies. Table 34.3 shows the results of these studies, including two cohort studies which allowed for oral contraceptive use (associated with both smoking and inflammatory bowel disease, Vessey *et al.* 1986). Current smokers have about half the risk of ulcerative colitis compared to never-smokers and more than twice the risk of Crohn's disease, though the risk is higher in women than in men (Table 34.4). It is estimated that about one-third of all cases of Crohn's disease could be attributed to smoking (Logan 1990). In ex-smokers, whilst the risk for Crohn's disease is lower than that in current smokers (former vs. never; relative risk 1.5, 95% CI 1.1–1.9 and current vs. never; relative risk 2.4, 95% CI 2.0–2.9), the association with ulcerative colitis is unclear; there seems to be an increased risk. The pooled result in the eight case–control studies is 1.9 (95% CI 1.6–2.3) and it is similarly raised, though not so greatly, in the cohort study by Vessey *et al.* 1986 (relative risk 1.25). If similar results are found in further cohort studies it would indicate that the timing of smoking plays some part in the development of ulcerative colitis.

The biological mechanism for inflammatory bowel disease and its association with smoking are not yet fully understood, and it is still unclear why current smoking would have opposite effects on these two disorders, that is, it seems to promote Crohn's disease but protect against ulcerative colitis. Nicotine (in the form of patches or chewing gum) has been proposed as a possible treatment for ulcerative colitis though its effectiveness remains to be confirmed. Reviews of smoking and inflammatory bowel disease can be found in Ashley (1997), Logan (1990), and Rubin and Hanauer (2000).

Table 34.3 Studies that reported results on Crohn's disease and smoking*

Study	Country	Total number of subjects with Crohn's disease	Gender	Relative risk in current smokers compared to never-smokers (95% CI)
Case–control				
Logan et al. 1984, 1986	UK	131	Men and women	4.2 (2.5–6.8)
Tobin et al. 1987	UK	127	Men and women	3.2 (1.9–5.5)
Franceschi et al. 1987	Italy	109	Men and women	2.9 (1.8–4.9)
Lindberg et al. 1988	Sweden	144	Men and women	2.2 (1.4–3.3)
Benoni and Nilsson 1987	Sweden	155	Men and women	2.0 (1.3–3.1)
Calkins et al. 1984	USA	132	Men and women	2.1 (1.2–3.5)
Sandler and Holland 1988	USA	298	Men and women	1.9 (1.3–2.8)
Combined	**–**	**1096**	**Men and women**	**2.4 (2.0–2.9)**
Cohort				
Vessey et al. 1986	UK	18/17 032	Women	3.0 (1.0–9.0)[#]
Logan et al. 1986, 1989	UK	42/>20 000	Women	1.75 (0.93–3.3)[#]

*Adapted from Logan (1990).

[#]Current smokers compared to never and ex-smokers (relative risk adjusted for age, social class, and oral contraceptive use).

Table 34.4 Studies that reported results on ulcerative colitis and smoking*

Study	Country	Gender	Total number of subjects with ulcerative colitis	Relative risk in current smokers compared to never-smokers (95% CI)
Case–control				
Logan et al. 1984, 1986	UK	Men and women	175	0.23 (0.14–0.38)
Tobin et al. 1987	UK	Men and women	131	0.18 (0.10–0.33)
Franceschi et al. 1987	Italy	Men and women	124	0.61 (0.35–1.00)
Lindberg et al. 1988	Sweden	Men and women	258	0.64 (0.45–0.90)
Benoni & Nilsson 1987	Sweden	Men and women	173	0.33 (0.21–0.53)
Calkins et al. 1984	USA	Men and women	85	0.62 (0.29–1.30)
Boyko et al. 1987	USA	Men and women	212	0.64 (0.41–1.00)
Sandler and Holland 1988	USA	Men and women	170	0.80 (0.46–1.40)
Combined	–	**Men and women**	**1328**	**0.47 (0.39–0.56)**
Cohort				
Vessey et al. 1986	UK	Women	31/17 032	0.65 (0.25–1.70)[#]
Logan et al. 1986, 1989	UK	Women	78/>20 000	0.68 (0.41–1.1)[#]

*Adapted from Logan (1990).

[#]Current smokers compared to never and ex-smokers (relative risk adjusted for age, social class, and oral contraceptive use).

Gallbladder (gallstone) disease

The evidence for smoking as a cause has been less consistent compared to inflammatory bowel disease, partly because there is only a modest increase in risk (about a 30% increase in risk in smokers compared to non-smokers). Whilst cohort studies seem to consistently show an increased risk (Table 34.5), other studies, namely surveys and case–control studies, suggest no association or even a decreased risk. Given the consistency between the cohort studies and that they all allowed for several known or potential confounding factors (for example, alcohol intake and body mass index), smoking does seem to be a risk factor. The subject is reviewed by Ashley 1997 and Logan and Skelly 2000.

Skin

Psoriasis

The prevalence of psoriasis is generally high (about 1 in 50). It is associated with several risk factors, both genetic and environmental, including those that are also strongly associated with smoking (for example, alcohol and stress). For many years there has been speculation over whether smoking is a cause, and few studies have been designed to address the issue directly. Most of the epidemiological studies have had a case–control design (see Naldi 1998 for a summary of several studies) and few have allowed for confounding factors. Findings from such studies and a large cohort study suggest that there is a two- to three-fold (100–200%) increase in risk in women (Table 34.6) and a 30–40% increase in risk in men. There is also a dose–response relationship. In the study by Naldi et al. (1999), it was concluded that smoking was a more important risk factor for psoriasis in women than alcohol, but the opposite may be true in men. This observation is consistent with the well-known anti-oestrogenic effects of smoking. However, there is some evidence that once acquired, those who quit smoking do not seem to benefit much (Naldi et al. 1999), the risk in ex-smokers was still increased.

It is possible that stress plays a part in the observed association. Stress could result in the onset of psoriasis, after which the subject takes up smoking; smoking would therefore not be a risk factor. This has, to some extent, been allowed for by basing the results of studies on smoking habits before the onset of disease (Poikolainen et al. 1994; Naldi et al. 1999); both report an increased risk in smokers.

It is estimated that perhaps one in five cases of psoriasis could be due to smoking. Recent reviews of this topic can be found in Naldi (1998) and Higgins (2000).

Neurological system

Parkinson's disease

Smoking and its possible protective effect on Parkinson's disease was reported as far back as 1959 (Dorn et al. 1959), and there have since been numerous studies that have consistently shown smokers to have a lower risk of developing or having this disorder

Table 34.5 Cohort studies that reported results on gallbladder (gallstone) disease and smoking*

Study	Country	Number of subjects	Total number of subjects with gallstone disease	Gender	Relative risk in current smokers compared to never-smokers (95% CI)#
Layde et al. 1982	UK	17 000	227	Women	1.63 (p-value <0.004)[2]
Kato et al. 1992	USA (Hawaii)	7831	471	Men	1.6 (1.2–2.0)[1]
Stampfer et al. 1992	USA	90 300	2122	Women	1.3 (1.0–1.7)[1]
Murray et al. 1994	UK	23 000	1087	Women	1.19 (1.06–1.34)[2]
Misciagna et al. 1996	Italy	2472	104	Men and Women	2.15 (1.3–3.5)[1]
Sahi et al. 1998	USA	16 785	685	Men	1.52 (1.03–2.24)[1]
Leitzmann et al. 1999	USA	42 882	1016	Men	1.40 (1.14–1.72)[1]

*Partly adapted from Logan and Skelly (2000); some information taken from the individual publications.

#Adjusted for: (1) age, alcohol, body mass index, and other factors; (2) age, body mass index, oral contraceptive use, and other factors.

Table 34.6 Studies that reported results on psoriasis and smoking

Study	Country	Total number of subjects with psoriasis	Gender	Cigarette consumption	Relative risk in current smokers compared to never-smokers (95% CI)
Case–control					
Naldi et al. 1999	Italy	219	Men	1–15 cigs/day	1.3 (0.7–2.0)*
				>15	1.4 (0.9–2.2)*
		185	Women	1–15 cigs/day	1.7 (1.0–2.7)*
				>15	3.9 (1.9–7.9)*
Poikolainen et al. 1994[1]	Finland	55	Women	≥20 cigs/day	3.3 (1.4–7.9)#
Cohort					
Vessey et al. 2000[2]	UK	92/17 032	Women	≥15 cigs/day	1.9 (1.0–3.6)+

[1]Based on smoking habits before onset of psoriasis.

[2]Based on first hospital referral for psoriasis.

*Adjusted for age and alcohol.

#Alcohol and smoking had independent effects.

than non-smokers; they have about half the risk. Morens *et al.* (1995) reviewed 35 studies (cohort and case–control) and all showed a decreased risk. Table 34.7 shows the results from the cohort studies some of which, for example Hirayama (1985), Doll *et al.* (1994), and Hernan *et al.* (2001), reported that risk decreased with increasing number of cigarettes smoked. Gorell *et al.* (1999) also showed a clear relationship in ex-smokers, in which those who gave up relatively recently (1–20 years) had a much lower risk compared to never-smokers than those who had given up for a longer time (>20 years); relative risk 0.4 versus 0.9. Several mechanisms have been proposed to explain the association; nicotine stimulates an increase in dopamine, the anti-oxidant effect of carbon monoxide in cigarette smoke is protective and smoking offers some protection against neuronal damage. There have been several reviews including Marmot (1990), Morens *et al.* (1995), and Fratiglioni and Wang (2000).

Alzheimer's disease

Because Alzheimer's disease accounts for most cases of dementia in the elderly, there was interest in the early studies that, like Parkinson's disease, suggested a decreased risk in smokers. In an early meta-analysis (Lee 1994), the estimated risk in ever smokers was almost half that in never smokers (relative risk 0.64, 95% CI 0.54–0.76). However, unlike Parkinson's disease, the evidence was not so consistent between studies. Many were relatively small case–control studies that relied on information from surrogates and suffered from several limitations (see Doll *et al.* 2000 for a discussion). A recent comprehensive meta-analysis of both case–control and cohort studies showed conflicting results according to study type (Almeida *et al.* 2002). In 21 case–control studies (based on a total of 1143 affected subjects) the pooled relative risk was 0.74 (95% CI 0.66–0.84). The pooled estimate from eight cohort studies (1156 affected individuals) was 1.10 (95% CI 0.94–1.29); the results from these studies are shown in Table 34.8. Smoking does not seem to be protective against this disorder; previous results showing a benefit are likely to be artefactual. On the contrary, there is evidence that it in fact increases risk (Doll *et al.* 2000; Almeida *et al.* 2002), though this is yet to be established.

Eyes

Studies have suggested that smoking may be a risk factor for several diseases of the eye, some of which can lead to irreversible blindness. However, the evidence for many has not been strong, for example glaucoma and diabetic retinopathy. It is likely that smoking has some direct effects on the lens and retina because of its well-known thrombotic and atherosclerotic effects. Reviews of this subject can be found in Solberg *et al.* (1998), Cheng *et al.* (2000), and Evans (2001).

Cataracts

Cataracts are a major cause of blindness and visual impairment in developed countries and their removal is the most common reason for eye surgery. Table 34.9 shows the

Table 34.7 Cohort studies that reported results on Parkinson's disease and smoking*

Study	Country	Number of subjects	Total number of subjects with Parkinson's disease	Gender	Relative risk in current smokers compared to never-smokers (95% CI)
Kahn 1959	USA	~250 000	40	Men	0.23 (not reported)
Hammond 1966	USA	~1 million	123	Men and women	0.76 (age 45–64) and 0.80 (age 65–79)
Hiryama 1985	Japan	–	–	Men and women	0.57
Doll et al. 1994	UK	34 439	152	Men	0.75 (not reported)
Morens 1966	USA (Hawaii)	8006	92	Men	0.40 (0.26–0.61)
Hernan et al. 2001	USA	51 529	92	Men	0.3 (0.1–0.8)
		121 700	102	Women	0.4 (0.2–0.7)

*Adapted from Fratiglioni and Wang (2000), except Hernan (2001) (from which the results were obtained directly).

Table 34.8 Cohort studies that reported results on Alzheimer's disease and smoking*

Study	Country	Number of subjects	Total number of subjects with Alzheimer's disease	Gender	Relative risk in current smokers compared to never-smokers (95% CI)
Doll et al. 2000	UK	24 133	370	Men	0.99 (0.78–1.25)
Hebert et al. 1992	USA	513	76	Men and women	0.7 (0.3–1.4)
Hirayama et al. 1992	Japan	265 118	120	Men and women	1.61 (1.01–2.56)
Katzman et al. 1989	USA	434	32	Men and women	0.27 (0.11–0.61)
Launer et al. 1999	Europe#	16 334	277	Men and women	1.74 (1.21–2.50)
Merchant et al. 1999	USA	2128	142	Men and women	1.02 (0.60–1.50)
Ott et al. 1998	Netherlands	6870	105	Men and women	1.70 (0.60–1.50)
Wang et al. 1999	Sweden	343	34	Men and women	1.1 (0.5–2.4)

*Adapted from Almeida et al. 2002.

#Denmark, France, Netherlands, and UK.

Table 34.9 Cohort studies that reported results on cataracts and smoking

Study	Country	Number of subjects	Total number of subjects with cataracts	Gender	Cigarette consumption	Relative risk* in current smokers compared to never-smokers (95% CI)
Klein et al. 1993	USA	2164	261, diagnosis	Men		1.09 (1.05–1.14)
		2762	547, diagnosis	Women		1.09 (1.04–1.16)
Christen et al. 2000	USA	20907	1118, diagnosis 662, extraction	Men		1.49 (1.30–1.72) 1.52 (1.26–1.85)
Hankinson et al. 1992	USA	50828	480, extraction	Women	1–14 cigs/day 15–24 25–34 ≥35	0.71 (0.46–1.11) 1.33 (0.99–1.79) 1.40 (0.93–2.10) 1.58 (0.96–2.60)
Weintraub et al. 2002	USA	77749	1900, extraction	Men and women	1–14 cigs/day ≥15	1.12 (0.75–1.68) 1.53 (1.39–1.69)
Hiller et al. 1997	USA	660	381, diagnosis	Men and women	1–19 cigs/day ≥20	1.65 (0.82–3.34) 2.84 (1.46–5.51)

Some of the women in Hankinson et al. (1992) are included in Weintraub et al. (2002).

*All adjusted for at least age.

Table 34.10 Cohort studies that reported results on age-related maculopathy and smoking

Study	Country	Number of subjects	Total number of subjects with age-related maculopathy	Gender	Cigarette consumption	Relative risk in current smokers compared to never-smokers (95% CI)
Christen et al. 1996	USA	21157	268	Men	1–20 cigs/day ≥20	1.18 (0.57–2.42) 2.57 (1.70–3.90)
Seddon et al. 1996	USA	31843	215	Women		1.9 (1.3–2.6)
Klein et al. 1998	USA	632	81	Men		1.69 (0.96–2.98)
		1200	112	Women		0.80 (0.48–1.33)

results from cohort studies. There is about a 50% increase in risk in current smokers compared to never-smokers, with some studies showing clear dose–response relationships. In ex-smokers, however, it is unclear whether there is a marked reduction in risk (Hankinson *et al.* 1992; Christen *et al.* 2000).

Age-related maculopathy

Like cataracts, this disorder is an important cause of blindness and visual impairment; once acquired there is no cure. There are several case–control and cohort studies and they show that smokers are more likely to have or develop age-related maculopathy (Evans 2001). Table 34.10 shows the results from cohort studies; there is about a two-fold increase in risk in smokers compared to never-smokers.

Bones

Hip fracture

Hip fracture is an important disorder in the elderly, in particular in post-menopausal women. Many studies have reported on the association between smoking and bone mineral density and smoking and the risk of hip fracture. A meta-analysis of 29 cross-sectional studies based on a total of 2156 smokers and 9705 non-smokers (Law and Hackshaw 1997) showed that there was practically no difference in bone density between smokers and non-smokers before the menopause, but post-menopause the extent of bone loss was greater than in non-smokers and this increased with age. For every increase in age by 10 years, bone density loss was 2% greater in smokers, so that by age 80 there is a 6% difference between smokers and non-smokers. This is consistent with the evidence that the risk of hip fracture in post-menopausal women also increases with age; these studies are shown in Fig. 34.1 (taken from Law and Hackshaw 1997). At age 60, the excess risk in smokers is 17% rising to 108% at age 90. The limited data in men suggest a similar effect. It is estimated that one in eight hip fractures is attributable to smoking. Several biological mechanisms have been proposed including a direct effect of smoking on bone and that smokers have a reduction in calcium. The studies also suggest that in smokers who quit, further bone loss is prevented. Certainly, those who stop at the time of menopause may avoid much of the excess risk associated with smoking.

Reproduction and pregnancy

Despite many attempts to encourage women to quit smoking before conception and during pregnancy, there is still a relatively high prevalence of smokers (about 15–20%). Smoking is an established cause of several disorders associated with fertility and complications in pregnancy (UK Department of Health 1988; US Surgeon General 1989), some of which shall be presented here.

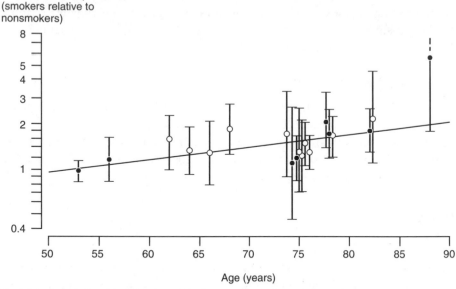

Fig. 34.1 The relative risk of having a hip fracture in smokers compared to non-smokers in 19 studies of post-menopausal women according to age (cohort studies are indicated by solid circles and case–control studies by open circles). Taken from Law and Hackshaw (1997).

Infertility

About 25% of women of reproductive age experience some degree of infertility. It is defined in several ways, but it is generally accepted to be when conception has not occurred after 12 consecutive months of unprotected intercourse. Women who smoke are less likely to conceive or take longer to conceive. A meta-analysis of eight cohort studies (based on 20 059 women) showed that women who smoked were 42% (95% CI 27–58%) more likely to be infertile than non-smokers (Augood *et al.* 1998). It is likely that such a relationship exists because the risk also increases with increasing cigarette consumption and in several studies the risks were still raised after allowing for several potential confounding factors (such as alcohol and coffee intake and oral contraception use). The subject is reviewed by Augood *et al.* (1998) and Baird (1992), both of which describe the evidence and the limitations to determining causality.

Miscarriage

It is well established that women who smoke are more likely to have a miscarriage, and that the association is causal. A meta-analysis of seven cohort studies (based on 86 633 pregnancies) yields a 24% increase in risk (95% CI 19–30%) in smokers compared to non-smokers; all of the individual studies yielded statistically significant results. It is estimated that 3–7.5% of miscarriages can be attributable to smoking

(DiFranza and Lew 1995). The results from case–control studies were similar. There is also a dose–response relationship (the higher the cigarette consumption the higher the risk of miscarriage) and the association remains after allowing for the effects of maternal age, previous miscarriage, alcohol consumption, education, and ethnicity.

Low birthweight

Smoking is also an established cause of low birthweight, a major factor associated with infant morbidity and mortality. Babies from mothers who smoke weigh, on average, 150–250 g less than those from non-smoking mothers (UK Department of Health 1988). From a meta-analysis of 22 studies (based on 347 553 pregnancies), women who smoke were 82% more likely (95% CI 67–97%) to give birth to a baby that weighs <2500 g compared to non-smokers (DiFranza and Lew 1995); all but one study reported statistically significant results. The results from case–control studies were similar. It was also estimated that 11–21% of babies with low birthweight is attributable to smoking. The association is certainly causal because randomized trials of smoking cessation during pregnancy have shown that birthweight is increased when the mother quits (UK Department of Health 1988).

Limb reduction defects

Because toxins in tobacco smoke can cross the placenta, there is likely to be a teratogenic effect on the fetus during development. Several studies have suggested a link between smoking in women during pregnancy and limb reduction defects in their babies, in which part or all of one or more limbs fail to develop. However, most studies are based on a relatively small number of affected cases and the results are not statistically significant. The results of some of the larger studies are shown in Table 34.11, three of which report dose–response relationships (Czeizel et al. 1994; Wasserman et al. 1996; Kallen 1997). Whilst there does seem to be an association, there needs to be

Table 34.11 Studies that reported results on limb reduction defects and smoking

Study	Country	Total number of babies with limb reduction defects	Relative risk in current smokers compared to never-smokers (95% CI)*
Case–control			
Aro et al. 1984	Finland	329	1.7 (1.0–2.8)[1]
Czeizel et al. 1994	Hungary	537	1.68 (1.26–2.24)[2]
Wasserman et al. 1996	USA	175	1.19 (0.82–1.74)[3]
Cohort			
Kallen 1997	Sweden	610 (out of ~1.1 million births)	1.26 (1.06–1.50)[4]

*Adjusted for: (1) alcohol, maternal age; (2) education, birth order; (4) year of birth, maternal age, parity; (3) Crude estimate (the estimate adjusted for race, parity, and alcohol was reported to be similar but not published).

large well-conducted studies, with adequate allowance for possible confounding factors such as alcohol before a causal link can be firmly established.

Hormonal system

Diabetes

Studies have shown that smokers are more likely to develop type II (non-insulin dependent) diabetes mellitus than never-smokers. Table 34.12 shows the results from some cohort studies; they indicate that men who smoke more than 20 or 25 cigarettes per day have about a two-fold increase in risk while women in this smoking category have about a 50% increase. The risks remain high after adjustment for other factors that are associated with both smoking and diabetes, such as body mass index (an indicator of obesity) and alcohol intake. The risk also increases with increasing cigarette consumption. These studies show that the risk is reduced in ex-smokers, indicating the importance of quitting, especially considering that diabetes is itself a risk factor for cardiovascular disease, renal disease, and retinopathy. It has been shown that smoking can promote insulin resistance and that smokers tend to have higher glucose concentrations, both of which can contribute to development of the disorder. Reviews of this subject can be found in Dierkx *et al.* (1996) and Haire-Joshu *et al.* (1999).

Oral cavity

There is now much evidence showing that smoking is associated with various oral disorders. As well as the common side effects of halitosis and teeth discolouration, there are more serious consequences such as periodontal disease, caries, and acute ulcerative gingivitis (for a review, see Allard *et al.* 1999; Winn 2001).

Periodontitis

Periodontitis is a common chronic disorder amongst adults and there have been many studies that have reported on the association with smoking. Although the biological mechanism for the effect of smoking on periodontal disease is uncertain the epidemiological data is clear. The studies, cross-sectional and cohort, have looked at the risk of having a diagnosis of periodontitis or measuring markers of it (such markers are used in diagnosis). Table 34.13 shows some of the studies in which relative risks were reported. Smokers have about a four-fold increase in risk (Tomar and Asma 2000). It has been postulated that smokers only have a poorer oral hygiene (which itself is a cause of periodontitis) and so the observed associations are due to confounding factors. However, several studies have adjusted for this factor, as well as other confounding factors (such as income), and there is still an effect of smoking. Smoking is also associated with more severe disease and it can delay the healing process. Reviews can be found in Qandil *et al.* (1997) and Salvi *et al.* (1997).

Table 34.12 Cohort studies that reported results on type II (non-insulin dependent) diabetes and smoking*

Study	Country	Number of subjects	Total number of subjects with type II diabetes	Gender	Cigarette consumption	Relative risk in current smokers compared to never-smokers (95% CI)*
Rimm et al. 1995	USA	41 810	509	Men	15–24 cigs/day	2.38 (1.57–3.59)
					≥25	1.94 (1.25–3.03)
Feskens and Kromhout 1989	Netherlands	841	58	Men		3.3 (1.4–7.9)
Kawakami et al. 1997	Japan	2312	41	Men	1–15 cigs/day	1.13 (0.30–4.26)
					16–25	3.27 (1.18–9.09)
					≥26	3.21 (1.05–9.83)
Rimm et al. 1993	USA	114 247	233	Women	1–14 cigs/day	0.95 (0.76–1.20)
					15–24	1.19 (0.99–1.43)
					≥25	1.42 (1.18–1.72)
Manson et al. 2000	USA	21 068	770	Men	1–20 cigs/day	1.5 (1.0–2.2)
					≥20	1.7 (1.3–2.3)

*All studies except for Feskens and Kromhout (1989) allowed for several confounding factors such as alcohol intake, body mass index, and family history of diabetes or cardiovascular disease. Feskens and Kromhout (1989) reported that smoking was an independent risk factor from other factors.

Table 34.13 Studies that reported results on periodontitis and smoking

Study	Country	Number of subjects	Total number of subjects with periodontitis or marker of it	Gender	Cigarette consumption	Relative risk in current smokers compared to never smokers (95% CI)
Periodontitis						
Haber et al. 1993	USA	95	32	Men and women		8.6 (2.7–27.8)[5]
Tomar and Asma 2000	USA	13 652	1256	Men and women		3.94 (3.20–4.93)[1]
Ismail et al. 1990	USA	165	22	Men and women		6.26 (2.42–16.20)
Marker of periodontitis						
Grossi et al. 1995[2]	USA	1361	194	Men and women	0.1–5.2 pack years 5.3–15 16–30 >30	1.48 (1.02–2.14) 3.25 (2.33–4.54) 5.79 (4.08–8.27) 7.28 (5.09–10.31)
Beck et al. 1990[3]	USA	381	–	Men and women Men and women		2.8 (1.71–4.70)[6] 6.7 (3.17–14.02)[7]
Mullaly 1996[4]	Ireland	100	–	Men and women		4.6 (2–10.6)

[1] Adjusted for age, sex, ethnic origin, income, education.

[2] Severe alveolar bone loss.

[3] Attachment loss and pocket depth.

[4] Molar furcation.

[5] Adjusted for age.

[6] Afro-caribbeans aged ≥65 years

[7] Caucasions aged ≥65 years

Caries and tooth loss

Because periodontitis is a cause of tooth loss, a few studies, have assessed the effect of smoking on tooth loss, primarily in the elderly, those who are edentulous. Although the evidence is not as strong as with periodontitis there is a suggestion of an effect (Table 34.14). Amongst the elderly, smokers are about twice as likely to have no teeth left than non-smokers.

Table 34.15 shows the results from one study that looked at differences between smokers and non-smokers with regards to indicators of caries. There are clear associations that smokers tend to have more missing teeth and more decayed, missing, or filled surfaces.

Conclusion

The literature on smoking and the disorders briefly described in this section is extensive. Many disorders have long been regarded as partly caused by smoking. Whilst most studies have provided evidence for an association, establishing causality has required careful consideration, and in some cases still does. Many studies showed dose–response relationships (risk of the disorder increased with increasing cigarette consumption) and that ex-smokers had a lower risk than current smokers. Allowing for factors that may artificially produce a relationship with smoking and risk has also been addressed, particularly in the more recent and large studies. This has been important when there are established confounding factors, such as alcohol, which is associated with both smoking and several disorders (for example, psoriasis and gallstones). Study design has also been of importance. Cohort studies of disease incidence can overcome many of the limitations of cross-sectional or case–control studies. A good example is Alzheimer's disease, which had been thought by some to be less common in smokers. After careful analysis of the published studies it is clear now that at best there is no association; in fact it may increase the risk. Biological plausibility can, in many instances, only be postulated due to the multi- factorial nature of the disorders. This is unsurprising given the number of toxins and chemicals in tobacco smoke and the many biological pathways associated with disease.

Table 34.16 provides approximate estimates of the effect of smoking on the population assuming that all the disorders listed are caused in part by smoking (as mentioned before, this is yet to be established for some such as Alzheimer's disease, but the estimates are presented for interest). For disorders, such as Crohn's disease in women and periodontitis, as much as half of all diagnosed cases may be due to smoking. For others, though this proportion is relatively low, smoking can account for several hundred or several thousand extra cases amongst smokers (for example, hip fracture and miscarriage).

In summary, smoking is a risk factor for many disorders other than cancer, respiratory, and cardiovascular disease. It is associated with significant morbidity in society much of which can be avoided.

Table 34.14 Studies that reported on tooth loss and smoking

Study (first author)	Country	Number of subjects	Number of subjects with tooth loss	Gender	Cigarette consumption	Relative risk in current smokers compared to never-smokers (95% CI)
Holm 1994	Sweden	149	–	Men	1–15 cigs/day	2.07 (1.2–3.5)[1]
					≥15	3.18 (1.9–5.5)[1]
		124		Women	1–15 cigs/day	0.95 (0.5–1.7)[1]
					≥15	1.7 (0.7–4.1)[1]
Locker 1992	Canada	907	137[2]	Men and women[3]	1–9 cigs/day	1.95 (1.2–3.3)
					≥20	2.57 (1.5–4.3)
Jette et al. 1993	USA	1156	~433[2]	Men[4]		1.68 (1.16–2.44)
				Women[4]		1.70 (1.12–2.57)

[1] Lost at least one tooth during past 10 years.

[2] Number that are edentulous.

[3] ≥50 years of age.

[4] ≥70 years of age.

Table 34.15 The effect of smoking on tooth health in 808 adults (adapted from Axelsson et al. 1998)

Age (years)	Number of subjects	Difference between smokers and non-smokers in relation to:			
		Mean number of missing teeth	Mean number of decayed surfaces	Mean number of missing surfaces	Mean number of filled surfaces
35–49	127	+0.6	+0.6	+2.8	+6.9*
50–64	369	+1.5*	+0.1	+6.8*	+0.7
65–74	190	+3.5*	+0.3	+16.0*	–10.4*
75+	122	+5.8*	+0.07	+26.2*	–11.6*

*Statistically significant (p-value ≤0.05).

Table 34.16 Summary of disorders in which smoking is associated with an increased risk

Disorder	Gender (age if not all ages)	Approximate relative risk in current smokers compared to never-smokers	Percentage of all affected individuals that may be attributable to smoking (%)*	The number of affected individuals that may be attributable to smoking amongst 100 000 smokers#
Gastro-intestinal				
Peptic ulcer	Women	2	20	440
	Men	2	20	800
Crohn's disease	Men	2	20	80
	Women	4.5	47	190
Gallbladder disease	Men and women	1.3	7	100
Skin				
Psoriasis	Men	1.4	9	730
	Women	2.5	27	2180
Neurological				
Alzheimer's disease+	Men and women (≥65)	1.1	2	120
Eyes				
Cataract extraction	Women (≥45)	1.5	11	70
	Men (≥45)	1.5	11	135
Age-related maculopathy	Women (≥50)	2	20	55
	Men (≥40)	2	20	85

Table 34.16 (continued) Summary of disorders in which smoking is associated with an increased risk

Disorder	Gender (age if not all ages)	Approximate relative risk in current smokers compared to never-smokers	Percentage of all affected individuals that may be attributable to smoking (%)*	The number of affected individuals that may be attributable to smoking amongst 100 000 smokers#
Bones				
Hip fracture	Women (55–64)	1.2	5	10
	Women (≥85)	2.1	22	2420
Fertility and pregnancy				
Infertility	Women	1.4	10	9500
Miscarriage	Women	1.25	6	4700
Low birthweight (<2500 g)	Women	1.8	17	3330
Limb reduction defect	Women	1.5	11	30
Hormonal				
Type II diabetes mellitus	Men (≥40)	2	20	240
	Women (30–55)	1.2	5	35
Teeth				
Periodontitis	Men and women	4	43	17 140

*The population attributable proportion. It assumes that 25% of the population are current smokers. The actual percentage will be less if not all the increased risk observed in smokers is due to smoking.

#The absolute excess risk between smokers and non-smokers. Based on the incidence of the disorder (per 100,000 per year), except psoriasis and periodontitis (ba ed on the prevalence) and miscarriage, limb reduction defects and birthweight (based on 100,000 births).

†Included for interest; although there is a suggestion of an association there may not be one at all.

References

Allard, *et al.* (1999). Tobacco and oral diseases—Report of EU Working Group, 1999. *J. Irish Den. Assoc.*, **46**(1), 12–23.

Almeida, O. P., Hulse, G. K., Lawrence, D., and Flicker, L. (2002). Smoking as a risk factor for Alzheimer's disease: Contrasting evidence from a systematic review of case-control and cohort studies. *Addiction*, **97**, 15–28.

Anda, R. F., Williamson, D. F., Escobedo, L. G., and Remington, P. L. (1990). Smoking and the risk of peptic ulcer disease among women in the United States. *Arch. Intern. Med.*, **150**, 1437–41.

Aro, T., Haapakoski, J., and Heinonen, O. P. (1984). A multivariate analysis of the risk indicators of reduction limb defects. *Int. J. Epidemiol.*, **13**(4), 459–64.

Ashley, M. J. (1997). Smoking and diseases of the gastrointestinal system. An epidemiological review with special reference to sex differences. *Can. J. Gastroenterol.*, **11**(4), 345–52.

Augood, C., Duckitt, K., and Templeton, A. A. (1998). Smoking and female infertility: A systematic review and meta-analysis. *Human Reprod.*, **13**(6), 1532–9.

Axelsson, P., Paulander, J., and Lindhe, J. (1998). Relationship between smoking and dental status in 35-, 50-, 65- and 75-year old individuals. *J. Clin. Periodont.*, **25**, 297–305.

Baird, D. D. (1992). Evidence for reduced fecundity in female smokers. In: *Effects of smoking on the fetus, neonate and child* (ed. D. Poswillo and E. Alberman). Oxford University Press, Oxford.

Beck, J. D., Koch, G. G., Rozier, G., and Tudor, G. E. (1990). Prevalence and risk indicators for periodontal attachment loss in a population of older community dwelling blacks and whites. *J. Periodonal.*, **61**, 521–8.

Benoni, C. and Nilsson, A. (1987). Smoking habits in patients with inflammatory bowel disease— a case-control study. *Scandinavian Journal of Gastroenterology*, **22**, 1130–6.

Borody, T. J., George, L. L., Brandl, S., Andrews, P., Jankiewicz, E., and Ostapowicz, N. (1992). Smoking does not contribute to duodenal ulcer relapse after *Helicobacter pylori* eradication. *Am. J. Gastroenterol.*, **87**(10), 1390–3.

Boyko, E. J., Koepsell, T. D., Perera, D. R., and Inui, T. S. (1987). Risk of ulcerative colitis among former and current cigarette smokers. *New England Journal of Medicine*, **316**, 707–10.

Calkins, B., *et al.* (1984). Smoking factors in ulcerative colitis and Crohn's disease in Baltimore. *American Journal of Epidemiology*, **120**, 498A.

Chan, F. K. L., Sung, J. J. Y., Lee, Y. T., Leung, W. K., Chan, L. Y., Yung, M. Y., and Chung, S. C. S. (1997). Does smoking predispose to peptic ulcer relapse after eradication of *Helicobacter pylori*? *Am. J. Gastroenterol.*, **92**(3), 442–5.

Cheng, A. C. K., Pang, C. P., Chua, J. K. H., Fan, D. S. P., and Lam, D. S. C. (2000). The association between cigarette smoking and ocular diseases. *Hong Kong Med. J.*, **6**(2), 195–202.

Christen, W. G., Glynn, R. J., Manson, J. E., Ajani, U. A., Buring, J. E., and Hennekens, C. H. (1996). A prospective study of cigarette smoking and risk of age-related macular degeneration in men. *JAMA*, **276**, 1147–51.

Christen, W. G., Glynn, R. J., Ajani, U. A., Schaumberg, D. A., Buring, J. E., Hennekens, C. H., and Manson, J. E. (2000). Smoking cessation and risk of age-related cataract in men. *JAMA*, **284**, 713–6.

Czeizel, A. E., Kodaj, I., and Lenz, W. (1994). Smoking during pregnancy and congenital limb deficiency. *BMJ*, **308**, 1473–6.

Dierkx, R. I. J., van de Hoek, W., Hoekstra, J. B. L., and Erkelens, D. W. (1996). Smoking and diabetes mellitus. *Neth. J. Med.*, **48**, 150–62.

DiFranza, J. R. and Lew, R. A. (1995). Effect of maternal cigarette smoking on pregnancy complications and sudden infant death syndrom. *J. Family Practice*, **40**(4), 385–94.

Doll, R., Peto, R., Wheatley, K., Gray, R., and Sutherland, I. (1994). Mortality in relation to smoking: 40 years' observations on male British doctors. *BMJ*, **309**, 901–11.

Doll, R., Peto, R., Boreham, J., and Sutherland, I. (2000). Smoking and dementia in male British doctors: Prospective study. *BMJ*, **320**, 1097–102.

Eastwood, G. L. (1997). Is smoking still important in the pathogenesis of peptic ulcer disease? *J. Clin. Gastroenterol.*, **25**(Supp 1), S1–7.

English, D. R., Holman, C. D. J., and Milne, E. (1995). *The quantification of drug-caused morbidity and mortality in Australia, 1992.* Commonwealth Department of Human Services and Health, Canberra.

Evans, J. R. (2001). Risk factors for age-related macular degeneration. *Progress Retinal Eye Res.*, **20**(2), 227–53.

Feskens, E. J. M. and Kromhout, D. (1989). Cardiovascular risk factors and the 25-year incidence of diabetes mellitus in middle-aged men. *Am. J. Epidemiol.*, **130**(6), 1101–8.

Fratiglioni, L. and Wang, H.-X. (2000). Smoking and Parkinson's and Alzheimer's disease: Review of the epidemiological studies. *Behav. Brain Res.*, **113**, 117–20.

Franceschi, S., Panza, E., La Vecchia, C., Parazzini, F., Decarli, A., and Bianchi Poro, G. (1987). Non-specific inflammatory bowel disease and smoking. *American Journal of Epidemiology*, **125**, 445–52.

Gorell, J. M., Rybicki, B. A., Johnson, C. C., and Peterson, E. L. (1999). Smoking and Parkinson's disease: A dose-response relationship. *Neurology*, **52**, 115–9.

Grossi, S. G., Genco, R. J., Machtei, E. E., Ho, A. W., Koch, G., Dunford, R., Zambon, J. J., and Hausmann, E. (1995). Assessment of risk for periodontal disease. II. Risk indicators for alveolar bone loss. *J. Periodontol.*, **66**, 23–9.

Haber, J., Wattles, J., Crowley, M., and Mandell, R. (1993). Evidence for cigarette smoking as a major risk factor for periodontitis. *J. Periodontol.*, **64**, 16–23.

Haire-Johnson, D., Glasgow, R. E., and Tibbs, T. L. (1999). Smoking and diabetes. *Diabetes Care*, **22**(11), 1887–98.

Hankinson, S. E., Willett, W. C., Colditz, G. A., Seddon, J. M., Rosner, B., Speizer, F. E., and Stampfer, M. J. (1992). A prospective study of cigarette smoking and risk of cataract surgery in women. *JAMA*, **268**, 994–8.

Hebert, L. E., Scherr, P. A., Beckett, L. A., Funkenstein, H. H., Albert, M. S., Chown, M. J., and Evans, D. A. (1992). Relation of smoking and alcohol consumption to incident Alzheimer's disease. *American Journal of Epidemiology*, **135**, 347–55.

Hernan, M. A., Zhang, S. M., Rueda-de Castro, A. M., Colditz, G. A., Speizer, F. E., and Ascherio, A. (2001). Cigarette smoking and the incidence of Parkinson's disease in two prospective studies. *Ann. Neurol.*, **50**(6), 780–6.

Higgins, E. (2000). Alcohol, smoking and psoriasis. *Clin. Exp. Dermatol.*, **25**, 107–10.

Hiller, R., Sperduto, R. D., Podger, M. J., Wilson, P. W. F., Ferris, F. L., Colton, T., D'Agostino, R. B., Roseman, M. J., Stockman, M. E., and Milton, R. C. (1997). Cigarette smoking and the risk of development of lens opacities. *Arch. Ophthalmol.*, **115**, 1113–8.

Hirayama, T. (1992). Large cohort study on the relation between cigarette smoking and senile dementia without cerebrovascular lesions. *Tobacco Control*, **1**, 176–9.

Holm, G. (1994). Smoking as an additional risk for tooth loss. *J. Periodontal.*, **65**, 996–1001.

Ismail, A. I., Morrison, E. C., Burt, B. A., Caffesse, R. G., and Kavanagh, M. T. (1990). Natural history of periodontal disease in adults: Findings from the Tecumseh Periodontal Disease study, 1959–87. *J. Dent. Res.*, **69**(2), 430–5.

Jette, A. M., Feldman, H. A., and Tennstedt, S. L. (1993). Tobacco use: A modifiable risk factor for dental disease among the elderly. *Am. J. Pub. Health*, **83**, 1271–6.

Johnsen, R., Forde, O. H., Straume, B., and Burhol, P. G. (1994). Aetiology of peptic ulcer: a prospective study in Norway. *J. Epidemiol. Comm. Health*, **48**, 156–60.

Kadayifci, A. and Simsek, H. (1997). Does smoking influence the eradication of *Helicobacter pylori* and duodenal ulcer healing with different regimes. *Int. J. Clin. Pract.*, **51**(7), 516–7.

Kallen, K. (1997). Maternal smoking during pregnancy and limb reduction malformations in Sweden. *Am. J. Pub. Health*, **87**, 29–32.

Kato, I., Nomura, A., Stemmermann G. N., and Chyou, P. -H. (1992). Prospective study of clinical gallbladder disease and its association with obesity, physical activity, and other factors. *Dig Dis Sci*, **37**, 784–90.

Katzman, R., Aronson, M., Fuld, P., Kawas, C., Brown, T., and Morgenstern, H. (1989). Development of dementing illness in an 80-year-old volunteer cohort. *Annals of Neurology*, **25**, 317–24.

Kawakami, N., Takatsuka, N., Shimizu, H., and Ishibashi, H. (1997). Effects of smoking on the incidence of non-insulin-dependent diabetes mellitus. *Am. J. Epidemiol.*, **145**(2), 103–9.

Klein, B. E. K., Linton, K. L. P., Klein, R., and Franke, T. (1993). Cigarette smoking and lens opacities: The Beaver Dam Eye Study. *Am. J. Prev. Med.*, **9**, 27–30.

Klein, R., Klein, B. E. K., and Moss, S. E. (1998). Relation of smoking to the incidence of age-related maculopathy. The Beaver Dam Eye Study. *Am. J. Epidemiol.*, **147**, 103–10.

Kurata, J. H. and Nogawa, A. N. (1997). Meta-analysis of risk factors for peptic ulcer. *J. Clin. Gastroenterol.*, **24**(1), 2–17.

Kurata, J. H., Nogawa, A. N., Abbey, D. E., and Petersen, F. (1992). A prospective study of risk for peptic ulcer disease in Seventh-Day Adventists. *Gastroenterology*, **102**, 909–909.

Launer, L. J., Anderson, K., Dewey, M. E., Letenneur, L., Ott, A., and Amaducci, L. A. (1999). Rates and risk factors for dementia and Alzheimer's diseaase: results from EURODEM pooled analysis. *Neurology*, **52**, 78–84.

Law, M. R. and Hackshaw, A. K. (1997). A meta-analysis of cigarette smoking, bone mineral density and risk of hip fracture: Recognition of a major effect. *BMJ*, **315**, 841–6.

Layde, P. M., Vessey, M. P., and Yeates, D. (1982). Risk factors for gall bladder disease: a cohort study of young women attending family planning clinics. *J Epidemiol Community Health*, **36**, 274–8.

Leitzmann, M. F., Rimm, E. B., Spiegelman, D., Willett, W. C., Stampfer, M. J., Colditz, G. A., *et al.* (1999). Smoking and the risk of symptomatic gallstone disease in men [Abstract]. *Am J Epidemiol* **149**, S4.

Lindberg, E., Tysk, C., Jarnerot, G., and Anderson, K. (1998). Smoking and inflammatory bowel disease. *Gut*, **29**, 352–7.

Locker, D. (1992). Smoking and oral health in older adults. *Can. J. Pub. Health*, **83**(6), 429–32.

Logan, R. F. A. (1990). Smoking and inflammatory bowel disease. In: *Smoking and hormone-related disorders* (ed. N. J. Wald and J. Baron), pp. 122–33. Oxford University Press, Oxford.

Logan, R. F. A. and Kay, C. (1989). Oral contraception, smoking and inflammatory bowel disease— findings in the RCGP oral contraception study. *International Journal of Epidemiology*, **18**, 105–7.

Logan, R. F. A. and Skelly, M. M. (2000). Smoking and hepato-biliary disease. *Eur. J. Gastroenterol.*, **12**, 863–7.

Logan, R. F. A., Edmond, M., Somerville, K. W., and Langman, M. J. S. (1984). Smoking and ulcerative colitis. *British Medical Journal*, **288**, 751–3.

Logan, R. F. A., Katschinski, B., Somerville, K. W., Pearson, J. C. G., and Langman, M. J. S. (1986). Smoking and inflammatory bowel disease. *Gastroenterology*, **90**, 1525.

Manson, J. E., Ajani, U. A., Liu, S., Nathan, D. M., and Hennekens, C. H. (2000). A prospective study of cigarette smoking and the incidence of diabetes mellitus among US male physicians. *Am. J. Med.*, **109**, 538–42.

Marmot, M. (1990). Smoking and Parkinson's disease. In: Smoking and hormone-related disorders (ed. N. J. Wald, and J. Baron), pp. 133–41. Oxford University Press, Oxford.

Marshall, B. J., Goodwin, C. S., Warren, J. R., Murray, R., Blincow, E. D., Blackbourn, S. J., Phillips, M., Waters, T. E., and Sanderson, C. R. (1988). Prospective double-blind trial of duodenal ulcer relapse after eradication of *Campylobacter pylori*, *Lancet*, **8626**, 1437–41.

Merchant, C., Tang, M. X., Albert, S., Manly, J., Stern, Y., and Mayeux, R. (1999). The influence of smoking on the risk of Alzheimer's disease. *Neurology*, **52**, 1408–12.

Misciagna, G., Leoci, C., Guerra, V., Chiloiro, M., Elba, S., Petruzzi, J., *et al.* (1996). Epidemiology of cholelithiasis in southern Italy. Part II: risk factors. *Eur J Gastroenterol Hepatol*, **8**, 585–93.

Morens, D. M., Grandinetti, A., Reed, D., White, L. R., and Ross, G. W. (1995). Cigarette smoking and protection from Parkinson's disease. *Neurology*. **45**, 1041–51.

Mullaly, B. H. (1996). Molar furcation involvement associated with cigarette smoking in periodontal disease. *J. Clin. Periodont.*, **23**, 658–61.

Murray, F. E., Logan, R. F. A., Hannaford, P. C., and Kay, C. R. (1994). Cigarette smoking and parity as risk factors for the development of symptomatic gall bladder disease in women: results of the Royal College of General Practitioners' oral contraception study. *Gut*, **35**, 107–11.

Naldi, L. (1998). Cigarette smoking and psoriasis. *Clin. Dermatol.*, **16**, 571–4.

Naldi, L., Peli, L., and Parazzini, F. (1999). Association of early-stage psoriasis with smoking and male alcohol consumption. *Arch. Dermatol.*, **135**, 1479–84.

O'Connor, H. J., Kanduru, C., Bhutta, A. S., Meehan, J. M., Feeley, K. M., and Cunnane, K. (1995). Effect of *Helicobacter pylori* on peptic ulcer healing. *Postgrad. Med. J.*, **71**, 90–3.

Ott, A., Slooter, A. J. C., Hofman, A., Van Harskamp, J. C. M., Witteman, J. C. M., and Van Broeckhoven, C. (1998). Smoking and risk of dementia and Alzheimer's disease in a population-based cohort study: the Rotterdam Study. *Lancet*, **351**, 1840–3.

Paffenberger, R. S., Wing, A. L., and Hyde, R. T. (1974). Chronic disease in former college students. *Am. J. Epidemiol.*, **100**(4), 307–15.

Parasher, G. and Eastwood, G. L. (2000). Smoking and peptic ulcer in the *Helicobacter pylori* era. *Eur. J. Gastroenterol. Hepatol.*, **12**, 843–83.

Poikolainen, K., Reunala, T., and Karvonen, J. (1994). Smoking, alcohol and life events related to psoriasis among women. *Br. J. Dermatol.*, **130**, 473–7.

Qandil, R., Sandhu, H. S., and Matthews, D. C. (1997). Tobacco smoking and periodontal diseases. *J. Canad. Den. Assoc*, **63**(3), 187–95.

Rimm, E. B., Manson, J. E., Stampfer, M. J., Colditz, G. A., Willett, W. C., Rosner, B., Hennekens, C. H., and Speizer, F. E. (1993). Cigarette smoking and the risk of diabetes in women. *Am. J. Pub. Health*, **83**, 211–4.

Rimm, E. B., Chan, J., Stampfer, M. J., Colditz, G. A., and Willett, W. C. (1995). Prospective study of cigarette smoking, alcohol use and the risk of diabetes in men. *BMJ*, **310**, 555–9.

Rubin, D. T. and Hanauer, S. B. (2000). Smoking and inflammatory bowel disease. *Eur. J. Gastroenterol.*, **12**, 855–62.

Salvi, G. E., Lawrence, H. P., Offenbacher, S., and Beck, J. D. (1997). Influence of risk factors on the pathogenesis of periodontitis. *Periodontol.*, [2000] **14**, 173–201.

Sahi, T., Paffenbarger, R. S. Jr., Hsieh, C. -C., and Lee, I. -M. (1998). Body mass index, cigarette smoking, and other characteristics as predictors of self-reported, physician-diagnosed gallbladder disease in male college alumni. *Am J Epidemiol*, **147**, 644–51.

Sandler, R. and Holland, K. (1998). Smoking and inflammatory bowel disease. *Gastroenterology*, **94**, A398.

Seddon, J. M., Willett, W. C., Speizer, F. E., and Hankinson, S. E. (1996). A prospective study of cigarette smoking and age-related macular degeneration in women. *JAMA*, **276**, 1141–6.

Solberg, Y., Rosner, M., and Belkin, M. (1998). The association between cigarette smoking and ocular diseases. *Surv. Ophthalmol.*, **42**, 535–47.

Stampfer, M. J., Maclure, K. M., Colditz, G. A., Manson, J. E., and Willett, W. C. (1992). Risk of symptomatic gallstones in women with severe obesity. *Am J Clin Nutr*, **55**, 652–8.

Stemmermann, G. N., Marcus, E. B., Buist, A. S., and MacLean, C. J. (1989). Relative impact of smoking and reduced pulmonary function on peptic ulcer risk. *Gastroenterol.*, **96**, 1419–24.

Tobin, M. V., Logan, R. F. A., Langman, M. J. S., McConnell, R. B., and Gilmore, I. T. (1987). Cigarette smoking and inflammatory bowel disease. *Gastroenterology*, **93**, 316–21.

Tomar, L. and Asma, S. (2000). Smoking-attributable periodontitis in the United States: Findings from NHANES III. *J. Periodontol.*, **71**, 743–51.

UK Department of Health (1988). *Fourth report of the independent scientific committee on smoking and health*. HMSO, London.

US Surgeon General Report (1989). *Reducing the health consequences of smoking: 25 years of progress*. US Department of Health & Human Services, DHHS Publication number (CDC) 89-8411.

Vessey, M. P., Villard-Mackintosh, L., and Painter, R. (1992). Oral contraceptives and pregnancy in relation to peptic ulcer. *Contraception*, **46**, 349–57.

Vessey, M. P., Painter, R., and Powell, J. (2000). Skin disorders in relation to oral contraception and other factors including age, social class, smoking and body mass index. Findings in a large cohort study. *Br. J. Dermatol.*, **143**, 815–20.

Vessey, M., Jewell, D., Smith, A., Yeates, D., and McPherson, K. (1986). Chronic inflammatory bowel disease, cigarette smoking, and use of oral contraceptives: findings in a large cohort study of women of childbearing age. *British Medical Journal*, **292**, 1101–3.

Wang, H. X., Fratiglioni, L., Frisoni, G. B., Vitanen, M., and Winblad, B. (1999). Smoking and the occurrence of Alzheimer's disease: cross-sectional and longitudinal data in a population-based study. *American Journal of Epidemiology*, **149**, 640–4.

Wasserman, C. R., Shaw, G. M., O'Malley, C. D., Tolarova, M. M., and Lammer, E. J. (1996). Parental cigarette smoking and risk for congenital anomalies of the heart, neural tube or limb. *Teratology*, **53**, 261–7.

Weintraub, J. M., Willett, W. C., Rosner, B., Colditz, G. A., Seddon, J. M., and Hankinson, S. E. (2002). *Am. J. Epidemiol.*, 155, 72–9.

Winn, D. M. (2001). Tobacco use and oral disease. *J. Dental Educ.*, **65**(4), 306–12.

Part 10

Genetics, nicotine addiction, and smoking

Chapter 35

Genes, nicotine addiction, smoking behaviour, and cancer

Michael Murphy, Elaine C. Johnstone, and Robert Walton

One of the most frustrating mistakes to be made is to be right for the wrong reasons. RA Fisher made many seminal contributions to statistical genetics. His instincts did not entirely mislead him in relation to smoking and (lung) cancer risk but have probably contributed to stunting the growth of behavioural genetic research. The resurgent interest in the relationship between genetic influences, smoking behaviour, and cancer has required both the laying of Fisher's ghost (that some of the same genes determine both smoking behaviour and cancer risk) and depended on the recognition of the addictive principle, nicotine, lying at the heart of much tobacco use (Swan 1999a, 1999b). The story has unfolded since the 1950s, in fits and starts at first but more smoothly recently. This chapter reviews the advances that have taken place in understanding the genetic contribution to individual variation in nicotine addiction and smoking behaviour, and, more briefly the contribution of genotype to risk of cancer, conditional upon being a smoker, since this topic is also considered in the cancer-specific chapters.

A variety of evidence, from animal models and observational and experimental studies in humans, has contributed to our reaching our present point of understanding. We are poised to be able to improve control of tobacco usage, not only through society wide actions but also through direct approaches which exploit differences in individual susceptibility to nicotine addiction and cancer risk.

Evidence for genetic contribution

Understanding the genetic contribution to a condition really requires three kinds of advance. The first is that there needs to be evidence that the condition or trait has components that appear to cluster within genetically related individuals, or more explicit vertical evidence of inheritability of the trait. The second (almost universally observed) is that there is interindividual variation to be explained. The third, and perhaps hardest, is to define the genes, and proteins for which they code, that mediate these influences, and the biological processes underlying the occurrence of the disease or trait.

The tobacco plant is beautiful but deadly (Doll and Peto 1976; Peto *et al.* 2000); recognizing that nicotine is the active principle which maintains (oral or smoked) dependence on tobacco for many people has helped to focus attention on this third area. Other chapters in the book deal with the neuropharmacology and structural biology of the nervous system pathways (mainly in the central nervous system) which underlie dependence. These provide the clues, to which we return later, in this third area of investigating exactly how genotype influences smoking behaviour. The first and second areas—heritability and individual variation—we consider first.

Even now, despite profound declines in the numbers of people who smoke, smoking remains a commonly observed behaviour, and is in that sense taken for granted as a feature of every day life. In the UK, however, the number of ex-smokers approximately equals the numbers who report themselves as current smokers (somewhat more than 10^7 in each case) (RCP 2000). What distinguishes them? It has been suggested that the average level of nicotine dependence increases amongst those who remain smokers, as others quit and this may plausibly define the size of the problem which remains in helping smokers give up (although it should be remembered that most of the 10^7 ex-smokers did so without the aid of any drugs). Certainly, even amongst those who do manage to quit, there is a range of variation in the success rate of their quit attempts.

In a recent follow-up survey of 850 participants in a randomized placebo-controlled trial of the nicotine patch conducted in general practices in the early 1990s, 'The PATCH study', the range of attempts to quit reported in those who remained smokers in 1999 was substantial (Yudkin *et al.* 2003, 2004 In Press) (Johnstone *et al.* In Press). In eight years more than a third had made no serious attempts, about a third had made 1 or 2 attempts and the remainder had made between 3 and 30. Similarly amongst smokers participating in a different general practice trial of health checks conducted in the late 1980s ('OXCHECK') for any given level of reported smoking, there was a considerable range of variation in the blood cotinine (and by implication nicotine levels) measured. We know that smokers adjust the way they smoke to obtain the level of nicotine that suits them best (interindividual compensation) and it seems that different individuals, have a wide range of set points to which they adjust their individual intakes.

Figure 35.1 shows cotinine levels measured by gas chromatography, obtained for a random sample of 173 smokers in the OXCHECK study, according to the amount they reported smoking (McKinney *et al.* 2000). There is obviously digit preference in the reporting, which may blur the distinction between smokers, but their biochemistry reveals how much variation there is in the total intake and/or metabolism of nicotine. Difficulty quitting and nicotine intake are probably the clearest measures of interindividual variation. Smoking initiation provides less discriminatory power. Conditional upon exposure to tobacco, most who become smokers do so in adolescence (in the UK 80% by 18, 90% by 19 years of age). There may be differences in susceptibility, conditional upon exposure, but this has so far been the subject of little investigation (in man) (Overstreet 1995; Overstreet *et al.* 1995; Perkins 1995; Pomerleau 1995; Rosecrans 1995).

There is similarly little doubt about the general size of contribution genotype makes to the behaviour. Animal models (particularly rat and mouse, the latter having 80% overlap with the human genome) have not only helped us to understand the anatomy,

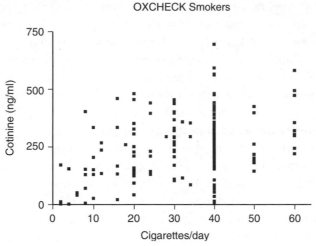

Fig. 35.1 Plasma cotinines measured in those reporting particular levels of cigarette consumption per days

pharmacology, and biology of the actions of nicotine which underlie human use of the drug, but also help to demonstrate the amount of genetic variation that exists in the way nicotine achieves its effects. The work of Collins and Marks in particular has demonstrated that inbred strains of animals (who therefore became increasingly homozygotic and invariant for, albeit anonymous, alleles) differ markedly between strains (in the relevant but unknown genes) contributing to:

*nicotine sensitivity

*nicotine receptor density

*tolerance development

*cross tolerance

*nicotine self administration

Even more telling is the evidence from human studies (mostly of twins, but some singleton adoption studies) which estimate the likely size of the contributions of genotype and environment, defined in the broadest sense, to determining smoking behaviour (Sullivan and Kendler 1999; Hall *et al.* 2002). Many of the twin panels whose results contribute to these estimates were established to answer the questions posed originally by Fisher's hypothesis that the same genes may determine not only that a smoker does so but their risk of disease also. The evidence from these studies unequivocally supported the alternative idea that smoking delivers toxic and carcinogenic products that determine disease risk directly. They have however also provided reliable evidence about the balance of contributions to smoking behaviour.

The Table 35.1 combines data from the Nordic Twin Studies of concordance of cancer risk (Lichtenstein *et al.* 2000) and from pooled analyses of the large number of twin studies which have examined smoking (Li *et al.* 2003). The estimates of heritability from about 20 studies each for smoking behaviours (initiation and tobacco use) are both about 50%, with quite a narrow confidence interval, also implying that environmental (non-genetic) factors contribute about the same amount to the variation in the behaviour observed in pairs of identical and non-identical twins. When examined individually, the studies which contribute to this meta analysis are quite consistent for both smoking phenotypes, for men and women, and despite the panels being assembled from twins in a number of different countries, and time periods in which population smoking prevalence varied (Sullivan and Kendler 1999). From the same table we can see that the heritability estimates for cancer risk from twin studies with the same design flaws and strengths are lower in general, even for those cancers such as breast and colorectal where genetic variation is known to contribute significantly to the risk of the disease (even though the environmental component may be greater) and for which a broader range of genotypic contribution almost certainly remains to be discovered. This comparison gives us no clue about the type of genetic contribution to smoking behaviour and cancer risk but suggests that it is substantial.

The twin study results point out another important aspect of the genetic epidemiology of smoking behaviour, namely that the behaviour has several distinct components, to which different amounts and types of genetic contribution may be made, and that smoking is best seen as a career or process. The figure indicates the component stages of the process, as we conventionally understand it, and genetic studies of the process need to distinguish between the different phenotypes that are examined, the definitions

Table 35.1 Heritability estimates and 95% confidence intervals (CI) of smoking behaviours and common cancers obtained from twin studies

Condition	Heritability	Genes
Smoking initiation	47% (41–53%)	
Smoking (tobacco use)	53% (44–63%)	
Bladder	31% (0–45%)	
Stomach	28% (0–51%)	
Pancreas	36% (0–53%)	
Lung	26% (0–49%)	
Cervix	0 (0–42%)	
Uterus	0 (0–35%)	
Ovary	22% (0–41%)	
Leukaemia	21% (0–54%)	
Prostate	42% (29–50%)	
Colorectum	35% (10–48%)	FAP/HNPCC
Breast (women)	27% (0–54%)	BRCAI/2

Cancers from Lichenstein *et al.* 2000 (3 Nordic cohorts).
Smoking from Li *et al.* 2003 (19–20 Twin studies).

of those phenotypes and the nature of the control/contrast phenotypes to which the smoking phenotype is compared. Overlaps in genotypic contribution because of mis-classification of the phenotypes might provide an important source of bias and confusion

Smoking Career
Tobacco Exposure
↓
Experimentation
↓
Initiation
↓
Progression
↓
Quitting (Relapse)
↓
Abstinence

The model of genetic variation contributing to such a complex behaviour as smoking, even when isolated into the component parts of the process for study, must necessarily itself be complex. The genetic variants involved may be completely different at different parts of the process, i.e. depending upon how smoking behaviour is defined. Or they may overlap (substantially) and their effects may be more or less important at different stages, e.g. in relation to initiation, determining how much a smoker smokes, the diffi-culty they have in giving up, and separately the way in which they respond to the drugs which are known to aid smokers to give up. Moreover the genetic contribution might be more or less direct. Thus there is evidence that genotypic variation is related to varia-tions in the extent to which measured personality traits are exhibited. There is separate evidence that some personality traits are associated with smoking behaviour, more specifically with smoking initiation rather than other elements of the process (Munafò *et al.* 2001). Similarly there is considerable evidence that genotypic variation affects mood, and there are separate associations between mood states and smoking behaviour. In particular the relation between smoking, quitting, and depression appears to be sub-stantial. Alternatively there may be direct effects of genotypic variation on nicotine neuropharmacology and metabolism, affecting why smokers smoke because of effects on the biochemical mechanisms affecting reward, withdrawal, and dependence (Breslau 1995; Gilbert and Gilbert 1995; Heath *et al.* 1995; Leonard 1999).

The neurochemistry and pharmacology of these latter processes is dealt with else-where and will not be reprised here, except to say that as the neurobiology of addiction to drugs of abuse generally and to nicotine specifically unfolds in animal models and human studies, an extensive set of proposed candidate genes is emerging (Crabbe 2002; Picciotto and Corrigall 2002; Watkins *et al.* 2000). The biological sub-strates of personality and mood are even less well understood, but nonetheless quite well studied. A recent systematic review (Munafò *et al.* 2003) identified 79 published studies conducted in 18 countries between 1995 and 2002 of candidate gene variation and measured personality attributes. Many of the genetic variants in neurochemical pathways hypothesized to be involved for personality associations are separately objects of direct interest in nicotine addiction, e.g. serotonergic, dopaminergic, noradrenergic, and GABAergic pathways. Again there is separate overlap with the neurochemical pathways thought to be involved in susceptibility to mood disorder and generation of mood state. The twin studies which have demonstrated strong evidence for heritable components of smoking behaviour also suggest some overlaps in the genetic contribution to smoking, personality, and mood, though classical twin studies cannot help to pinpoint the particular contribution of individual genes (Sullivan and Kendler 1999).

The evidence suggests therefore that in examining the genetic contribution to smoking behaviour we are looking for the cumulative effect of multiple genes exhibiting relatively common allelic variations, which each confer only small variations in risk or liability to the particular aspect of smoking behaviour. They may be differentially important in different populations, they may exert their effect through a wide range of mechanisms, they may contribute to different parts of the smoking process, and the same overall level of risk or liability may arise from many different combinations (i.e. heterogeneity of genotypic contributions) (Rutter and Plomin 1997).

Figure 35.2 illustrates some of the implications of different hypothetical models of the population distribution of additive genotypic relative risk under different assumptions of the number of genetic loci at which a small increase in risk is conferred by possession of particular allelic variants, and the prevalence of these alleles in the population. Integrating the notions of heritability and attributable risk is not yet easily possible, but would serve communication about genotypic contribution to smoking behaviour risk well if it were. As the figure shows the effects of the fixed small increases in

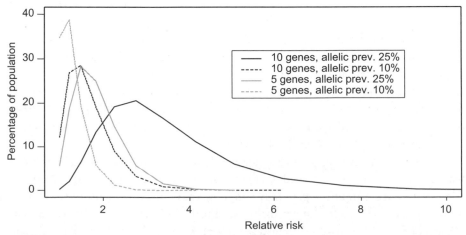

Fig. 35.2 Hypothetical population distributions of additive genotypic relative risk. For each gene locus: RR homozygous wildtype = 1; heterozygous variant = 1.22; homozygous variant = 1.5.

risk associated with possession of increasing numbers of alleles at increasing numbers of loci and their increases in prevalence both mean that an increasing proportion of the population starts to be at an important level of liability, e.g. to acquisition of nicotine dependence, but comparatively few are at very low or very high risk, which might be a reasonable, but entirely hypothetical, description of the population's liability. If so it would suggest the numbers of genes to be interested in are numbered in the tens if not hundreds when assessing genetic contribution.

Thus all of the usual difficulties of investigating a complex genetic trait to define the quantitative trait loci (QTL) which contribute to the phenotype are evident in the study of smoking behaviour. Nevertheless the strength of the evidence that genes are important, the potential rewards from identifying even some of the factors which contribute to variation in smoking behaviour, the grip exerted by tobacco use, and the ways in which it might be lessened, are potent incentives to regard the problem of understanding the genetics of smoking behaviour as a potentially tractable one

Identifying genes contributing to smoking behaviour

The usual approaches to identify the potential genes of interest in smoking—familial clustering, pedigree-based linkage studies, affected relative (usually sibling) pair studies, and candidate gene association studies have all contributed though most effort has been concentrated on the latter. Results from only four genome scan studies have so far been published (in some shape or form), dealing with different smoking phenotypes. A fifth (the largest to date and conducted amongst female non-identical twin pairs) has recently been conducted but is, as yet, unpublished (Munafò *et al.* personal communication).

Duggirala *et al.* (1999) looked at the phenotype 'cigarettes per day' and found some evidence of linkage on chromosomes 4, 5,15, and 17. Bergen *et al.* (1999) contrasted 'ever/never smokers' and found evidence for linkage to 6, 9, and 14. Straub *et al.* (1999) studied 'nicotine dependence' and incriminated regions on chromosomes 2, 10, 16, and 17. Wang *et al.* (1997) reported weak evidence for linkage of 'smoking behaviour' to genes on chromosomes 1, 9, 10, 13, 14, and 20. Unpublished findings (Munafò *et al.* personal communication) suggest no strong evidence of linkage for 'ever/never' smokers (i.e. initiation) or for 'ex-/current' smokers (i.e. cessation), but quite good evidence of linkage to chromosomes 7 and 8 for, 'age at initiation' and to 7, 8, and also 18 for 'cigarettes/day'.

There is not obviously a lot of consistency between these findings, and in none of the individual studies was the strength of the evidence for linkage absolutely compelling for any of the regions identified, though some of the measures of association were certainly sufficiently strong to be hypothesis generating. Some further progress might be made by meta-analytic pooling of the datasets to maximize the power to detect linkage, but the variation in definition of the phenotypes considered may argue against the value of this.

Table 35.2 shows the human chromosomal map location of the genes controlling expression of the major components of the dopaminergic, serotonergic, and noradrenergic pathways, the nicotinic acetyl cholinergic receptor subunits and the enzymes thought to be involved in nicotine metabolism. Biological reasoning suggests some of these genes might be important for smoking behaviour. They are distributed widely across the genome, and though it is possible to identify some map locations which broadly correspond to the areas of linkage interest, finer detail mapping in larger samples, with very well-defined phenotypes may be necessary to provide significant clues to the genetic contribution to smoking behaviour, using this approach.

Far more attention has been paid to candidate gene association studies. A systematic review of such studies in relation to a variety of smoking behaviour phenotypes has revealed at least 20 relevant studies published to end 2002 (Munafò *et al.* in press).

Table 35.2 Gene map

Chromosome no.	Gene	Map location
1	nAChRβ2	1q21.3
	5HTID	1p34.3–36.3
	5HT6	1p35–36
2	AHH(CYP1A1)	2q31-2pter
	5HT2B	2q36.3–37.1
	5HT5B	2q11–13
	ADRα2B	2
3	DRD3	3q13.3
	5HT1F	3q11
4	DRD5	4p16.1
	ADRα2C	4p16.1
5	DAT1	5p15.3
	DRD1	5q35.1
	5HT1A	5q11.2–13
	5HT4	5q31–33
	ADRB2	5q32–34
	ADRα1A	5
	ADRα1B	5q31.1 (long arm)
6	5HT1B	6q13
	5HT1E	6q14–15
7	5HT5A	7q36
8	nAChRα2	8p21
	nAChRβ3	8p11.2
	nAChRα6	8p22
9	DBH	9q34.1
10	5HT7	10q21–24
	ADRβ1	10q24–26
	ADRα2A	10q24–26
11	TH	11p15.5
	TPH	11p15.3–p14
	DRD2	11q21–q22

Table 35.2 (continued) Gene map

Chromosome no.	Gene	Map location
	DRD4	11q23
	5HT3A	11
	5HT3B	11
12		
13	5HT2A	13q14–q21
14		
15	nAChRβ,α3,α5	15q24
	nAChR α7	15q13–q14
16	NET1	16q12.2
17	5HTT	17q11.2
	PNMT	17q21q22
18		
19	CYP2A6	19q13.2
	CYP2β6	19q13.2
20	nAChRα4	20q13.2–q13.3
	ADRαD	20
21		
22	CYP2D6	22q13.1
	COMT	22p11.2
X	MAOa,MAO6	Xp11.3
	5HT2C	Xq24
Y		

Most of the allelic variants studied were at the loci shown in the gene map above, because the same biological reasoning about the process of addiction generally and smoking behaviour particularly, led to the specification of these pathways as important. However, many of the genes studied have been looked at by only a few investigators, the phenotypes again vary considerably or are not well defined, individual sample size and characteristics are imperfect, and the models of genetic action are poorly specified. All of these factors hamper pooling and interpretation (Walton *et al.* 2001).

Two examples from our own work may illustrate the difficulties of deciding whether particular genes are important candidates or not.

Candidate genes—false start?

Catechol O Methyl Tranferese (COMT) is a plausible candidate gene for involvement in smoking behaviour. It catalyses the inactivation of amine neurotransmitters such as dopamine and noradrenaline within the synapse, terminating their action. It is polymorphic, the variants are common and functional, increasing the extraneuronal enzyme activity, and have been linked to substance abuse. Amongst the OXCHECK sample of smokers, who attended a health check in the early 1990s (mentioned earlier in the chapter), there was no effect observed in two separate studies. Allele presence did not appear to influence the number of self-reported cigarettes/day or heavy smoking amongst a random sample of 226 smokers (McKinney *et al.* 2000) nor was it associated with smoking status (current, ex-, never smokers) when three age–sex matched groups of 270 subjects were compared to one another (David *et al.* 2002). Should further studies be done?

Candidate genes—false promise?

Dopamine β Hydroxylase (DBH) converts dopamine to noradrenaline, exhibits common silent polymorphisms which are tightly linked to variants which probably reduce enzyme activity and has been linked to substance abuse. In the same first OXCHECK sample of 226 smokers referred to for COMT, allele presence was associated with a significantly reduced number of self-reported cigarettes per day (especially in women) (McKinney *et al.* 2000). When we tried to replicate this finding in all the remaining 1275 smokers for whom we had data in the OXCHECK cohort, allele presence was only associated with slightly reduced consumption in men and women (Johnstone *et al.* 2002). However it may be associated with response to NRT particularly in women (see later) so perhaps there is a case for further studies (Johnstone *et al.* 2004, In Press; Yudkin *et al.* In Press).

Systematic review—hope?

The clearest results from all the studies combined and examined in the systematic review suggest a relationship between possession of the Dopamine D2 receptor Taq1A1 allele and polymorphisms in the Dopaminergic Transporter (DAT1), but the summary estimates of genotypic risk associated with allelic possession are always less than 2 whatever the hypothesized mode of gene action examined (for which there is currently little good evidence to choose between, e.g. dominant, codominant, recessive etc.) (Walton *et al.* 2001). They reinforce the prevailing notion that the genetic variants that will be identified may be common (possessed by one person in three, say) but uniformly of small effect. The results provide a 'scoping' study, which allied to advance in neurobiological understanding should define the principal target of interest (Munafò *et al.* In Press).

The levels and types of evidence that these (and many other) genetic variants contribute to overall genetic liability with respect to smoking behaviour are various. There is 'analogy' in the sense that debate still rages about whether the DRD2 Taq1A1 allele is related to alcohol use and abuse. Possession of the same allele has also now been linked to associated or surrogate measures of the smoking behaviour phenotype in (at least) 3 pre-clinical studies. Gilbert *et al.* demonstrated that smokers carrying at least one copy of the allele exhibited greater EEG slowing over one month after quitting smoking than non-carriers (SRNT Savannah abstract 2002). The same authors also demonstrated that smokers possessing at least one copy of the allele benefited less from negative affect (mood) reducing effects of nicotine than non-carriers, when undergoing tests of attention/distractibility (SRNT Savannah abstract 2002). Finally David *et al.* (In Press) demonstrated that smokers possessing at least one copy of the allele benefit less from the action of bupropion on smoking withdrawal symptoms than non-carriers.

Another type of evidence for involvement of the DRD2 gene in smoking behaviour (and from the point of view of cancer prevention perhaps at present the most important study results to obtain) is whether and how genetic variation underpins some of the variation in difficulty smokers have in quitting. As yet there is little direct evidence on this; two studies only have investigated drug–genotype interaction in helping smokers to quit with respect to the DRD2 Taq1A1 allele (amongst others). One cautionary note in these drug-effectiveness studies is that, in hypothesizing candidate genes for interaction to explain the variation in effectiveness observed, one might expect most effect to be seen with genes that directly contributed to the pharmacological mechanism of action of the drug rather than in the more general neural systems involved in smoking behaviour, but we remain uncertain about how the drugs work to exert their effect on smokers 'ability to quit'. Hence the DRD2 Taq1A1 allele may not be the genetic variant of primary interest, though the general evidence to date suggests it needs to be examined.

The PATCH studies (Yudkin *et al.* 2003; Johnstone *et al.* 2004, In Press; Yudkin *et al.* In Press) enrolled 1685 heavy smokers in 19 general practices in Oxfordshire, England in 1991–2, to a randomized placebo-controlled trial of the nicotine patch and demonstrated a significant effect on quitting rates to one year. In 1999–2000, 1532 of the 1612 smokers still available were contacted, and 840 returned detailed questionnaires and 755 gave DNA. Exactly half of this sample (378 vs. 377) had originally used active patch and placebo. Cessation rates on NRT were higher amongst those smokers possessing the DRD2 Taq1A1 allele and lower amongst those possessing the allele who used placebo, resulting in significantly increased effectiveness odds of quitting for active drug use amongst those possessing the DRD2 Taq1A1 allele. Amongst those who possessed not only the variant DRD2 allele, but also possessed the variant DBH allele, the odds were greater still, suggesting that both genetic variants might play a part in smoking behaviour, particularly quitting. It is of interest that possession of both alleles appears to be a common phenomenon (30% in smokers).

In the only other reported study of drug–gene interaction for smoking cessation, so far, Lerman *et al.* (2002, 2003) examined the effect of bupropion in a placebo-controlled trial of 555 USA smokers of 10 cigarettes or more/day, genotypic analysis being restricted to 426 European Caucasians. There was no clear main effect of the DRD2 Taq1A1 allele (or DAT1) on prolonged abstinence to the end of the treatment phase, and bupropion's effects were comparable in groups defined by DRD2 or

DAT genotype. However there was some evidence of effect in those who possessed allelic variants of the cytochrome enzyme CYP2B6 (which may play a part in metabolizing nicotine and is responsible for metabolizing bupropion to other active compounds).

The subject of genetic contribution to smoking behaviour is clearly still in its infancy, and the promises and pitfalls of unravelling the contribution are similar to those involved in the hunt for many other 'disease' genes. However the subject is finally on the agenda in the search for how to reduce the toll tobacco takes.

Some possible implications of improving our understanding of the genetic contribution to smoking behaviour might be speculated on:

♦ How will the tobacco industry react if genetic susceptibility is demonstrated? Will it try to argue that responsibility for nicotine addiction lies with the individual because of their genetic make-up?

♦ How will the pharmaceutical industry, who make the effective smoking cessation aids respond to the notion that not all smokers should be considered part of the market for their drug if another might suit them better?

♦ How will professionals respond to the notion of individualizing therapy, based on treatments preferred for smokers with a particular genotype?

♦ How will smokers react to the notion that their wish to smoke stems partly from their genetic make up, having become tobacco dependent in the first place?

Investigations in these areas will be needed.

We now turn to a brief overview of the state of understanding of how a smoker's genotype may alter their risk of developing cancer. More detailed consideration of genotype and specific cancer risk amongst active smokers is provided in the cancer specific chapters elsewhere in this book.

Smoking-related cancer

Cigarette smoking has an aetiological link with several types of cancer, predominantly solid tumours of the lung, larynx, pharynx, oesophagus, bladder, kidney, and pancreas but also including myeloid leukemia. Although a large number of cancer deaths are caused by smoking (in 1999, 22% of all cancer deaths were of lung cancer), only a proportion of smokers ultimately develop lung cancer (Mattson *et al.* 1987). The precise reasons for this remain unclear, but the discrepancy most likely results from the combination of variation in carcinogen exposure and genetic susceptibility. (Zang and Wynder) The Table 35.1 earlier in the chapter indicates that lung, and the other smoking-related cancers, have heritability estimates that, whilst not as great as for some other cancers, are nonetheless substantial. Current studies focus on genetic susceptibilities to lung cancer in particular, and how they modify the effects of tobacco smoke carcinogens. Studies on bladder cancer have also been performed but other cancers are less well studied in this area.

Steps to carcinogenesis

Exposure to smoke

The harmful consequences of smoking are well known. The smoking of tobacco is an efficient method of delivering nicotine to the brain where it elicits rewarding effects. However tobacco smoke also carries more than 50 carcinogens direct to the lungs, including polycyclic aromatic hydrocarbons (PAHs) such as benzo[*a*]pyrene and several nitrosamine-based compounds that are specific to tobacco. Actual doses of nicotine, carcinogens, and toxins will vary, depending on an individual's intensity and method of smoking and also on the smoking device. Genetic predisposition to nicotine addiction (discussed previously) will also contribute to risk via modulation of both amount smoked and ability to stop smoking.

Activation of procarcinogens

Tobacco carcinogens are metabolized by complex enzyme systems and involve both activation and detoxification. Phase 1 enzymes such as those from the cytochrome P450 family are primarily responsible for the activation (via oxidation) of procarcinogens. Many genes encoding CYP enzymes are polymorphic and this inherited variation will influence the activity of specific CYP isozymes, resulting in individual differences in exposure to activated carcinogens. CYP1A1 (on chromosome 2, see gene map earlier in chapter) is the principal enzyme that metabolizes PAHs and possessing polymorphic variant alleles seems to confer elevated risk of lung cancer, in certain ethnic populations (Vineis *et al.* 1999).

Adduct formation

Smoking-related DNA adducts (long-lasting aggregates of tobacco carcinogens and genetic material) have been detected by a variety of analytical methods in respiratory tract, bladder, cervix. DNA adducts are found at higher levels in tissues of smokers compared to non-smokers (Perera *et al.* 1987). Biomarker data provide convincing evidence that carcinogen uptake, activation, and binding to cellular macromolecules (including DNA) are higher in smokers than non-smokers (Randerath and Randerath 1993).

Failure of DNA repair

DNA repair plays a crucial role in maintenance of genome stability by removing these kinds of lesions, thus diminished DNA repair capacity may increase susceptibility to smoking-related cancers. Reduced DNA repair has been shown in lymphocytes from lung cancer patients *in vitro* compared to age-matched controls (Wei *et al.* 2000), although poor repair is thought to be independent of smoking status. Whilst DNA repair is undertaken, cell cycle checkpoints will arrest the growth of the cell, and if the damage is too severe to repair, apoptosis occurs. A key-player in deciding the cell's fate is p53, and mutation of this gene is a common event in tumour cells. Thus variation in p53 activity (and that of other proteins involved in these checkpoints) will also have an important role in the long-term effects of adduct formation on the cell. If not repaired, such damage can result in gene mutations and instability, which may in turn result in malignant transformation.

Individual variation

Many studies have shown a relationship between tobacco smoke exposure, carcinogen-DNA adduct formation, DNA repair capacity, and cancer risk. An individual's susceptibility is a complex interplay of (a) exposure to tobacco smoke and (b) response to exposure, and inherited variation in key (and possibly overlapping) genes in both cases will modulate both smoking behaviour (exposure) and detoxification and repair (response). The hypothesis under test is that a smoker with low capacity to detoxify carcinogens (or who has enhanced activation), and/or low capacity to repair damaged DNA will be at higher risk of tobacco-related cancers.

Detoxification

There are a large number of studies examining metabolic susceptibility genes, and the most conspicuous aspect is the lack of a consistent role for this group of enzymes as cancer risk factors. This is perhaps not surprising given the low penetrance of these genes, and their indirect involvement in the complex process of cellular malignant transformation.

The Phase II enzyme superfamily of glutathione S-transferases (GSTs) plays an important role in the detoxification of smoke-derived carcinogen metabolites and people who have variant alleles of GSTM1 in particular appear to have increased susceptibility to lung cancer after exposure to tobacco smoke (Vineis *et al.* 1999). The *N*-acetyl transferases (NAT1 and NAT2) are responsible for inactivation of various aromatic amines and several allelic variants of both genes have been detected some of which contribute to reduced enzyme function. Several studies have found a significant association between NAT2 slow acetylation and bladder cancer after smoking or occupational exposure. As a susceptibility locus for lung cancer the risk associated with NAT2 variants is inconsistent (Vineis *et al.* 1999). A recent large study suggested the NAT2 slow acetylator phenotype as a risk factor for lung cancer only in heavy smokers (80 pack-years) (Zhou *et al.* 2002). The sulfotransferases, which catalyse the sulfation of numerous carcinogenic and mutagenic compounds, have recently also been implicated as risk factors for lung cancer. The variant allele of SULT1A1 (SULT1A1*2), which encodes for low activity, is more commonly found in lung cancer cases, compared to age, sex, and smoking-status matched controls (Wang *et al.* 2002). Furthermore, this modest increase in risk was significantly higher in current smokers.

DNA repair

As previously alluded to, variation between individuals in DNA repair capacity may be a risk factor for cancer. There are several processes (and associated genes) involved in DNA repair including detection of DNA damage (TP53), nucleotide excision repair (XPD and XPF) and double-strand/recombination repair (XRCC1 and XRCC3). A recent paper by Wu *et al.* (2002) extensively examined three polymorphisms in p53 and found each variant, along with variant haplotypes, to be associated with an increased risk of lung cancer. Functional effects of variant alleles were tested *in vitro*, and lymphoblastoid cell lines with all wild type alleles had significantly higher apoptotic indices and DNA repair capacity, than those with at least one variant, suggesting the effect of the polymorphisms may be to inhibit p53 function. Despite their low penetrance, these variant alleles are quite prevalent in the population (albeit ethnicity dependent), leading to a high population attributable risk.

Several polymorphisms in DNA repair enzymes have been examined, XRCC1 and XPD being the most frequently studied. XRCC1 variant alleles have reduced base excision repair capacity and are associated with increased population-dependent risks of bladder cancer (Stern *et al.* 2001) and breast cancer (Duell *et al.* 2001), but conflicting results for lung cancer (Park *et al.* 2002). A number of fairly prevalent (~30%) polymorphisms in XPD have been described and until recently their influence on function was unclear. The functional effect of variation within this gene has now been associated with increased levels of aromatic adduct, and also with increased lung cancer risk.

Other targets

Other targets to consider include enzymes involved in tumour invasion and metastasis, such as collagenases. Variation in the matrix metalloproteinase-1 gene (MMP-1) promoter region partially regulates gene expression and appears to increase risk of lung cancer; this risk was also further elevated in smokers (Zhu *et al.* 2001). The association was also less evident in former smokers and more evident in heavy smokers.

Summary

In conclusion conditional upon becoming a regular smoker, which may itself be genetically influenced, there are several key areas which may impact on the genetic susceptibility of an individual. The complex multistage process that leads a smoker to develop cancer will no doubt involve multiple (low penetrant) gene effects both dictating exposure and the host response. Gene–environment interactions are of particular interest, i.e. for a given environmental exposure (smoking) does the risk of cancer differ with respect to polymorphic variation? We have examined here only those genes thought to contribute to risk, not the myriad of genes involved in cellular changes prior to progression to malignancy. Using a candidate gene approach, the importance of haplotypes will also become more evident particularly when relating variation with protein function or expression.

References

Bergen, A. W., Korczak, J. F., Weissbecker, K. A., and Goldstein, A. M. (1999). A genome-wide search for loci contributing to smoking and alcoholism. *Genet Epidemiol Suppl*, 17, S55–S60.

Breslau, N. (1995). Psychiatric comorbidity of smoking and nicotine dependence. *Behav Genet*, 25, 95–101.

Crabbe, J. C. (2002). Genetic contributions to addiction. *Annu Rev Psychol*, 53, 435–62.

David, S. P., Johnstone, E., Griffiths, S. E., Murphy, M., Yudkin, P., and Walton, R. (2002). No association between functional Catechol O-Methyl Transferase Polymorphism (COMT A1947G) and smoking initiation, maintenance or cessation. *Pharmacogenetics*, 12, 265–8.

David, S. P., Niaura, R. S., Papandonatos, G. D., Shadel, W. G., Burkholdes, G. J., Britt, D. M., Day, A., Stumpff, J., Hutdrinson, K., Murphy, M., Johnstone, E., Griffiths, S.-E., and Walton, R. T. (2004 inpress). Does the DRD2-Taq1A polymorphism influence treatment response to bupropion hydrochloride for reduction of the nicotine withdrawal syndrome? *Nicotine and Tobacco Research*.

Doll, R. and Peto, R. (1976). Mortality in relation to smoking: 20 years' observations on male British doctors. *Br Med J*, 2(6051), 1525–36.

Duell, E. J., Millikan, R. C., *et al.* (2001). Polymorphisms in the DNA repair gene XRCCI and breast cancer. *Cancer Epidemiol Biomarkers Prev*, 11, 23–7.

Duggirala, R., Almasy, L., and Blangero, J. (1999). Smoking behaviour is under the influence of a major quantitative trait locus on human chromosome 5q. *Genet Epidemiol Suppl*, 17, S139–44.

Gilbert, D. G. and Gilbert, B. O. (1995). Personality, psychopathology, and nicotine response as mediators of the genetics of smoking. *Behav Genet*, 25, 133–47.

Hall, W., Madden, P., and Lysnskey, M. (2002). The genetics of tobacco use: Methods, findings and policy implications. *Tobacco Control*, 11(2), 119–124.

Heath, A. C., Madden, P. A. F., Slutske, W. S., and Martin, N. G. (1995). Personality and the inheritance of smoking behavior: A genetic perspective. *Behav Genet*, 25, 103–17.

Johnstone, E., Munafò, M., Neville, M., Griffiths, S., Murphy, M., and Walton, R. (2002). Pharmacogenomics of Tobacco Addiction. Chapter 22 In: *Pharmacogenomics: The search for individualised therapeutics* (ed. J. Licinio, and M-L. Wong), pp. 443–60. Wiley Verlag, Weinheim Germany.

Johnstone, E., Clark, T., Griffiths, S. E., Murphy, M. F. G., and Walton, R. T. (2002) Polymorphisms in dopamine metabolic enzymes and tobacco consumption in smokers—seeking confirmation of the association in a follow-up study. *Pharmacogenetics*, 12(7), 585–7.

Johnstone, E. C., Yudkin, P. L., Hey, K., Roberts, S. J., Welch, S. J., Murphy, M. F. G., Griffiths, S. E., and Walton, R. T. (2004 in press). Genetic variation in dopaminergic pathways and short term effectiveness of the nicotine patch. *Pharmacogenetics*.

Leonard, B. E. (1999). Neuropharmacology of antidepressants that modify central noradrenergic and serotonergic function: A short review. *Hum Psychopharmacol Clin Exp*, 14, 75–81.

Lerman, C., Shields, P. G., Wileyto, E. P., Audrain, J., Hawk, L. H. Jr, Pinto, A., Kucharski, S., Krishnan, S., Niaura, R., and Epstein, L. H. (2002). Effects of dopamine transporter and receptor polymorphisms on smoking cessation in a bupropion clinical trial. *Health Psychol*, Sept 22(5), 541–8.

Lerman, C., Shields, P. G., Wileyto, E. P., Audrain, J., Hawk, L. H. Jr, Pinto, A., Krishnan, S., Niaura, R., and Epstein, L. H. (2002). Pharmacogenetic investigation of smoking cessation treatment. *Pharmacogenetics*. Nov 12(8), 627–34.

Li, M. D., Cheng, R., Ma, J. S., and Swan, G. E. (2003). A meta-analysis of estimated genetic and environmental effects on smoking behavior in male and female adult twins. *Addiction*, 98, 23–32.

Lichtenstein, P., Holm, N. V., Verkasalo, P. K., Iliadai, A., Kaaprio, J., Kodkenvuo, M., *et al.* (2000). Environmental and heritable factors in the causation of cancer. Analyses of cohorts of twins from Sweden, Denmark and Finland. *NEJM,* **343,** 78–85.

Mattson, M. E., Pollack, E. S., and Cullen, J. W. (1987). What are the odds that smoking will kill you? *Am J Public Health,* **77(4),** 425–31.

McKinney, E., Walton, R., Marshall, S., Yudkin, P., Fuller, A., Haldar, *et al.* (2000). Association between polymorphisms in dopamine metabolic enzymes and tobacco consumption in smokers. *Pharmacogenetics,* **10,** 483–91.

Munafò, M., Johnstone, E., Murphy, M. F. G., and Walton, R. (2001). New directions in the genetic mechanisms underlying nicotine addiction. *Addict Biol,* **6,** 109–17.

Munafò, M. R., Clark, T. G., Moore, L. R., Payne, E., Walton, R., and Flint, J. (2003). Genetic polymorphisms and personality: A systematic review and meta-analysis. *Molecular Psychiatry,* **8,** 471–84.

Munafò, M. R., Clark, T. G., Johnstone, E. C., Murphy, M. F. G., and Walton, R. (in press). The genetic basis for smoking behavior: A systematic review and meta-analysis. *Nicotine and Tobacco Research.*

Overstreet, D. H. (1995). Differential effects of nicotine in inbred and selectively bred rodents. *Behav Genet,* **25,** 179–85.

Overstreet, D. A., Karan, L., and Rosecrans, J. A. (1995). Genetic, environmental, and situational factors mediating the effects of nicotine—an introduction. *Behav Genet,* **25,** 93–4.

Park, J. Y., Lee, S. Y., Jeon, H. S., Bae, N. C., Chae, S. C., Joo, S., *et al.* (2002). Polymorphism of the DNA repair gene XRCC1 and risk of primary lung cancer. *Cancer Epidemiol Biomarkers Prev,* **11(1),** 23–7.

Perera, F. P., Santella, R. M., Brenner, D., Poirier, M. C., Munshi, A. A., Fischman, H. K., *et al.* (1987). DNA adducts, protein adducts, and sister chromatid exchange in cigarette smokers and nonsmokers. *J Natl Cancer Inst,* **79(3),** 449–56.

Perkins, K. A. (1995). Individual variability in responses to nicotine. *Behav Genet,* **25,** 119–132.

Peto, R., Darby, S., Deo, H., *et al.* (2000). Smoking, smoking cessation, and lung cancer in the UK since 1950: Combination of national statistics with two case-control studies. *BMJ,* **321(7257),** 323–9.

Picciotto, M. R. and Corrigall, W. A. (2002). Neuronal systems underlying behaviors related to nicotine addiction: Neural circuits and molecular genetics. *J Neurosci,* **22,** 3338–41.

Pomerleau, O. F. (1995). Individual differences in sensitivity to nicotine: Implications for genetic research on nicotine dependence. *Behav Genet,* **25,** 161–77.

Randerath, E. and Randerath, K. (1993). Monitoring tobacco smoke-induced DNA damage by 32P-postlabelling. *IARC Sci Publ,* **(124),** 305–14.

Rosecrans, J. A. (1995). The psychopharmacological basis of nicotine's differential effects on behavior: Individual subject variability in the rat. *Behav Genet,* **25,** 187–96.

Rutter, M. and Plomin, R. (1997). Opportunities for psychiatry from genetic findings. *Br Journal of Psychiatry,* **171,** 209–19.

Stern, M. C., Umbach, D. M., van Gils, C. H., Lunn, R. M., and Taylor, J. A. (2001). DNA repair gene XRCC1 polymorphisms, smoking, and bladder cancer risk. *Cancer Epidemiol Biomarkers Prev,* **10,** 125–31.

Straub, R. E., Sullivan, P. F., Ma, Y., Myakishev, M. V., Harris-Kerr, C., Wormley, B., *et al.* (1999). Susceptibility genes for nicotine dependence: A genome scan and follow-up in an independent sample suggest that regions on chromosomes 2,4,10,16,17 and 18 merit further study. *Molecular Psychiatry,* **4,** 129–144.

Sullivan, P. F. and Kendler, K. (1999). The genetic epidemiology of smoking. *Nicotine Tob Res,* Volume 1, Supplement 2, **1,** S51–S57.

Swan, G. E. (1999a). Implications of genetic epidemiology for the prevention of tobacco use. *Nicotine and Tobacco Research*, Volume 1, Supplement 1, S49–56.

Swan, G. E. (1999b). Multiple risk factors for the initiation of smoking: the public health imperative for multidisciplinary genetic epidemiological investigations of nicotine addiction. *Nicotine Tob Res*, Volume 1, Supplement 2, S71–3

Tobacco Advisory Group of the Royal College of Physicians (2000). Nicotine Addiction in Britain. London. RCP.

Vineis, P., Malats, N., Lang, M., D'Errico, A., Caporaso, N., Cuzick, J., *et al.* (1999). Metabolic polymorphism and susceptibility to cancer. *IARC Sci Publ.*

Walton, R., Johnstone, E., Munafò, M., Neville, M., and Griffiths, S. (2001). Genetic clues to the molecular basis of tobacco addiction and progress towards personalized therapy. *Trends in Molecular Medicine*, 7(2), 70–6.

Wang, Y.-F., Gillanders, E., Wang, S., Sun, C., Freas-Lutz, D., Zhang, Y.-J., Korrtge, T. E., Gunsolley, J. C., Schenkein, H. A., and Diehl, S. R. (1997). Mapping genes influencing smoking behaviour and IgG2 levels in early onset periodontitis families. *Journal of Dental Research*, 76, 409.

Wang, Y., Spitz, M. R., Tsou, A. M., Zhang, K., Makan, N., and Wu, X. (2002). Sulfotransferase (SULT) 1A1 polymorphism as a predisposition factor for lung cancer: a case-control analysis. *Lung Cancer*, 35, 137–42.

Watkins, S. S., Koob, G. F., and Markou, A. (2000). Neural mechanisms underlying nicotine addiction: Acute positive reinforcement and withdrawal. *Nicotine Tob Res*, 2, 19–37.

Wei, Q., Cheng, L., Amos, C. I., Wang, L. E., Guo, Z., Hong, W. K., *et al.* (2000). Repair of tobacco carcinogen-induced DNA adducts and lung cancer risk: A molecular epidemiologic study. *J Natl Cancer Inst*, 92(21), 1764–72.

Wu, X., Zhao, H., Amos, C. I., Shete, S., Makan, N., Hong, W. K., *et al.* (2002). p53 Genotypes and haplotypes associated with lung cancer susceptibility and ethnicity. *J Natl Cancer Inst*, 94(9), 681–90.

Yudkin, P., Hey, K., Roberts, S., Welch, S., Johnstone, E., Murphy, M. F. G., Griffiths, S. -E., Jones, L., Munafò, M., and Walton, R. Sex-specific differences in genotypic response to NRT. *BMJ, in press.*

Yudkin, P., Hey, K., Roberts, S., Welch, S., Johnstone, E., Murphy, M. F. G., Jones, L., and Walton, R. (2003). Abstinence from smoking 8 years after participation in randomised controlled trial of nicotine patch. *BMJ*, 327, 28–9.

Zang, E. A. and Wynder, E. L. (1996). Differences in lung cancer risk between men and women: Examination of the evidence. *J Natl Cancer Inst*, 88(3–4), 183–92.

Zhou, W., Liu, G., Thurston, S. W., Xu, L. L., Miller, D. P., Wain, J. C., *et al.* (2002). Genetic polymorphisms in N-acetyltransferase-2 and microsomal epoxide hydrolase, cumulative cigarette smoking, and lung cancer. *Cancer Epidemiol Biomarkers Prev*, 11(1), 15–21.

Zhu, Y., Spitz, M. R., Lei, L., Mills, G. B., and Wu, X. (2001). A single nucleotide polymorphism in the matrix metalloproteinase-1 promoter enhances lung cancer susceptibility. *Cancer Res*, 61, 7825–9.

Part 11

Tobacco and alcohol

Chapter 36

Tobacco and alcohol interaction

Albert B. Lowenfels and Patrick Maisonneuve

Introduction

Throughout the world, tobacco and alcohol abuse are responsible for an appreciable proportion of avoidable deaths. Alcohol has been used in all cultures throughout recorded history, but tobacco only became widely available after the discovery of the New World. At first, tobacco use was restricted to the wealthy class, but by the beginning of the seventeenth century, combined exposure to alcohol and tobacco was common in all classes (Figure 36.1). Both agents are addictive, although nicotine, the major addictive compound contained in tobacco, is probably more so than alcohol. Both agents are widely used: nearly 80% of Americans over age 12 have consumed alcohol at some time, which is similar to the percentage of persons who report ever using tobacco. However, less than one-third of adults are current smokers—much smaller than the proportion of current alcohol users.

Tobacco use creates an enormous health burden because of its well-known association with numerous diseases, but increased consumption of alcohol is also known to have deleterious health effects and there are several diseases where exposure to both substances can be harmful. Table 36.1 lists background information and societal covariates for these two substances. Since both substances are so widely used and since tobacco users often consume alcohol, some of the adverse health effects of tobacco may be caused by drinking. Furthermore, there is a real possibility that combined exposure to these two substances may be more harmful than a single exposure to only one of these agents.

Combined use of tobacco and alcohol

Epidemiology

We can estimate the frequency of the combined use of tobacco and alcohol at the population level from survey data. For the United States, the 1997 National Household Survey on Drug Abuse (1997) provides age-specific estimates of exposure to these agents. Overall, as shown in Table 36.2, smoking is much more common in alcohol consumers than in teetotalers: this difference is striking in the younger age groups. With respect to the combined use of alcohol and tobacco, approximately 20% of responders to the survey report exposure to both substances during the month prior to the survey.

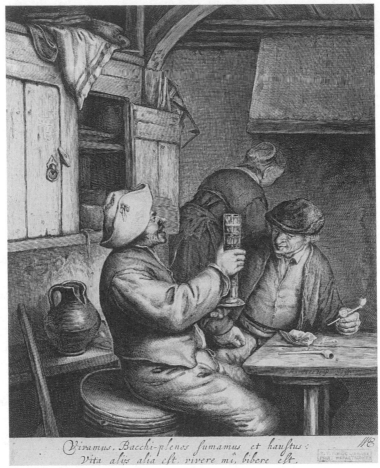

Viramus, Bacchi-plenos fumamus et hauftus:
Vita aliis alia eft, vivere mi, bibere eft.

Fig. 36.1 By the early 17th century exposure to both alcohol and tobacco was common. Jonas Suyerdof, *Three peasants in an interior*. With permission, from the print collection, Mirian and Ira D. Wallach Division of Art, Prints and Photographs, The New York Public Library, Astor, Lenox and Tilden Foundations.

The major effect of alcohol when viewed at the population level relates to increased morbidity and mortality from injuries—usually affecting younger age groups. Alcohol also contributes to a somewhat lesser extent to degenerative diseases and to cancer. The major effect of tobacco is to increase the risk of cardiovascular disease as well as many types of cancer.

Biologic aspects

Experimental and human data are beginning to clarify the damaging effect resulting from combined exposure to these two substances. In animal experiments, tissue-specific DNA alterations have been discovered after combined exposure to alcohol

Table 36.1 Comparison of alcohol and tobacco use

Variable	Tobacco	Alcohol
History of early use	Brought back to Europe from the Americas by Columbus. Widespread use by 1700s.	Mentioned in Old Testament
Minimum legal age (USA)	18 or 19, depending on locality	21
Estimated deaths per year in USA (Miller and Gold 1998)	400 000	100 000
Taxable substance?	Yes	Yes
Current use by persons ≥18 yrs in 1999 (USA)		
Males	26%	70%
Females	22%	56%
Estimated % with addiction	High proportion	5–10%
Recommended 'safe' level for consumption	No 'safe' level	Recommended upper limit: Males ≤ 2 units per day Females ≤ 1 unit per day
Known carcinogens present?	Yes	No
Impact on fetus	Lowers birth weight	Causes fetal alcohol syndrome
Cost/yr	60 Billion (1994)	148 Billion (1998)
Number web sites (Google)[1]	Smoking 5 630 000 Tobacco 3 540 000	Drinking 4 490 000 Alcoholism 625 000
Number medline retrivals[1]	Smoking 83 291 Tobacco 32 514	Drinking 58 163 Alcoholism 48 226

[1] February 2002.

Table 36.2 Association between use of tobacco and alcohol during past month in 24 505 persons responding to National USA Household Survey on drug abuse, 1997

Age group	N	% Smokers	% Smokers in non-drinkers	% Smokers in drinkers	% Smokers and drinkers
12–17	7844	19%	9.5%	57%	11%
18–25	6239	36%	19%	50%	28%
26–34	4387	34%	25%	40%	24%
35+	6035	29%	24%	33%	17%
Total	24 505	28%	20%	36%	19%

Data from Table 8.7, Ref #1. Drinking refers to any consumption of alcohol in past month.

and cigarette smoke. Target organs included the esophagus, the lung, and the heart. At each organ site, the damage induced by combined exposure to alcohol and cigarette smoke was greater than the DNA damage induced by smoke or alcohol alone (Izzotti *et al.* 1998). In human studies, both alcohol consumption and tobacco are associated with p53 mutations in non-small cell lung cancer, compatible with the possibility that alcohol enhances mutagenicity induced by tobacco smoke (Ahrendt *et al.* 2000).

Alcohol is not considered to be a carcinogen, but more likely acts as a co-carcinogen or a tumor promoter to increase the toxic effects of tobacco-specific carcinogens such as *N*-nitrosoamines (Hecht 1999). Another mechanism of action of alcohol metabolism possibly leading to cancer relates to the formation of acetaldehyde and to highly reactive free radicals. Acetaldehyde has greater cellular toxicity than alcohol and could induce DNA damage or interfere with DNA repair mechanisms (Homann *et al.* 2000)

For some organs, such as the mouth or the esophagus, alcohol could increase the permeability of mucous membranes to tobacco-specific carcinogens (Du *et al.* 2000). Finally, heavy consumption of alcohol can be associated with nutritional deficiencies such as vitamin A and selenium, which could enhance tumor development (Seitz *et al.* 1998).

Genetic factors

There is abundant evidence reminding us that at all levels of consumption smoking patterns correlate with alcohol consumption. This association is especially true for higher consumption categories (Gulliver *et al.* 1995). A natural question pertains to the reason for this association: Is there a genetic component? If so, how strong is the association, and what gene(s) might be implicated?

Swan and associates in a multivariate analysis of Caucasian male twins identified a genetic factor that explained the link between smoking, alcohol, and coffee use (Swan *et al.* 1996). In a group of adolescent twins, Han *et al.* (1999) estimated the heritable factor for tobacco and alcohol to be, respectively, 59 and 60% in males, and 11 and 10% in females. The data could be explained by a common underlying substance abuse factor. Koopmans and colleagues (1997) in a study of 1266 young adult Dutch twins noted that alcohol and tobacco use was associated due to the same genetic risk factors.

Since about 1990, evidence has been accumulating implicating a dopamine receptor gene (DRD2) as a major factor in addictive disorders, including alcohol addiction and smoking (Noble 1998; Noble 2000*a*, *b*). The prevalence of the A1 allele of the D_2 dopamine receptor (DRD2) gene appears to be increased in both alcoholics, and smokers. DRD2 may act as a reward or 'pleasure' gene; exposure to alcohol, tobacco, or other addictive drugs, in conjunction with alterations in the DRD2 gene, might result in an increase in brain dopamine levels, leading to enhanced feelings of reward and satisfaction. These genetic defects could be important because they are potentially associated with early age of onset of smoking or alcoholism (Comings *et al.* 1996; Kono *et al.* 1997; Spitz *et al.* 1998).

Although gene therapy has rarely been successful in humans, Thanos and co-workers report that delivering the DRD2 gene into the brain of rats trained to self-administer alcohol, markedly reduces their intake of alcohol (Thanos *et al.* 2001). This type of study strengthens the link between the DRD2 gene and sensitivity to alcohol.

Medical consequences

Malignant disease

Cancer of the upper aero-digestive tract (UAT)

UAT tumors provide strong evidence that tobacco and alcohol interact to yield an excess risk of cancer in these sites. One mechanism might be that mucosal damage induced by alcohol, acts synergistically with carcinogens contained in tobacco smoke to induce cancer. Beverages containing higher concentrations of alcohol are more likely to induce epithelial damage than low content beverages. This could explain why some studies have found that fortified wines and spirits yield higher risks of cancer than weaker beverages (Jaber *et al.* 1999).

Using the World Health Association mortality database, Macfarland and co-workers (1996) assessed current trends in male mortality from UAT tumors, relating country-specific frequency to past national alcohol consumption and tobacco exposure. Previous alcohol consumption was a strong predictor of deaths from UAT cancer and the increased death rate from these cancers in the 90s could be explained by increased alcohol consumption during the 60s and 70s.

Oro-pharyngeal cancer

The oral cavity is exposed to high concentrations of both alcohol and tobacco, explaining why these two risk factors are important etiologic factors for oral cancer (Schlecht *et al.* 1999). Predictably, both agents also are associated with pre-malignant lesions in this area (Gupta, 1984; Macigo *et al.* 1996; Jaber *et al.* 1999; Hashibe *et al.* 2000).

Since oropharyngeal cancers are aggressive lesions with a poor long-term survival, successful efforts to prevent these tumors depends upon recognition of pre-malignant lesions such as leukoplakia and erythroplasia. Both these lesions are known to be associated with alcohol and tobacco, including the increasingly common use of smokeless tobacco. Effective counseling for managing pre-malignant oropharyngeal cancers must include information about the contributory role of alcohol.

Larynx

Alcohol and tobacco are predictors of risk for laryngeal cancer, but there are site-specific differences in the impact of these two substances. Alcohol is more strongly related to supraglottic laryngeal tumors than to glottic tumors, whereas smoking is related to both types (Brugere *et al.* 1986). The probable reason is that both parts of the larynx will be exposed to tobacco smoke, but that the glottis is unlikely to be exposed to ingested alcohol.

Esophageal cancer

Esophageal cancer is an excellent example of a tumor caused by exposure to tobacco and alcohol (Figure 36.2). Pioneering work by Tuyns and co-workers (Tuyns 1970; Tuyns et al. 1977) carried out over several years have emphasized the importance of both alcohol and tobacco as etiologic agents for this aggressive cancer. Much of this research was carried out in the northwest of France, where the incidence of esophageal cancer is exceptionally high. Case–control studies revealed that both alcohol and tobacco are major risk factors and a greater than addictive effect was noted following exposure to both agents. It was shown from an early study in France (Tuyns 1982) that smoking in light consumers of alcohol carries less of a risk than smoking in heavy drinkers. In the subgroup of persons that are heavily exposed to both agents, the risk of esophageal cancer is nearly 40–50 times greater than in lightly exposed populations (Figure 36.3). These data imply that control of both smoking and drinking will be required to reduce the burden of esophageal cancer.

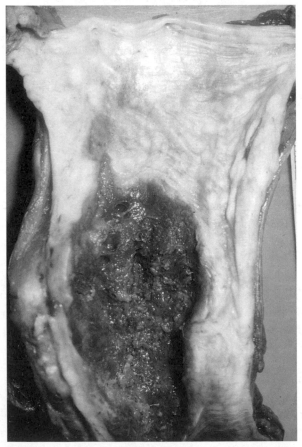

Fig. 36.2 Squamous cell cancer of the esophagus is one of the best examples of a tumor related to exposure to both alcohol and tobacco.

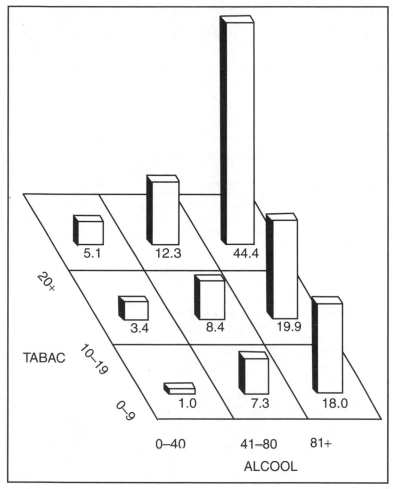

Fig. 36.3 The effects of combined exposure to alcohol and tobacco on the risk of esophageal cancer. (From Tuyns 1982.)

Most patients with esophageal cancer have been exposed to both tobacco and alcohol, so it is difficult to estimate the independent impact of each single risk factor. But in his study 743 esophageal cancers from the Calvados region of Normandy, France, Tuyns found 19 non-drinkers and 75 non-smokers (Tuyns 1983). The relative risk of esophageal cancer in non-drinking smokers was approximately 5, compared to a relative risk of 11 in non-smoking heavy alcohol consumers. It appears that both agents can act independently and that their relative effect will to some extent depend upon the level of population exposure. One report suggests that for tobacco, a moderate intake over a long time period poses a higher risk than a high intake over a short period. For alcohol, high intake over a shorter period is more likely to induce esophageal cancer than a low intake over a longer period. (Launoy *et al.* 1997).

Stomach cancer

Several studies have examined smoking and alcohol consumption as risk factors for gastric cancer (Kabat *et al.* 1993; D'Avanzo *et al.* 1994; Hansson *et al.* 1994; Vaughan *et al.* 1995; Ji *et al.* 1996; de Stefani *et al.* 1998; Chow *et al.* 1999, 40; Zaridze *et al.* 2000; Wu *et al.* 2001) (Table 36.3). Nearly all show that although smoking increases the risk of gastric cancer; alcohol, in contrast, unless consumed in large quantities, does not.

Table 36.3 Case–control studies of association between alcohol and stomach cancer

Author, Year	Study location	Study size	Results
Wu *et al.* (2001)	USA, California	Population-based. 277 gastric cardia, 443 distal stomach, 1356 controls	Alcohol use not associated with an increased cancer risk.
Zaridze *et al.* (2000)	Moscow, Russia	448 cases, 610 hospital controls	Alcohol, particularly vodka increased risk of gastric cancer, especially for gastric cardia.
Ye (1999)	Sweden	Population-based. 514 cases, 1164 controls	No association with alcoholic beverages
Chow *et al.* (1999)	Warsaw, Poland	Population-based. 464 cancers, 480 controls	No relation between alcohol consumption and risk of gastric cancer
De Stefani *et al.* (1998)	Montevideo, Uruguay	331 cases, 622 hospitalized controls	Alcohol associated with about a twofold increased risk of gastric cancer
Ji (1996)	China	Population-based case control study. 1124 cases, 1451 controls.	Alcohol a risk factor only for distal stomach cancer and only in heavy drinkers.
Vaughan *et al.* (1995)	Washington State	Population based. Includes esophageal squamous-cell cancer and adenocarcinoma of gastric cardia.	Alcohol a significant risk factor for both types
D'Avanzo *et al.* (1994)	Northern Italy	746 stomach cancer patients, 2053 hospital controls	No convincing evidence for alcohol as a risk factor, except possible in very heavy drinkers.
Hansson *et al.* (1994)	Central Sweden	Population-based study. 338 cases, 679 controls.	Alcohol not associated with gastric cancer
Kabat *et al.* (1993)	USA	Hospital-based study of 194 patients with adenocarcinoma of the distal esophagus or cardia, 4544 controls.	Moderate-heavy alcohol consumption ($\geq$ 4 drinks per day caused a 2.3 increased risk compared to non-drinkers.

Heavy drinking is known to cause gastritis of the stomach, a possible explanation why heavy drinking raises the risk of gastric cancer.

Non-malignant disease

Cardiovascular system

Consumption of alcohol and tobacco has important implications for the heart and for the entire vascular system. There is strong evidence that high levels of exposure to either of these agents damages the heart, leading to both increased morbidity and mortality. The main impact of tobacco relates to the increased risk of atherosclerosis, causing narrowing of coronary arteries and, eventually to myocardial infarction. Large amounts of alcohol are cardiotoxic, causing cardiomyopathy, and in some heavy drinkers, fatal cardiac arrhythmias.

The interaction of these agents has been studied in healthy volunteers. Ethanol and nicotine increased heart rate, and also increased the product of heart rate times blood pressure. The combination of exposure to both drugs could contribute to serious arrhythmias and sudden death, especially in persons with pre-existing coronary heart disease (Benowitz et al. 1986).

In patients with pre-existing heart disease, both alcohol and tobacco are independent risk factors for disease progression. Evangelista and co-workers (Evangelista et al. 2000) conducted a longitudinal study of 753 patients previously hospitalized with heart disease. In a multivariate analysis current smoking (odds ratio 1.8, 95% confidence interval 1.2–2.8) and current drinking (odds ratio 5.8, 95% confidence interval 3.8–9.1) were independent predictors of readmission for heart disease.

The deleterious effects of tobacco on the heart are dose-related, with no demonstrable 'safe' level of exposure to tobacco. But for alcohol, there are several longitudinal studies suggesting that persons consuming low levels of alcohol—generally about 1 or perhaps two drinks per day, have a lower risk of cardiac disease than abstainers or than persons consuming larger quantities of alcohol do (Fuchs et al. 1995; Thun et al. 1997). The overall impact on large populations is questionable and if there is a benefit from light drinking, it is likely to affect males more than females, and older persons rather than younger persons.

Pancreatitis

The pancreas, unlike the mouth, the larynx, the esophagus or the stomach, does not come into direct contact with ingested alcohol. Alcohol reaches the pancreas via the blood stream, where it stimulates pancreatic secretion, either directly or via activation of the secretin mechanism. Moderate consumption of alcohol does not usually cause pancreatic injury, but heavy drinking is a major cause of both acute and chronic pancreatitis.

There is evidence from many sources that the combination of heavy drinking and smoking is especially injurious to the pancreas. Individuals who drink heavily tend to be heavy smokers, so it can be difficult to separate the effects of these two agents on the pancreas. However, several studies have now reported that smoking in addition to alcohol is a separate risk factor for pancreatitis. (Lowenfels *et al.* 1987; Talamini *et al.* 1996; Hartwig *et al.* 2000; Lin *et al.* 2000). Chronic pancreatitis is an example of a digestive tract disorder where exposure to both addictive substances leads to the onset of a debilitating, painful disease.

Dupuytren's contracture

Dupuytren's contracture (William Dupuytren, French surgeon 1777–1835), has long been known to be associated with moderate to heavy alcohol consumption. The lesion, which occurs in the palmar or plantar fascia, is characterized by the development of strong fibrous bands, which restrict digital mobility. Recent studies have demonstrated that smoking, in addition to alcohol, is a risk factor for this disease. One case-control study based on 222 operated patients, revealed that smoking nearly tripled the risk of developing this Dupuytren's contracture: adjusted odd ratio 2.8, 95% CI = 1.5–5.2.) Alcohol was an additional risk factor, resulting a twofold increased risk (Burge *et al.* 1997). In another study, the findings were nearly identical (An *et al.* 1988). The mechanism might be related to microvascular occlusion with subsequent development of fibrosis, leading to disabling contractures.

Other conditions

Trauma

The combination of drinking and smoking can cause serious injury—particularly burns. A frequent scenario is as follows: after two or three drinks, a person smokes a final cigarette in bed, falls asleep with the cigarette still burning, wakes up only after sustaining a major burn. Both smoking and drinking are modifiable risk factors that can significantly reduce the frequency of domestic fires (Warda *et al.* 1999).

Pregnancy

Despite the well-known adverse effects of smoking and drinking during pregnancy, many women continue to smoke and drink even though they are pregnant. Estimated exposure figures, based on actual interviews, are 34% for tobacco and 25% for alcohol (Jones-Webb *et al.* 1999).

The main effect of smoking exposure and moderate alcohol intake seems to be a reduction in fetal birth weight (Olsen *et al.* 1983), whereas heavy alcohol exposure causes fetal alcohol syndrome, characterized by distinct facial abnormalities, hyperirritability, and persistent cognitive impairment (Streissguth *et al.* 1994). Both smoking and drinking may interact with specific genetic alterations to cause cleft lip and/or cleft palate (Romitti *et al.* 1999). Clearly, both smoking and drinking have adverse effects on the fetus; efforts at intervention should be included as an integral part of pre-conception planning (Barrison and Wright 1984).

Treatment issues and co-dependence

Effective smoking cessation programs will be necessary to reduce the global burden of tobacco-related disease. Does alcohol play a role in determining the success of smoking intervention programs? The evidence strongly suggests that drinking reduces the already low success rate in smoking intervention programs. This is especially so for heavy drinkers, and less so for light or moderate drinkers. Binge drinking, loosely defined as consuming at least five or more drinks on one or more occasions in the previous month, reduces the probability of success by as much as 50% (Murray *et al.* 1995; Dawson 2000). The reason might be that binge drinkers are more likely to have a genetic defect leading to a more serious addiction problem to both alcohol and tobacco than moderate drinkers (see above).

Prevention of alcohol and tobacco-related diseases is even more important than treatment, especially in adolescents and young adults. There is solid evidence that the use of both substances begins at an early age, implying that efforts to promote a healthy lifestyle must begin early in life (Burke *et al.* 1988).

Summary

Both tobacco and alcohol contribute greatly to the global burden of disease. In the United States, an estimated 20% of the population has had recent exposure to both drugs, but at high levels of consumption of either substance, dual exposure is common, perhaps because of genetic susceptibility to addictive agents. At the biologic level, alcohol, although not a carcinogen, could enhance carcinogenicity of substances such as N-nitrosoamines contained within tobacco smoke, implying that exposure to both drugs will have a greater deleterious effect than exposure to either single agent. Malignancies of the mouth, throat, larynx, and esophagus where there is direct exposure to tobacco smoke and to alcohol are known to be related to exposure to both agents.

Of the several non-malignant diseases associated with dual exposure to these two substances, cardiac disease is clearly the most important: both heavy drinking and heavy smoking increase the risk of heart disease.

Smoking and alcohol consumption adversely effect pregnancy; regrettably, even though the deleterious impact of these substances on the fetus is well documented, exposure rates are still high.

Effective smoking cessation programs will be required to reduce the frequency of smoking-related disease. Unfortunately, smoking cessation programs are less effective in heavy drinkers; effective treatment of these individuals will require specially designed intensive therapeutic protocols.

References

1994. Medical-care expenditures attributable to cigarette smoking—United States, 1993. *MMWR Morb Mortal Wkly Rep*, **43**, 469–72.

National Household Survey on Drug Abuse: Main Findings (1997). National Clearinghouse for Alcohol and Drug Information. 1997. 2-26-2002. Ref Type: Electronic Citation.

Economic Costs of Alcohol and Drug Abuse estimated at $246 Billion in the United States. National Institute on Alcohol Abuse and Alcoholism. 1998. Ref Type: Electronic Citation.

Ahrendt, S. A., Chow, J. T., Yang, S. C., Wu, L., Zhang, M. J., Jen, J., and Sidransky, D. (2000). Alcohol consumption and cigarette smoking increase the frequency of p53 mutations in non-small cell lung cancer. *Cancer Res,* **60**, 3155–9.

An, H. S., Southworth, S. R., Jackson, W. T., and Russ, B. (1988). Cigarette smoking and Dupuytren's contracture of the hand. *J Hand Surg [Am],* **13**, 872–4.

Barrison, I. G. and Wright, J. T. (1984). Moderate drinking during pregnancy and foetal outcome. *Alcohol Alcohol,* **19**, 167–72.

Benowitz, N. L., Jones, R. T., and Jacob, P. III. (1986). Addictive cardiovascular effects of nicotine and ethanol. *Clin Pharmacol Ther,* **40**, 420–4.

Brugere, J., Guenel, P., Leclerc, A., and Rodriguez, J. (1986). Differential effects of tobacco and alcohol in cancer of the larynx, pharynx, and mouth. *Cancer,* **57**, 391–5.

Burge, P., Hoy, G., Regan, P., and Milne, R. (1997). Smoking, alcohol and the risk of Dupuytren's contracture. *J Bone Joint Surg Br,* **79**, 206–10.

Burke, G. L., Hunter, S. M., Croft, J. B., Cresanta, J. L., and Berenson, G. S. (1988). The interaction of alcohol and tobacco use in adolescents and young adults: Bogalusa Heart Study. *Addict Behav,* **13**, 387–93.

Chow, W. H., Swanson, C. A., Lissowska, J., Groves, F. D., Sobin, L. H., Nasierowska-Guttmejer, A., *et al.* (1999). Risk of stomach cancer in relation to consumption of cigarettes, alcohol, tea and coffee in Warsaw, Poland. *Int J Cancer,* **81**, 871–6.

Comings, D. E., Ferry, L., Bradshaw-Robinson, S., Burchette, R., Chiu, C., and Muhleman, D. (1996). The dopamine D2 receptor (DRD2) gene: a genetic risk factor in smoking. *Pharmacogenetics,* **6**, 73–9.

D'Avanzo, B., La Vecchia, C., and Franceschi, S. (1994). Alcohol consumption and the risk of gastric cancer. *Nutr Cancer,* **22**, 57–64.

Dawson, D. A. (2000). Drinking as a risk factor for sustained smoking. *Drug Alcohol Depend,* **59**, 235–49.

de Stefani, E., Boffetta, P., Carzoglio, J., Mendilaharsu, S., and Deneo-Pellegrini, H. (1998). Tobacco smoking and alcohol drinking as risk factors for stomach cancer: a case–control study in Uruguay. *Cancer Causes Control,* **9**, 321–9.

Du, X., Squier, C. A., Kremer, M. J., and Wertz, P. W. (2000). Penetration of N-nitrosonornicotine (NNN) across oral mucosa in the presence of ethanol and nicotine. *J Oral Pathol Med,* **29**, 80–5.

Evangelista, L. S., Doering, L. V., and Dracup, K. (2000). Usefulness of a history of tobacco and alcohol use in predicting multiple heart failure readmissions among veterans. *Am J Cardiol,* **86**, 1339–42.

Fuchs, C. S., Stampfer, M. J., Colditz, G. A., Giovannucci, E. L., Manson, J. E., Kawachi, I., *et al.* (1995). Alcohol consumption and mortality among women. *N Engl J Med,* **332**, 1245–50.

Gulliver, S. B., Rohsenow, D. J., Colby, S. M., Dey, A. N., Abrams, D. B., Niaura, R. S., and Monti, P. M. (1995). Interrelationship of smoking and alcohol dependence, use and urges to use. *J Stud Alcohol,* **56**, 202–6.

Gupta, P. C. (1984). Epidemiologic study of the association between alcohol habits and oral leukoplakia. *Community Dent Oral Epidemiol,* **12**, 47–50.

Han, C., McGue, M. K., and Iacono, W. G. (1999). Lifetime tobacco, alcohol and other substance use in adolescent Minnesota twins: univariate and multivariate behavioral genetic analyses. *Addiction,* **94**, 981–93.

Hansson, L. E., Baron, J., Nyren, O., Bergstrom, R., Wolk, A., and Adami, H. O. (1994). Tobacco, alcohol and the risk of gastric cancer. A population-based case-control study in Sweden. *Int J Cancer,* **57**, 26–31.

Hartwig, W., Werner, J., Ryschich, E., Mayer, H., Schmidt, J., Gebhard, M. M., Herfarth, C., and Klar, E. (2000). Cigarette smoke enhances ethanol-induced pancreatic injury. *Pancreas*, **21**, 272–8.

Hashibe, M., Mathew, B., Kuruvilla, B., Thomas, G., Sankaranarayanan, R., Parkin, D. M., and Zhang, Z. F. (2000). Chewing tobacco, alcohol, and the risk of erythroplakia. *Cancer Epidemiol Biomarkers Prev*, **9**, 639–45.

Hecht, S. S. (1999). DNA adduct formation from tobacco-specific N-nitrosamines. *Mutat Res*, **424**, 127–42.

Homann, N., Tillonen, J., Meurman, J. H., Rintamaki, H., Lindqvist, C., Rautio, M. *et al.* (2000). Increased salivary acetaldehyde levels in heavy drinkers and smokers: a microbiological approach to oral cavity cancer. *Carcinogenesis*, **21**, 663–8.

Izzotti, A., Balansky, R. M., Blagoeva, P. M., Mircheva, Z. I., Tulimiero, L., Cartiglia, C., and De Flora, S. (1998). DNA alterations in rat organs after chronic exposure to cigarette smoke and/or ethanol ingestion. *FASEB J*, **12**, 753–8.

Jaber, M. A., Porter, S. R., Gilthorpe, M. S., Bedi, R., and Scully, C. (1999). Risk factors for oral epithelial dysplasia—the role of smoking and alcohol. *Oral Oncol*, **35**, 151–6.

Ji, B. T., Chow, W. H., Yang, G., McLaughlin, J. K., Gao, R. N., Zheng, W., Shu, X. O., *et al.* (1996). The influence of cigarette smoking, alcohol, and green tea consumption on the risk of carcinoma of the cardia and distal stomach in Shanghai, China. *Cancer*, **77**, 2449–57.

Jones-Webb, R., McKiver, M., Pirie, P., and Miner, K. (1999). Relationships between physician advice and tobacco and alcohol use during pregnancy. *Am J Prev Med*, **16**, 244–7.

Kabat, G. C., Ng, S. K., and Wynder, E. L. (1993). Tobacco, alcohol intake, and diet in relation to adenocarcinoma of the esophagus and gastric cardia. *Cancer Causes Control*, **4**, 123–32.

Kono, Y., Yoneda, H., Sakai, T., Nonomura, Y., Inayama, Y., Koh, J., *et al.* (1997). Association between early-onset alcoholism and the dopamine D2 receptor gene. *Am J Med Genet*, **74**, 179–82.

Koopmans, J. R., van Doornen, L. J., and Boomsma, D. I. (1997). Association between alcohol use and smoking in adolescent and young adult twins: a bivariate genetic analysis. *Alcohol Clin Exp Res*, **21**, 537–46.

Launoy, G., Milan, C. H., Faivre, J., Pienkowski, P., Milan, C. I., and Gignoux, M. (1997). Alcohol, tobacco and oesophageal cancer: effects of the duration of consumption, mean intake and current and former consumption. *Br J Cancer*, **75**, 1389–96.

Lin, Y., Tamakoshi, A., Hayakawa, T., Ogawa, M., and Ohno, Y. (2000). Cigarette smoking as a risk factor for chronic pancreatitis: a case–control study in Japan. Research Committee on Intractable Pancreatic Diseases. *Pancreas*, **21**, 109–14.

Lowenfels, A. B., Zwemer, F. L., Jhangiani, S., and Pitchumoni, C. S. (1987). Pancreatitis in a Native American Indian population. *Pancreas*, **2**, 694–7.

Macfarlane, G. J., Macfarlane, T. V., and Lowenfels, A. B. (1996). The influence of alcohol consumption on worldwide trends in mortality from upper aerodigestive tract cancers in men. *J Epidemiol Community Health*, **50**, 636–9.

Macigo, F. G., Mwaniki, D. L., and Guthua, S. W. (1996). Influence of dose and cessation of kiraiku, cigarettes and alcohol use on the risk of developing oral leukoplakia. *Eur J Oral Sci*, **104**, 498–502.

Miller, N. S. and Gold, M. S. (1998). Comorbid cigarette and alcohol addiction: epidemiology and treatment. *J Addict Dis*, **17**, 55–66.

Murray, R. P., Istvan, J. A., Voelker, H. T., Rigdon, M. A., and Wallace, M. D. (1995). Level of involvement with alcohol and success at smoking cessation in the lung health study. *J Stud Alcohol*, **56**, 74–82.

Noble, E. P. (1998). The DRD2 gene, smoking, and lung cancer. *J Natl Cancer Inst*, **90**, 343–5.

Noble, E. P. (2000a). Addiction and its reward process through polymorphisms of the D2 dopamine receptor gene: a review. *Eur Psychiatry*, 15, 79–89.

Noble, E. P. (2000b). The DRD2 gene in psychiatric and neurological disorders and its phenotypes. *Pharmacogenomics*, 1, 309–33.

Olsen, J., Rachootin, P, and Schiodt, A. V. (1983). Alcohol use, conception time, and birth weight. *J Epidemiol Community Health*, 37, 63–5.

Romitti, P. A., Lidral, A. C., Munger, R. G., Daack-Hirsch, S., Burns, T. L., and Murray, J. C. (1999). Candidate genes for nonsyndromic cleft lip and palate and maternal cigarette smoking and alcohol consumption: evaluation of genotype–environment interactions from a population-based case–control study of orofacial clefts. *Teratology*, 59, 39–50.

Schlecht, N. F., Franco, E. L., Pintos, J., Negassa, A., Kowalski, L. P., Oliveira, B. V., and Curado, M. P. (1999). Interaction between tobacco and alcohol consumption and the risk of cancers of the upper aero-digestive tract in Brazil. *Am J Epidemiol*, 150, 1129–37.

Seitz, H. K., Poschl, G., and Simanowski, U. A. (1998). Alcohol and cancer. *Recent Dev Alcohol*, 14, 67–95.

Spitz, M. R., Shi, H., Yang, F., Hudmon, K. S., Jiang, H., Chamberlain, R. M., *et al.* (1998). Case–control study of the D2 dopamine receptor gene and smoking status in lung cancer patients. *J Natl Cancer Inst*, 90, 358–63.

Streissguth, A. P., Barr, H. M., Sampson, P. D., and Bookstein, F. L. (1994). Prenatal alcohol and offspring development: the first fourteen years. *Drug Alcohol Depend*, 36, 89–99.

Swan, G. E., Carmelli, D., and Cardon, L. R. (1996). The consumption of tobacco, alcohol, and coffee in Caucasian male twins: a multivariate genetic analysis. *J Subst Abuse*, 8, 19–31.

Talamini, G., Bassi, C., Falconi, M., Frulloni, L., Di Francesco, V., Vaona, B., *et al.* (1996). Cigarette smoking: an independent risk factor in alcoholic pancreatitis. *Pancreas*, 12, 131–7.

Thanos, P. K., Volkow, N. D., Freimuth, P., Umegaki, H., Ikari, H., Roth, G., *et al.* (2001). Overexpression of dopamine D2 receptors reduces alcohol self-administration. *J Neurochem*, 78, 1094–103.

Thun, M. J., Peto, R., Lopez, A. D., Monaco, J. H., Henley, S. J., Heath, *et al.* (1997). Alcohol consumption and mortality among middle-aged and elderly U.S. adults. *N Engl J Med*, 337, 1705–14.

Tuyns, A. J. (1970). Cancer of the oesophagus: further evidence of the relation to drinking habits in France. *Int. J. Cancer*, 5, 152–6.

Tuyns, A. J. (1982). Prevention et Depistage Precoce du Cancer de L'Oesophage. *Ouest Med*, 35[20], 1189–91. Ref Type: Journal (Full)

Tuyns, A. J. (1983). Oesophageal cancer in non-smoking drinkers and in non-drinking smokers. *Int. J Cancer*, 32, 443–4.

Tuyns, A. J., Pequignot, G., and Jensen, O. M. (1977). [Esophageal cancer in Ille-et-Vilaine in relation to levels of alcohol and tobacco consumption. Risks are multiplying]. *Bull Cancer*, 64, 45–60.

Vaughan, T. L., Davis, S., Kristal, A., and Thomas, D. B. (1995). Obesity, alcohol, and tobacco as risk factors for cancers of the esophagus and gastric cardia: adenocarcinoma versus squamous cell carcinoma. *Cancer Epidemiol Biomarkers Prev*, 4, 85–92.

Warda, L., Tenenbein, M., and Moffatt, M. E. (1999). House fire injury prevention update. Part I. A review of risk factors for fatal and non-fatal house fire injury. *Inj Prev*, 5, 145–150.

Wu, A. H., Wan, P., and Bernstein, L. (2001). A multiethnic population-based study of smoking, alcohol and body size and risk of adenocarcinomas of the stomach and esophagus (United States). *Cancer Causes Control*, 12, 721–32.

Zaridze, D., Borisova, E., Maximovitch, D., and Chkhikvadze, V. (2000). Alcohol consumption, smoking and risk of gastric cancer: case–control study from Moscow, Russia. *Cancer Causes Control*, 11, 363–71.

Part 12

Tobacco control: Successes and failures

Chapter 37

Global tobacco control policy

Nigel Gray

Introduction

Tobacco control policy has evolved over time and will continue to do so. To every action by the tobacco industry there has been a reaction by public health authorities and vice versa. As a result there has been a continuing struggle between those committed to market expansion (the industry) and those committed to market shrinkage (public health authorities). As a result the market is shrinking in most developed countries while it expands in many, but not all, developing countries. Between 1997 and 1999 world tobacco leaf sales went from 7 975 360 tonnes to 6 341 430 tonnes (United States Department of Agriculture 2001), while world cigarette production went from 5 614 830 million pieces in 1996 to 5 573 464 million pieces in 2000 (United States Department of Agriculture 2001). If public health is winning, it is winning very slowly. Fifty years of obstruction and obfuscation has maintained industry profits and has seen a steady increase in global mortality (Peto 1994). To be effective, tobacco control policy must be comprehensive and global.

Making tobacco policy is not the same as implementing it and the time lag between the two processes is often decades. Tobacco use is, and will remain, one of the most difficult health issues facing society in the twenty-first century. It is worth reflecting on the history of the major infectious diseases and the disappearance from developed countries within a decade or less of smallpox, measles, diphtheria, tetanus, whooping cough, rubella, and scarlet fever. These diseases were conquered by the discovery, and use, of penicillin and vaccines that both worked and were used. Some of these diseases persist in developing countries for reasons related to social organisation and money but NOT to organized opposition, which explains the slow progress against the tobacco epidemic. The single reason for the dominance of the tobacco problem is that someone is selling it, whereas no one is selling diphtheria or tuberculosis. This fact is unique to tobacco which has been, until very recently, the subject of a 50-year campaign of denial. There was never a serious suggestion that asbestos did not cause asbestosis or that drunken driving was merely a pleasurable habit.

That the environment has changed is due to the effects of litigation, mainly within the United States, which has led to the arrival in the public domain of over 33 million documents which revealed what the tobacco industry knew and when it knew it. The outcome of this process has been, at least in the case of Philip Morris (newly named Altria), a policy reversal which led to the admission set out in the following paragraph, which is a quote from their web site (Philip Morris USA 2002),

'Cigarette Smoking and Disease in Smokers: We agree with the overwhelming medical and scientific consensus that cigarette smoking causes lung cancer, heart disease, emphysema, and other serious diseases in smokers. Smokers are far more likely to develop serious diseases, like lung cancer, than non-smokers. There is no 'safe' cigarette. These are and have been the messages of public health authorities worldwide. Smokers and potential smokers should rely on these messages in making all smoking-related decisions.

Choose from the following for more detailed information from public health authorities on cigarette smoking and disease in smokers:'

This volte-face, accompanied as it is by a worldwide decline in the credibility of the industry, means that policy makers are working in a completely different environment and that the task of proving the seriousness of the situation is less complicated, is more related to its magnitude, can focus on what needs to be done and is much less of a debate. It does not mean that suggestions to governments go unopposed, or that the objective of market expansion has been abandoned by the industry.

This chapter will deal primarily with the cigarette, which is the most widely used and best-studied product. It should be noted that the remarkable mix of tobacco products that are smoked and chewed often in bizarre mixtures, pose singular difficulties, as they are usually regional, based on cottage industries and frequently not subject to tax, counting or inclusion in national statistics.

Key policy issues include prevention of initiation; management of addiction; regulation of the cigarette, the way it is sold, its nicotine content and its emissions; protection of non-smokers from secondhand smoke; public education and control of labelling and trademarks; disincentives to purchase (tax) and restrictions on sales to minors. Many of these topics are covered in detail in the relevant chapters. This chapter will summarize what is, in effect, modern comprehensive policy.

Prevention of initiation

Tobacco smoking is a *learned* habit. *Initiation* of smoking is a psycho-social phenomenon discussed in detail by Hill and Pierce (Chapter 18). *Maintenance* is sustained by the development of *addiction* (Chapters 6, 7, 8, 9).

Prevention of initiation requires removal of all the positive stimuli to take up smoking and the provision of effective education which warns teenagers of the dangers of smoking without triggering a desire to experiment. This is not easy to do.

Removal of all forms of tobacco promotion is also not easy to do. Many countries have passed effective legislation to prohibit all forms of advertising down to and including point of sale advertising. This was achieved by straightforward legislation in Norway and Finland but in Australia (which is a federation) separate legislation (sometimes at state level, sometimes federal) was required for health warnings; broadcast media; billboards; print media; and point of sale. Sponsorship of sport was eliminated indirectly by prohibition of advertising of brand names, which also covered 'brand stretching' (or sale of other products using the brand name, and often trade mark) of the cigarette. Ultimately overall Federal legislation brought all these individual pieces together over two decades after the first law was passed for health warnings.

Not all countries have the power to totally abolish tobacco promotion. Both the United States and the European Union probably lack the powers to do so. No country can prohibit transnational advertising such as accompanies the formula one grand prix, both car and motor cycle, although individual countries can prohibit exhibition of brand names but then face the possibility that such events will be moved elsewhere. International sports advertising is ubiquitous and uses sports of wide interest such as car and motorcycle racing, cricket, golf, and soccer.

Voluntary codes for advertising restriction have not been successful. However, if global advertising is to cease it can probably only be achieved by negotiation with the international tobacco industry under the sort of litigation-induced duress that brought about negotiations for a settlement in the United States in 1997 (Gray 1997). Such negotiations are only conceivable within a framework which envisages acceptance by both sides that the global tobacco market should shrink. Negotiation with the international television industry is another conceivable option but similarly difficult, though not impossible, to achieve.

The relationship between promotion and chemistry

While the contribution of advertising to initiation is undoubted, it is now evident (Wayne and Connolly 2002) that changes to cigarette design, particularly during the eighties, led to the cigarettes intended for the 'young adult smoker' (YAS) and the 'first usual brand young adult smoker' (FUBYAS) being made significantly 'smoother' with characteristics of less 'harshness', greater 'mildness' and 'lightness', among other features. Camel, in particular, developed an advertising campaign using Joe Camel, the 'smooth character' in parallel with significant design changes that sent the cigarette's chemistry in the direction desired by YAS and FUBYAS. Thus the cigarette became easier to smoke and easier to learn to smoke, and, as it had higher yields of nicotine, it may have become more addictive. Between 1987 and 1993, Camel's market share among 18-year-olds grew from 2.5% to 14%.

Competitive marketing

The market for cigarettes, and other forms of tobacco, is intensely competitive. While this persists abolition of promotion will remain extremely difficult. As a matter of policy, consideration needs to be given to replacing the open marketplace with a centralized, government-controlled wholesale purchaser for cigarettes, similar to the systems which operate in many countries for the purpose of purchasing pharmaceutical drugs.

Such a body would then be in a position to specify what products it is willing to place on the retail market.

The role of packet labelling

The branded and trade-marked cigarette packet is a potent advertisement (Wakefield *et al.* 2000), whether featured on a billboard or as observable in almost any streetscape where a smoker, or a teenager, offers a friend a cigarette from a well-known packet. The packet is also a potent opportunity to give information ranging from the explicit, research-based health warnings in Australia to the graphic and similarly explicit warnings in Canada. In the longer term a generic packet with suitable warnings is the only possible policy objective. This means abolition of trade marks, an objective that will not be easily attained.

Labelling with 'tar' and nicotine yields has been shown to be misleading in that the Federal Trade Commission (FTC) method of measurement does not represent the dose of smoke actually taken in by the smoker, and compensatory smoking is a frequent occurrence (Benowitz 2001; Jarvis *et al.* 2001; Kozlowski *et al.* 2001). For this reason alone use of these terms on the packet should be prohibited.

A second reason for abolishing these terms is the credible body of evidence suggesting that switching to low-yield cigarettes has been seen by smokers as a viable alternative to quitting (Weinstein 2001). Further they have been used as justification for the use of terms such as 'Light' and 'Mild' (Pollay and Dewhirst 2002) which have, rightly, been prohibited by the European parliament (Council of the European Union 2000) (the legislation is under legal challenge at the time of writing).

The management of addiction—smoking cessation

This topic is covered by Kunze in Chapter 43. There can be no doubt that modern techniques of counselling, associated with Nicotine Replacement Therapy (NRT) can substantially increase quit rates. The current position is unsatisfactory in most countries in that NRT is more expensive and less available than the cigarette. A further problem is posed by the failure of the health professions to use available knowledge and therapy in a widespread way (Boyle *et al.* 2000).

This situation is regrettable and represents a seriously missed opportunity as cessation offers the most immediate return for health expenditure in terms of mortality reduction.

Harm reduction

The concept of harm reduction is a logical approach to tobacco use. While abstinence from smoking is clearly the optimal approach, there is little excuse for the current legislative failure, worldwide, to regulate what goes into the cigarette and what comes out of it.

The first attempt to reduce the harmfulness of the cigarette was the policy of reducing tar and nicotine yields. This was logical at the time (the late sixties) and should have been more successful than it was. Tar and nicotine reduction was subverted by the changes in design of the modern cigarette described by Hoffmann (Hoffmann *et al.* 2001). These changes involved increases in nitrates and consequently, tobacco-specific nitrosamines (TSNAs) which have been associated with increases in the relative and absolute risk of adenocarcinoma of the lung. Together with other design changes (Kozlowski *et al.* 2001) which contributed to compensatory smoking the modern, low-yield cigarette, has not proven substantially less dangerous than its predecessor of 30–50 years (Thun and Burns 2001).

The fact that the low-yield program was not successful is no reason not to persist with attempts to regulate the content of cigarette smoke. Two areas of regulation attract interest. Control of smoke levels of carcinogens and toxins, and control of the driver to inhalation, nicotine.

Control of carcinogens and toxins

The policy objective is to reduce as far as practical the levels of known carcinogens and toxins in smoke. Such control is best focussed on smoke content rather than the constituents of the cigarette although certain substances, such as nitrosamines, may be best controlled at source—the nitrate levels in tobacco and the curing process.

Hoffmann has listed 15 major toxins and 69 carcinogens known to be in cigarette smoke (Hoffmann and Hoffmann 2001). Clearly these substances are the prime candidates for reduction. A system has been proposed, based on analysis of cigarettes actually on the market now, whereby the median of the market levels would become, over time, the maximum permitted (Gray and Boyle 2002), with the process repeated over time. Such a regulatory system is practical now as brands already on the market meet these criteria. There can be no justification for the continued marketing of cigarettes that are unnecessarily dangerous. If this form of regulation were to limit the number of brands available substantially, no harm would be done, cigarettes could still be sold profitably, and the harmfulness of cigarettes should be reduced. This in no way suggests that the cigarette would be 'safe' but it should certainly be less dangerous. Such an approach has been taken, successfully, to motor car exhausts.

Control of nicotine

Nicotine yields are currently measured by the FTC system, or something analogous. This system does not represent actual smoking patterns. A comparison of actual smoking patterns with the FTC method (Hoffmann and Hoffmann 2001) showed that smokers actually inhale between approximately one and a half to two and a half times as much nicotine, carbon monoxide, benz(*a*)pyrene and 4-(methylnitrosamine)-1-(3-pyridyl)-1-butanone (NNK) than would be inhaled if the cigarette was smoked according to the FTC parameters.

Clearly, if nicotine dose is to be regulated, a better measuring system is needed. For regulatory purposes a simple measure of the amount of nicotine in the cigarette tobacco should suffice. However, if the smoker is to be informed of the dose he or she is getting, something much more complex would be needed.

Until now the dose given to the smoker has been determined by the cigarette manufacturer. The result is the carefully engineered (Kozlowski *et al.* 2001) modern cigarette which is smoked in a compensatory way. The degree of compensation occurring with this cigarette has not been meaningfully compared with the degree of compensatory inhalation that occurred three and more decades ago. It is probably greater. Clearly compensatory smoking delivers greater amounts of carcinogens and toxins to the lung and one object of regulation should be to reduce this.

The intricacies of nicotine policy are discussed elsewhere and require consideration of nicotine in cigarettes and nicotine available in other forms. It is enough to canvass here the possible options for the cigarette. The first policy requirement is that nicotine becomes the object of regulation. The options then become:

♦ *Increase the amount of nicotine.* Providing a 'satisfying' amount of nicotine (which may mean an increase) has the advantage that it could be presumed to reduce compensation and therefore carcinogen/toxin dose (Russell 1976). The disadvantage is that it does nothing to reduce (and may enhance) dependence on the cigarette as a source of nicotine. Regulatory authorities are unlikely to be comfortable with this approach after several decades of struggle to reduce the dose.

♦ *Allow the status quo.* This has the disadvantage of leaving decision making to the tobacco industry, leaves today's level of compensatory smoking, and does nothing to reduce the addictiveness of the cigarette.

♦ *Reduce the amount of nicotine.* First proposed in 1994 (Benowitz and Henningfield 1994) this has the potential to reduce the addictiveness of the cigarette and the disadvantage that compensatory smoking might increase. It could only be done in parallel with a determined attempt to provide more widely available and efficacious NRT which might, used separately or together with cigarettes, replace the cigarette as the prime delivery system for nicotine. Clearly a major requirement would be a concerted comprehensive public education campaign. This option has possibilities in the long term but remains in the realm of the theoretical until nicotine levels in cigarettes are more universally captured by regulatory systems. The possibility of 'more efficacious' NRT being, or becoming, addictive, also needs to be faced.

Real control of dose and compensation

The above discussion of carcinogens/toxins and nicotine is aimed at reducing the amounts of the substances available per unit dose of smoke and need to be based on some form of standard measuring technique. The FTC system, or the various modifications of it, allows comparison across brands for regulation of carcinogens and toxins per litre of smoke. Reduction of the amount by weight of nicotine only means that the smoker must take more smoke to achieve the same physiological dose. Kozlowski (Kozlowski and O'Connor 2002) quotes a Philip Morris study which demonstrated that smoke intake may be remarkably large in the case of a smoker seeking more nicotine. He records an individual smoke intake of 1397 mls from a single cigarette (Carlton) for which the mean smoke volume seen was 713 mls and the machine (FTC) volume was 315 ml. Thus smokers are capable of taking fourfold increases in smoke dose from a low-yield cigarette. This is related to the amount of filter ventilation in the cigarette. Clearly regulation of cigarettes needs to take account of this and consideration needs to be given to prohibiting filter ventilation, which would lead to a less 'elastic' cigarette (one with which compensation is more difficult). Not only is it desirable that cigarettes deliver a more uniform dose of nicotine, this dose should be known to the consumer, which it cannot be in a cigarette designed to facilitate compensation.

Secondhand smoke—the role of the smoke-free environment

The issue of exposure to secondhand smoke has more public health significance than is indicated by its direct effects on health. Since early publications indicating that such exposure was associated with increased disease risk (Colley *et al.* 1974; Harlap and Davies 1974; Hirayama 1981; Trichopoulos *et al.* 1981; Chilmonczyk *et al.* 1993) the non-smoking public has been a significant force in supporting reduction of such exposures. To a considerable degree, smokers have been compliant with attempts to restrict smoking opportunities and have even been shown to favour smoke-free workplaces (Hocking *et al.* 1991) and public places.

The policy of reduction of exposure to secondhand smoke has several important effects. The most important is that it contributes to reduction in smoking and in smoking rates (Chapman *et al.* 1999). The second is that it can be expected to reduce disease in those susceptible, particularly to asthma. The third is reduction in lost work-time (Borland *et al.* 1997). An important factor in the establishment of the smoke-free environment has been successful litigation by employees suffering compensable diseases induced by secondhand smoke (Chapman 2001; Stewart and Semmler 2002). In Australia in 1997, 28% of smokers did not smoke at home (Borland *et al.* 1999). The insurance industry is an important ally in this area, as courtcases involving the tobacco industry have been extremely expensive and settling out of court can be cheaper. Further, after successful litigation, insurance of workplaces where employees are exposed to smoke becomes more expensive and may even be unobtainable.

Taxation policy

This issue is covered in detail in Chapter 42. Tax policy is an important part of overall policy as it can be a strong disincentive to initiation as well as to the amount smokers smoke and to quitting (Manley *et al.* 1993). Taxes should be high to be as large a deterrent as possible, and may be responsible for a significant proportion of total government tax revenues. For example they provided, in 1994–95, 4.34% of total tax in Argentina, 3.38% in Australia, 2.79% in China and 2.43% in India (Sunley *et al.* 2000). Earmarking of a proportion of tax for health purposes is sensible and may be popular. Increasing tax to a point where it equals three quarters to two-thirds of the price of cigarettes is regarded as achievable and appropriate (Chaloupka *et al.* 2000).

Public education

There is a clear relationship between levels of consumer information and tobacco use, so the process of public education is an important element of comprehensive policy. In its simplest form, the provision of a health warning on the packet, provides a basis for further and more specific education campaigns. All available means should be used, including mass media (Friend and Levy 2002; Wakefield and Chaloupka 2000), and the best programs are based on relevant research in the population in question. Major educational interventions such as technical reports have important if short lived effects (Kenkel and Chen 2000).

Availability

Sales to children, aged 16–18 are prohibited in many countries. Such prohibition is sensible but is rarely policed. Attempts are underway in the United States to remedy this. Until these attempts are shown to fail the policy remains important and should be seriously considered by developing countries.

What works

What works is all of the above, together, as part of a comprehensive, planned, regularly re-inforced and expensive exercise based on research within the society in which it is delivered, and constantly re-evaluated.

Acknowledgement

This work was conducted within the framework of support from the *Associazione Italiana per la Ricerca sul Cancro* (Italian Association for Cancer Research).

References

Benowitz, N. L. (2001). Compensatory smoking of low yield cigarettes. In: *Anonymous Risks Associated with Smoking Cigarettes with Low Machine-measured Yields of Tar and Nicotine*, Bethesda MD: US Department of Health and Human Services, National Institutes of Health, National Cancer Institute, pp. 39–63.

Benowitz, N. L. and Henningfield, J. E. (1994). Establishing a nicotine threshold for addiction. The implications for tobacco regulation. *N Engl J Med*, **331**, 123–5.

Borland, R., Cappiello, M. and Owen, N. (1997). Leaving work to smoke. *Addiction*, **92**, 1361–8.

Borland, R., Mullins, R., Trotter, L., and White, V. (1999). Trends in environmental tobacco smoke restrictions in the home in Victoria, Australia. *Tob Control*, **8**, 266–71.

Boyle, P., Gandini, S., Robertson, C., Zatonski, W., Fagerstrom, K., Slama, K., *et al.* (2000). Characterisics of smoker's attitudes towards stopping. *European Journal of Public Health*, **10**, 5–14.

Chaloupka, F. J., Hu, T., Warner, K. E., Jacobs, R., and Yurekli, A. (2000). The taxation of tobacco products. In: *Anonymous Tobacco Control in Developing Countries*, pp. 237–72. Oxford University Press, Oxford.

Chapman, S. (2001). Australian bar worker wins payout in passive smoking case. *BMJ*, 2001. May. 12;322.(7295):1139. **322**, 1139.

Chapman, S., Borland, R., Scollo, M., Brownson, R.C., Dominello, A., and Woodward, S. (1999). The impact of smoke-free workplaces on declining cigarette consumption in Australia and the United States. *Am J Public Health*, **89**, 1018–23.

Chilmonczyk, B. A., Salmun, L. M., Megathlin, K. N., Neveux, L. M., Palomaki, G. E., Knight, G. J., *et al.* (1993). Association between exposure to environmental tobacco smoke and exacerbations of asthma in children. *N Engl J Med*, **328**, 1665–9.

Colley, J. R., Holland, W. W., and Corkhill, R. T. (1974). Influence of passive smoking and parental phlegm on pneumonia and bronchitis in early childhood. *Lancet*, **2**, 1031–4.

Council of the European Union (2000). Proposal for a Directive of the European Parliament and of the Council on the approximation of the laws, regulations and administrative provisions of the member states concerning the manufacture, presentation and sale of tobacco products (recast).

Friend, K. and Levy, D. T. (2002). Reductions in smoking prevalence and cigarette consumption associated with mass-media campaigns. *Health Educ Res, 2002.Feb.;17.(1.):85.-98.* **17**, 85–98.

Gray, N. (1997). The global settlement—a global view. *J Surg Oncol*, **66**, 79–80.

Gray, N. and Boyle, P. (2002) Regulation of cigarette emissions. *Ann Oncol*, **13**, 19–21.

Harlap, S. and Davies, A. M. (1974). Infant admissions to hospital and maternal smoking. *Lancet*, **1**, 529–32.

Hirayama, T. (1981). Non-smoking wives of heavy smokers have a higher risk of lung cancer: a study from Japan. *Bull.World Health Organ. 2000.;78.(7.):940.-2*, **78**, 940–2.

Hocking, B., Borland, R., Owen, N., and Kemp, G. (1991). A total ban on workplace smoking is acceptable and effective. *J Occup Med*, **33**, 163–7.

Hoffmann, D. and Hoffmann, I. (2001). The changing cigarette: chemical studies and bioassays. In: Anonymous *Risks Associated with Smoking Cigarettes with Low Machine-measured Yields of Tar and Nicotine*, Bethesda: US Department of Health and Human Services, National Institutes of Health, National Cancer Institute, pp. 159–191.

Hoffmann, D., Hoffmann, I., and El-Bayoumy, K. The less harmful cigarette: a controversial issue. A tribute to Ernst L. Wynder. *Chem Res Toxicol, 2001 Jul.;14.(7.):767.-90*, **14**, 767–90.

Jarvis, M. J., Boreham, R., Primatesta, P., Feyerabend, C., and Bryant, A. (2001). Nicotine yield from machine-smoked cigarettes and nicotine intakes in smokers: evidence from a representative population survey. *J Natl Cancer Inst*, **93**, 134–8.

Kenkel, D. and Chen, L. (2000). Consumer information and tobacco use. In: Jha, P. and Chaloupa, F.J., (Eds.) *Tobacco Control in Developing Countries*, pp. 177–236. Oxford University Press, Oxford

Kozlowski, L. T. and O'Connor, R. J. (2002). Cigarette filter ventilation is a defective design because of misleading taste, bigger puffs, and blocked vents. *Tob Control, 2002.Mar.;11 Suppl 1.:I40–50*, **11 Suppl 1:I40–50**, I40-50.

Kozlowski, L. T., O'Connor, R. J., and Sweeney, C. T. (2001). Cigarette Design. In: Anonymous *Risks Associated with Smoking Cigarettes with Low Machine-measured Yields of Tar and Nicotine*, pp. 13–37. Bethesda MD: US Department of Health and Human Services, National Institutes of Health, National Cancer Institute.]

Manley, M., Glynn, T. J., and Shopland, D. (1993). *The Impact of Cigarette Excise Taxes on Smoking among Children and Adults: Summary Report of a National Cancer Institute Expert panel*, Bethesda MD: National Cancer Institute.

Peto, R. (1994). Smoking and Death: the past 40 years and the next 40 years. *BMJ*, **309**, 937–9.

Philip Morris U.S.A. (2002). Health Issues for Smokers. Philip Morris U.S.A. http://www.philipmorrisusa.com/DisplayPageWithTopic.asp?ID=60

Pollay, R. W. and Dewhirst, T. (2002). The dark side of marketing seemingly 'Light' cigarettes: successful images and failed fact. *Tob.Control, 2002.Mar.;11.Suppl.1.:I18.-31.* **11 Suppl 1:I18–31**, I18–31

Russell, M. A. (1976). Low-tar medium-nicotine cigarettes: a new approach to safer smoking. *Br Med J*, **1**, 1430–3.

Stewart, B. W. and Semmler, P. C. (2002). Sharp v Port Kembla RSL Club: establishing causation of laryngeal cancer by environmental tobacco smoke. *Med J, Aust 2002 Feb 4 ;176.(3.):113.-6*, **176**, 113–16.

Sunley, E. M., Yurekli, A., and Chaloupa, F. J. (2000). The design, administration, and potential revenue of tobacco excises. In: *Tobacco Control in Developing Countries*, (ed. P. Jha, and F. J. Chaloupa), pp. 409–26. Oxford University Press, Oxford.

Thun, M. J. and Burns, D. M. (2001). Health impact of 'reduced yield' cigarettes: a critical assessment of the epidemiological evidence. *Tob Control*, **10 Suppl 1:** 14–11.

Trichopoulos, D., Kalandidi, A., Sparros, L., and MacMahon, B. (1981). Lung cancer and passive smoking. *Int J Cancer*, **27**, 1–4.

United States Department of Agriculture. Tobacco World Markets and Trade. United States Department of Agriculture 2001. http://www.fas.usda.gov/tobacco/circular/2001/0109/index.htm

Wakefield, M. and Chaloupka, F. (2000). Effectiveness of comprehensive tobacco control programmes in reducing teenage smoking in the USA. *Tob Control, 2000 Jun.;9.(2.):177.-86*, **9**, 177–86.

Wakefield, M., Morley, C., Horan, J. K., and Cummings, K. M. (2000). The cigarette pack as image: new evidence from tobacco industry documents. *Tob.Control 2002.Mar.;11.Suppl.1.:I73.-80.* **11 Suppl 1:I73–80**, I73–80.

Wayne, G. F. and Connolly, G. N. (2002). How cigarette design can affect youth initiation into smoking: Camel cigarettes 1983–93. *Tob.Control, 2002 Mar.;11.Suppl.1.:I32.-9.* **11 Suppl 1:I32–9**, I32–9.

Weinstein, N. D. (2001). Public Understanding of Risk and Reasons for Smoking a Low-yield Product. In: Anonymous *Risks Associated with Smoking Cigarettes with Low Machine-measured Yields of Tar and Nicotine*, Bethesda MD: US Department of Health and Human Services, National Institutes of Health, National Cancer Institute, pp. 193–235.

Chapter 38

Lessons in tobacco control advocacy leadership

Michael Pertschuk

There are, of course, volumes of lessons in policy advocacy. Indeed, there are available through GOBALink and other tobacco control web-sites sound strategic and tactical guides on every conceivable advocacy challenge. Here, then, in these few pages, let us look at a few of the central strategic issues in building, sustaining, and *winning* a national or regional tobacco control policy campaign.

Fight

Perhaps the most important lesson so many of us have learned—painfully—over the nearly half-century of the tobacco wars is simply that tobacco control, unlike most public health struggles, is a *war* with a opposing enemy, the tobacco industry. This very fact has disabled or neutralized our most common public health strategies: the dissemination of scientific consensus; public health education; the presentation of science-based policy initiatives to the responsible public officials.

Indeed, we have had science, truth, and public health firmly on our side. But none of these suffices in the face of the economic and political power of the tobacco lobby—and its willingness to corrupt science, lie, and avoid even the most elemental responsibility for the human misery and avoidable death it causes.

So we have had to learn to fight, not only fiercely, but skillfully. We have had to learn the lobbyist's trade—and to understand that lobbying in the public interest cannot only be justified, but noble. We have learned to approach the mass media—not fearfully or timidly—but as perhaps our most important resource in the public exposure of the industry's corrupt practices and the public shaming of public officials who have shunned their fundamental responsibilities for the public health.

An outside–inside strategy

We have also learned that an effective political fight requires many different leadership roles. None have proved to be more essential, or effective, than the strategic complementarity of 'outside sparkplugs' and 'inside' advocates.

Outside sparkplugs. Sparkplugs are agitators: unabashed tellers of truth to power. They operate outside of conventional, political (or other) establishments, free of the ties that bind 'inside' players, and capable of holding our governments and other established organizations up to their own rhetoric of mission and commitment. Sparkplugs can kick-start a movement, coalition, or organization, and keep energy flowing through it. A community may be concerned, even outraged, but it may not be moved to action without a fiery goad. In their more exalted incarnations, sparkplugs echo the Old Testament prophets—lone, difficult, impossible—voices, churning up our collective conscience, annoying us into action.

As Stanton A. Glantz and Edith D. Balbach demonstrate persuasively in their important book, *Tobacco War; Inside the California Battles* (University of California Press, Berkeley 2000), 'Tobacco control advocates need to seek ways to keep the public informed and involved on the tobacco issue. If advocates instead retreat to playing only the inside political game, they will probably fail. They must be willing to withstand and embrace the controversy that the tobacco industry and its allies will generate.'

But the key to this counsel is the word, 'only'. To gain significant public policy successes, even the most potent outside advocacy must be coupled with effective 'inside' advocacy. By 'inside,' we are actually referring to two distinct categories of advocate:

1. Those who actually serve inside the corridors of power—political leaders, senior bureaucrats, and, in surprisingly many cases, the junior staff persons close to, and trusted by them, and

2. Those in the non-government sector who have earned the respect and trust of key government decision makers.

Inside advocates. Inside Advocates are wise in the ways of the political process, they are skilled negotiators, and positioned to influence key policy makers. Whether they occupy seats of power or have established an open door to those who do, they intuit the approaches and arguments that resonate with policy makers, and press them in ways that are not easily dismissed.

There is a needed caution to be added: while outside and inside advocates ideally play complementary roles, they can also play dysfunctional roles.

The Outside Sparkplug can get intoxicated on protest; let the passion of righteous outrage flash angrily at colleagues seen to be insufficiently militant; let the adrenaline of battle replace the pursuit of concrete policy goals and objectives; demand too much; come away with nothing. The Outside Sparkplug can come to disdain even sound, strategic compromise.

The inside advocate walks a very fine line—the line between the faithful representation of those he or she speaks for and the seizing of opportunities that don't allow for broad participation and full deliberation. The inside advocate can be seduced by the game of negotiation and the lure of the deal; cherish agreement for its own sake; develop entangling relationships with negotiators on the other side; accept too little; come away with next to nothing.

A tobacco control leadership 'taxonomy'

Fighters, both inside and outside, are essential to achieving policy objectives, but they cannot do this alone. Effectively to challenge and overcome the resistance of the tobacco lobby, a national tobacco control movement usually needs to fill several distinct, complementary, leadership roles. We have come to call such a diverse cabinet of leaders a 'tobacco control movement taxonomy'—a taxonomy that incorporates: Visionaries, Strategists, Statespersons, Experts, Strategic Communicators, and Movement Builders—as well as 'Inside' Advocates, and 'Outside Sparkplugs'.

Leaders who make up such complementary Leadership roles each bring to tobacco control a special skill set. Visionaries raise our view of the possible. Statespersons elevate the cause in the minds of both the public and decision-makers. Strategists chart our road maps to victory. Communicators deploy the rhetoric to inflame and direct public passion toward the movement's objectives. Inside Advocates understand how to turn power structures and established rules and procedures to advantage. Movement Builders are generators of optimism and good will, with the ability to infect others with dedication to the common good. The happy confluence of each of these leadership roles is the hallmark of a successful movement.

Visionaries. Tobacco control advocacy campaigns take flight through visionaries. Visionaries lift the horizons of others, setting goals that have never before been imagined or seen as realistic. Visionaries challenge the conventional view of the possible, aim high, take risks, and rethink priorities. Vision often comes from outsiders unencumbered by habitual thinking. It has been tobacco control visionaries who have seen the need to abandon traditional public health education for lobbying—policy advocacy—as the central strategic path to tobacco control.

Strategists. Strategists sort out that part of the vision that is realistically attainable, and develop a road map to get there. Strategists anticipate obstacles, including those laid by unruly coalition members, and provide guidance to insure that the movement remains headed in the right direction.

Statespersons. Statespersons raise the tobacco control flag for decision-makers and the larger public. They are the 'larger than life' public figures, scientific, medical, political who embody authority and public trust. Statespersons radiate credibility for the movement far beyond its core supporters.

Experts. There is a latter day tendency to disdain credentialed expertise as 'elitist', but the tobacco control movement has been built on a solid foundation of science—economic as well as bio-medical science—whose banner is held aloft by authoritative experts. With Experts as part of the tobacco control leadership team, ensuring that all new discoveries and public policy positions are grounded it facts and well reasoned, it becomes much easier to convince the public that the tobacco industry is wrong when they call us 'unthinking zealots'.

Strategic communicators. Strategic Communicators are public teachers, masters of the 'sound bite' as the concentrated encapsulation of potent messages. They translate complex scientific data, complex public policy, and basic concepts of truth and justice into accurate, powerful metaphorical messages, the significance of which can be instantly grasped by the broad public.

Movement builders (community organizers plus). The quiet heroes of any successful tobacco control movement, Movement Builders reach out to draw in new allies; they recruit new leaders and make them feel welcome, valued, and heeded. They do the same for longtime movement members as well. They know that a movement is weakest when it shuns diversity and seeks only a narrow, homogeneous base. Builders bridge generations, link local with national, even international advocacy, create space for the knowledge gained through experience to be passed on, and initiate new approaches to participation so that diverse voices are heard and their demands heeded.

Builders also heal. They circumvent organizational turf hurdles, they convene and facilitate, seek to explore differences through civil discourse and debate, and eschew rancorous division.

Again, a caution: While the combination of the leadership roles delineated in the taxonomy may be essential to the success of most national tobacco control campaigns, they are not automatically complementary—as we have seen with the vulnerabilities of outside and inside advocates: Visionaries can lose touch with reality and clash with Strategists; Statespersons can become blinded by ego. Communicators can degenerate into propagandists, manipulators of science and the truth, giving Experts a bad reputation. These leadership conflicts, if not acknowledged and addressed, can arrest tobacco control momentum, transforming a potentially dynamic and complementary leadership taxonomy into a nightmare taxonomy of dysfunctional conflict, sending a national movement on a downward spiral of distrust, frustration, and anger.

We have learned, together, that internal balance and self-knowledge are needed in all of our leaders to assure that their very strengths don't morph into undermining weaknesses. And we learn that each leader needs to strive to balance advocacy and detachment. Sociologist John Lifton encapsulates these essential qualities as such: 'Sufficient detachment to bring to bear one's intellectual discipline on the subject, and sufficient moral passion to motivate and humanize the work'.

Flexibility

Fight has proved a sound rule. It has served well in many tobacco control battles in many countries. But no rule, however sound, is without exception; and the most successful country advocates deeply understand the social and political cultures in which they must operate.

Among the most important advocacy leadership lessons we have learned is that what is absolutely the right strategy at one stage of tobacco control development in one place on the Globe, may be absolutely wrong for another country at a different stage.

When Witold Zatonski almost single-handedly launched his campaign to persuade the Polish government to enact a national advertising ban, the international experts told him there were two immutable rules he must follow: (1) Make the corruption of the transnational tobacco companies the central theme of your advocacy, and (2) Accept no compromises—if your parliament is not willing to enact a total ban on advertising, oppose their bill.

But Zatonski took the pulse of his country's new-found freedom from Soviet dominance and politely rejected this advice. Instead of attacking the tobacco companies, he chose not to make industry the central theme, but to embrace the affirmative theme of public health as a transcendent democratic value. And when, in 1995, the parliament was prepared to enact only modest tobacco control measures—far short of a total ad ban—he judged that such a bill would not foreclose stronger legislation later, but would open the door for future strengthening.

And six years later, December 5, 2002, Zatonski sent out this message on GLOBALink:

> It gives me great pleasure to impart to you perhaps one of the most important news for good health of Poles. Last night I looked over Polish newspapers and magazines. I did not find any tobacco ad. A year before (on 5th of December) tobacco ads disappeared off billboards throughout Poland, and yesterday tobacco ads disappeared off all written mass media in our country.
>
> Poland has become one more country free of tobacco advertising. Besides, tobacco companies are now banned from sponsoring sports, cultural, educational, health, and socio-political activities and events. (This included a ban on political contributions from tobacco companies).

Then, He graciously added:

> I should like to thank all our friends all over the world, who made our success possible.
>
> Thank you, thank you, and thank you.

Similarly, in South Africa, after the end of racial Apartheid, Health Minister Zuma [full name] was faced with an initial tobacco control bill with little more than a series of modest label warnings. Again, the international experts cautioned that such labels were worse the useless.

But she and other South African advocates decided otherwise. She believed that the passage of legislation itself and the creation of the warning labels would generate opportunities for broad media attention to the hazards of tobacco use—and the need for banning cigarette advertising. She was right. She reported that even illiterate smokers noted that something had changed on the package label and demanded to know what the change was about. Public awareness and support grew, and South Africa enacted an advertising ban three [years] later.

Opportunism

In policy advocacy, opportunism is not a character-flaw—but a virtue—and even apparent disaster may be turned into opportunity.

For example, in the Geneva negotiations on WHOs proposed Framework Convention on Tobacco Control, the US delegation's opposition to a ban on advertising in the pending WHO FCTC has been a true outrage. But surging international resentment at the US heavy handed bullying provoked developing regions to react by taking a strong stand in support of ad bans, including the Indian government, which had previously shown little interest in pursuing such a ban internally.

In India, tobacco control advocates seized upon this opportunity to press the government to introduce comprehensive national legislation, including a total ban on tobacco product advertising and broad smoke-free policies in public places.

But opportunism needs to function within an existing strategic framework—without which, opportunism can easily lead advocates astray from their priority objectives.

In the US from the turn of the century, state tobacco control coalitions, with technical assistance and funding from national tobacco control organizations, had building the capacity to launch campaigns for massive tobacco excise tax increases.

For three years, little progress was made. Conservative governors, campaigning against all tax increases, vowed never to raise the taxes—including tobacco taxes. Then came an economic recession, and the governors suddenly faced terrifying budget deficits.

The coalitions and the national organizations were ready:

- Their research teams deployed state of the art soft-ware to calculate state-specific tax revenue benefits from large excise tax increases.

- They conducted carefully public opinion polls in key states finely attuned to each state's political environment. The polls didn't stop at demonstrating popular support for tax hikes, they were designed to show—and DID show that cigarettes tax hikes were very good politics—particularly popular among the very 'swing' voters that all elected officials covet.

- To convey this message, the coalitions held press conferences, issued editorial board memoranda, developed state-specific news releases—featuring localized sound bites from prominent state leaders.

For three years, Nebraska's staunchly conservative Governor, when asked about the possibility of Cigarette excise tax increases, had growled, 'NO way; NO how!' After meeting with the pollster hired by the tobacco control advocates, he proposed a 50 cent a pack cigarette excise tax increase.

- 15 other governors—including several rabid anti-tax crusaders—proposed similar massive tobacco tax increases.

Thus, when the opportunity arose, they were ready and prepared to seize it. This is testament to strategic planning; putting the critical resources in place; keeping focused—and then, seizing the opportunity.

Realistic hope

Eric Fromm, the great social psychologist, wrote about 'hope' as 'a decisive element in any effort to bring about social change'.

But such hope, he added, is neither passive waiting ... nor the disguise of phrase making and adventurism, of disregard for reality, and of forcing what cannot be forced'.

True hope, wrote Fromm, 'is like the crouched tiger, which will jump only when the moment for jumping has come'.

That is, perhaps, the most profound lesson for tobacco control leaders in any country!

Chapter 39

A brief history of legislation to control the tobacco epidemic

Ruth Roemer

The protection and promotion of the health and welfare of its citizens is considered to be one of the most important functions of the modern state (Rosen 1958).

In no sense is this more true than with respect to the role of governments in combating the world-wide tobacco epidemic.

This chapter seeks to trace the evolution of tobacco legislation in the second half of the twentieth century, from 1950 to 2002. Our object is to analyse the progress made, the deficits still existing, and the challenges facing the countries of the world in the future.

The world has suffered many epidemics from the plagues in the time of Justinian in 543 and in the Middle Ages, from smallpox, malaria, and many infectious diseases, to the contemporary HIV/AIDS epidemic, but the tobacco epidemic is the first one in which the cause is not bacterial or viral but corporate—a multinational industry bent on profits from selling its lethal product.

The history of modern tobacco control legislation can be divided into five periods: (1) early legislation during the period 1890–1960; (2) legislation enacted in the 1960s and early 1970s in response to the proven connection between smoking and disease and regulating specific, categorical aspects of tobacco promotion and use; (3) the first comprehensive laws in the 1970s; (4) the decade of the 1980s when additional countries enacted legislation, both categorical and comprehensive; and (5) beginning in the 1990s the wide enactment of comprehensive legislation or greatly strengthened laws dealing with multiple aspects of tobacco production, marketing, and use.

Early research and reports

The modern story of laws to control the promotion and use of tobacco began with the science base for legislation. In 1938, Raymond Pearl documented dramatically the association between tobacco use and shortened duration of life, but his work failed to activate the health authorities (Pearl 1938). In 1950, the research of Wynder and

Graham in the United States (Wynder and Graham 1950) and that of Doll and Hill in the United Kingdom (Doll and Hill 1950) provided irrefutable epidemiological evidence on the grave health hazards of tobacco.

Following this ground-breaking research, two landmark reports linked smoking to lung cancer and launched the anti-smoking campaign in earnest. In 1962, the first report of the Royal College of Physicians of London (1962) established the association of smoking with serious morbidity and mortality. In 1964, Doll and Hill published their studies showing lower mortality among British physicians who had stopped smoking (Doll and Hill 1964). And in 1964, the Advisory Committee to the United States Surgeon General established a clear link between cigarette smoking and lung cancer and other disabling or fatal diseases and pronounced cigarette smoking 'a health hazard of sufficient importance to warrant appropriate remedial action' (U.S. Public Health Service 1964).

In 1970, the World Health Organization began its long and courageous campaign to translate the scientific evidence on the health risks of tobacco into programs and policies to protect the people of the world against this scourge. In May 1970, the World Health Assembly passed the first of many resolutions on tobacco (WHA 23.32). Reading this resolution after 32 years of experience with tobacco control legislation, we find this early policy remarkably prescient. It called for making the health consequences of smoking the subject of World Health Day, urged countries to limit smoking, recommended convening an expert group to propose further actions, emphasized education of young people not to begin smoking, and suggested that the Food and Agriculture Organization study crop substitution in tobacco-producing countries. The many resolutions of the World Health Assembly that followed noted the indisputable scientific findings on the harmful effects of tobacco use, condemned the aggressive promotion of tobacco in developed and developing countries, and proposed new and strengthened strategies to protect smokers and non-smokers.

Early legislation, 1890–1960

Early legislation concerned mainly prohibiting cigarette sales to minors, as in Norway (1899), Japan (1900), Canada (1908), New Zealand (1927), and Scotland (1908 and 1937) (Roemer 1993).

Another type of early legislation consisted of bans on smoking in places of entertainment, apparently designed to prevent fires. Examples of such legislation existed in Alexandria, Egypt (1908), Sao Paulo, Brazil (1950), and the State of New Delhi, India (1953) (Roemer 1993).

Legislation of the 1960s and early 1970s

Despite the wide dissemination of the findings of the 1962 report of the Royal College of Physicians of London and the 1964 report of the US Surgeon General's Advisory

Committee, mentioned above, little tobacco control legislation was enacted in the 1960s. There were two notable exceptions: (1) In 1962, Italy became the first country in western Europe to prohibit the advertising of tobacco—a measure dictated not so much by health considerations as by the need to protect the Italian State monopoly in tobacco (Roemer 1993). (2) In 1965, the United States Congress passed the Federal Cigarette Labeling and Advertising Act, which banned tobacco advertising on radio and television and required health warnings on cigarette packages. The act was subsequently amended in 1969 to include warning notices on little cigars and smokeless tobacco. This legislation was impelled by the effective strategy of a young lawyer, John Banzhaf, who petitioned the Federal Communications Commission to allow equal time for antismoking ads under the 'fairness doctrine,' which allowed free time on the broadcast media for opposing views on controversial issues. With powerful antismoking ads authored by the American Cancer Society and a subsequent decline in cigarette sales, the tobacco industry preferred a legislative ban to continued antismoking ads on the electronic media, and it wanted to avoid different health warnings required by the states (Warner 1979). Congress voted to ban tobacco advertising on television and radio and to require a national health warning.

Comprehensive laws of the 1970s

In the 1970s, a wealth of legislation was enacted in various countries restricting advertising on radio and television, requiring health warnings on cigarette packages and advertising, banning smoking in hospitals, indoor supermarkets, and other public places, and in workplaces. Countries that enacted legislation dealing with multiple aspects of tobacco control rather than single-issue, categorical laws are Singapore (1970), Norway (1973), Finland (1976), and France (1976) (Roemer 1993). All these laws were designed to make one measure potentiate another and to express more forcefully than single-issue laws the political will of the government to control the tobacco epidemic.

A prototype for a comprehensive law was the law of Finland, enacted in 1976. Concern about the death rate of adult males in Finland led to a finding that tobacco was the culprit. The Finnish Parliament consequently banned all advertising of tobacco, prohibited smoking in public places, and allocated a part of tobacco tax revenue to antismoking activities. But tobacco prices were raised only slightly so that tobacco became a cheap luxury. In 1985, the Advisory Committee on Health Education of Finland issued a landmark report, announcing that

> Every tobacco price decision is also a health policy decision: a decision as to the amount of tobacco-related illness and premature deaths in the future. In making such a decision, the needs of the State Budget, developments in the profitability of the tobacco industry, and inflation control objectives have all traditionally come before public health objectives, despite the fact that purely economic viewpoints also speak for a reduction in smoking.

The Finnish Committee concluded that unless the real price of cigarettes is raised and unless the price is raised repeatedly and keeps pace with inflation, there will be no decline in smoking (Finland, Advisory Committee on Health Education 1985).

Contributing to the movement for stronger legislation was the support of international bodies that had joined WHO in calling for restrictions on promotion of tobacco. In 1972, the Nordic Council of Ministers had recommended to its members— Denmark, Finland, Iceland, Norway, and Sweden—that cigarette advertising be banned and public information campaigns on the dangers of tobacco be launched, with special attention to preventing smoking by young people (Nordic Council of Ministers 1972). In 1973, the Council of Europe recommended that advertising of tobacco and alcohol in newspapers, on television and radio, and in theatres be banned (Council of Europe 1973). The movement for regional action continued. In 1986, the Council of the European Communities, in adopting a program of action against cancer, called for development of measures to limit and reduce the use of tobacco as a first priority (Council of the European Communities 1986). Following up on this resolution, in 1989 the Council of Ministers of Health of the Member States of the European Community urged Member States to ban smoking in public places and public transport (Council of the European Communities 1989). A historic but failed advance occurred in July 1988 when the European Parliament voted to ban all tobacco advertising and sponsorship in the 15 countries of the European Union, effective 2006, but on 5 October 2000 the Court of Justice of the European Community annulled this directive (*Federal Republic of Germany* vs. *European Parliament and Council of the European Union* 2000).

The greatest breakthrough in achieving the international cooperation that WHO had long sought was the decision of major specialized agencies of the United Nations—principally the Food and Agriculture Organization and the World Bank—to throw their influence behind programs of tobacco control. In 1979, the Food and Agriculture Organization, which in the past had actively promoted tobacco production, adopted a policy of encouraging tobacco cultivation only 'in such cases where overriding economic considerations so warrant' (Cunningham 1996). In 1991, the World Bank adopted a clear policy against support of tobacco production and in favor of tobacco control. Its policy consists of the following five measures:

1. The Bank's activities in the health sector discourage the use of tobacco products.

2. The Bank does not lend directly for, invest in, or guarantee investment or loans for tobacco production, processing, or marketing. In a few countries heavily dependent on tobacco as a source of income, the Bank aims to help these countries diversify away from tobacco.

3. The bank does not generally lend indirectly to tobacco production activities.

4. Tobacco and its related processing machinery and equipment cannot be included among imports financed under loans.

5. Tobacco and tobacco-related imports may be exempt from borrowers' agreements with the Bank to liberalize trade and reduce tariffs (Jha and Chaloupka 2000, p. 345).

Legislation of the 1980s

In the 1980s, the movement for strengthened tobacco control legislation spread and accelerated. It was greatly encouraged by increasingly urgent resolutions of WHO, calling for legislative action and cooperation with specialized agencies of the United Nations (WHA 24.48), urging Member States to identify the health problems associated with smoking in their countries and strengthen health education on smoking (WHA 29.44), and requesting the Director General to intensify WHO's action to control tobacco smoking (WHA 31.56). In 1983, a report of a WHO Expert Committee strongly backed legislation as essential to effective tobacco control. It states:

> It may be tempting to try introducing smoking control programmes without a legislative component, in the hope that relatively inoffensive activity of this nature will placate those concerned with public health, while generating no real opposition from cigarette manufacturers. This approach, however, is not likely to succeed. A genuine broadly defined education programme aimed at reducing smoking must be complemented by legislation and restrictive measures (WHO Expert Committee 1983).

In 1986, WHO took a bold step and adopted a resolution (WHA 39.14) calling for comprehensive tobacco control legislation. It defined such legislation as containing the following nine elements:

1. protection from involuntary exposure to tobacco smoke in enclosed public places, restaurants, transport, and places of work and entertainment

2. protection of children and young people from becoming addicted

3. ensuring that a good example is set in all health-related premises and by all health personnel

4. measures towards progressive elimination of socioeconomic, behavioral, and other incentives that maintain and promote the use of tobacco

5. prominent health warnings, including the statement that tobacco is addictive, on all types of tobacco products

6. establishment of programs of education and public information on tobacco-related diseases, and effectiveness of national smoking control programs

7. monitoring trends in smoking and other forms of tobacco use, tobacco-related diseases, and effectiveness of national smoking control action

8. promotion of viable economic alternatives to tobacco production, trade, and taxation

9. establishment of a national focal point to stimulate, support, and coordinate all tobacco control activities (World Health Organization 1997).

In the wake of these initiatives by WHO and actions by other international and regional agencies, more Member States of WHO acted in the decade of the 1980s to adopt legislation restricting advertising, requiring health warnings, curbing smoking in public places and workplaces, and increasing public education on the risks of tobacco.

Moreover, instead of categorical laws limited to one or another aspect of tobacco control, an increasing number of countries continued to adopt comprehensive laws dealing with various aspects of tobacco control, notably Iceland (1984), Ireland (1986), and Canada (1988) (Roemer 1993). By the end of the 1980s or early in the 1990s, Australia, New Zealand, France, Sweden, and Thailand had enacted comprehensive legislation (World Health Organization 1997). Here we give accounts of the experiences of four countries—Canada, Thailand, Poland, and South Africa—in achieving comprehensive tobacco control legislation.[1]

The experience of Canada[2]

The experience of Canada in achieving effective, comprehensive tobacco control legislation is particularly significant because it shows the necessity for continued and persistent political will in the face of strong industry opposition. As early as 1969, a committee of the Canadian House of Commons called for comprehensive tobacco control measures—a complete ban on advertising, strong health warnings, setting maximum levels of tar and nicotine contents. But legislation was not passed until 1988. The tobacco companies immediately challenged the legislation in the courts, contending that the advertising ban was an unconstitutional restriction of freedom of expression protected by the Canadian Charter of Rights and Freedoms. The Quebec trial court invalidated the legislation on the grounds urged by the industry. On appeal, the Quebec Court of Appeal reversed the lower court's decision and upheld the legislation. In September 1995, however, the Supreme Court of Canada, by a vote of 5 to 4, struck down the ban on advertising, indicating that it would uphold a partial ban on lifestyle

---

[1] These accounts are based on case studies appended to a report submitted to the World Health Organization entitled *Strengthening Enactment, Enforcement, and Evaluation of Tobacco Control Legislation* by Ruth Roemer and Barbara Berman, April 2002. The contents of this report are incorporated in the excellent book by D. Douglas Blanke, *Tobacco Control Legislation, An Introductory Guide: Tools for Advancing Tobacco Control in the 21st Century* (2003).

[2] Based on Rob Cunningham, *Smoke and Mirrors: The Canadian Tobacco War*. Ottawa: International Development Research Centre, 1996.

advertising and advertising related to minors. It also invalidated unattributed health warnings and the ban on tobacco trademarks on non-tobacco goods.

The response of the government of Canada was prompt and strong. Three months later, in 1995, the Minister of Health issued a report outlining the legislative directions that the federal government proposed to take (Marleau 1995).

In the years between 1989 when the Tobacco Products Control Act, C-51, took effect and 1995, when the Canadian Supreme Court struck down major portions of the Act, many actions occurred to strengthen tobacco control, including stronger rotating warnings, a ban on smoking in the federal public service, a requirement for smoke-free flights on Canadian carriers, local ordinances restricting smoking in public places and workplaces, and substantial tax increases (an increase of US $4 a carton in 1987 and US $6 a carton in 1991).

The tax increases were followed by smuggling of Canadian cigarettes into the United States and back into Canada through a reservation of Native Americans that straddled both countries, among other means. Thus, the Canadian tax was not paid, and the cigarettes sold for US $2.50 per pack instead of US $4.50 per pack. Despite efforts by health groups to urge an export tax to control smuggling, the federal and five provincial governments elected to reduce tobacco taxes—an action that led to an increase in smoking among young people (Cunningham 1996).

On April 25, 1997, the Canadian Parliament adopted a new tobacco control law— Bill C-71, an Act to Regulate the Manufacture, Sale, Labeling, and Promotion of Tobacco Products. The Act gives sweeping powers to the government to regulate the contents of tobacco products, bans sales to persons under 18, requires posting of signs by retailers that the sale or giving of tobacco products to persons under 18 is illegal, prohibits sale of cigarettes in packages other than packages of 20, prohibits sales from vending machines, mandates health warnings and authorizes package inserts about the health hazards of tobacco, prohibits tobacco advertising except for product information and brand preference advertising that is not lifestyle, misleading, or appealing to persons under 18, prohibits the distribution and promotion of tobacco products if any brand elements appear on a non-tobacco product associated with youth or lifestyle, and restricts sponsorship until October 2003 when all sponsorship advertising is prohibited.

In 2000, Canada strengthened its tobacco control legislation further. It requires one of 16 strong, large, picture-based rotated warnings on the top 50 per cent of the front and back of cigarette packages. Inside the package one of the 16 rotated warnings is required either on an insert or on the 'slide' of 'slide and shell' packages. Nine of the 16 messages provide advice on quitting, and seven provide detailed health information.

In 2002, Canada pioneered another innovation. It launched an attack on deceptive descriptors of tobacco products. Exposing the deception in promotion of 'light' and 'mild' cigarettes, the Ministerial Council on Tobacco Control recommended to the Canadian Minister of Health that a complete ban be placed on these misleading descriptors and others that may also be misleading. This ban should be promulgated through new regulations, the Council urged, as the quickest and most effective route to protect the health of Canadians (Ministerial Advisory Council of Canada 2002).

The Canadian tobacco-control legislation, obtained against strong opposition from the tobacco industry, is a model for other countries. Persistent political will on the part of the government led to success. Health Canada, the national department of health, received support from other departments of the federal government—Labour, Treasury, Transport, Justice, and Finance. Non-governmental agencies and the media provided important help. A critical component was research on the prevalence of smoking, taxation, costs of tobacco use, and other matters—research essential to inform Parliamentarians and the people. Above all, the ability, imagination, and commitment of the leadership of the tobacco-control movement in Canada led to its successful, comprehensive legislation.

The experience of Thailand[3]

The assault of the transnational tobacco companies on Thailand in the 1990s set in motion a series of events that led to Thailand's enactment in 1992 of two laws: the Tobacco Products Control Act and the Nonsmokers' Health Protection Act (Chitanondh 2000). When Thailand was charged with violation of international agreements by its attempt to exclude foreign tobacco companies (and their advertising) from the country, a panel of the General Agreement on Tariffs and Trade (predecessor of the World Trade Organization) ruled that Thailand was in violation but, under a clause allowing protection of the health of the people, Thailand could restrict the sale and promotion of tobacco on condition that the restrictions applied to all tobacco, both domestic and imported.

Following this decision, the Minister of Public Health appointed a committee to draft legislation, using the model of the Tobacco Control Act of Norway. Throughout this process and as the legislation went before the Parliament, the tobacco companies criticized and opposed the legislation on the grounds that it duplicated existing laws, it interfered in business operations, it opened the way to abuse of power, and it failed to give an opportunity to the business affected by the legislation to express its opinion. During a meeting of the Standing Committee on Health and the Environment, the manager of Philip Morris of Thailand, in violation of Parliamentary rules, entered a closed door meeting of the committee considering the legislation (Chitanondh 2000).

Under the leadership of Dr Hatai Chitanondh, Deputy Permanent Secretary of the Ministry of Health, both bills passed the Parliament. The Tobacco Products Control Act (the supply side law) prohibits the sale of tobacco products to persons under 18, the sale of tobacco products in vending machines, use of tobacco products for entry to games

---

[3] Based on Hatai Chitanondh, *The Passage of Tobacco Control Laws: Thai Davids versus Transnational Tobacco Goliaths*, Thailand Health Promotion Institute, the National Health Foundation, Bangkok, 2000.

or shows, and distribution of free samples. Most importantly, the legislation prohibits advertising and sponsorship and sale of tobacco products without required labels and health warnings. It requires one of ten warnings with white background and black letters.

The Nonsmokers' Health Protection Act (the demand side law) bans smoking in a wide range of public places designated by the Minister of Public Health. Strict enforcement has followed enactment of the laws.

The tobacco-control program of Thailand has resulted in a decline in smoking prevalence for men from 63.2% of the population in 1981 to 42.2% in 1999; for women from 5.4% in 1981 to 2.6% in 1999, and for both sexes from 35.2% in 1981 to 22.4% of the population in 1999.

The experience of Poland[4]

In response to the frighteningly increasing morbidity and mortality from tobacco-related diseases, Polish tobacco control advocates, encouraged by international contacts with the International Union against Cancer (UICC) and WHO and with help from Finnish and UK health experts, undertook systematic studies of the tobacco and cancer epidemics in the Polish population. These studies estimated that 58% of all malignant tumors in middle-aged men were due to cigarette smoking, and 42% of cardiovascular deaths and 71% of respiratory deaths among middle-aged men were due to smoking (Peto *et al.* 1994).

Once the legislation was drafted, a conference entitled 'A Tobacco-Free Europe,' was held at Kazimierz, Poland in 1990. There a framework for cooperation on tobacco control between central and eastern Europe was developed, and education and training for public health workers on tobacco control was planned for the region.

The legislation was introduced in the upper chamber of the Parliament, the Senate, to which a considerable number of physicians had been elected. Supporters of the bill emphasized the health arguments and stressed the catastrophic state of adult health in Poland. Despite strong opposition from the tobacco industry and delays in action caused by the industry's contention that 'a parliamentary act, which is, after all, a piece of paper' cannot improve the health of the nation, the legislation passed by an overwhelming majority in November 1995.

After the law was passed, investigations were undertaken of the effect of tobacco price policies on prevalence of smoking. As a result, in 1999 and 2000, the tobacco tax was increased by 30% and again in 2001 by 20%. Not until 1999 did tobacco control activities succeed in convincing Parliament to amend the law to provide for a total ban on tobacco advertising and to allocate 5% of tobacco excise taxes to the national tobacco program.

---

[4] Based on 'Case Study of Poland's Experience in Tobacco Control' by Professor Witold Zatonski, MD, ScD, Director, Department of Cancer Epidemiology and Prevention, the Maria Sklodowska-Curie Memorial Cancer Center and Institute of Oncology and WHO Collaborating Centre, Warsaw, 2001.

The Polish law protects the right of non-smokers to live in a smoke-free environment, creates legal and economic conditions to encourage reduction in tobacco use, informs the public about the adverse effects of smoking and the levels of harmful substances in tobacco by messages on tobacco packages and advertisements (in magazines for adults), provides for decreasing the maximum levels of harmful substances in tobacco products, provides treatment of tobacco-dependent persons free of charge in public health facilities, prohibits smoking in health and educational institutions and other public places, prohibits sales to minors, including sales through vending machines and in packages of fewer than 20 cigarettes, prohibits production and marketing of smokeless tobacco, prohibits advertising and promotion of tobacco products on television and radio, in cinemas, newspapers, magazines for children and teenagers, in educational and cultural institutions, and in sports facilities, and requires on each package of cigarettes two different warnings on health effects and on levels of tar and nicotine contents, with the messages covering 30% of each side of the cigarette pack.

Although the Polish law has been in force for only a few years, its effects are already apparent. Smokers in Poland have been reduced from 14 million at the end of the 1970s to 10 million in 2000, from 62% of adult men to 40%, and from 30% of adult women to 20%. The upward trend in mortality from lung cancer in the 1980s has been reversed, and by the end of the 1990s mortality had decreased by about 20% compared to the peak level. By comparison, Professor Zatonski points out, in Hungary, where trends in lung cancer had been the same as in Poland but effective tobacco-control activity has not occurred, incidence of lung cancer is still increasing (Zatonski 2001). Similarly, Poland has experienced a significant reduction in the burden of cardiovascular disease, part of which is attributed to reduced cigarette consumption.

Poland's success in enacting effective, comprehensive tobacco control legislation was due to several key elements in its campaign: extensive epidemiological investigation of smoking patterns in Poland; competent, dynamic persistent leadership, which generated and sustained political will to combat the serious premature adult morbidity and mortality from tobacco-related diseases; and adopting the strategy of first achieving what was possible and then amending the legislation to strengthen it.

The experience of South Africa[5]

South Africa's experience with tobacco control demonstrates the feasibility of obtaining effective legislation in stages, provided the necessary political will exists.

South Africa both grows and manufactures tobacco. Under apartheid the country's powerful tobacco sector had enormous production and profits. Smoking rates soared in the period between 1967 and 1991. Although the Health Ministry recognized the

---

[5] Based on speeches by Dr Yussuf Saloojee, Director, National Council Against Smoking of South Africa to a conference of cancer associations (2001) and to the WHO Meeting for the Development of Tool-kits for Tobacco Legislation and Economic Intervention, Geneva, 30–31 March 2000.

threat to the people's health, other priorities took precedence over tobacco control. In the dying days of apartheid, the policy on tobacco began to change. In 1993 the government of South Africa passed its first tobacco Products Control Act, a modest, limited law that provided only for control of smoking in enclosed public areas, labeling of tobacco packages and advertisements with health warnings and tar and nicotine contents, and prohibition of sales to children under 16.

In 1994, with the election of a new democratic government, the Minister of Health, Dr Nkosazana Zuma, strengthened the legislation and issued regulations mandating strong, prominent, rotating health warnings on tobacco packages and advertisements. Included on the cigarette packages are the benefits of stopping and a telephone number for advice on quitting.

Most importantly, the Ministry of Finance increased tobacco taxes specifically to protect the health of the people. Between 1994 and 1999, real tobacco excise taxes rose 149%, which increased real cigarette prices by 81%. The government's tobacco tax revenues doubled, while consumption decreased by 21%.

In March 1999 the South African Parliament enacted strengthened legislation—the Tobacco Control Amendment Act, effective April 1, 2001. This legislation prohibits all tobacco advertising, sponsorship, and promotion. Strong enforcement has resulted in regulations banning smoking in all enclosed places, including workplaces, in specifying the maximum amounts of nicotine, tar, and other ingredients in tobacco, in banning free distribution by the tobacco companies of tobacco products and awards or prizes to induce the purchase of tobacco, and in requiring supervision of vending machines to prevent children under 16 from obtaining cigarettes.

In achieving these wide-ranging controls in its 1999 legislation, the government had to overcome the strong opposition of the tobacco industry, which contended that it was not consulted, jobs would be lost, and 'freedom' was being attacked. Attempting to delay Parliamentary action, the industry sought a high court injunction asking that the Ministry of Health make available all information it used in preparing the bill and requesting time to study the information. The injunction was denied, and the denial was upheld on appeal. The industry also formed alliances with other businesses and labor unions that opposed the bill and claimed to be independent of the tobacco companies. The industry employed highly credentialed local and international 'experts' to testify to the Parliamentary Health Committee to attack the constitutionality of the legislation and the science involved, contending that the legislation would not be effective.

But the majority of the people supported the legislation. In commenting on the South Africa experience, Dr Yussuf Saloojee, Director of the National Council Against Smoking of South Africa, ascribed South Africa's success to the bold leadership of the Health Minister and of President Nelson Mandela and to the following factors:

◆ production of sound epidemiological and economic data

◆ effective advocacy by non-governmental organizations in support of the legislation to Parliamentarians and to the public and the media

- cooperation of the ministries of finance, agriculture, and sports with the health ministry
- international developments, such as the decision of the British government and the European Union to ban tobacco advertising and promotion, thus making South Africa's action part of a global trend (Saloojee 2001).

Judicial action

No account of tobacco-control legislation would be complete without recognition of the role of litigation as a tool to obtain the objectives of legislation and to seek damages for the vast illness and death inflicted by tobacco (Daynard 1993). In 1984, a brilliant young lawyer, Professor Richard A. Daynard of Northeastern University Law School in Boston, launched the Tobacco Products Liability Project (TPLP). Describing Daynard's development of the TPLP, the historian, Richard Kluger, explains the strategy of litigation as having arisen from Daynard's drafting of the first worksite smoking control statute in the town of Newton, Massachusetts. Kluger writes:

> Foreseeing an endless campaign to put across such measures in the state's 350 other such municipalities, Daynard sought a more telling way to combat the health problem. Given the tobacco industry's record of fierce resistance to legislative action against it, he honed a strategy relying on the judicial branch of government, which seemed less susceptible to the companies' infiltration (Kluger 1996, p. 559).

The mission of the Tobacco Products Liability Project was to force the media and the public to recognize the magnitude of the danger of tobacco 'by focusing on the suffering of particular individuals, thereby helping to counterbalance the $52 billion spent annually... which promoted this catastrophic epidemic' (Kluger 1996, p. 559).

As Daynard explained in 1993, these suits allege that the products are unreasonably dangerous in that their risks exceed any possible benefits, that the tobacco companies have failed to give full warnings, that they have lied about the dangers, and that they have failed to pursue safer product designs (Daynard 1993). Later, he would add that the tobacco companies denied the addictiveness of tobacco and targeted young people as their market.

At the time that Daynard launched the TPLP, no plaintiff had ever recovered damages from a tobacco company for the morbidity and mortality caused by tobacco. In the 18 years since then, many suits have been won or settled, and litigation has been pursued in many countries, including Canada, Finland, Australia, the United Kingdom, and others.

When Daynard established the TPLP, no one could have anticipated the powerful effect this movement would have. Initially, product liability suits were brought in the United States on behalf of individual plaintiffs. Then class action suits were filed. For example, *Broin* v. *Philip Morris* was a class action suit on behalf of 60 000 flight attendants who were sick from exposure to dense environmental tobacco smoke in airplane cabins.

The case was settled by an agreement with the defendant tobacco companies allowing all class members to proceed with their individual claims and providing payment of $300 million by the tobacco companies to establish the Broin medical research foundation which, in part, will help with early detection and cure of diseases associated with cigarette smoke suffered by flight attendants (*Tobacco on Trial* 1997).

But when the Attorney General of Mississippi filed the first lawsuit on behalf of a state against the tobacco companies to recover the costs incurred by the state for treating patients with tobacco-related diseases, the floodgates opened. Four state lawsuits were eventually settled. The Mississippi case was settled out of court on July 3, 1997, with tobacco companies agreeing to pay $3.3 billion over 25 years. Florida settled next on August 25, 1997 for $11.3 billion. Texas settled on January 16, 1998 for $15.3 billion. In Minnesota, the Attorney General refused to settle until all the evidence was on the record, so that millions of industry documents would be disclosed. The Minnesota case was settled on May 8, 1998 for $6.1 billion, with a requirement that the industry maintain depositories of 30 million documents and release an index to millions of previously released documents (Bloch *et al.* 1998). These documents reveal the duplicity of the industry, its targeting of children, its corrupt science, its deliberate enhancement of the nicotine contents of tobacco, its denial of the addictiveness of tobacco, and its concealment from the public of what it knew about the dangers to health caused by tobacco (Glantz *et al.* 1996). This evidence, together with depositories of industry documents in San Francisco, California and Guilford, England reveal the extent of the fraud and concealment by the industry, now available for use in other litigation (Rabin 2001).

A stormy period ensued in which a global settlement agreement was negotiated in 1997. It required approval by Congress because it would have affected the authority of the Food and Drug Administration to regulate tobacco and would have barred private litigation against the companies. No legislation passed because the industry insisted on immunity from further liability; and when this was unlikely, it withdrew its support for the global settlement (Bloch *et al.* 1998).

In November 1998 the suits of the remaining 46 states were settled in a Master Settlement in which the tobacco companies agreed to pay $206 billion over 25 years (the global settlement called for payment of $516 billion over 25 years), with each state receiving an average of $200 million annually (Daynard *et al.* 2001).

In addition, the Master Settlement commits the states to reduce underage tobacco use, prohibits gifts, credits, and coupons based on proof of purchase without documentation that the purchaser is adult, restricts free samples of cigarettes to adult only facilities, limits advertising by prohibiting cartoons and requiring removal of billboards, transit advertising, and other outdoor advertising, and bans four types of sponsorship (concerts, events of which the intended audience is a significant percentage of youth, events with paid youth participants, and certain athletic events). Moreover, the Master Settlement requires the industry to dissolve the Council for Tobacco Research—USA and the Tobacco Institute, although manufacturers may create new trade associations. Most importantly, the industry is required to fund a foundation to provide tobacco-control programs and undertake other activities to reduce tobacco use. The foundation is the American Legacy Foundation.

Although these provisions may seem at first blush to restrict some of the most egregious marketing and promotion policies of the industry, analysts are critical of the limitations and loopholes in the Settlement (Daynard *et al.* 2001). For example, no requirement is imposed on the states to spend their share of the settlement on prevention of smoking. In fact, the General Accounting Office, the investigative arm of Congress, found that only 7% of the settlement money was being used for new or expanded tobacco control programs, and many of the states were using all the funds for non-health related purposes (Janofsy 2001). The definitions of 'underage' and 'adult' are uncertain. No ban is imposed on self-service displays or sales through vending machines. The restriction on lobbying is limited to only certain issues.

Despite the weaknesses of the Master Settlement, the litigation of the State Attorneys General was important in shining a spotlight on the fraudulent, pernicious actions of the industry. The media's reporting of the litigation was a powerful public health lesson. The Master Settlement and the settlements of the four states led the tobacco companies to provide some compensation for the vast harm they had caused. Finally, the Master Settlement brought about some small changes in industry practices that advocates had long sought through legislation. As Daynard and his colleagues stated, 'tobacco litigation remains an important public health tool' (Daynard *et al.* 2001, p. 1970).

Legislation of the 1990s and beyond

In addition to litigation, other forces have contributed to the accelerated development of strong, comprehensive legislation. Most important has been the work of nongovernmental organizations in planning, supporting, and assisting the passage of legislation. The value of their work cannot be overestimated. They have provided insights from their research and experience. They have trained advocates and provided funding, and reached into communities to take public opinion polls on tobacco control, to rally support for legislation, and to assist in the implementation of legislation.

A wealth of research and reports has emerged from investigations worldwide. These reports have provided new insights and information that have become the scientific basis for legislative advocacy and programs of tobacco control. Dissemination of these findings has empowered countries at the national and subnational levels of government to seek and enact strong tobacco-control legislation. For example, in 1993 the report of the U.S. Environmental Protection Agency provided conclusive evidence of the danger of secondhand smoke. Tobacco was found to be a risk not only to smokers but to non-smokers, including spouses and children. The EPA concluded that

> ETS is a Group A human carcinogen, the EPA classification 'used only when there is sufficient evidence from epidemiologic studies to support a causal association between exposure to the agents and cancer' (US Environmental Protection Agency 1993, p. 170).

Another study by Harvard researchers found that secondhand smoke is not only a risk for cancer but it doubles the risk of heart disease (Grady 1977). These definitive studies have provided the most powerful evidence for the enactment of legislation banning smoking in public places and workplaces (Bayer and Colgrove 2002).

Much of this research has been presented at the eleven world conferences on tobacco or health that have mobilized and energized thousands of tobacco-control advocates from developed and developing countries. The papers presented at these conferences have served to inform and inspire activities all over the world. The resolutions adopted at these conferences have opened the way for new initiatives in the struggle to change the social culture from acceptance of tobacco to the goal of a smoke-free world.

The most important force impelling legislation has been the leadership of tobacco-control advocates. Some are governmental officials who see the benefits in human and economic terms of controlling the epidemic. Some are expert consultants who come for a time from other countries to share their knowledge and expertise, such as Judith Mackay of the Asian Consultancy on Tobacco or Health who has assisted many Asian countries and Dr Kjell Bjartveit of Norway, who provided expert testimony on the Canadian legislation. Key leaders are the in-country advocates, working day in and day out, who have become experts on the substantive issues in tobacco control and on the process of transforming their knowledge into effective legislation.

Challenges ahead

The success stories recounted in the experiences of Canada, Thailand, Poland, and South Africa are by no means universal. In many countries, the legislation to control the tobacco epidemic remains limited, weak, or not enforced. Even in a sphere in which legislation is common, such as restrictions on smoking in public places, the legislation is not commensurate with the enormous risk of cancer and heart disease from second-hand smoke. The statutes often list only a limited number of public places where smoking is banned or do not cover workplaces, where workers spend much more time than in a public building, or may not be enforced. The challenge is to make the policy fit the science.

Enforcement is a serious problem with various types of tobacco-control legislation. For example, in low-income countries, where children are selling individual cigarettes on the street, it is so difficult to enforce a ban on sales to minors that some tobacco-control experts in these countries advise deferring legislation on sales to minors until other laws, such as tax increases, have been enacted and implemented. The challenge is to put the same political will behind enforcement as is used in the process of enacting legislation.

Many countries face the need to strengthen legislation enacted before all the evidence was available on the magnitude of the danger from the industry's ruthless promotion of its product, before the addictiveness of tobacco was widely known, before effective strategies for combating the epidemic had been developed. For example, many countries still use the weak, hackneyed warning, 'tobacco is dangerous to your health' and have failed thus far to follow the examples of Canada, Sweden, Norway, Ireland,

Brazil, and other countries in requiring powerful, rotating, large, vivid warnings with pictures.

Another challenge is to equip tobacco-control advocates to combat the opposition of the tobacco companies to restrictive legislation. For example, one resort of the industry in the United States has been to seek limited laws at a state level preempting strong local ordinances, especially with respect to clean indoor air restrictions (Jacobson and Zapawa 2001, pp. 221–3). Thus, the less comprehensive state law prevents more stringent local restrictions.

The ultimate, basic challenge is to change the social culture in every country of the world to one that rejects tobacco as an addictive, lethal drug and that welcomes a tobacco-free society as the social norm.

Fortunately, WHO has taken a giant step towards this goal by its adoption of its first international convention. In May 2003, the World Health Assembly adopted by consensus the WHO Framework Convention on Tobacco Control (WHA.49.17). The FCTC is a binding treaty that commits its signatories in general terms to comprehensive tobacco control. It will be associated with or followed by protocols on specific topics that countries will adopt as they are ready for policy and action on that particular phase of tobacco control. The aspects of tobacco control covered by the treaty include the following.

- Prices. Harmonization of taxes on tobacco products at the international level in order to avoid excessive price differences among neighboring countries.

- Smuggling. Regulation of international transport of cigarettes to prevent a third of annual global exports becoming contraband, as at present.

- Tax-free tobacco products. Ending duty-free tobacco, which makes cigarettes available cheaply.

- Advertising and sponsorship. A worldwide ban on all tobacco advertising will prevent tobacco advertising in imported magazines and during broadcasting of national and international events.

- The Internet. End advertising on and trade in tobacco on the internet, which will affect all countries worldwide.

- Test methods. Base test procedures for the contents of tobacco products on internationally accepted methods. Require public disclosure of the toxic contents in tobacco and regulate the contents and emissions of tobacco.

- Package design and labeling. Agree on package design at the international level to improve trade relations and promote public health.

- Agriculture. Cease subsidies for tobacco production, which distort markets and encourage consumption in low-income countries through dumping of cheap tobacco.

- Information sharing. Agree on standardized approaches to information to facilitate global monitoring of the tobacco epidemic and evaluation of policies to control it (Joossens 1999, p. 11).

At the end of 2003, 83 countries have signed and five countries have ratified the WHO Framework Convention on Tobacco Control (ratification by 40 countries is required for the treaty to take effect). The support of country after country for the Framework Convention and its protocols will encourage other countries to enact or strengthen their tobacco control legislation and thus be part of the global movement for a tobacco free world.

References

Bayer, R. and Colgrove, J. (2002). Science, politics, and ideology in the campaign against environmental tobacco smoke. *American Journal of Public Health*, **92**(6), 949–54.

Blanke D. Douglas. (2003). *Tobacco control legislation, an introductory guide: Tools for Advancing Tobacco Control in the 21st Century.* Geneva: World Health Organization.

Bloch, M., Daynard R., and Roemer, R. (1998). A year of living dangerously: the tobacco control community meets the global settlement. *Public Health Reports*, November/December, **113**, 489–1607.

Chitanondh, Hatai (2000). The passage of tobacco control laws: Thai Davids versus transnational tobacco Goliaths. Bangkok: Thailand Health Promotion Institute, the National Health Foundation.

Council of Europe Consultative Assembly (1973). Recommendation 716 on the control of tobacco and alcohol advertising and on measures to curb consumption of these products.

Council of the European Communities and the Ministers of Health of the Member States on smoking in enclosed premises open to the public; 18 July 1989.

Council of the European Communities and the representatives of the governments of the Member States (1986). Resolution on a programme of action of the European Communities against cancer.

Cunningham, R. (1996). *Smoke and mirrors: the Canadian tobacco war.* Ottawa: International Development Research Centre.

Daynard, Richard A. (1993). *Judicial action for tobacco control.* In Roemer, R. Legislative action to combat the world tobacco epidemic. Geneva: World Health Organization, pp. 137–48.

Daynard, R. A., Parmet, W., Kelder, G., and Davidson, P. (2001). Implications for tobacco control of the multistage tobacco settlement. *American Journal of Public Health*, **91**(12), 1967–71.

Doll, R. and Hill, A. B. (1950). Smoking and carcinoma of the lung. *British Medical J*, **2**, 729–48.

Doll, R. and Hill, A. B. (1964). Mortality in relation to smoking: ten years' observations of British doctors. *British Medical J*, **1**, 1399–1410.

Federal Republic of Germany v. European Parliament and Council of the European Union, Case C375/87, October 5, 2000.

Finland Advisory Committee on Health Education (1985). An evaluation of the effects of an increase in the price of tobacco and a proposal for the tobacco price policy in Finland 1985–87. Helsinki; National Board of Health.

Glantz, S. A., Slade, J., Bero, L. A., Hanauer, P., and Barnes, D. E. (1996). *The Cigarette Papers.* California University Press, Berkeley, CA.

Grady, D. (1997). *Study finds secondhand smoke doubles risk of heart disease.* New York Times, May 20, pp. 1, A10.

Jacobson, P. D. and Zapawa, L. M. (2001). Clean indoor air restrictions: progress and promise. In: Rabin, R.L., Sugarman, S.D., *Regulating Tobacco.* Oxford University Press, New York, pp. 207–44.

Janofsky, M. (2001). *Little of settlement money is spent on tobacco control.* New York Times, August 11, p. A9.

Jha, P. and Chaloupka, F., editors. (2000). *Tobacco Control in Developing Countries*. Oxford University Press, Oxford.

Joossens, L. (1999). *Improving Public Health Through an International Framework Convention*. In Framework convention on tobacco control, technical briefing series, Paper 2, WHO/NCD/TFI/99.2. Geneva: Tobacco Free Initiative, World Health Organization.

Kluger, R. (1996). Ashes to ashes: America's hundred year cigarette war, the public health and the unabashed triumph of Philip Morris. Alfred A. Knopf, New York.

Marleau, D. (1995). *Tobacco control: a blueprint to protect the health of Canadians*. Health Canada, Ottawa.

Ministerial Advisory Council on Tobacco Control. Putting an end to deception: Proceedings of the International Expert Panel on Cigarette Descriptors. A report to the Canadian Minister of Health. Ottawa: Canadian Council for Tobacco Control; January 2002.

Nordic Council of Ministers. Recommendation Number 12. Helsingfors; 22 February 1972.

Pearl, R. (1938). Tobacco smoking and longevity. *Science*, **87**, 216–17.

Reto, R., *et al.* (1994). *Mortality from smoking in developed countries 1950–2000: Indirect estimates from national vital statistics*. New York, Oxford University Press.

Rabin, R. L. (2001). The third wave of tobacco tort litigation. In Rabin, R.L., Sugarman, S.D., eds. *Regulating tobacco*. Oxford University Press, New York.

Roemer, R. (1993). *Legislative action to combat the world tobacco epidemic, 2nd edition*. World Health Organization, Geneva.

Rosen, G. A. (1958). *A History of Public Health*. MD Publications, New York, p. 17.

Royal College of Physicians of London. (1962). *Smoking and health*. Summary report of the Royal College of Physicians of London on smoking in relation to cancer of the lung and other diseases. Pitman Medical Publishers, London.

Salooje, G. (2001) *The tobacco products act of South Africa, 1993, 1999*. Presentations to conference of cancer associations (2001) and to WHO Meeting for the Development of Tool-Kits for Tobacco Legislation and Economic Interventions, Geneva, 31 March 2000.

Tobacco on Trial. Environmental Tobacco Smoke Special Issue, November 1997. Northeastern University, School of Law, 400 Huntington Avenue, Boston, MA.

US Environmental Protection Agency. Respiratory health effects of passive smoking; lung cancer and other disorders. The report of the U.S. Environmental Protection Agency, U.S. Department of Health and Human Services. Public Health Service, National Institute of Health, NIH Publication No. 93-3605; August 1993.

U.S. Public Health Service (1964). *Smoking and health: report of the Advisory Committee to the Surgeon General of the Public Health Service*. Washington, DC: U.S. Department of Health, Education, and Welfare (PHS Publication No. 1103).

Warner, K. E. (1979). Clearing the airwaves: the cigarette ad ban revisited. *Policy Analysis Fall*, **5**(4), 435–49.

World Health Organization (1983). *Smoking control strategies in developing countries: report of a WHO Expert Committee*. Geneva: WHO Technical Report Series, No. 678.

World Health Organization (1997). *Tobacco or health: a global status report*. Geneva: World Health Organization.

Wynder, E. L. and Graham, E. A. (1950). Tobacco smoking as a possible etiological factor in bronchiogenic carcinoma. *JAMA*, **143**, 329–35.

Zatonski, W. (2001). *Case Study of Poland's experience in tobacco control*. Warsaw: Department of Cancer Epidemiology and Prevention, the Maria Skloclowska – Curie Memorial Cancer Center and Institute of Oncology and WHO Collaborating Centre (processed).

Chapter 40

Roles of tobacco litigation in societal change

Richard A. Daynard

Litigation plays at least six different roles in tobacco control. First, the most common and least dramatic role is ordinary enforcement of tobacco-control laws. Laws frequently ban sales to minors, smoking in public places, and certain types of advertising. The governments that impose these laws have the burden of enforcing them, which may involve litigation against violators. Second, too frequently governments enforce tobacco-control laws sporadically or not at all, creating the opportunity for NGOs either to bring law enforcement actions directly, or to sue their governments to force them to do their job, depending on whether courts will permit NGOs to take such actions. Third, tobacco companies increasingly use litigation to thwart effective tobacco control legislation and programs, typically arguing that constitutional provisions or other controlling law preempts such measures. Fourth, lawsuits and administrative proceedings have been brought by smoke-sensitive individuals against employers and places of public accommodation, seeking protection from secondhand smoke or compensation for illnesses caused or exacerbated by exposure to secondhand smoke. Fifth, many lawsuits have been brought by individuals, groups or classes of individuals, and third-party health care payers against the tobacco companies, seeking compensation for tobacco-caused illness, death, and/or out-of-pocket economic costs. Sixth, governments occasionally attempt to enforce general laws (e.g. against racketeering) against tobacco companies, alleging that deceptive and illegal practices by the industry have harmed the general public. Unlike ordinary law enforcement, these cases seek court orders requiring fundamental changes in the way these companies do business.

Each of these roles has implications for social change. Each will be discussed in turn, with the most attention devoted to the cases against the tobacco industry. We will then look at the role that legislation can play in encouraging or discouraging tobacco litigation. We will conclude with a brief discussion of how tobacco control would have been different in the twentieth century in the absence of litigation, and how litigation may affect the course and success of tobacco control in the twenty-first century.

Law enforcement

While many tobacco-control objectives can be achieved through legislation, legislation is effective only to the extent that it is enforced. This is a major issue because many legislative initiatives seek to change customary social behavior such as selling to minors and smoking in public places, while the tobacco industry has strong motivation and little compunction about evading legislative restrictions such as advertising bans and counter-smuggling measures on its own behavior. Both public education and active enforcement are often necessary if these laws are not to be 'dead letters'.

Enforcement can be accomplished through administrative measures (e.g. license suspensions or revocations) or through criminal or quasi-criminal (e.g. traffic summons-type procedures, civil fines) processes. Most enforcement activity does not involve extensive litigation, because the facts are usually easy for the authorities to establish, and the level of sanctions typically low enough that it is not worthwhile for the wrongdoer to fight the charges in court. The principal exceptions are where the defendant, often supported by the tobacco industry, refuses to comply in order to force a legal challenge to the validity of the tobacco- control legislation (discussed below in Section 'Industry counter-attacks'), or in smuggling and tax-avoidance cases where the penalties sought may be very large.

Litigation by NGOs to compel enforcement

Many tobacco-control laws and regulations are rarely if ever formally enforced. Occasionally this is a good sign, as with laws restricting smoking in public places in the United States that are informally but effectively enforced through social pressure. However, where public support has not been mobilized behind the policy underlying the law, the failure of public authorities to enforce the law results in its being flouted by anyone who has incentive to do so. This characterized, for example, the status of sales-to-minors bans in the United States until the 1990s, restrictions on smoking in Parisian restaurants and San Francisco bars around the year 2000, and bans on advertising in many countries since their adoption.

In the United States the doctrine of 'prosecutorial discretion' prevents private parties from forcing government action, but state consumer protection laws frequently allow parties to act as 'private attorneys general' in the public interest to require product manufacturers or sellers to obey the law. In Massachusetts, for example, a 1987 lawsuit brought by the Group Against Smoking Pollution of Massachusetts against Store 24, a local convenience store chain, alleging that they had sold cigarettes repeatedly to teenagers in violation of state law, resulted in Store 24 agreeing to demand positive identification from young people before selling them cigarettes as well as monitoring their own stores for compliance with the new policy. This was the first time that such a 'carding' requirement was imposed anywhere in the United States, and set a model for subsequent regulations. A similar approach was used in Bangladesh and in Mali, where

NGOs obtained sanctions against tobacco firms that were engaged in illegal promotion and advertising (Rendezvous with Mahamane Cisse 2000).

Some legal systems do permit NGOs to bring 'public interest' actions to require the government to enforce the law, including relevant constitutional provisions. The 1999 pioneering case in the Indian state of Kerala produced a judicial order applying the constitutional right to health protection by requiring the police to enforce a ban on smoking in public places. This was followed by a similar ruling by the Indian Supreme Court in November 2001, which led to action by governmental bodies throughout India banning smoking in public places (Murli *et al.* 2001). Another case in Uganda produced a settlement with the government to the same effect (The Environmental Action Network, Ltd. *et al.* 2000).

Industry counter-attacks

While the tobacco industry became increasingly litigious in the course of the 1990s, it threatened more litigation than it brought. It would typically send its lawyers to meetings of local legislative bodies that were considering strong tobacco-control measures. They would 'inform' the lawmakers that the measures they were considering were beyond their jurisdiction; were unconstitutional; and/or were 'preempted' by higher state or federal law that were expressly or implicitly inconsistent with the proposed regulations, or else that simply 'occupied the regulatory field,' leaving no room for local regulation. Sometimes the lawmakers would back down and pass ineffective measures instead. Often, they would go ahead with the strong measures, and the threatened lawsuits did not materialize. Occasionally the industry (typically acting through local stores, restaurants, or bars, whose legal bills they would cover) would actually file suit to restrain the enforcement of the measures: these cases came out both ways, typically depending on nuances of the local and state laws involved, as well as the disposition of the deciding judge.

The industry did score some high-level judicial victories that set back important tobacco control initiatives. In 1995 the Canadian Supreme Court invalidated Canada's cigarette advertising restrictions as a free-speech violation, reasoning that the government had not shown these restrictions to be necessary or effective as a public health measure (MacDonald 1995). The government later adopted even more sweeping restrictions on the industry's marketing behavior: a trial in Montreal in 2002 and subsequent appeals will test whether the evidence the government has gathered in support of its new law will assuage the Court's concerns. Similarly, a 2000 decision by the European Court of Justice invalidated a European Union (EU) advertising ban on the ground that it was not adopted through the appropriate EU processes. As with Canada, the European Commission has tried again, and the validity of their renewed efforts will again be tested through litigation brought by the industry.

In the United States, two major Supreme Court decisions based on legal challenges from the tobacco industry may have produced more lasting damage. In a 2000 decision, the Court invalidated FDA jurisdiction over tobacco products, reasoning that had Congress intended the agency to have such jurisdiction, it would have said so explicitly. While in principle this simply leaves it to Congress to establish FDA jurisdiction, as a practical political matter Congress has never taken affirmative action to effectively regulate the tobacco industry, and is not likely to do so in the foreseeable future. As a result, there is no central regulatory authority in the U.S. over cigarette design, packaging, or marketing. The second decision, in 2001, cut off state efforts to fill the void in marketing regulation. Massachusetts had attempted to prohibit outdoor tobacco advertising within 1000 feet of schools and playgrounds. Several cities had adopted similar regulations, which had been upheld by lower courts in the face of tobacco industry challenges. The Supreme Court ruled, however, that the state restrictions were preempted by federal law, and were in any event unconstitutionally violative of the free speech rights of tobacco marketers. Unlike the similar 1995 Canadian Supreme Court decision, it is not clear if any possible evidentiary showing by states could lead the U.S. Supreme Court to relent and permit effective advertising restrictions (Daynard in press).

The tobacco industry also uses litigation and the threat of litigation to harass and discourage tobacco control researchers and activists. The authors of 1991 articles exposing 'Joe Camel's' appeal to young children were required to hand their drafts and research materials over to the tobacco companies as 'discovery' in cases not involving the authors in which these articles were cited, or under state 'freedom of information' acts. Similar orders were issued to authors of landmark studies of the synergy between asbestos and tobacco exposure, and of the adverse effects of secondhand smoke exposure (Sweda and Daynard 1996). The industry has also used the freedom of information acts to harass state and local tobacco control programs, requiring them to produce voluminous materials for copying by industry lawyers (Aguinaga and Glantz 1995). Defamation actions were filed against advocates and NGOs in several countries including the Netherlands, Sweden, and Switzerland. These actions usually resulted in vindication for the tobacco control supporters, but not until their energies were absorbed for many months in defending the cases, and they had been subjected to 'a good scare.'

Secondhand smoke cases

Two types of cases exert pressure to change social norms in the direction of protecting nonsmokers from exposure to secondhand smoke. Some cases, such as those brought under laws protecting disabled individuals, seek judicial orders requiring particular employers or proprietors of places of public accommodation either to ban smoking outright, or at least to ensure that nonsmokers can avoid exposure to secondhand smoke. Other judicial or administrative proceedings, such as workers' compensation cases, achieve change indirectly by attaching a high price tag to neglecting to protect employees from secondhand smoke exposure.

In a 1980s case, a nonsmoking social worker, supported by an NGO, sued the Commonwealth of Massachusetts to require it to provide her with a safe, i.e. smoke-free working environment. A court ruled preliminarily that the common law right to a safe workplace would support injunctive relief: the state settled the case by providing nonsmoking workplaces to all its employees. Actions brought under the Americans with Disability Act, the Rehabilitation Act, and various state and federal regulations imposing similar obligations upon governmental bodies and regulated industries, have established that workers and patrons of public accommodations whose medical conditions require smoke-free environments are entitled to them, and have ordered employers and proprietors to change their rules accordingly. Other American decisions have conditioned custody orders in divorce cases upon the custodial spouse not smoking, and not permitting smoking, in places where the child is present (Edward 2001).

Cases seeking financial compensation from employers, whether for illness or disability caused by exposure to secondhand smoke or for lost wages as a result of needing to leave a smoky workplace (or both), are more numerous and widespread. Successful cases have been brought in Sweden, Britain, and Australia, as well as the U.S. Even a prior history of smoking has not disqualified claimants, so long as the secondhand smoke exposure was a substantial contributing cause of their illness or disability. In this area a few successful cases can have a broad-scale social impact. A 2001 Australian jury award of Aus$466 000 to a bartender who contracted throat cancer, combined with a handful of earlier less generous awards, led to a movement throughout Australia to ban smoking in restaurants, bars, and casinos. In Britain a few modest awards led the government to rethink occupational safety rules and mandate protections for non-smokers (Daynard *et al.* 2000). In the U.S. the fear of such awards has resulted in insurers, legal counsel for employers, and groups representing building owners and managers urging their insureds, clients, and members to eliminate indoor smoking.

A number of cases have required disability insurers and pension plans to cover employees who were forced to leave the workplace because smoke-related medical conditions. Others have required employers to pay back wages to employees who were fired for complaining about smoky working conditions or for refusing to work in these conditions. These have added to the impression among employers and their insurers and counsel that prudence requires a smoke-free workplace.

Lawsuits against tobacco companies seeking money damages

The power of the tobacco industry to block most forms of effective tobacco control legislation in the United States led advocates to seek other venues in which the industry could be held accountable and pressured to change its behavior. Money damage lawsuits at first seemed an odd strategic choice, since the connection with societal change was not obvious. Nonetheless, the Tobacco Products Liability Project began advocating for such lawsuits as a tobacco control strategy in 1984, and gradually persuaded the public health community of its merits (Daynard 1988).

Tobacco products liability suits offer at least six potential social benefits. First, since smoking causes over $100 billion in health care and lost income costs (and untold billions more in suffering by the victims and their families) each year in the U.S. alone, shifting any substantial fraction of this burden to the manufacturers through successful lawsuits would force them to raise prices dramatically. Since the demand for cigarettes is somewhat price-elastic, especially among children and teenagers, increased prices would result in reduced consumption, especially among youth. This is precisely what has happened as a result of the settlements in 1997 and 1998 of lawsuits against the industry brought by state attorneys general seeking reimbursement of state-borne tobacco-caused health-care expenditures. Consumption among 12ths grade students in the United States since 1996 has declined by more than one third (Fountain 2001).

Second, the publicity from these lawsuits would dramatize for the public the fact that smoking injures and kills real people, not just statistics. This has been enhanced by the industry's public relations response to these cases—that anyone so heedless as to smoke cigarettes after the Surgeon General warned of the dangers has only himself or herself to blame for whatever grave illness ensues. This response has until recently been quite effective for the industry in discouraging adverse jury verdicts, but it severely undercuts their marketing campaign to confuse and distract smokers and potential smokers from thinking about the deadly consequences of using their products.

Third, fear of such lawsuits, and especially of large punitive damage awards, might motivate tobacco executives to change the way they do business. Indeed, the threat of punitive damages is now very real, with a $145 billion punitive damage verdict in a class action in Florida, and a $3 billion verdict (later reduced to $100 million) in an individual California case. Concern about product liability awards is frequently cited by manufacturers of other products as reasons for including graphic warnings, altering product designs, or even withholding particularly dangerous products from the market. In the case of cigarette manufacturers, such concern might lead them to stop denying that smoking causes addiction, disease, and death, or stop targeting their marketing efforts at young people, or perfect and implement cigarette designs that would be somewhat less deadly. Although tobacco liability suits began in 1954, it was not until such cases started winning in 1996 that the industry's behavior began to change. The 'voluntary' changes to date have been modest and mostly cosmetic, but movement is finally perceptible. The companies no longer deny the connections between smoking and various diseases, and actually admit the connection on their websites; but they do nothing else to publicize these connections, and continue to vigorously deny the relationships between secondhand smoke exposure and disease. They have refocused their marketing target from children and teenagers to college-age young adults. They have also actively embarked on research and development of less toxic cigarettes.

Fourth, the 'discovery' process, which permits parties in lawsuits to demand copies of relevant internal documents from opposing parties and even nonparties, has unearthed millions of pages of industry documents, many of which are quite incriminating. In particular, they demonstrate that the companies knew since the 1950s that smoking caused cancer and other diseases, yet continued to pretend the contrary, actively suppressing or refuting reports that they believed to be true (Glantz *et al.* 1996). Since these documents became available in the mid-1990s largely as a result of aggressive discovery by the lawyers for the State of Minnesota's case against the industry (as well as the heroic, if illegal, removal and dissemination of documents by a tobacco company paralegal named Merrell Williams), they have been instrumental in persuading juries to focus on the misdeeds of the industry rather than the weakness-of-will of the smokers. Equally important, their wide availability on the Internet and in public depositories and publication in numerous media stories has helped make the industry a political pariah, making antitobacco legislation possible in many states. Nor has the effect been limited to the United States: major document-based studies of industry misbehavior in Britain, the Middle East, and with respect to the World Health Organization, among others, has increased the determination and effectiveness of tobacco control advocates throughout the world (Zeltner *et al.* 2000).

Fifth, the money from verdicts and settlements can be used to reimburse individuals and third-party health-care payers for injuries and expenses caused by the tobacco industry and its products. Some money from the states' settlements of their Medicaid reimbursement cases is being devoted to tobacco-control activities. Although this represents only a small percentage of the approximately $10 billion per year that the states are receiving from the industry, it has nonetheless greatly increased the total amounts that the states are spending for tobacco control. An additional $1.5 billion resulting from the 1998 'Master Settlement Agreement' between 46 states and the industry has gone to the American Legacy Foundation which funds tobacco-control activities on the national level.

Sixth, the fact that, at least in the United States, cigarettes annually produce far more financial harm than revenue creates the ongoing possibility that a flood of individual cases or class actions will bankrupt the industry. While the consequences of bankruptcy are somewhat unpredictable, it is likely that a bankruptcy court would not permit the companies to continue selling cigarettes as part of a reorganization plan if the new cigarettes were likely to create as much liability as the ones that sent the companies into bankruptcy. This would create an important opening for public health organizations, which could advise the court of changes in cigarette design and marketing necessary to reduce the potential for future liability (Mark and Daynard 2002).

While the most cases continue to be brought by individuals, since 1994 both class actions and third-party reimbursement cases have also been filed. Class actions permit a large number of similarly situated individuals to be represented by a few named plaintiffs: any legal judgment on the common issues rendered in the case applies equally to the named and unnamed class members. The only tobacco class action settled in the twentieth century was on behalf of a nationwide class of flight attendants who had been exposed on the job to secondhand smoke. The settlement provided $300 million for a foundation to fund medical research on smoke-related illnesses, and eased the legal burden for flight attendants to seek individual damages (Master Settlement Agreement 1988). Another case, on behalf of Florida smokers who contracted tobacco-caused diseases, produced three landmark jury verdicts: the first found that smoking caused 20 diseases, and held the industry liable on a number of grounds, including conspiracy to defraud their customers and to fraudulently conceal health information (Engle and Reynolds Tobacco Co. 1999); the second awarded an average of $4 million in compensatory damages to each of three named smokers; the third awarded the class $145 billion in punitive damages. As of 2002, the appeals process was just beginning, and the process for awarding compensatory damages to the hundreds of thousands of unnamed class members was still in the future. While the tobacco industry had successfully discouraged most lawyers from bringing cases in the past by its scorched earth litigation tactics, these two class actions brought by the same husband-and-wife team (Stanley and Susan Rosenblatt) demonstrated that the industry could be defeated by talented, determined, but only modestly funded attorneys.

Other class actions have been brought seeking funds for monitoring the medical condition of smokers and former smokers, and seeking refunds of money spent by smokers who were induced to smoke 'low tar' cigarettes on the fraudulent representation that they were safer. One medical monitoring case was tried unsuccessfully, and another will be tried in 2002. Five 'low tar' consumer fraud cases have thus far been judicially certified for class action status in three states, with similar cases pending elsewhere.

Third party reimbursement cases are predicated on the fact that the tobacco industry knows that most smoking-induced medical costs are not paid by the smokers themselves. Since the companies know that they cause financial injury to third parties (states, health insurers, etc.), they should be liable for the costs that flow from the design of their products and their deceptive conduct. Litigation pioneered by Mississippi and Minnesota, and later brought by most other U.S. states as well, resulted in mostly-favorable judicial decisions and the resulting multi-billion dollar settlements already mentioned. Unfortunately, American courts have almost uniformly rejected all subsequent cases brought on the same theory, ruling that the third party's financial injuries were too 'indirect', and distinguishing the opposite decisions in the state cases on unconvincing (but nonetheless authoritative) grounds. Thus, private health insurers, union health and welfare funds, foreign governments, and even the U.S. federal government, have all had their reimbursement claims rejected.

The tobacco industry has not always been content to take its chances in court. In the United States the industry has been a prime—but usually hidden—sponsor of 'tort reform' efforts, which seek enactment of state or federal laws changing the legal principles applied by the court so as to make lawsuits against the industry more difficult or even impossible. Such a statute prevented tobacco litigation in California for 10 years, until it was repealed in 1998. The industry also supports procedural changes with similar effects, such as: (1) laws providing only a modicum of regulation, while 'preempting' claims that could otherwise be brought against the industry; (2) proposed federal legislation that would remove class actions against them from state courts, where they have sometimes been successful, to federal courts where they are quickly dismissed; (3) proposed state legislation to prevent public airing of documents obtained in discovery; (4) proposed bans on the use of class actions or punitive damages in litigation against the industry; and (5) state or federal laws limiting attorneys fees in tobacco litigation so as to discourage competent practitioners from taking these cases.

On the other hand, laws facilitating the state lawsuits against the industry were passed in Florida, Massachusetts, and Maryland in the mid-1990s. The proposed Framework Convention on Tobacco Control may also have provisions on liability and compensation that would make lawsuits against the industry viable in most countries.

Enforcement of laws prohibiting deceptive conduct

Tobacco companies, like all other legal entities, are subject to general restrictions against obtaining money dishonestly. In the state context these generally include laws outlawing 'unfair or deceptive acts or practices in commerce.' State attorneys general, and often private litigants as well, may bring lawsuits to enjoin tobacco companies from continuing to engage in such behavior. Indeed, the state lawsuits, though they principally sought money damages for Medicaid reimbursement, almost all sought injunctive relief under these state consumer protection acts. In response to these claims, the resulting settlements, including the November 1998 Master Settlement Agreement, contained several provisions restricting various tobacco industry marketing techniques. These included bans on outdoor advertising and the distribution of merchandise that advertised tobacco products, as well as limitations on sponsorship of concerts and other public events (Daynard *et al.* 2001). Similarly, the class actions addressing 'low tar' cigarettes seek, in addition to refunds, injunctions against the companies' continuing the deceptive practice of labeling cigarettes 'low tar' when they are no less dangerous than 'regular' cigarettes.

Federal law has an even more powerful instrument against businesses like the tobacco companies whose success depends on deceiving their customers. The Racketeer-Influenced and Corrupt Organizations Act (RICO) allows the United States Department of Justice to seek judicial orders fundamentally changing the way the industry does business, as well as disgorgement of all 'ill-gotten gains.' Expert reports filed in 2001 in a case brought by the Department of Justice against the tobacco industry indicate that such ill-gotten gains amount to more than $200 billion, and by some calculations almost $1 trillion. Private RICO actions are also available to compensate for economic losses but not illness or death.

Furthermore the discovery, mostly through documents uncovered in the Minnesota litigation, of the industry's deep involvement in smuggling cigarettes to many countries was, at century's end, leading to an exploration by lawyers working for European, Canadian, and Latin American governments of possible avenues of judicial redress for the billions of dollars of lost tax revenues.

Conclusion

The twentieth century ended with most types of tobacco litigation on the upswing. Some already had a major impact on tobacco control. The Canadian and American Supreme Court decisions invalidating tobacco advertising restrictions and FDA jurisdiction over tobacco products halted important tobacco-control efforts that had been well underway. On the other hand, the state lawsuits against the industry made public millions of pages of internal industry documents, many quite damning, thereby feeding tobacco-control efforts around the globe. The settlements of these cases led to dramatic price increases, greatly reducing youth consumption; some of the settlement payments supported aggressive new state and national tobacco-control campaigns; and the agreed-upon advertising and marketing restrictions at least put a crimp on the industry's preferred techniques for maintaining and expanding their markets.

Litigation in the twenty-first century is likely to spread world-wide, raising consciousness of the dangers of tobacco use and of exposure to tobacco smoke, and of the nefarious role played by cigarette manufacturers, even in countries where tobacco use and marketing is currently uncontroversial. Litigation will be increasingly used by NGOs to force governments and tobacco companies to take existing laws seriously, and to obtain judicial orders making public places smoke-free. NGOs and health departments will become increasing adept at drafting laws that can withstand industry legal attacks, and defending them when these attacks arrive. Countries other than the United States will begin holding tobacco companies responsible for the health care costs attributable to their products and conduct. As a result, prices will increase, consumption will decline, and some of the damages paid will fund tobacco-control programs. Some tobacco companies will probably find their way into bankruptcy court, giving public health authorities and NGOs new opportunities to shape how tobacco products get manufactured and marketed. Finally, more vigorous efforts can be expected to require tobacco manufacturers and their executives to avoid illegal conduct, and a wide range of legal sanctions, civil and criminal, can be anticipated.

References

Aguinaga, S. and Glantz, S. A. (1995). The use of public records acts to interfere with tobacco control. *Tob Control*, **4**, 222–30.

Daynard, R. A. (1995). Resisting tobacco industry abuse of the legal process. *Tob Control*, **4**, 209.

Daynard, R. A., Bates, C., and Francey, N. (January 2000). Tobacco Litigation Worldwide, 320 *British Medical Journal* 111.

Daynard, R. A., Parmet, W., Kelder, G., and Davidson, P. (2001). Implications for tobacco control of the multistate tobacco settlement. *Amer J of Public Health*, **91**, 1967–81.

Daynard, R. A. (in press). Regulating tobacco or why we need a public health judicial decision-making Canon. *J. Law, Medicine and Ethics*.

Daynard, R. A. (1988). Tobacco liability litigation as a cancer control strategy. *J National Cancer Institute*, **80**, 9–13.

Engle v. R.J. Reynolds Tobacco Co., Verdict Form For Phase I, 14.3 Tobacco Products Litigation Reporter 2.101 (1999).

Glantz, S. A., Slade, J., Bero, L. A., *et al.* (2002). *The Cigarette Papers.* Berkeley, California: University of California Press, 1996; Hurt R and ??, JAMA; Ciresi M and Walburn R, ??, John Marshall L. Rev.; Special supplement I, *Tobacco Control*, 11.

Gottlieb, M. and Daynard, Richard A. (2002). Will Big Tobacco Seek Bankruptcy Protection? William and Mary Environmental Policy Review, No. 1.

John, W. Fountain, Study Finds Teenagers Smoking Less; Campaign Is Cited, New York Times, December 20, 2001, p. A24.

MacDonald, R. J. R. Inc. v Attorney General of Canada, 127 DLR 4th, 1 91 (1995).

Master Settlement Agreement, November 1998 (viewable at http://www.naag.org/tobac/cigmsa.rtf).

Murli, S. and Deora V. *Union of India et al.*, Supreme Court of India Writ Petition No. 316 of 1999, November 2, 2001.

'Rendezvous with Mahamane Cisse', August 10, 2000, http://www.tobacco.org/News/rendezvous/cisse.html; David Simpson, Bangladesh: voyage of disdain sunk without trace. *Tobacco Control*, **9**, 129–135;130.

The Environmental Action Network, Ltd. (2000). The Attorney General, *et al.* High Court at Kampala.

Sweda, E. L. and Daynard, R. A. (1996). Tobacco Industry Tactics. *Br. Med Bull*, **52**(1), 183–92.

Sweda Edward, L. Jr., Summary of Legal Cases Regarding Smoking in the Workplace and Other Places, 16.2 Tobacco Products Litigation Reporter 4.1–4.79 (2001).

Zeltner, T., *et al.* (2000). *Tobacco Industry Strategies to Undermine Tobacco Control Activities at the World Health Organization.* World Health Organization.

Chapter 41

Impact of smoke-free bans and restrictions

Ron Borland and Claire Davey

Introduction

This chapter reviews the progress that is being made in protecting people from exposure to tobacco smoke in their environments, and on the impact that these changes are having on tobacco use. In doing so we attempt to explain the reasons for apparent differences in progress in different countries, and make some predictions as to future trends.

Environmental tobacco smoke (ETS) is also known as passive smoking, involuntary smoking, or secondhand smoke. The terminology used varies, but all are intended to refer to pretty much the same thing, although subtle distinctions can usefully be made. It is easier to use ETS when referring to what is actually in the environment; passive smoking (or involuntary smoking) when referring to exposures of individuals; and secondhand smoke to what the smoker produces. Thus 'the secondhand smoke produced by smokers increases the level of environmental tobacco smoke which results in higher levels of passive smoking by those in that area'. In this context we use the term secondhand smoke to refer to both the smoke exhaled by smokers and the smoke coming directly from the cigarette into the environment. We also describe the smoke as coming from cigarettes but note that smoke from other forms of burnt tobacco is likely to be equivalently toxic, but as it is much less common in almost all countries, it is easier to simply refer to cigarettes.

Tobacco use has not always resulted in problems with passive smoking. Historically, in Victorian England after the introduction of tobacco from the Americas, smoking was initially an activity of the rich and they engaged in it in special smoking rooms to protect women and children from the odours. These niceties gradually disappeared until for much of the twentieth century smokers in most places came to assume a right to smoke virtually wherever and whenever they choose. Non-smokers put up with the smells which most found mildly unpleasant because to do otherwise would seem impolite.

Modern moves to reduce passive smoking have come in the light of strong evidence about the harmfulness of these exposures to health.

Health effects of ETS

Information about the damaging effects of ETS began to appear in the 1970s for children (e.g. Colley 1974) and for adults in the early 1980s (Hirayama 1981). In the mid-1980s a number of governmental reports and reviews, of which the US Surgeon-General's report was the most influential (U.S. Department of Health and Human Services 1986) had confirmed findings of the harmful effects of ETS for non-smokers. Subsequent reviews have confirmed and extended these conclusions (e.g. United States Environment Protection Agency 1992; California Environment Protection Agency 1997; Tobacco Free Initiative 1999).

The more serious adult conditions linked to passive smoking include chronic respiratory symptoms, lung cancer, cardiovascular disease (CHD), and disorders of the nose and sinus (Benninger 1999; Wiebel 1997). Infants, children, and those with chronic conditions such as respiratory disorders are more susceptible to harm from ETS exposure than adults (Davis 1998). Adverse effects of passive smoking on children, include a causal role in respiratory diseases such as bronchitis, pneumonia, asthma (as well as triggering bouts), and reduced lung function, plus increases in middle ear infections and SIDS. ETS has also been causally linked to lower birth weight. There is also evidence of harmed neural development *in utero* (Samet 1999).

Immediate reactions to ETS include sore eyes, itching, sneezing, coughs, and wheezing. The financial cost of treating coughs, phlegm, and wheeze in children exposed to ETS is estimated to be 14% higher in homes with one smoker and 25% higher in homes with two smokers compared to children not exposed to ETS (Peters *et al.* 1998).

Voluminous evidence now attest to the adverse health effects of ETS on non-smokers, with both long term and immediate health effects constituting a clear threat to public health. Further, it is likely that passive smoking adds to the risks of active smoking in smokers. However, the nature of the dose–response relationship is less well documented. Studies showing adverse effects of ETS exposure have used crude exposure measures, such as spouse smoking and rarely have there been more than two categories of exposure (e.g. for children's exposure: neither, one, or both parents smoking). Extrapolating from the active smoking literature where dose–response effects are clearly present and detectable at low exposures, plus the reality that ETS exposures are almost always lower than active smoking exposures, it is reasonable to assume that there is no safe level of exposure. For many conditions, chronic exposure seems to be critical; however, there are conditions, which can be triggered or exacerbated by acute exposure such as asthma attacks and problems for those with major respiratory problems like cystic fibrosis. That said, from what we know the bulk of the serious harm comes from prolonged (chronic) exposure, so this should be the focus of public policy and public education.

The magnitude of the adverse health consequences caused by passive smoking while comparable to other environmental toxins are small compared with those associated with active smoking. The strong societal responses to reduce passive smoking summarized in this chapter, is evidence that society is prepared to take stronger measures against risks imposed on others than risks taken on by the individual. This is so even in the case with smoking, even though the risk of active smoking is not purely voluntary, given the dependence–forming nature of tobacco use. One major aim of this chapter is to explore the impact of progress in controlling ETS on active smoking, as it is possible that such effects may contribute at least as much to population health as the reduction in disease caused by passive smoking. The other major aim is to describe the scope and the consequences of smoking restrictions and issues surrounding their implementation. In doing this we have tried to paint a representative picture of what is known rather than attempt a comprehensive review of all published literature.

Determinants of exposure to ETS

Passive smoking only occurs because there is active smoking. Potentially the most effective way of eliminating passive smoking would be to eliminate active smoking. While this is not practical, any programme of measures to reduce passive smoking should consider the potential impact on active smoking, and wherever possible use the measures to help reduce smoking overall.

People can be exposed to ETS anywhere that smoking occurs. Most adults spend about 90% of their time at work or home, thus most at risk of exposure to ETS are those who live or work with smokers. Homes are likely to be even more important for children. However, consideration of ETS should not be restricted to work and home, because some people spend considerable periods in other places, most notably recreational venues. If those places are smoky it can contribute significantly to overall exposures for people who spend extended time in them.

Exposure to ETS is a function of the amount of active smoking, how much time the person spends in the enclosed space, the size of the space, and the degree of ventilation. Proximity to the smoker(s) varies in importance for different components, being greater for exposure to the particulate than to those toxins in the gaseous phase. However, for most practical purposes it is reasonable to assume fairly even diffusion of smoke into any particular room.

While there continues to be active smoking, protecting non-smokers from passive smoking involves changing when and where smokers smoke. This involves encouraging the appropriate evolution of smoker behaviour in the context of non-smokers. This should include voluntarily not smoking around non-smokers, or in enclosed areas they frequent, and compliance with rules about when and where smoking is allowed.

Smokers in making a decision not to smoke in a particular situation are doing so in the context of a choice about alternative options about them smoking. The smoker may choose to forego completely or delay a cigarette that they would have liked to smoke or they may seek an alternative acceptable place to smoke it. Over time they may adopt some combination of the two. They may also choose to smoke, and/or forget the existence of the rule and smoke without any volitional intent of violating a ban. The potential benefits to non-smokers are a function of the extent to which smokers desist from smoking in situations where exposures of others are likely, and the effect on the smokers themselves will vary as a function of how it affects their total consumption.

The evidence is overwhelming that bans on smoking when complied with result in reduction in ETS exposures for those who spend time in those places. Research shows that the number of smokers in a household or hours exposed to ETS at work is significantly associated with metabolic nicotine (serum cotinine) (Davis 1998). Similarly, research shows that bans on workplace smoking can result in less reported ETS as well as lower continine levels in non-smokers (Heloma *et al.* 2001; Hopkins *et al.* 2001), and bans in homes can reduce exposures of children (Biener and Nyman 1999). Indeed, bans on smoking in bars in California have been shown to lead to improved respiratory health of bartenders (Eisner *et al.* 1998). The impact of smoking bans on ETS might be most dramatically shown in the skies. Measures of respirable particles before and after smoking bans were introduced on intercontinental flights reduced dramatically from a mean of 66 to $3\,\mu g/m^3$ (Wieslander *et al.* 2000).

Rates of exposure in different environments will vary both as a function of the prevalence of smoking and the nature and compliance with any restrictions. Estimates will also vary as a function of the measurement tool. This all means that in the absence of comparable measures for a broad range of countries, preferably with time trends, it is not particularly useful to report on the small number of published point estimates.

Home is where most people spend most of their time, but some of this time is spent sleeping. While smokers are sleeping they are not adding to ETS. However, where ventilation is poor, exposure can accumulate considerably during sleep due to smoke lingering. Where there are no regular smokers living in the home or the amount smoking in the home is low actual exposures may be less than in other venues.

Work is the other major source of potential high exposures if smoking is allowed and smoking prevalence among the workforce is significant. In industrialized countries over three quarter of workers work primarily in indoor settings (Chapman *et al.* 1999; MMWR 2000), and while percentages are likely to be lower in more agrarian societies, workplace exposure remains a potential hazard for those who work in enclosed spaces.

Exposure to ETS can also occur in other public places such as public transport, hospitals, cinemas and theatres, and shopping centres, indeed anywhere where smoking occurs. Apart from the issue of exposure to staff, exposures to patrons of recreational venues, is of some concern. The concern is primarily for those who are very susceptible to acute exposure, and for those who frequent such venues regularly. For others, the intermittent exposures are likely to be more nuisance value than significant risks to health. Regardless of the magnitude of the risks, it is both prudent and desirable to create contexts where the possibility of passive smoking is minimized.

What drives the introduction of, and compliance with, bans?

Under what conditions will there be action to reduce passive smoking? The answer to this question can best be answered by attempting to understand the diversity of responses to the problem both within and between jurisdictions. First of all, a necessary condition for action is awareness of the evidence of harm at levels that warrant action. The awareness could be at the level of the informed public or the general public, and may or may not include institutional acceptance of the risk. There is no doubt that authoritative government sponsored reviews can play a major role. For example, the Australian NHMRC (1987) led to immediate government administrative action to control smoking in government offices, but not to legislative moves to restrict smoking in other workplaces.

The likelihood of government action (where it has jurisdiction) will be a function of the nature of the proposed action and of the views of key stakeholders. In particular, it will be more difficult to enact rules where there is an expectation that it will compel behaviour change than where the rules are more symbolic.

Cultural expectations surrounding laws or policies appears to be a major factor influencing compliance. In some countries rules are put in place to announce a new aspiration or goal of policy makers. Any public education and/or moves to enforce compliance follows formal implementation. A major role for activists is to encourage compliance. By contrast other countries only impose laws when they believe that there is public support for high compliance, and in these cases public education precedes implementation and there are strong expectations about high compliance at the point of implementation and typically enforcement mechanisms to ensure this happens. French tobacco-control expert Gerard Dubois has observed that countries influenced by anglo-saxon legal traditions tend to follow the latter path, while much of the rest of the world, most notably those influenced by southern European traditions, favour the former. Thus in a country like France, a law restricting smoking in enclosed places was passed with a minimum of fuss because there was no real expectation that it would be enforced (at least in the short term), while in countries like the US, new laws are often strongly opposed by vested interests, because the expectation is that they will be enforced.

Compliance with smoke-free legislation and bans can likewise vary substantially between countries. In countries such as North America, Australasia, and northern Europe, changes to smoking regulations that have used a combination of legislation and efforts to modify public attitudes have generally decreased exposure to environment tobacco smoke. However, the existence of legislation in some countries has not had the same impact and this may reflect the variety of cultural and sociological factors alluded to above (Serra *et al.* 2000). Serra *et al.* concluded that the most effective interventions for preventing smoking in public places were those where the institutions concerned developed, resourced and supported comprehensive programmes to achieve compliance with their policy decisions to ban smoking.

Likelihood of legislative action is also likely to be determined by the views of stakeholders, of which the key ones are general community views, those of commercial interests, special interest groups, bureaucrats, and lastly of decision-makers themselves. Strong opposition at any level can be enough to prevent action, while strong support at least one level is probably necessary to stimulate action. The tobacco industry and its allies have a long record of vigorously opposing actions to increase restrictions on smoking, especially where they believe they will be enforced.

In countries, or eras when bans on smoking are not mandated by government the main factors driving increased restriction on smoking imposed by employers seems to be a mix of awareness of the risks (with associated concern for staff health), threat of litigation, and pressure from staff. Experience in Australia suggests that government instrumentalities were prepared to act for their own employees purely on the basis of authoritative knowledge, but that a mix of fear of litigation and staff demands was required to get action in most other places. For example, the landmark Australia legal case where a judge for the first time declared the evidence in the harms of passive smoking overwhelming (the Morling decision: (Everingham and Woodward 1991)) led to a significant upsurge in interest in smoking bans, as did publicity for out-of-court settlements (Palin and Young 1994). In the early days of restrictions, non-smokers, while supportive of bans on the whole, were not typically strong advocates. While they did not like the exposure, they were used to it and seemed reluctant to demand protection. As more and more places become smoke-free and non-smokers got to enjoy the benefits, and they saw that the restrictions on smokers were not unreasonable, they have become more militant. Now unions representing workers in areas where smoking is still prevalent are taking a leading role in advocating bans.

It is useful to consider the process from the perspective of diffusion of innovation theory (Rogers 1995). This model describes several stages of uptake of new product or ideas, which we will simplify to three: an early innovation stage where uptake is slow, an intermediate period where uptake is rapid, then a third slow period where some of those resistant to change (laggards) are gradually won over. The early innovation period is characterized by people who either have an unusual need for the innovation and/or a high level of interest in trying new things. Rogers divides them into two subgroups; the innovators, the first 2.5% to change, and the early adopters (the next 13.5%). In the social arena, they are people who are prepared to act in the face of normative pressures to preserve the status quo. This is a period when effective restrictions on smoking are few and most smokers see no need to change their behaviour, and few are prepared to make changes on their own initiative. Non-smokers, used to the smoke, for the most part continue to tolerate it. Restrictions may be seen as an-in-principle good idea, but one that may not prove practical in some situations. There is likely to be concern over whether smokers will comply, indeed over whether they will be able to comply or should be expected to comply. Those attempting to implement bans or ensure compliance will often be faced with strong resistance.

Once a critical level of adoption has occurred (around one-sixth of all units according to the theory), the period of rapid introduction occurs. This tends to sweep up all those with only modest potential gains and no major perceived costs of changing. This is accompanied by a change in norms which seem to be critical for getting non-smokers to begin to collectively work toward and/or actively support action to introduce bans. Previously in the innovation phase, it was left to activists. During this period not smoking becomes normative. Opposition to change declines and/or becomes centred in areas where there are perceived to be disadvantages.

The third period is about convincing laggards. These are typically jurisdictions, organizations, or individuals who perceive relative disadvantage from smoke-free places. Jurisdictions least likely to act are those with strong tobacco industries, those where the harms associated with passive smoking are dwarfed by other health concerns, and those where smoking rates are high among key decision-makers. For organizations or businesses, most of those are in the hospitality section, where the concerns are typically about reduced custom, and associated adverse economic costs. For individuals, moves to smoke-free homes will be least likely where there are only smokers in the home; those who live in accommodation (e.g. apartments) where it is structurally difficult to always smoke outside; and those who have responsibilities that might keep them from going outside to smoke. Unfortunately, this last group includes parents who smoke, and who need to supervise children (Ashley and Ferrence 1998).

To move the laggards either involves demonstrating to them that their fears are groundless (where they are) or changing the pattern of incentives such that they are either compensated for losses or stand to lose even more if they fail to introduce policies (for organizations) or comply with expectations (for individuals). Fortunately, all the evidence reviewed in the following sections show that most of the fears about the costs of implementing smoking bans are exaggerated.

Diffusion of innovation is not a passive process. It occurs as a result of understanding of potential benefits and positive experiences with the change being communicated to those who have not yet changed. Apart from awareness of the harms and associated desire to protect non-smokers, other factors that are important for driving action are threat of litigation, and the social acceptability of imposing restrictions, including demands from exposed individuals for action. Threat of litigation is made more salient by precedents, and is made more certain where the act of allowing smoking is specifically prohibited rather than relying on generic legislation and/or on the need for individuals to sue after they have experienced some disease associated with passive smoking. Social acceptability in something that builds up in the light of successful implementation of bans and the experience of the benefits by non-smokers and even, in many cases, smokers.

In summary, for change to occur key individuals and/or organizations need to accept that ETS is harmful enough to warrant action, to believe that institutional change is a reasonable part of the solution, believe that the change is practical (it can be done) and that it will be acceptable (enough) to affected parties. In addition, it helps if the individual or organization believes that they have an obligation to act either out of fear of personal injury litigation (for domestic restrictions) or to protect vulnerable loved ones. As innovation progresses, these move from being desirable outcomes through to becoming general expectations as to what is acceptable.

Change does not all occur at once. In some of the countries that have been at the forefront of actions to control passive smoking (e.g. USA, Canada, Australia), the moves to smoke-free places have been first in workplaces, then in private homes, and last of all in hospitality venues, especially bars. Somewhere along the way, bans are often imposed in public transport and in crowded places like cinemas and public halls, and even in crowded outdoor sporting stadiums. In most places, bans in these places have been enacted with a minimum of fuss. In other countries (e.g. Singapore) where action is reputedly strong, less information has appeared in the international literature, and so to the pattern by which change was, and is occurring. In the following sections we review knowledge on implementation and compliance with bans in the workplace; then in other public places, especially hospitality venues; and finally consider the home as the issues there are quite different to those in public places. Consideration of the effects on smoking prevalence and consumption are considered separately. In reviewing this material, it needs to be realized that the bulk of the empirical work comes from three countries: the USA, Canada, and Australia, all who have been innovators in ETS control and all have low and declining smoking prevalence by world standard (Corrao *et al.* 2000). The reader is encouraged to exercise caution in extrapolating from this research to their own country's situation, especially where the social conditions are quite different. We have tried to be sensitive to these issues, but the lack of good data and our lack of understanding of the diversity of world cultures means that we cannot be certain that we have taken all important issues into consideration.

The introduction of smoke-free environments

Smoke-free workplaces

In principle, as for other contexts, workplaces can be smoke-free because they have no smokers, or because smokers all voluntarily do not smoke there, or because smokers comply with rules not to smoke. In most countries initial moves to smoke-free workplaces has come from employers, followed by legislation mandating such practices, at least legislation where there is strong expectations of compliance. In these cases legislation has followed, largely as a way of forcing laggards to act.

Following the early authoritative reviews on the harmfulness of passive smoking, employers in some places began to voluntarily implement restrictions in workplaces. In some places voluntary introduction of bans was quite rapid. For example, reported prevalence of such bans in parts of Australia in the late 1980s was under 20%, but this rose to around 65% by the middle of the 1990s (Borland *et al.* 1997*a*). Such self report measures tend to at least partly take into account compliance, with many workers not reporting total bans where they are mandated but not complied with. In 1999, a national US study found 69% of all indoor workers reported smoke-free policies at work (Shopland *et al.* 2001). The type and level of coverage has varied overtime within and between countries. In the United States, Shopland *et al.* found that there was about a 35% absolute difference between the State with the highest (84%) and lowest (49%) levels of coverage suggesting that states in the USA are in or at the end of the main uptake phase for workplace protection.

Studies that have used the existence of legislative requirements provide a somewhat difficult picture. A review of smoking restrictions in different countries found that the majority of countries (with data about ETS ordinance) had laws restricting smoking in some form, but this may not reflect the amount of ETS exposure experience by workers (Brownson *et al.* 2002). The most common form of restriction was national legislation prohibiting smoking in the workplace, which included designated smoking areas. This policy applied to half of nearly 100 countries for which there was data available, but notable countries without such bans include the USA and Australia which are among the few countries with any published data on population-wide levels of smoke-free workplaces. Anecdotal reports from at least some countries with legislative bans suggests that compliance varies greatly, probably related to the cultural difference in when legislative approaches are implemented and societal traditions of compliance. We suspect that many of these countries have lower levels of actual protection than for some of the countries without legislative bans, but with strong social movements encouraging local action. Indeed Chapman (1998) gathered together brief commentaries from 11 countries that demonstrate this for a limited range of countries at least. A couple of examples will suffice. Poland introduced smoke-free legislation in 1996; however, in reality it was virtually impossible to spend a day in Poland without being exposed to tobacco smoke in the year or so afterwards (at least). Few public places are smoke-free with corridors of hospitals and parliament full of smoke and enforcement dependent on whether the boss smokes or not (Chapman 1998). Italy has laws that restrict smoking but were not commonly applied. For example, a survey of three hospitals in 1996 found that 87% of employees were exposed to ETS inside the hospital especially in cooking areas, information desks, and corridors (Zanetti *et al.* 1998). Within countries, there is a relationship between strength of laws and worker exposure in the expected direction (Pederson *et al.* 1996; Shopland *et al.* 2001). Legislation clearly has an important role to play; whether it is about motivating laggards or about providing the conditions to stimulate action in the first place.

Research indicates that compliance with smoking bans and restrictions in the workplace can be very high (Borland *et al.* 1990*a*; Wakefield *et al.* 1996). However, compliance is not guaranteed. It should not be assumed that regulatory action is self-enforcing even in countries where there is public acceptance of the need to comply (Brownson *et al.* 2002). A high level of compliance with workplace smoking bans is related to the consultative process used with employees. The literature indicates that use of a consultative process that involves employees is related to employee acceptance of bans and to high compliance with them. For example, a survey of clerical workers comparing methods of implementing workplace smoking bans found acceptance was enhanced by providing thorough information about why the bans were required before they were imposed and doing this in a social sensitivity manner which acknowledged the inconvenience and difficulties for smokers. The survey also found that smokers showed the most incremental gain in accepting bans after exposure to comprehensive information presented in a highly sensitive manner and that all employees valued the fairness associated with the process (Greenberg 1994). Kemp *et al.* (1993), in an Australian study of pockets of non-compliance with a total indoor workplace ban, found that non-compliance was largely due to poor management practice, not to any characteristics of the smokers. Management support may be more important than the specific approach used to implement smoking restrictions and bans. However, regardless of how bans are implemented, a subgroup of smokers may require additional help in the form of quit programmes or assistance with cravings to help them adjust to bans.

Overall, studies have consistently shown support for workplace bans and that the level of support improves after implementation especially where compliance is high (Borland *et al.* 1990*a*; Hocking *et al.* 1991; Daughton *et al.* 1992; Brownson *et al.* 2002). There is also data from Japan that supports strong acceptance and high compliance with bans (Mizoue *et al.* 1999).

Research indicates that even though heavy smokers may find it harder to comply with bans than lighter smokers (Daughton *et al.* 1992), a substantial number of smokers approve and accept bans in a context of almost universal compliance (Owen *et al.* 1991; Stave and Jackson 1991; Daughton *et al.* 1992; Emont *et al.* 1995). This finding is consistent with the notion that many smokers are ambivalent about their smoking and that they adjust attitudes in line with behaviours, even when the behaviour change is not voluntary (Borland *et al.* 1990*a*).

The nature of the restrictions affect their effectiveness in ways that are entirely predictable. Research indicates that smoking bans are more effective than partial smoking restrictions in reducing ETS (Hopkins *et al.* 2001). Compliance is higher for total bans (Sorensen *et al.* 1991; Wakefield *et al.* 1996) and satisfaction with smoking regulations appear highest when employees report the least amount of exposure to environmental tobacco smoke (Sorensen *et al.* 1991). This has also been found in Germany (Brenner *et al.* 1997). The next most effective restriction is ventilated smoking lounges, but is more costly and can elevate lung cancer risk in smokers. The least effective restriction in reducing ETS being designated smoking area without ventilation (Brownson *et al.* 2002). Japanese research (Mizoue *et al.* 1999) supports the finding that complete bans are complied with better suggesting considerable generality of this phenomenon. There is a tendency to support the level of restriction to which you are subject, but this does not hold for some levels of partial ban (Borland *et al.* 1992) suggesting that such things as smoking rooms can be problematic.

Research from industrial countries indicates that workers are more likely to be protected from ETS if they are employed in firms with 50 or more people, have a higher level of education, are female, and worked indoors. Those workers more likely to be exposed to ETS included blue-collar workers, self employed, service occupations (e.g. bar workers), and lower skill occupations which tend to have higher prevalence of smokers than higher skilled groups (Borland *et al.* 1997*a*; Brownson *et al.* 2002). Larger companies are more likely to have organized occupational health and safety policies and are less likely to have policy affected by one influential person (e.g. the boss).

All of the evidence points to the net effect of workplace bans being positive. The health and well-being of non-smokers (at least) is improved. In addition, the workplace is made more attractive without the unpleasant smells of tobacco smoke, and cleaning costs are reduced. The only potential downside is possible loss of productivity among smokers. One of the most notable features of workplace smoking bans is the phenomenon of smokers leaving their workplace to have a cigarette (Borland *et al.* 1997*b*). This exiled smoking seems to persist and serves social as well as dependence-serving functions. While some exiled smoking occurs in work breaks, some smokers take extra breaks, which can place extra demands on their co-workers and/or reduce their productivity. One effect of exiled smoking is that it results in lots of workers smoking on city streets. This can create nuisance value to non-smokers exposed to the smoke, and by being so public may contribute to perception that smoking prevalence is higher than it actually is, a known risk factor for uptake among adolescents (U.S. Department of Health and Human Services 1994). It is also not clear to what extent it affects productivity of those smokers who take breaks during work time. However, some organizations have taken action to minimize such adverse effects by either banning such practices or having workers clock-off and make up the time spent.

Smoking bans in other public places

In this section we consider movement toward implementation of bans in other public places, with a special emphasis on hospitality venues.

Partly because most public venues are also workplaces and partly to protect patrons, there is strong movement towards increased bans or smoking in public places. These range from shops to enclosed arcades, residential business such as hospitals and hotels, public transport, and indoor or enclosed sporting facilities. Public places such as transport, hospitals, cinemas, and theatres have commonly become smoke-free in many countries (Melihan-Cheinin and Hirsch 1997). There is very little published about bans in these areas. In some cases the implementation of bans in such places occurs in concert with legislation to ban smoking in workplaces (as most are also workplaces), but in some cases they are subject to special regulations that may come into place before rules mandating all workplaces be smoke-free, or in the case of hospitality venues (in particular), might be specifically exempted from generic workplace legislation. One interesting extension of bans is to crowded outdoor spectator areas at sporting venues. Bans are increasingly been implemented and acceptance and compliance can be high (Pikora *et al.* 1999). There seems to be little doubt that in most places bans can be readily complied with, and come to be appreciated by smokers as well as non-smokers in the same way as for workplaces in general. The few more contentious issues are discussed below.

An interesting area of research regarding smoking restrictions in public places was initiated by Bonfill *et al.* (1997) in Spain. They simulated violations of public area laws and observed bystander interventions. They found that only in a small percentage of cases did violations lead to any action to discourage the smoking. A replication in Australia (Salmon and Rissel 1999) found similar low levels of intervention, but also noted some disapproving looks. Poland *et al.* (1999) explored public reactions to violations and found reluctance to directly confront violators. Options ranged from 'Grin and bear it', though moving away, an appeal to a third party (i.e. someone in authority), to overt signs of displeasure. In no case is direct confrontation likely to be easy. In areas where smoking in public is still normative, a request not to smoke may be seen as inappropriate, while in areas where it is normative, violators may be more likely to be anti-social and thus likely to respond to warnings in an aggressive manner. In our view this work shows that it is not appropriate to rely on the bystander to enforce laws. If there is a problem with compliance, public education coupled with enforcement by trained staff should be considered. That said, where norms are appropriate, compliance is likely to be close to complete.

Residential facilities where bans could have marked impact on residents' capacity to smoke have a range of unique issues. For example, prisoners are restricted in where they can go, and hospital patients and nursing home residents are sometimes incapacitated and unable to readily move to areas where smoking may be permitted. There is not much systematic research on these settings. However, it is notable that an observational study of smoking areas at a hospital found that only 10% of users were patients (Nagle *et al.* 1996), suggesting that in some cases concern for clients is exaggerated.

One area that has been studied is psychiatric patients, who along with drug and alcohol services often have very high smoking rates. Restrictions in residential facilities for these conditions are less than for other types of hospital patients (Longo *et al.* 1998). Even though studies of implementation of bans show little adverse effect, and most of that transitory (Velasco *et al.* 1996) it is not clear to what extent these patients had access to places where they could smoke or were forced to not smoke. Related to this, Rigotti *et al.* (2000) found high levels of reported cravings among in-patient residents of a general hospital, with one quarter reporting smoking, although only a minority of these admitting to smoking where it was banned. Where in-patients cannot readily go to smoking areas alternatives will be needed for those smokers who cannot readily or will not take advantage of the situation to attempt to quit. There is a need to explore the utility of nicotine replacement therapy as a substitute for cigarettes in these contexts, not just as a cessation aid.

The main area where there appears to be strong resistance to the implementation of smoke-free policies is in hospitality venues, particularly those that also serve alcohol, but also extending to restaurants of all kinds and gaming venues. Of these restaurants and bars have been most studied. It seems to be the case that implementing smoking bans in bars is the area that arouses the most apposition. Arguments against bans are based on presumed preferences of users of such venues. Proprietors fear loss of patronage from smoking clients with no clear expectations of increased patronage from non-smokers. All of the evidence to date indicates that proprietors fears are misplaced. Indeed for the hospitality sector overall the net effect seem to be beneficial. A recent systematic review of the economic impact of bans on the hospitality industry showed that virtually all the evidence of adverse effect came from studies with weak designs and/or reliance or opinion measures (Scollo *et al.* 2003). Studies with strong designs and actual expenditure measures found either no impact or a small positive impact of bans. It was notable that all studies showing adverse effects used weaker designs and were also funded by the tobacco industry or sources close to them. It is now certain that there are no overall adverse economic consequences of bans on smoking in hospitality venues. A minority of individual business may be adversely affected if they are unable to adapt, but overall there are potential economic benefits as well as the social and health benefits of maintaining clear air. For the most part, proprietors have nothing to fear. It seems that much of the concern has been whipped up by the tobacco industry who may have more to fear as such bans may affect tobacco use (see later).

Bans in restaurants when implemented are complied with and accepted without need for coercive measures at least in some jurisdictions (Hyland *et al.* 1999; Chapman *et al.* 2001). Furthermore, complete bans do not lead to infrastructure costs associated with implementation of separately ventilated smoking rooms. Less is known about bans in bars, but in the limited number of places where they have been implemented both compliance and acceptance seem to be high (August and Brooks 2000). For all that is known, the only area where there appears to be any need for significant compensatory efforts is in residential facilities, and here opportunities to go outside and use of NRT are likely to be adequate solutions in most cases.

Smoke-free homes

Smoking in homes can be done by residents and/or visitors. Clearly there are different challenges involved in implementing bans when residents smoke than when it is only a matter of discouraging visitors. Further, the issue of having a ban only really emerges when there is a possibility of somebody smoking. As a consequence surveys of the prevalence of smoking bans in non-smoking households may underestimate the true prevalence of smoke-free homes because some of the homes without bans may never the less have no smoking. Even given this, surveys consistently find that prevalence of bans in non-smoker households is higher than when there are smokers living there.

Like for institutions, mere awareness of the harm has not been sufficient to motivate mass action in most places. For example in Victoria, Australia, acceptances of the harmfulness of passive smoking was high by the mid-1980s and has risen little more since then, yet the main movement to voluntarily restrict smoking in homes did not occur until the mid-1990s (Borland *et al.* 1999). The growing awareness of the harm of ETS and the benefits of clean air has shifted public attitudes on smoking from one of it being just a personal behaviour to a key social concern.

At present not smoking in the home and around their children appears to have only become normative in some countries. The expectation is or was that smokers could smoke when and where they wanted to. In this context attempting to enforce a smoking ban on others was likely to have been seen as unnecessary and thus unreasonable. Further, from the perspective of smokers, even if they personally believed in the need not to smoke around others, to act on such a belief would have been seen as unusual by others. As the social climate changes, the environment becomes one where the expectation is that smokers will not smoke in their homes, or especially in those of others, and it now requires a radical stance to smoke. The patterns of change in expected behaviours have meant that it is now easy to institute bans in societies which have moved to restrictions being normative, but it is likely to be much harder where this is not yet the case.

The vast majority of people (including many smokers) find ETS unpleasant, both the direct experience and the residual smell (e.g. on clothes). ETS can lead to irritation of the eyes, throat, and, in susceptible individuals, acute respiratory problems (e.g. asthma attacks). Smoking in the home causes significant mess, from dropped ash and smoke settling on surfaces. This increases cleaning needs and contributes to the stale odour of rooms that have been smoked in. Drawing smokers' attention to these effects can help them to see immediate benefits of their decisions not to smoke and will provide benefits that might not have, of themselves, justified restricting when and where smoking occurs.

Engaging in ETS control behaviours at home can sometimes be inconvenient for the smoker. Smoking outside in inclement conditions can be unpleasant, as can having to interrupt valued activities to go outside. In addition, having to move away from children or other non-smokers to find somewhere to smoke can be difficult at times. Under almost all circumstances it is not desirable to have doors opened as it is likely to result in at least some of the smoke being blown back into the house. If the smoker is responsible for supervision of, for example, children, it is impossible to smoke outside if the children cannot be seen or cannot be supervised from outside (no acceptable line of sight), or where the children actively seek close contact. This analysis explains why the task of ETS exposure reduction seems to be harder for smoking parents, especially for single parents where there is reduced opportunity to go 'off duty' (Ashley and Ferrence 1998).

For a smoker who lives alone or with non-smokers and has few smoker friends who visit, ETS control is largely a personal choice. For most other smokers the task is more of a collective one. In all houses where it is consequential, there is more than one person involved within the household. Even if the household agrees to eliminate smoking inside there is the problem faced in dealing with friends who visit and the need for smokers to maintain behavioural consistency if it is going to be feasible to expect friends not to smoke when they visit. Take the case of a smoker who reluctantly agrees to have his household smoke-free, but then goes and smokes at a friend's place whom subsequently visits and goes to light up. What does the person do? Asking the person not to smoke violates the principle of reciprocity, yet allowing it violates an agreement with his/her family. This highlights the fact that a ban on smoking in one's home can change the nature of a person's relationships with all affected people (e.g. smokers who visit). In social context where smoking around others is not implicitly accepted as an issue, negotiating such a change in relationships with a range others is likely to be difficult as there may be no shared reason to justify the act. However, as the social context changes to where most smokers expect not to smoke around others, the opposite would be the case, and it would be difficult to smoke in others homes, as it would be likely to threaten relationships.

Research or strategies to increase home-based smoking restrictions demonstrates that focused 'clinical' interventions find it difficult to gain much change in home-smoking unless they are quite intense, and even here effects are modest (Borland *et al.* 1999; Hovell *et al.* 2000). For example, Hovell *et al.* (2000) used seven counselling sessions to find a modest effect. By contrast, in communities that are aware of the risks and where there has been mass public education to encourage smoke-free homes, there can be rapid increases in the rates of smoke-free homes (Borland *et al.* 1999). If we are to action high levels of smoke-free homes, the best strategy would seem to be changing community norms about what is acceptable. To do this requires innovators, who will often be parents of children at high risk (e.g. asthmatics). In our view, clinical style interventions have a limited role in protecting children from ETS. A case can be made for developing better clinical interventions to help parents of high risk children move ahead of social trends. A further possible role for intense interventions may be among those who have special problems in enacting home restrictions; for example, single parents in high rise apartments, but even here environmental change may be more important than any form of skills training.

In cases where not smoking in the home is not practical, there is a need to explore which exposure reduction strategies are likely to be most effective. Wakefield *et al.* (2000*a*) have shown that lesser restrictions lead to lower cotinine levels than no restrictions, even though levels are greater than for total bans. Wakefield *et al.* found that smoking in rooms the child rarely frequents was associated with lower exposures, but it is not clear if this is a benefit of where the smoking occurs or related to lower levels of smoking. More research is needed to find ways to help smokers for whom the implementation of smoke-free homes is structurally difficult.

Effects of restrictions on smoking

Although the primary objective of smoking bans and restriction in work-sites and public places is to reduce exposure to environmental tobacco smoke particularly of non-smokers, bans have other effects, mainly on smokers, and it is these effects to which we now turn. In theory there could be effects on tobacco use on non-smokers and ex-smokers as well as on smokers. Restrictions on smoking could effect the rate of uptake among non-smokers. Among ex-smokers it may affect likelihood of resuming tobacco use and among current smokers it may lead to reduction in a number of cigarettes smoked and puffing characteristics of cigarettes smoked, which together affect total intake; and perhaps effect rates of complete cessation.

The extent of change in consumption and thus potential exposure following introduction of rules will to some extent vary as a function of choices the smoker makes, as well as other contingencies. This all means that estimates of effect size of studies of the imposition of bans on smoking represent average effects rather than some underlying 'true' effect. Understanding differences in effect sizes is a legitimate and important area for research.

Effects on daily cigarette consumption

When people cannot smoke for prolonged periods in their workplace, on public transport, and other public locations some may be stimulated to attempt to quit, or smoke less. However, smokers may compensate for restrictions by smoking more in other places and times when they can smoke (Chapman et al. 1999). The change in daily cigarette consumption due to bans or other restrictions is a function of the total number of cigarettes not smoked that otherwise would have been in the situation subject to the ban, minus any extra cigarettes smoked at other times to compensate.

There is consistent evidence that smoke-free workplaces decrease cigarette consumption. (Eriksen and Gottlieb 1998; Chapman et al. 1999; Hopkins et al. 2001). This evidence comes from community surveys of workers, retrospective surveys, prospective cross-sectional work-site studies, and prospective cohort studies (Chapman et al. 1999). This decline in consumption has been found in a variety of workplaces (Eriksen and Gottlieb 1998), including in Germany (Brenner and Fleischle 1994) and Japan (Mizoue et al. 2000).

The precise effect on consumption varies with studies showing a decrease ranging up to about 5 cigarettes per day, compared to those workplaces with no restrictions. A number of reviews (using different definitions of methodological robustness) have estimated that the decline in consumption resulting from smoking bans to be 1.2 cigarettes (Hopkins et al. 2001), 3.5 cigarettes (Chapman et al. 1999), and 3.4 cigarettes

(Eriksen and Gottlieb 1998). The main difference between the Hopkins *et al.* finding and that of the other two was that the Hopkins review relied on quasi randomized trials whereas the other two included before–after comparison studies. In our view, this is a situation where the use of comparison groups is not the strongest method for estimating the size of consumption changes. This is because the introduction of restrictions on smoking is a social phenomenon, and the organizations introducing bans are likely to differ in important and relevant ways to those not (yet) introducing them. For example, several of the comparison studies used hospitals as the workplace where bans were implemented. These are not typical environments. Many staff refrained from smoking around patients before bans were implemented and other refrained from smoking while on duty (smoking is unhealthy and health care workers should set a good example). To the extent this happened, bans on smoking would be likely to have a smaller effect on overall consumption. Further, prior to the moves to restrict smoking, estimates of tobacco consumption were very stable, and the effects of bans so big (in some cases) that there is no other plausible alternative explanation for the observed drop in consumption. Indeed, unpublished work from our group is tracking a small group of smokers close to the introduction of a total workplace bans. This found a drop in consumption. This decrease occurred from the workday before the bans were introduced to the first day of the bans. This effect is very similar to the observed effect on the larger population studied before and some months after the bans (Borland *et al.* 1990*b*). We believe that the average estimate of between 3 and 4 cigarettes per day is the most valid.

That said, there is no magic amount that one should expect when bans are implemented. Indeed a small number of studies have found no effects of bans on consumption, while others have found large effects (Eriksen and Gottlieb 1998). Understanding what influence the magnitude of effects is of considerable interest. Variance in effect on consumption may be due to the type of smoking restriction, the amount of consumption before the restrictions, the ability to access places where smoking is allowed, number and length of legitimate work breaks, degree of compliance, and implementation issues.

Evidence indicates that more restrictive workplace policies have a greater impact on consumption (Farrelly *et al.* 1999; Mizoue *et al.* 2000). Farrelly *et al.* (1999), in a large study concluded that partial restrictions (allowing smoking areas) cut the level of reduction by about half.

A characteristic of the decline in cigarette consumption has been that heavy smokers report the largest reductions (Borland *et al.* 1990*b*; Borland and Owen 1995; Owen and Borland 1997; Hopkins *et al.* 2001). However, this might vary as a function of ease of cutting down. Borland and Owen (1995) found that heavy smokers who no longer felt the need to smoke cut down a lot, but those heavy smokers with a strong need to smoke were less likely to change as they were prepared to put in the effort to find places where smoking was allowed (Borland and Owen 1995).

More controversial, there is weak evidence that declines in consumption dissipate over time (Owen and Borland 1997; Levy *et al.* 2001). For example, the Owen and Borland (1997) study which found a decline, was of a group who initially changed more than average. However, another study (Borland *et al.* 1991) found no declines in other workplaces with smaller initial declines 18 months after bans were implemented. Declines in reduction in consumption should not be assumed, but if they occur they are likely to relate to changing opportunities for compensatory smoking.

Compensatory smoking will effect overall consumption effects. Some studies report that smoking bans have not increased compensatory smoking (e.g. Olive and Ballard 1996) whilst others indicate considerable compensation (e.g. Parry *et al.* 2000). The degree of compensatory smoking is likely to be affected by the ease with which smokers can find acceptable places to smoke. Leaving work to smoke can be common. A survey of workers in Victoria, Australia found that half of smokers reporting leaving work to smoke, with one-fourth leaving work more than three times a day (Borland *et al.* 1997*b*). If these opportunities are curtailed, consumption reduction should increase, but if new opportunities to smoke emerge, consumption might increase.

Most of the research has looked at reported cigarette consumption rather than measures of tobacco intake. Gomel *et al.* (1993) in a small study found that workers reduced their overall and daily consumption of cigarettes after a total ban was imposed. However, biological measures indicated that contrary to the self-report, consumption reverted to baseline levels after an initial decrease. It is possible that some smokers come to compensate by getting more from each cigarette they smoke. Chapman *et al.* (1997) observed that workers puffed longer on cigarettes than other people who were on city streets. Reductions in consumption of number of cigarettes should not be assumed to translate into comparable reductions in exposure to tobacco-related toxins.

Regardless of the effects on smokers, reductions in consumption can have adverse effect on tobacco companies. Approximately, 22.3% of the 2.7 billion decrease in cigarettes consumed in Australia between 1988 and 1995 has been attributed to smoke-free workplaces as has 12.7% of the 76.5 billion decrease in the USA over a similar time (Chapman *et al.* 1999). This is almost certainly the main reason tobacco companies spend so much effort trying to discourage restrictions.

Even if some of the reductions in consumption do not result in reduced exposure, there is some evidence that reduced consumption can make quitting easier (Pierce *et al.* 1998) and it reduces the amount they spend on cigarettes. It seems safe to conclude that these are clear benefits to smokers as a result of the effects of bans in leading to many of them smoking less.

Little is known about the effects of consumption on bans outside the workplace. It is likely that they will add to consumption declines. The limiting factor for dependent smokers is likely to be the amount they need to satisfy their addiction. As it becomes more difficult for smoker to smoke, it is possible that more will break their addictions and either quit altogether or become non-addicted users. Indeed, in California, a place that has moved as far as anywhere to becoming smoke-free, there has been an increase in the prevalence of non-daily smoking, even as daily smoking has declined (Pierce *et al.* 1998).

Effects on cessation

The evidence on the impact of bans on smoking cessation is less clear. Chapman *et al.* (1999) concluded no clear evidence of any effect, but Hopkins *et al.* (2001) relying on studies with comparison groups concluded that there is an effect for cessation but acknowledge studies that have looked at smoking prevalence have been equivocal. Biener and Nyman (1999) found evidence of increased cessation associated with bans over a three-year period, but only where the evidence suggested the bans were effectively enforced. There is some evidence that the onset of bans is associated with an increase in quitting, with the event being used by some smokers as a good time to quit (Chapman *et al.* 1999). The frequency of this and whether such actions increase overall quitting or merely change its timing is unclear. Further, in the period when workplace bans were becoming most prevalent in Australia, the USA, and some other countries, was a period where there was little or no change in population smoking prevalence (Hill *et al.* 1995; MMWR 1999).

Related to the possible effects on quitting, bans should reduce relapse in ex-smokers by providing an increased range of safe places. However, there is no clear empirical evidence to show that this is a real benefit to those trying to stay stopped, but that is because of a lack of studies rather than a failure to find effects.

Based on all of this work, we tentatively conclude that while these may be small positive effects of bans on cessation, they are unlikely to be of a magnitude to make a major contribution to reducing population smoking prevalence. However, as restrictions become more prevalent in homes and in recreational venues, it seems likely that effects on cessation are likely to increase in magnitude.

Possible effect on smoking uptake

One of the most intriguing possible effects of smoke-free places impact is on uptake of regular tobacco use. Theories around possible effects vary by the type of restriction. The example bans set and what they say about social norms should have a positive effect, as should the reduction in opportunities to smoke. The only possible adverse effect relates to exiled smoking. As restrictions on smoking often result in smokers going out into outdoor public areas to smoke, their smoking becomes more noticeable by bystanders. There is no evidence that this activity entices non-smokers in the workplace to smoke (Clarke *et al.* 1997), but it may affect the bystanders if it effects their perceptions of the prevalence of smoking (U.S. Department of Health and Human Services 1994). On the other hand, if those smokers are perceived negatively (e.g. as slightly desperate), it might act to discourage smoking, by making it seem less attractive.

Smoke-free workplaces for non-smokers may reduce internal pressure to uptake by not having smoking as part of the workplace. This effect may also influence experimental smokers, making them more likely to quit. Bans should create a barrier that might slow down progress from social smoking, which typically occurs later in the day from being transformed into the levels of addictive smoking typified by smoking soon after waking. Bans in recreational venues and other public places are likely to have their effect by removing situations which used to be strongly linked to smoking (e.g. dance venues) into places where smoking is no longer normative. Home bans effects are likely to be largely through the messages they provide about parental attitudes.

The limited research available to date is supportive of a positive contribution of all kinds of smoke-free places on inhibiting uptake of regular smoking, but in no case is the evidence definitive, because it is largely based on cross-sectional data, or on professed intentions.

The evidence for effects in the home is strongest, with three studies finding effects (Farkas *et al.* 2000; Proescholdbell *et al.* 2000; Wakefield *et al.* 2000*b*). It is of note that two of these found the strongest effects in homes with no adult smokers, suggesting the importance of smoke-free homes for conveying parental attitudes. Where one or more parents smoke, there are likely to be a range of other ways by which their attitudes to smoking are conveyed.

The workplace studies (Farkas *et al.* 2000; Wakefield *et al.* 2000*b*) are also consistent with hypothesized effects, with one (Wakefield *et al.* 2000) finding an effect only on the transition from experimental to regular smoking.

There is also potential for benefits of bans in recreational venues with Philpot *et al.* (1999) reporting that many young social smokers who frequent pubs and nightclubs saying that smoking bans in those venues would lead them to quit altogether. As such venues are ones where social smokers are more likely to smoke (Trotter *et al.* 2002), such effects are plausible, but yet to be demonstrated.

We conclude that smoke-free places have potential to discourage uptake of smoking, including reducing the transition from experimental to regular smoking. There is no evidence of any negative effects. Nothing is known of the size of any effects or of the factors that might effect their size except for the plausible finding that poorly enforced policies, are likely to have lesser or no positive effects.

Predictions for the future

There seems to be little doubt that the world is moving to a situation where the responsibility to protect non-smokers from passive smoking will take priority over whatever needs smokers have to smoke. In some jurisdictions we are getting very close to this in 2004, but for much of the world there is still an enormous amount of work to do. Unfortunately, lack of data means that we do not have any precise estimate as to what is required, except in a small number of places that are probably among the most advanced. Although in countries like the USA where the most is known there is considerable variation in the current situation (Shopland *et al.* 2001).

The strategy to progress will need to include both public education, legislative measures, and compliance systems. The order in which the first two are introduced will vary by jurisdiction, and if the public education component is adequate, there is unlikely to be a major need for large scale compliance measures as the rules are likely to be self-enforcing. At least, that has been the experience where appropriate mixes of education and rules have been introduced.

But what will the future look like? Enclosed public places and workplaces will be all smoke-free. Some facilities will have separately ventilated smoking rooms, especially where suitable outdoor smoking venues are not available. These rooms will need to be places where people do not need to work for extended periods (they will need to be cleaned), and they should not have alcohol served or available given the interactive health harms between tobacco and alcohol (IPCS (International Programme on Clinical Safety) 1999). The alternative to smoking areas is to force addicts into areas where they can 'sneak' a smoke. Some of these areas may create other risks, such as of fire and/or risks to the physical security of the smokers. We do not think that such smoking rooms will be needed at most workplaces, they clearly will not, but there will be a need for some in crowded business areas and such places as airports where people sometimes need to spend extended periods.

For private environments, the move towards smoke-free rooms are likely to depend more on public education and changing social norms than on legislation. As smoking is restricted in public places, pressure to implement restrictions in homes (and cars) is likely to build. Not smoking in homes will become normative, but in a small number of cases smoking will persist, most notably in multi-floor dwelling without balconies. At least in richer countries, it is likely that building regulations will be modified to ensure at least some exposure reduction mechanisms are available for these situations, but in poorer countries, such solutions may be too costly.

Tobacco smoking will retreat to being a private activity engaged in alone or among consenting adults. This social marginalization of smoking is likely to encourage cessation and reduce uptake, contributing to other efforts that will help to create what is effectively a smoke-free world for most of its inhabitants. The overwhelming majority of non-smokers will be able to live their lives free of harmful and annoying exposure to ETS. The movement to control ETS is one of the great successes of public health already in some countries, and we expect it to become the case in the rest of the world quite quickly.

References

Ashley, M. J. and Ferrence, R. (1998). Reducing children's exposure to environmental tobacco smoke in homes: issues and strategies. *Tob Control*, **7**(1), 61–5.

August, K. and Brooks, L. (2000). Support for smoke-free bars grows stronger in California. California Department of Health Service, CA.

Benninger, M. S. (1999). The impact of cigarette smoking and environmental tobacco smoke on nasal and sinus disease: a review of the literature. *Am J Rhinol,* **13**(6), 435–8.

Biener, L. and Nyman, A. L. (1999). Effect of workplace smoking policies on smoking cessation: results of a longitudinal study. *J Occup Environ Med,* **41**(12), 1121–7.

Bonfill, X., Serra, C., and Lopez, V. (1997). Employee and public responses to simulated violations of no-smoking regulations in Spain. *Am J Public Health,* **87**(6), 1035–7.

Borland, R., Cappiello, M., and Owen, N. (1997*b*). Leaving work to smoke. *Addiction,* **92**(10), 1361–8.

Borland, R., Chapman, S., Owen, N., and Hill, D. (1990*b*). Effects of workplace smoking bans on cigarette consumption. *Am J Public Health,* **80**(2), 178–80.

Borland, R., Morand, M., and Mullins, R. (1997*a*). Prevalence of workplace smoking bans in Victoria. *Aust N Z J Public Health,* **21**(7), 694–8.

Borland, R., Mullins, R., Trotter, L., and White, V. (1999). Trends in environmental tobacco smoke restrictions in the home in Victoria, Australia. *Tob Control,* **8**(3), 266–71.

Borland, R. and Owen, N. (1995). Need to smoke in the context of workplace smoking bans. *Prev Med,* **24**(1), 56–60.

Borland, R., Owen, N., Hill, D., and Chapman, S. (1990*a*). Changes in acceptance of workplace smoking bans following their implementation: a prospective study. *Prev Med,* **19**(3), 314–22.

Borland, R., Owen, N., and Hocking, B. (1991). Changes in smoking behaviour after a total workplace smoking ban. *Aust J Public Health,* **15**(2), 130–4.

Borland, R., Pierce, J. P., Burns, D. M., Gilpin, E., Johnson, M., and Bal, D. (1992). Protection from environmental tobacco smoke in California. The case for a smoke-free workplace. *JAMA,* **268**(6), 749–52.

Brenner, H., Born, J., Novak, P., and Wanek, V. (1997). Smoking behavior and attitude toward smoking regulations and passive smoking in the workplace. A study among 974 employees in the German metal industry. *Prev Med,* **26**(1), 138–43.

Brenner, H. and Fleischle, B. (1994). Smoking regulations at the workplace and smoking behavior: a study from southern Germany. *Prev Med,* **23**(2), 230–4.

Brownson, R. C., Hopkins, D. P., and Wakefield, M. (2002). Effects of smoking restrictions in the workplace. *Annul Review of Public Health,* **23**, 333–48.

California Environment Protection Agency. (1997). *Health effects of exposure to environmental tobacco smoke-final report and appendices.* Sacramento: CA: Office of Environmental Health Hazard Assessment.

Chapman, S. (1998). Bans on smoking in public become more commonplace. *BMJ,* **316**(7133), 727–30.

Chapman, S., Borland, R., and Lal, A. (2001). Has the ban on smoking in New South Wales restaurants worked? A comparison of restaurants in Sydney and Melbourne. *Med J Aust,* **174**(10), 512–5.

Chapman, S., Borland, R., Scollo, M., Brownson, R. C., Dominello, A., and Woodward, S. (1999). The impact of smoke-free workplaces on declining cigarette consumption in Australia and the United States. *Am J Public Health,* **89**(7), 1018–23.

Chapman, S., Haddad, S., and Sindhusake, D. (1997). Do work-place smoking bans cause smokers to smoke 'harder'? Results from a naturalistic observational study. *Addiction,* **92**(5), 607–10.

Clarke, J., Borland, R., and McGartland, M. (1997). The effects of smoking outside workplaces on non-regular smokers. *J Occup Environ Med,* **39**(8), 734–9.

Colley, J. R. T. (1974). Respiratory symptoms in children and parental smoking and phlegm production. *BMJ,* **2**(5912), 201–4.

Corrao, M. A., Guindon, G. E., Sharma, N., and Shokoohi, D. F. (2000). *Tobacco control country profiles.* Atlanta Georgia: American Cancer Society.

Daughton, D. M., Andrews, C. E., Orona, C. P., Patil, K. D., and Rennard, S. I. (1992). Total indoor smoking ban and smoker behavior. *Prev Med*, 21(5), 670–6.

Davis, R. M. (1998). Exposure to environmental tobacco smoke: identifying and protecting those at risk. *JAMA*, 280(22), 1947–9.

Eisner, M. D., Smith, A. K., and Blanc, P. D. (1998). Bartenders' respiratory health after establishment of smoke-free bars and taverns. *JAMA*, 280(22), 1909–14.

Emont, S. L., Zahniser, C. C., Marcus, S. E., Trontell, A. E., Mills, S., Frazier, E. L., *et al.* (1995). Evaluation of the 1990 Centers for Disease Control and Prevention smoke-free policy. *Am J Health Promot*, 9(6), 456–61.

Eriksen, M. P. and Gottlieb, N. H. (1998). A review of the health impact of smoking control at the workplace. *Am J Health Promot*, 13(2), 83–104.

Everingham, R. and Woodward, S. (ed.). (1991). *Tobacco Litigation: The case against passive smoking*. Sydney: Legal Books.

Farkas, A. J., Gilpin, E. A., White, M. M., and Pierce, J. P. (2000). Association between household and workplace smoking restrictions and adolescent smoking. *JAMA*, 284(6), 717–22.

Farrelly, M. C., Evans, W. N., and Sfekas, A. E. (1999). The impact of workplace smoking bans: results from a national survey. *Tob Control*, 8(3), 272–7.

Gomel, M., Olderburg, B., Lemon, J., Owen, N., and Westbrook, F. (1993). Pilot study of the effects of a workplace smoking ban on indices of smoking, cigarette craving, stress and other health behaviours. *Psychology and Health*, 8, 223–9.

Greenberg, J. (1994). Using socially fair treatment to promote acceptance of a work site smoking ban. *J Appl Psychol*, 79(2), 288–97.

Heloma, A., Jaakkola, M. S., Kahkonen, E., and Reijula, K. (2001). The short-term impact of national smoke-free workplace legislation on passive smoking and tobacco use. *Am J Public Health*, 91(9), 1416–8.

Hill, D., White, V. M., and Schollo, M. M. (1995). Smoking behaviours of Australian adults in 1995: trends and concerns. *Medical Journal of Australia*, 168, 209–13.

Hirayama, T. (1981). Non-smoking wives of heavy smokers have a higher risk of lung cancer: A study from Japan. *Br Med J*, 282, 183–5.

Hocking, B., Borland, R., Owen, N., and Kemp, G. (1991). A total ban on workplace smoking is acceptable and effective. *J Occup Med*, 33(2), 163–7.

Hopkins, D. P., Briss, P. A., Ricard, C. J., Husten, C. G., Carande-Kulis, V. G., Fielding, J. E., *et al.* (2001). Reviews of evidence regarding interventions to reduce tobacco use and exposure to environmental tobacco smoke. *Am J Prev Med*, 20(2 Suppl), 16–66.

Hovell, M. F., Zakarian, J. M., Wahlgren, D. R., and Matt, G. E. (2000). Reducing children's exposure to environmental tobacco smoke: the empirical evidence and directions for future research. *Tob Control*, 9(Suppl 2), II40–47.

Hyland, A., Cummings, M., and Wilson, M. P. (1999). Compliance with the New York City Smoke-Free Air Act. *J Public Health Manag Pract*, 5(1), 43–52.

IPCS (International Programme on Clinical Safety). (1999). *Health effects of interactions between tobacco use and other agents*. WHO, Geneva.

Kemp, G., Hocking, B., and Borland, R. (1993). Managing implementation of a no smoking policy. *Asia Pacific Journal of Human Resources*, 31(1), 92–9.

Levy, D. T., Friend, K., and Polishchuk, E. (2001). Effect of clean indoor air laws on smokers: The clean air module of the SimSmoke computer simulation model. *Tob Control*, 10(4), 345–51.

Longo, D. R., Feldman, M. M., Kruse, R. L., Brownson, R. C., Petroski, G. F., and Hewett, J. E. (1998). Implementing smoking bans in American hospitals: results of a national survey. *Tob Control*, 7(1), 47–55.

Melihan-Cheinin, P. and Hirsch, A. (1997). Effects of smoke-free environments, advertising bans and price increases. In: *The tobacco epidemic. Prog Respir Res* (Vol. 28) (ed. C. T. Bollinger and K. O. Fagerstrom), Karger, Basel.

Mizoue, T., Reijula, K., Heloma, A., Yamato, H., and Fujino, Y. (2000). Impact of workplace smoking restrictions on smoking behaviour and attitudes toward quitting in Japan. *Tob Control*, 9, 435.

Mizoue, T., Reijula, K., Yamato, H., Iwasaki, A., and Yoshimura, T. (1999). Support for and observance of worksite smoking restriction policies—A study of municipal employees at a city office in Japan. *Prev Med*, 29(6 Pt 1), 549–54.

MMWR (1999). Tobacco use—United States, 1990–1999. *MMWR Morb Mortal Wkly Rep*, 48, 986–93.

MMWR (2000). State-specific prevalence of current cigarette smoking among adults and the proportion of adults who work in a smoke-free environment—United States, 1999. *MMWR Morb Mortal Wkly Rep*, 49(43), 978–82.

Nagle, A. L., Schofield, M. J., and Redman, S. (1996). Smoking on hospital grounds and the impact of outdoor smoke-free zones. *Tob Control*, 5(3), 199–204.

NHMRC. (1987). *Effects of passive smoking on health. Report of National Health and Medical Research Council working party on the effects of passive smoking on health.* Canberra ACT: Australian Government Publishing Service.

Olive, K. E. and Ballard, J. A. (1996). Changes in employee smoking behavior after implementation of restrictive smoking policies. *South Med J*, 89(7), 699–706.

Owen, N. and Borland, R. (1997). Delayed compensatory cigarette consumption after a workplace smoking ban. *Tob Control*, 6(2), 131–5.

Owen, N., Borland, R., and Hill, D. (1991). Regulatory influences on health-related behaviours: the case of workplace smoking-bans. *Australian Psychologist*, 26(3), 188–91.

Palin, M. and Young, M. (1994). The impact of smoking litigation on Australian workplaces. *Tobacco Control*, 7, 61–5.

Parry, O., Platt, S., and Thomson, C. (2000). Out of sight, out of mind: workplace smoking bans and the relocation of smoking at work. *Health Promotion International*, 15(2), 125–33.

Pederson, L. L., Bull, S. B., and Ashley, M. J. (1996). Smoking in the workplace: do smoking patterns and attitudes reflect the legislative environment? *Tob Control*, 5(1), 39–45.

Peters, J., McCabe, C. J., Hedley, A. J., Lam, T. H., and Wong, C. M. (1998). Economic burden of environmental tobacco smoke on Hong Kong families: scale and impact. *J Epidemiol Community Health*, 52(1), 53–8.

Philpot, S. J., Ryan, S. A., Torre, L. E., Wilcox, H. M., Jalleh, G., and Jamrozik, K. (1999). Effect of smoke-free policies on the behaviour of social smokers. *Tob Control*, 8(3), 278–281.

Pierce, J. P., Gilpin, E. A., and Farkas, A. J. (1998). Can strategies used by statewide tobacco control programs help smokers make progress in quitting? *Cancer Epidemiol Biomarkers Prev*, 7(6), 459–64.

Pikora, T., Phang, J. W., Karro, J., Corti, B., Clarkson, J., Donovan, R. J., *et al.* (1999). Are smoke-free policies implemented and adhered to at sporting venues? *Aust N Z J Public Health*, 23(4), 407–9.

Poland, B. D., Stockton, L., Ashley, M. J., Pederson, L., Cohen, J., Ferrence, R., and Bull, S. (1999). Interactions between smokers and non-smokers in public places: a qualitative study. *Can J Public Health*, 90(5), 330–3.

Proescholdbell, R. J., Chassin, L., and MacKinnon, D. P. (2000). Home smoking restrictions and adolescent smoking. *Nicotine Tob Res*, **2**(2), 159–67.

Rigotti, N. A., Arnsten, J. H., McKool, K. M., Wood–Reid, K. M., Pasternak, R. C., and Singer, D. E. (2000). Smoking by patients in a smoke-free hospital: prevalence, predictors, and implications. *Prev Med*, **31**(2 Pt 1), 159–66.

Rogers, E. M. (1995). *Diffusion of Innovation 4th Ed*. Free Press, NY.

Salmon, A. M. and Rissel, C. (1999). Smoking in enclosed shopping centres: employee and public responses to simulated violation. *Tob Control*, **8**(4), 440.

Samet, J. (1999). *Synthesis The health effects of tobacco smoke exposure on children*. Geneva: WHO.

Scollo, M., Lal, A., Hyland, A., and Glantz, S. (2003). Review of the quality of studies on the economic effects of smoke-free policy on the hospitality industry. *Tob Control*, **12**(1), 13–20.

Serra, C., Cabezas, C., Bonfill, X., and Pladevall-Vila, M. (2000). *Interventions for preventing tobacco smoking in public places (Cochrane Review)* (Vol. 4). Oxford: Update Software.

Shopland, D. R., Gerlach, K. K., Burns, D. M., Hartman, A. M., and Gibson, J. T. (2001). State-specific trends in smoke-free workplace policy coverage: the current population survey tobacco use supplement, 1993 to 1999. *J Occup Environ Med*, **43**(8), 680–6.

Sorensen, G., Rigotti, N. A., Rosen, A., Pinney, J., and Prible, R. (1991). Employee knowledge and attitudes about a work-site nonsmoking policy: rationale for further smoking restrictions. *J Occup Med.*, **33**(11), 1125–30.

Stave, G. M. and Jackson, G. W. (1991). Effect of a total work-site smoking ban on employee smoking and attitudes. *J Occup Med*, **33**(8), 884–90.

Tobacco Free Initiative (1999). *International consultation on environmental tobacco smoke (ETS) and child health*. Geneva: WHO.

Trotter, L., Wakefield, M., and Borland, R. (2002). Socially cued smoking in bars, nightclubs, and gaming venues: a case for introducing smoke-free policies. *Tob Control*, **11**(4), 300–304.

U.S. Department of Health and Human Services (1994). *Preventing Tobacco use among young people: A report of the Surgeon General*. Atlanta: US Department of Health and Human Services, Public Health Service, Centres for Disease Control and Prevention, National Centre for Chronic Disease Prevention and Health Promotion, Office on Smoking and Health.

U.S. Department of Health and Human Services (1986). *The health consequences of involuntary smoking: A report of the Surgeon General*. Rockville MD: U.S. Department of Health and Human Services.

United States Environment Protection Agency (1992). *Respiratory health effects of passive smoking: Lung cancer and other disorders*. Rockville MD: U.S. Department of Health and Environment Assessment.

Velasco, J., Eells, T. D., Anderson, R., Head, M., Ryabik, B., Mount, R., and Lippmann, S. (1996). A two-year follow-up on the effects of a smoking ban in an inpatient psychiatric service. *Psychiatr Serv*, **47**(8), 869–71.

Wakefield, M., Banham, D., Martin, J., Ruffin, R., McCaul, K., and Badcock, N. (2000a). Restrictions on smoking at home and urinary cotinine levels among children with asthma. *Am J Prev Med*, **19**(3), 188–92.

Wakefield, M., Roberts, L., and Owen, N. (1996). Trends in prevalence and acceptance of workplace smoking bans among indoor workers in South Australia. *Tob Control*, **5**(3), 205–8.

Wakefield, M. A., Chaloupka, F. J., Kaufman, N. J., Orleans, C. T., Barker, D. C., and Ruel, E. E. (2000b). Effect of restrictions on smoking at home, at school, and in public places on teenage smoking: cross sectional study. *BMJ*, **321**(7257), 333–7.

Wiebel, F. J. (1997). Health effects of passive smoking. In: *The Tobacco Epidemic. Prog Respir Res.* (ed. C. T. Bollinger and K. O. Fagerstrom), (Vol. 28, pp. 107–121). Basel: Karger.

Wieslander, G., Lindgren, T., Norback, D., and Venge, P. (2000). Changes in the ocular and nasal signs and symptoms of aircrews in relation to the ban on smoking on intercontinental flights. *Scand J Work Environ Health*, **26**(6), 514–22.

Zanetti, F., Gambi, A., Bergamaschi, A., Gentilini, F., De Luca, G., Monti, C., and Stampi, S. (1998). Smoking habits, exposure to passive smoking and attitudes to a non-smoking policy among hospital staff. *Public Health*, **112**(1), 57–62.

Chapter 42

Effective interventions to reduce smoking

Prabhat Jha, Hana Ross, Marlo A. Corrao and
Frank J. Chaloupka

Introduction

Cigarette smoking and other tobacco use currently accounts for one of every ten adult deaths world wide. Given current trends, about 500 million people alive today will die prematurely as a result of tobacco use, with one billion deaths from tobacco expected during this century (WHO 1997; Peto and Lopez 2001). Future tobacco mortality depends largely on current smoking patterns. The increase in tobacco deaths is the result of both increases in the susceptible population size and increases in age-specific disease rates. Low-income countries will pay the biggest toll in this respect, accounting for 87 per cent of the increase in tobacco-attributable deaths between 1990 and 2020 (Murray and Lopez 1997). Even though reducing smoking initiation will reduce the burden associated with smoking in the long run, the most immediate reduction in tobacco related mortality would be achieved by encouraging cessation among current smokers (Peto and Lopez 2001; Donald *et al.* 2002).

Given the public health consequences of smoking, governments have a strong incentive for intervening to reduce tobacco use. However, many governments have resisted taking strong action because of concerns that effective interventions would have harmful economic consequences. Recent efforts by the World Bank, in partnership with the World Health Organization (WHO), have addressed these concerns. A team of over 40 economists, epidemiologists, and other tobacco control experts examined the state of knowledge about tobacco use and tobacco control strategies. A summary of this work was published in 1999 (Jha and Chaloupka 1999), and the background papers contributing to this work were published in 2000 (Jha and Chaloupka 2000*a*, *b*).

This chapter reviews and updates the findings from these global analyses. It begins with an overview of trends in global tobacco use and its consequences, followed by a review of the evidence for the effectiveness of tobacco control policies and their impact on smoking initiation and cessation. A description of the types and comprehensiveness of policies currently in place and a discussion of some of the factors correlated with the strength and comprehensiveness of these policies follows. Finally, the constraints against implementing tobacco control policies and global efforts to overcome these constraints are discussed.

Tobacco use and its consequences

Our estimates indicate that over 1.1 billion people smoke worldwide, with about 82 per cent of the world's smokers residing in low- and middle-income countries (Table 42.1). Smoking prevalence is highest in the European/Central Asia region and in the East Asia/Pacific region where over one-third of the population smokes. As Table 42.1 indicates, smoking prevalence is significantly higher among men in low- and middle-income countries, with the difference between smoking prevalence among men and women being smaller in high-income countries (Jha *et al.* 2002).

The release of information linking smoking to poor health reversed the upward trend in smoking prevalence in most high-income countries. On the other hand, smoking continues to increase in many low- and middle-income countries, in part due to increasing income and trade liberalization (Taylor *et al.* 2000).

The impact of smoking on health has been extensively documented elsewhere (Peto *et al.* 1994; Gajalakshmi *et al.* 2000). Data from both high-income and low- and middle-income countries suggest that about half of all long-term regular smokers are killed by their addiction. Half of these deaths occur during productive middle age (35–69 years old) (Peto *et al.* 1994). Currently, about half of all tobacco-related deaths occur in high-income countries, while the others occur in low- and middle-income countries. Recent major studies from China (Liu *et al.* 1998; Niu *et al.* 1998), and emerging studies from

Table 42.1 Estimated smoking prevalence (by gender) and number of smokers, 15 years of age and over, by World Bank region, 1995

World Bank region	Smoking prevalence			Total smokers	
	Males (%)	Females (%)	Overall (%)	(millions)	(% of all smokers)
East Asia and Pacific	62	5	34	429	38
Europe and Central Asia	53	16	34	122	11
Latin America and Caribbean	39	22	31	98	9
Middle East and North Africa	38	7	23	37	3
South Asia (cigarettes)	20	1	11	84	7
South Asia (bidis)	20	3	12	94	8
Sub-Saharan Africa	28	8	18	56	5
Low and middle income	49	8	29	919	82
High income	37	21	29	202	18
World	47	11	29	1121	100

Note: Country economics are divided according to 1999 GNI per capita, calculated using the World Bank Atlas method. The groups are: low income, $755 or less; lower middle income, $756–$2995; upper middle income, $2996–$9265; and high income, $9266 or more (http://www.worldbank.org/data/databytopic/class.htm# Definitions_of_groups).
Source: Jha *et al.* 2002.

India (Gupta and Mehta 2000; Gajalakshmi *et al.* 2003), indicate that the overall risks of smoking are about as great as in high-income countries such as the United States and the United Kingdom (about one in two risk of death with persistent smoking). However, the pattern of smoking-related diseases in these nations is substantially different. A recent study in Chennai, India (Gajalakshmi *et al.* 2003) suggested that smoking accounted for about half of the tuberculosis deaths. Smoking caused 12 per cent of male tuberculosis deaths in China, but—in contrast to Western high-income countries, it caused few deaths from ischemic heart disease (Liu *et al.* 1998). Given the recent trends in smoking and the lags between smoking and disease onset, approximately 70 per cent of the 10 million tobacco-attributable deaths expected in 2030 will take place in low- and middle-income countries.

Smoking is more common among poor men than among rich men in nearly all countries. In developed countries, smoking accounts for approximately half of the mortality gap between rich and poor males (Bobak *et al.* 2000). For women, who have generally been smoking in large numbers for a shorter period, the relationship between smoking, smoking-attributable mortality, and socioeconomic status is more variable.

Interventions to reduce smoking

Tobacco use generates social costs that provide the rationale for government intervention in the tobacco market. Poor understanding of the addictive nature of tobacco products, particularly at the time of smoking initiation, coupled with insufficient information about the health consequences of smoking gives additional reason for government involvement (Warner *et al.* 1995; Jha *et al.* 2000c), particularly in low- and middle-income countries where general awareness of the health risks is even lower (Kenkel and Chen 2000).

In addition to preventing tobacco consumption among children, comprehensive approaches focusing on smoking cessation are critical to near-term improvements in public health. As illustrated by Fig. 42.1, a mix of tobacco control policies that is effective *only* in reducing smoking initiation would have little impact on smoking-attributable deaths during the first half of the twenty-first century. The vast majority of tobacco-attributed deaths over the next 50 years will occur among current smokers (Peto and Lopez 2001). Studies in western populations have documented the enormous benefits of quitting smoking, particularly before the onset of major diseases (Donald *et al.* 2002). Thus, cessation among today's smokers is key to progress in tobacco control over the next few decades (Fig. 42.1).

Interventions in the tobacco market can be classified as demand side or supply side interventions.

Demand side interventions

The effect of demand side interventions has been mostly examined in high-income countries. Recent studies from low- and middle-income countries provide additional

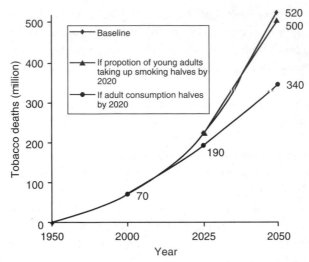

Fig. 42.1 Unless current smokers quit, tobacco deaths will rise dramatically in the next 50 years. Sources: Peto and Lopez (2001), and Peto *et al.* 1994.

Note: Peto and others estimate 60 million tobacco deaths between 1950 and 2000 in developed countries. We estimate an additional 10 million between 1990 and 2000 in developing countries. We assume no tobacco deaths before 1990 in developing countries and minimal tobacco deaths worldwide before 1950. Projections for deaths from 2000 to 2050 are based on Peto and Lopez (2000).

information on the possible impact of these interventions in different economic circumstances (Abedian *et al.* 1998).

Tobacco taxation

Historically levied to generate revenues, tobacco taxes have recently become an important tool to reduce smoking.

There are significant differences across countries in the level of tobacco taxes. As illustrated in Fig. 42.2, taxes tend to be absolutely higher and to account for a greater share of price in high-income countries. In low- and middle-income countries, taxes are generally much lower, accounting for less than half of the price of cigarettes.

Numerous studies from high-income countries demonstrate that increases in tobacco taxes lead to significant reductions in cigarette smoking and other tobacco use. This occurs as the combination of increased smoking cessation, reduced relapse, slower progression towards nicotine addiction, and decreased consumption among continuing tobacco users. The impact of price on consumption is measured by the price elasticity of demand, where the elasticity is defined as the percentage change in the quantity consumed resulting from a one-per cent increase in price.

Cigarette price elasticity estimates from high-income countries range from −0.3 to −0.5, indicating that a 10 per cent increase in cigarette prices will reduce overall

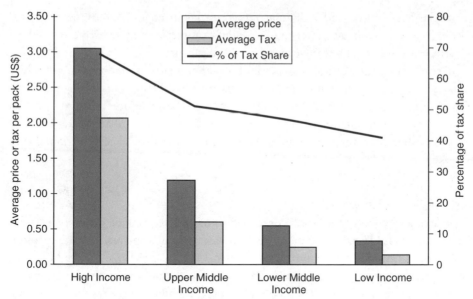

Fig. 42.2 Average cigarette price, tax, and percentage of tax share per pack, by income group, 1996.
Source: World Bank; and authors' calculations

cigarette smoking by 3–5 per cent (Chaloupka and Warner 2000; Chaloupka *et al.* 2000; USDHHS 2000). The theory of addiction accounting for slower response among addicted smokers suggests that long-run price elasticities are approximately twice as high as those in the short-run, with the long-run estimates centered on −0.8 (Becker *et al.* 1994). In addition, research confirmed an inverse relationship between price elasticity and age, with estimates for youth price elasticity of demand up to three times those obtained for adults (Harris and Chan 1999; Gruber 2000; Ross and Chaloupka 2001). Several recent studies indicate that cigarette price increases are particularly effective in reducing youth smoking uptake, preventing moving from experimentation into regular, addictive smoking (Douglas 1998; Emery *et al.* 2001; Ross *et al.* 2001; Tauras *et al.* 2001).

Several studies have explored differences in the price sensitivity of cigarette demand by income, education, and/or socioeconomic status (Chaloupka and Warner 2000; Chaloupka *et al.* 2000; USDHHS 2000). They demonstrated that less-educated persons (Chaloupka 1991), lower-income individuals (CDC 1994), and people with lower socioeconomic status (Townsend *et al.* 1994) reduce their tobacco consumption more in response to price increases than people who are more educated, have higher-income levels, and have higher socioeconomic status.

Higher price responsiveness among lower-income groups is supported by research in low- and middle-income countries (Chaloupka *et al.* 2000). In general, estimates of price elasticity for low- and middle-income countries are about double those estimated for high-income countries, implying that significant increases in tobacco taxes in these countries would be very effective in reducing tobacco use.

In summary, the empirical evidence indicates that increases in tobacco taxes reduce tobacco use by preventing initiation (and subsequent addiction), increasing the likelihood of cessation among current users, reducing relapse among former users, and reducing consumption among continuing users. Thus, higher tobacco taxes will lead to substantial improvements in public health and to lower social costs attributable to smoking.

Restrictions on smoking

Increased awareness of the health consequences of passive smoking exposure, particularly among children, has led many governments as well as private entities to adopt restrictions on smoking. While the rationale for these restrictions is to reduce non-smokers' exposure to environmental tobacco smoke, the policies also reduce smokers' opportunities to smoke. In Western populations, comprehensive restrictions on smoking lead to 5–15 per cent reductions in population smoking rates (Evans *et al.* 1999; Emont *et al.* 1992; Ohsfeldt *et al.* 1998; Hopkins *et al.* 2001; Levy and Friend 2003) and to the changes in social norms regarding smoking behavior, especially among youth (Woolery *et al.* 2000). Smoking bans in workplaces generally reduce quantity smoked by 5–25 per cent, and prevalence rates up to 20 per cent (Fichtenberg and Glantz 2002; Levy and Friend 2002). The no-smoking policies seem to be most effective when strong social norms against smoking help to make smoking restrictions self-enforcing (Jacobson and Wasserman 1997).

Health information and counter advertising

The first reports linking smoking to lung cancer released in the US and the UK in the 1960s, followed by publicity about the health consequences of smoking led to significant reductions in cigarette smoking, with initial declines between 4 and 9 per cent, and longer-term cumulative declines of 15–30 per cent (Townsend 1993; Kenkel and Chen 2000). Similar declines accompanied information dissemination on tobacco harm in low- and middle-income countries several years later (Kenkel and Chen 2000). Even after the initial information shock, mass media antismoking campaigns still have potential to reduce smoking prevalence by 4–12 per cent if sufficiently funded and combined with other tobacco control policies, and school- or community-based programme (Hopkins *et al.* 2001; Farrelly *et al.* 2002; Friend and Levy 2002). The continuing discovery of new evidence about the harmful effects of tobacco use and inadequate understanding of these risks among members of the public (Weinstein 1998), particularly in the lowest, income countries implies, however, that there is still much to be done in terms of health education.

Bans on advertising and promotion

Econometric studies exploring the relationship between cigarette advertising and cigarette demand have produced mixed findings, with the majority of them concluding that advertising has, at most, a small positive impact on demand (Townsend 1993; Chaloupka *et al.* 2000). However, critics of these studies note that econometric methods, which estimate the impact of a marginal change in advertising expenditures on smoking, are ill suited for studying the impact of total advertising (Townsend 1993; Chaloupka *et al.* 2000; FTC 2001). All cigarette producers operate at a highly saturated level of advertising exposure where the effect of a small change in advertising expenditures is almost untraceable. Approaches employing qualitative methods to evaluate the impact of cigarette advertising do support the hypothesis that increased exposure leads to higher cigarette demand (UK Department of Health 1992; USDHHS 1994).

Studying the impact of advertising and promotion bans on cigarette smoking provides more direct evidence on the impact of advertising (Chaloupka and Warner 2000; Saffer 2000). For example, a recent study predicted that a comprehensive set of tobacco advertising bans in high-income countries could reduce tobacco consumption by over 6 per cent, adjusted for price effects (Saffer and Chaloupka 2000). The study also concludes that partial bans have little impact on smoking behavior, given that the tobacco industry can shift its resources from the banned media to those that are not banned.

Smoking initiation and cessation interventions

Preventions of smoking initiation is important for long-term reduction in tobacco consumption. However, smoking cessation is the key to reversing the current unfavorable trend in smoking-related mortality over the next few decades.

Several studies using data from the US and the UK have concluded that it is possible to slow down smoking uptake and to motivate individuals to quit smoking using demand side interventions. There is some evidence that higher cigarette prices reduce smoking initiation. One study predicts that a 10 per cent rise in cigarette prices reduces the probability of smoking initiation from 3 per cent to 10 per cent depending on how initiation is defined (Tauras *et al.* 2001). Higher tobacco taxes were linked both to more quit attempts and quit success. It is estimated that a 5 per cent increase in tax can lead to a reduction in smoking of approximately 6–9.5 months (Forster and Jones 1999), and that a 10 per cent increase in cigarette prices increases the percentage of successful cessation by 8.5 per cent and quit attempts by 2.8 per cent in one year (Levy and Romano 2002). Two economic analyses of US young adults data confirmed a positive and significant impact of higher cigarette prices on the probability of first-time cessation as well as on subsequent cessation for those individuals who were unable to remain smoke-free after at least one prior cessation attempt (Tauras 1999; Tauras and Chaloupka 1999). According to these studies, a 10 per cent increase in cigarette price increases the probability of smoking cessation success by 3.4 per cent.

Besides price, limits on smoking at home and at school that are relatively strong and are enforced can slow down smoking uptake (Pierce and Gilpin 2001). Restriction on smoking at workplaces and at home can also increase cessation attempts and lower rates of relapse among smokers who attempt to quit (Wakefield *et al.* 2000; Levy and Romano 2002). Smoking restrictions are often a reflection of antismoking social norms that make smoking behavior less attractive, thus reducing the motivation for smoking initiation and increasing the probability of smoking cessation (Nyborg and Rege 2000).

Tobacco advertising and marketing is linked to higher rate of smoking experimentation (Pierce *et al.* 1998). In addition, comprehensive antismoking media campaigns (Pierce and Gilpin 2001; Levy and Romano 2002) and long-term community-wide programs (Korhonena *et al.* 1999; Farrelly *et al.* 2002) lead to more quit attempts and higher smoking abstinence rates.

Along with population-based cigarette demand interventions, there are individual-level efforts relying on behavioral treatments of smoking cessation. They range from self-help manuals and on-line quit guides to clinical interventions (USDHHS 2000). Recently, pharmacological treatments, including nicotine replacement therapies (NRTs) and antidepressants such as bupropion, have become widely available in high-income countries (Novotny *et al.* 2000; USDHHS 2000). There is mixed evidence on the impact of behavioral therapies on successful smoking cessation (Novotny *et al.* 2000; USDHHS 2000). Nevertheless, pharmacological treatment is linked to greater likelihood of quitting, with success rates two times those when this aid is not employed (Raw *et al.* 1999; Novotny *et al.* 2000; USDHHS 2000). The demand for NRT and other pharmacological therapies is related to economic factors, including their price (Tauras and Chaloupka 2001). Policies that decrease the cost of NRT and increase its availability would likely lead to substantial increases in the use of these products. The evidence from the US suggests that full coverage of a tobacco-dependence treatment benefit and/or their sale over-the-counter (OTC) are effective and relatively low-cost strategies for significantly increasing quit rates and quit attempts among adult smokers (Keeler *et al.* 2002). The net impact of NRT in low- or middle-income countries has been less well studied.

Table 42. 2 summarizes the current knowledge about the efficacy of various public health measures with respect to smoking initiation and smoking cessation.

Even though the recent attention to smoking uptake and cessation begins to fill in the knowledge gap, there are still many aspects of this complex behavioral change that need to be investigated in order to design more effective public policies encouraging smoking cessation and preventing smoking initiation.

Effectiveness of demand side interventions

Research has demonstrated that demand side interventions are highly effective in reducing the demand for tobacco products and that their widespread adoption would generate substantial reductions in the public health toll from tobacco.

Table 42.2 The effect of public health measures with respect to smoking initiation and cessation

Intervention	Initiation	Cessation

Price/tax increases	Evidence of negative effects
	Higher effect on initiation
	  of regular smoking then on
	  experimentation (social sources)
	10% increase in price: 3–9.5%
	  lower probability of
	  smoking initiation
		Evidence supports positive effect on
		  no. of attempts and on the success
		10% increase in price: 11–13%
		  shorter smoking duration; or
		  3.4% higher probability of cessation
		5% increase in tax: 6–9.5 months
		  shorter smoking duration

Antismoking
  media campaigns
	Some evidence of negative
	  effects of aggressive and well-
	  funded campaigns; more
	  effective when complemented
	  with school- or community-
	  based programs
		Positive effect of health information on
		  no. of attempts and on the success
		Positive effect of comprehensive
		  campaigns on no.of
		  attempts and on the success
		Existence of cessation program
		  improves success
		Positive effect of community
		  level Interventions

Tobacco advertising
  and marketing
	Positive effect on female initiation
	Positive effect on susceptibility
	  to smoking and experimentation
	Total ban reduces initiation
		Total ban has positive effect
		  (6% reduced consumption)
		Partial ban not effective

Youth access
  restrictions
	Weak evidence of negative
	  effect on uptake progress,
	  initiation and experimentation
		No evidence of an effect, perhaps
		  due to weak enforcement

Smoking
  restrictions
	Negative effect of school and
	  household restrictions if
	  enforced and relatively strong
	Mixed results for public places
	  restrictions
		Positive effect (particularly work and
		  household restrictions)
		Clean indoor air laws improve
		  probability of successful quitting

NRT	No evidence	Positive effect on the efficacy of quit attempts Positive effect on no. of attempts

Source: Authors.

Table 42.3 summarizes findings from a recently updated simulation model that estimates the global impact of alternative policies aimed at reducing the demand for tobacco (Ranson *et al.* 2001). The assumptions underlying this simulation model are deliberately conservative. Nevertheless, the results indicate that substantial savings in human lives would result from the various policy changes. A 10 per cent price increase, for example, would reduce expected smoking-attributable deaths among current smokers globally by an estimated 5–16 million. Similarly, lives can be saved by increased use of NRT and by introducing a comprehensive set of nonprice measures. This analysis concludes that these interventions are highly cost-effective, particularly

Table 42.3 Potential impact of a price increase of 10%, increased NRT use, and a package of nonprice measures

Region	Smoking-attributable deaths (millions)	Change in number of deaths (millions)					
		10% price increase		NRT with effectiveness of		Nonprice interventions with effectiveness of	
		Low elasticity*	High elasticity*	0.5%	2.5%	2%	10%
Low-income and middle-income	303	−4.6 −(1.5%)	−13.7 −(4.5%)	−1.1 −(0.3%)	−5.3 −(1.7%)	−4.2 −(1.4%)	−21.2 −(7.0%)
High-income	67	−0.5 −(0.7%)	−2.0 −(3.0%)	−0.2 −(0.3%)	−1.2 −(1.7%)	−0.9 −(1.4%)	−4.7 −(7.0%)
World	370	−5.1 −(1.4%)	−15.7 −(4.2%)	−1.3 −(0.3%)	−6.5 −(1.7%)	−5.2 −(1.4%)	−25.9 −(7.0%)

*Low elasticity is −0.2 for high-income regions and −0.4 for low-income and middle-income regions. High elasticity is −0.8 for high-income regions and −1.2 for low-income and middle-income regions.
Source: Ranson et al. 2001.

for low- and middle-income countries, when compared to other public health interventions.

Supply side interventions

In contrast to the effectiveness of demand side interventions, interventions reducing the supply of tobacco were not found very effective in curbing the epidemic (WHO 1997). For example, limiting youth access to tobacco was not yet clearly linked to less tobacco use (USDHHS 2000; Woolery et al. 2000). The effective implementation and enforcement of these policies also requires infrastructure and resources that are difficult to secure. Crop substitution and diversification programs usually do not reduce tobacco supply (Jacobs et al. 2000). While trade liberalization has contributed to increases in tobacco use, particularly in low- and middle-income countries, restrictions on trade in tobacco that violate international trade agreements may result in retaliatory measures harming the whole economy (Taylor et al. 2000).

The key intervention on the supply side is the control of cigarette smuggling, currently estimated to amount for 6–8 per cent of global consumption (Merriman et al. 2000). While differences in taxes and prices across countries suggest a motive for smuggling, a recent analysis showed that corruption within countries is a stronger predictor of smuggling than price (Merriman et al. 2000). Effective anti-smuggling supply side measures are not very well studied, but are likely to include prominent tax stamps and warning labels in local languages, better methods for tracking cigarettes through the distribution chain, aggressive enforcement of antismuggling law, and stronger penalties for those caught violating these laws (Joossens *et al.* 2000).

Comprehensive programs to reduce tobacco use

Comprehensive programs to reduce tobacco use are based on an assumption that there is a synergy among various antismoking policies improving their individual effectiveness. In general, these programs have one or more of four key components: national and community interventions, counter marketing campaigns, policy and regulation, and surveillance and evaluation (USDHHS 2000). Recent evidence from the US and UK clearly indicate that these comprehensive efforts have been successful in reducing tobacco use and in improving public health (Townsend 1998; USDHHS 2000; Wakefield and Chaloupka 2000; Farrelly *et al.* 2001).

Coverage of effective tobacco control policies

While there is substantial evidence concerning the effectiveness of numerous policy interventions to reduce tobacco use, their implementation is uneven and limited. An analysis of legislative data abstracted from the *Tobacco Control Country Profiles* database (Corrao *et al.* 2000) indicates that the higher-income countries have more antismoking laws in place than the low- and middle-income countries. Evidence points to a positive relationship between the comprehensiveness of tobacco control policies and income level, but there are also wide differences among countries within an income group (Chaloupka *et al.* 2001). These differences were found not to be linked to the relative employment in tobacco agriculture, but may be affected by tobacco industry lobbying power, and other factors such as rule of law and government effectiveness. The country's overall commitment to tobacco controls is also reflected in active enforcement of tobacco control provisions (Chaloupka *et al.* 2001).

Political resistance to tobacco control usually comes from worries about the loss of budget income from tobacco tax. Often, governments do not realize that if tobacco disappears from the economy, there is no net tax loss, because other products can replace tobacco as a tax base. Providing evidence that tobacco control programs, including research, could be self-financing when funded by tobacco excise taxes, can diminish the opposition. Another political tool used to gain the political and civil society support for tobacco control is to earmark tobacco tax. Earmarking could secure funds for services that would not have existed otherwise.

The Framework Convention on Tobacco Control (FCTC) could help to overcome some of the concerns about tobacco control policies. The FCTC aims to be an international treaty that would commit 191 member states of the WHO to adopting strong, effective tobacco control policies (Taylor and Bettcher 2000). The FCTC could be most effective in addressing issues associated with tobacco industry globalization such as restricting tobacco advertising and promotion, controlling the smuggling of tobacco products, improving the sharing of information internationally, and more.

Conclusions

Tobacco use is a huge and growing cause of death worldwide. If the current consumption patterns continue, it will kill about 1 billion people in the twenty-first century. There is strong evidence that tobacco tax increases, the dissemination of information about the health risks from smoking, restrictions on smoking in public places and workplaces, comprehensive bans on advertising and promotion, and increased access to cessation therapies are effective in reducing tobacco use. Despite this evidence, these policies have been unevenly applied, partly due to political constraints and lack of awareness about the effectiveness and cost-effectiveness of these interventions. Tobacco control advocates and those conducting research in this area will play an important role in dealing with this global public health problem.

References

Abedian, I., van der Merwe, R., Wilkins, and Jha, P. (ed.) (1998). *The economics of tobacco control: Towards an optimal policy mix*. University of Cape Town, Cape Town.

Becker, G. S., Grossman, M., and Murphy, K. M. (1994). An empirical analysis of cigarette addiction. *American Economic Review*, **84** (3), 396–418.

Bobak, M., Jha, P., Nguyen, S., and Jarvis, M. (2000). Poverty and smoking. In: *Tobacco control in developing countries* (ed. P. Jha, and F.J. Chaloupka), Oxford University Press, 41–61.

Centers for Disease Control and Prevention (1994). Response to increases in cigarette prices by race/ethnicity, income, and age groups—United States, 1976–1993. *Morbidity and Mortality Weekly Report*, **43** (26), 469–72.

Chaloupka, F. J. (1991). Rational addictive behavior and cigarette smoking. *Journal of Political Economy*, **99** (4), 722–42.

Chaloupka, F. J. and Warner, K. E. (2000). The economics of smoking. In: *Handbook of health economics* (ed. A. J. Culyer, J. P. Newhouse), pp. 1539–627. North-Holland, Amsterdam.

Chaloupka, F. J., Hu, T.-W., Warner, K. E., Jacobs, R., and Yurekli, A. (2000). The taxation of tobacco products. In: *Tobacco control in developing countries* (ed. P. Jha, and F.J. Chaloupka), pp. 237–72. Oxford University Press, Oxford.

Chaloupka, F., Jha, P., Corrao, M., Costa e Silva, V. L., Ross, H., Czart, C., and Yach, D. (2001). *Smoking-related mortality*. WHO Commission on Macroeconomics and Health Working Paper Series, June 25.

Corrao, M. A., Guindon, G. E., Sharma, N., and Shokoohi, D. F. (ed.) (2000). *Tobacco control country profiles*. American Cancer Society, Atlanta, GA.

Donald, H., Taylor, Jr., Vic Hasselblad, S., Jane Henley, Michael J., Thun, and Frank, A. Sloan (2002). Benefits of smoking cessation for longevity. *Am. J. Public. Health*, **92**, 990–6.

Douglas, S. M. (1998). The duration of the smoking habit. *Economic Inquiry*, **vXXXVI n1**, 49–64.

Emery, S. L., White, M. M., and Pierce, J. P. (2001). Does cigarette price influence adolescent experimentation? *Journal of Health Economics*, **20** (2), 261–70.

Emont, S. L., Choi, W. S., Novotny, T. E., and Giovino, G. A. (1992). Clean indoor air legislation, taxation and smoking behavior in the United States: An ecological analysis. *Tobacco Control*, **2**, 13–7.

Evans, W. N., Farrelly, M. C., and Montgomery, E. (1999). Do workplace smoking bans reduce smoking? *American Economic Review*, **89** (4), 728–47.

Farrelly, M. C., Pechacek, T. F., and Chaloupka, F. J. (2003). The impact of tobacco control program expenditures on aggregate cigarette sales: 1981–2000. *Journal of Health Economics*, 22, 843–59.

Farrelly, M. C., Niederdeppe, J., and Yarsevich, J. (July 2002). Future directions in tobacco countrymarketing mass media campaign, Working paper. Presented at Innovations in Youth Tobacco Control Conference, Santa Fe.

Federal Trade Commission (2001). Cigarette Report for 1999. Federal Trade Commission, Washington DC.

Fichtenberg, C. M. and Glantz, S. A. (2002). Effect of smoke-free workplaces on smoking behaviour: Systematic review. *British Medical Journal*, 325, 188.

Forster, M. and Jones, A. M. (1999). The role of tobacco taxes in starting and quitting smoking: Duration analysis of British Date. Working Paper, University of York, September 3.

Friend, K. and Levy, D. (2002). Reductions in smoking prevalence and cigarette consumption associated with mass-media campaigns. *Health Education Research*, 17 (1), 85–98.

Gajalakshmi, C. K., Jha, P., Ranson, K., and Nguyen, S. (2000). Global patterns of smoking and smoking attributable mortality. In: *Tobacco control in developing countries* (ed. P. Jha, and F.J. Chaloupka), pp. 11–39. Oxford University Press, Oxford.

Gajalakshmi, V., Peto, R., Kanaka, S., and Jha, P. (2003). Smoking and mortality in India: Retrospective study of 43,000 adult male deaths and 35,000 controls. *Lancet*, 362, 507–15.

Gruber, J. (2000). Youth smoking in the US: Prices and policies. Working paper no. 7507. National Bureau of Economic Research, Cambridge (MA).

Gupta, P. C. and Mehta, H. C. (2000). Cohort study of all-cause mortality among tobacco users in Mumbai, India. *Bull World Health Organ*, 78(7), 877–83.

Harris, J. E. and Chan, S. W. (1999). The continuum-of-addiction: Cigarette smoking in relation to price among Americans aged 15–29. *Health Economics*, 8 (1), 81–6.

Hopkins, D. P., Briss, P. A., Ricard, C. J., Husten, C. G., Carande-Kulis, V. G., Fielding, J. E., *et al.* (2001). Task Force on Community Preventive Services. Reviews of evidence regarding interventions to reduce tobacco use and exposure to environmental tobacco smoke. *American Journal of Preventive Medicine*, 20 (2S), 16–52.

Jacobs, R., Gale, H. F., Capehart, T. C., Zhang, P., and Jha, P. (2000). The supply-side effects of tobacco-control policies. In: *Tobacco control in developing countries* (ed. P. Jha, and F.J. Chaloupka), pp. 311–41. Oxford University Press, Oxford.

Jacobson, P. D. and Wasserman, J. (1997). *Tobacco control laws: Implementation and enforcement.* RAND, Santa Monica.

Jha, P. and Chaloupka, F. J. (1999). *Curbing the epidemic: Governments and the economics of tobacco control.* World Bank, Washington, DC.

Jha, P. and Chaloupka, F. J. (2000a). *Tobacco control in developing countries.* Oxford University Press, Oxford.

Jha, P. and Chaloupka F. J. (2000b). The economics of global tobacco control. *British Medical Journal*, 321, 358–61.

Jha, P., Musgrove, P., Chaloupka, F. J., and Yurekli, A. (2000c). The economic rationale for intervention in the tobacco market. In: *Tobacco control in developing countries* (ed. P. Jha and F. J. Chaloupka), pp. 153–74. Oxford University Press, Oxford.

Jha, P., Kent Ranson, M., Nguyen, Son, N., Yach, Derek. (June 2002). Estimates of global and regional smoking prevalence in 1995, by age and sex. *American Journal of Public Health*, 92(6).

Joossens, L., Chaloupka, F. J., Merriman, D., and Yurekli, A. (2000). Issues in the smuggling of tobacco products. In: *Tobacco control in developing countries* (ed. P. Jha and F. J. Chaloupka), pp. 393–406. Oxford University Press, Oxford.

Keeler, T. E., *et al.* (2002). The benefits of switching smoking cessation drugs to over-the-counter status. *Health Economics*, **11**(5), 389–402.

Kenkel, D. and Chen, L. (2000). Consumer information and tobacco use. In: *Tobacco control in developing countries* (ed. P. Jha and F. J. Chaloupka), pp. 177–214. Oxford University Press, Oxford.

Korhonena, T., Urjanheimob, E.-L., Mannonenc, P., Korhonena, H. J., Uutelaa, A., and Puska, P. (1999). Quit and Win campaigns and a long-term anti-smoking intervention in North Karelia and other parts of Finland. *Tobacco Control*, **8**, 175–81.

Levy, D. and Friend, K. (August 2001). Clean air laws: A framework for evaluating and improving clean air laws. *Journal of Public Health Management and Practice*, **7**(5), 87–97.

Levy, D. and Friend, K. (2003). A review of the literature on clean air laws: Where do we go from here? *Health Education Research*, Oct **18**(5), 592–609.

Levy, D. T. and Romano, E. (2002). The relationship of smoking cessation to socio-demographic characteristics, smoking intensity and tobacco control policies. *Tobacco Control*.

Liu, L., Peto, R., Chen, Z., *et al.* (1998). Emerging tobacco hazards in China. I. Retrospective proportional mortality study of one million deaths. *British Medical Journal*, **317**(1), 411–22.

Merriman, D., Yurekli, A., and Chaloupka, F. J. (2000). How big is the world wide cigarette smuggling problem? In: *Tobacco control in developing countries* (ed. P. Jha and F. J. Chaloupka), pp. 365–92. Oxford University Press, Oxford.

Murray, C. J. and Lopez, A. D. (1997). Mortality by cause for eight regions of the world: Global Burden of Disease Study. *Lancet*, **349**, 1269–76.

Niu, S. R., Yang, G. H., Chen, Z. M., Wang, J. L., Wang, G. H., He, X. Z., Schoepff, H., Boreham, J., Pan, H. C., and Peto, R. (1998). Emerging tobacco hazards in China 2. Early mortality results from a prospective study. *British Medical Journal*, **317**(7170), 1423–4.

Novotny, T. E., Cohen, J. C., Yurekli, A., Sweaner, D., and de Beyer, J. (2000). Smoking cessation and nicotine-replacement therapies. In: *Tobacco control in developing countries* (ed. P. Jha and F. J. Chaloupka), pp. 287–307. Oxford University Press, Oxford.

Nyborg, K. and Rege, M. (July 2000). The evolution of considerate smoking behavior. Discussion Paper No. 279, Statistics Norway, Research Department, <http://www.ssb.no>.

Ohsfeldt, R. L., Boyle, R. G., and Capilouto, E. I. (1998). Tobacco taxes, smoking restrictions, and tobacco use. NBER Working Paper Series. National Bureau of Economic Research, Cambridge, MA. March NBER Working Paper 6486.

Peto, R. and Lopez, A. D. (2001). The future worldwide health effects of current smoking patterns. In: *Critical issue in global health* (ed. E. C. Koop, C. E. Pearson, and M. R. Schwarz), pp. 154–61. Jossey-Bass, New York.

Peto, R., Lopez, A. D., Boreham, J., Thun, M., and Health, C., Jr. (1994). *Mortality from smoking in developed countries, 1950–2000*. Oxford University Press, Oxford.

Peto, R., Darby, S., Deo, H., Silcocks, P., Whitley, E., and Doll, R. (2000). Smoking, smoking cessation, and lung cancer in the UK since 1950: Combination of national statistics with two case-control studies. *British Medical Journal*, **321**, 323–9.

Pierce, J. P. and Gilpin, E. A. (2001). New media coverage of smoking and health is associated with changes in population rates of smoking cessation but not initiation. *Tobacco Control*, **10**, 145–53.

Pierce, J. P., Gilpin E. A., Emery, S. L., *et al.* (1998). Has the California tobacco control program reduced smoking? *Journal of the American Medical Association*, **280**, 893–99.

Ranson, M. K., Jha, P., Chaloupka, F. J., and Nguyen, S. N. (2001). Global and regional estimates of the effectiveness and cost-effectiveness of price increases and other tobacco control policies. Working paper, Health Policy Unit, London School of Hygiene and Tropical Medicine.

Raw, M., Mc Neill, A., and West, R. (1999). Smoking cessation: Evidence-based recommendations for the healthcare system. *British Medical Journal*, **318**, 182–85.

Ross, H., Chaloupka, F. J., and Wakefield, M. (2001*a*). Youth smoking uptake progress: Price and public policy effects. Research paper no. 11. ImpacTeen, Health Research and Policy Centers, University of Illinois at Chicogo, Chicago.

Ross, H. and Chaloupka, F. J. (2001*b*). The effect of public policies and prices on youth smoking. Research paper no. 8. ImpacTeen, Health Research and Policy Centers, University of Illinois at Chicago, Chicago.

Saffer, H. (2000). Tobacco advertising and promotion. In: *Tobacco control in developing countries* (ed. P. Jha and F. J. Chaloupka), pp. 215–36. Oxford University Press, Oxford.

Saffer, H. and Chaloupka, F. (2000). Tobacco advertising: Economic theory and international evidence. *Journal of Health Economics*, **19**(6), 1117–37.

Tauras, J. A. (November 1999). The transition to smoking cessation: Evidence from multiple failure duration analysis. NBER Working Paper 7412.

Tauras, J. A. and Chaloupka, F. J. (July 1999). Determinants of smoking cessation: An analysis of young adult men and Women. NBER Working Paper 7262.

Tauras, J. A., and Chaloupka, F. J. (June 2001). The demand for nicotine replacement therapies. NBER Working Paper 8332.

Tauras, J. A., Johnston, L. D., and O'Malley, P. M. (June 2001). An analysis of teenage smoking initiation: The effects of government intervention. NBER Working Paper 8331.

Taylor, A. L. and Bettcher, D. W. (2000). WHO framework convention on tobacco control: A global 'good' for public health. *Bulletin of the World Health Organization*, **78**(7), 925.

Taylor, A. L., Chaloupka, F. J., Guindon, E., and Corbett, M. (2000). The impact of trade liberalization on tobacco consumption. In: *Tobacco control in developing countries* (ed. P. Jha and F. J. Chaloupka), pp. 343–64. Oxford University Press, Oxford.

Townsend, J. L. (1993). Policies to halve smoking deaths. *Addiction*, **88**, 43–52.

Townsend, J. (1998). UK smoking targets: Policies to attain them and effects on premature mortality. In: *The economics of tobacco control: Towards an optimal policy mix* (ed. I. Abedian, R. van der Merwe, N. Wilkins, and P. Jha), pp. 185–98. Applied Fiscal Research Centre, University of Cape Town, Cape Town.

Townsend, J. L., Roderick, P., and Cooper, J. (1994). Cigarette smoking by socio-economic group, sex, and age: Effects of price, income, and health publicity. *British Medical Journal*, **309**(6969), 923–6.

UK Department of Health (1992). Effect of tobacco advertising on tobacco consumption: A discussion document reviewing the evidence. UK Department of Health, Economics and Operational Research Division, London.

US Department of Health and Human Services (1994). Preventing tobacco use among young people. A report of the Surgeon General. US Department of Health and Human Services, Public Health Service, Centers for Disease Control, Center for Chronic Disease Prevention and Health Promotion, Office on Smoking and Health, Atlanta, Georgia.

US Department of Health and Human Services (2000). Reducing tobacco use. A report of the Surgeon General. US Department of Health and Human Services, Public Health Service, Centers for Disease Control, Center for Chronic Disease Prevention and Health Promotion, Office on Smoking and Health, Atlanta, Georgia.

Wakefield, M. A. and Chaloupka, F. J. (2000). Effectiveness of comprehensive tobacco control. Programs in reducing teenage smoking in the United States. *Tobacco Control*, **9**(2), 177–86.

Wakefield, M. A., Chaloupka, F. J., Kaufman, N. J., Orleans, C. T., Barker, D. C., and Ruel, E. E. (August 2000). Effect of restrictions on smoking at home, at school, and in public places on teenage smoking: Cross sectional study. *British Medical Journal*, **321**, 333–37.

Warner, K. E., Chaloupka, F. J., Cook, P. J., Manning, W. G., Newhouse, J. P., Novotny, T. E., *et al*, (1995). Criteria for determining an optimal cigarette tax. The economist's perspective. *Tobacco Control*, **4**, 380–86.

Weinstein, N. D. (1998). Accuracy of smokers' risk perceptions. *Annals of behavioral Medicine*, **20**, 135–40.

Woolery, T., Asma, S., and Sharp, D. (2000). Clean indoor-air laws and youth access. In: *Tobacco control in developing countries* (ed. P. Jha and F. J. Chaloupka), pp. 273–86. Oxford University Press, Oxford.

World Bank, The World Development Report (1993). *Investing in health*. Oxford University Press, New York, NY.

World Health Organization (1997). *Tobacco or health: A global status report*. World Health Organization, Geneva.

Part 13

Treatment of dependence

Chapter 43

Treatment of tobacco dependence

Michael Kunze and E. Groman

Introduction

This chapter will review the state of the art of treatment of tobacco dependence, based on recent international recommendations and will also point out to some additional findings, especially those generated by the Nicotine Institute Vienna, the first specialized institution in Austria, founded 1998 to reduce the burden of tobacco-related diseases (Groman *et al.* 1999*b*).

On the basis of the 1980 UICC Guidelines for Smoking Control (Gray and Daube 1980), we started our work on developing guidelines on diagnosis and treatment of tobacco dependence back in 1984 (Kunze and Wood 1984).

The US Surgeon General Report of 1990 came up with major conclusions, which were the basis for further research on how to improve treatment of tobacco dependence (US Department of Health and Human Services 1990).

The big problem for the implementation of treatment is the relation between candidate patients, who need treatment, and the availability of services, which can provide treatment. For the Austrian situation we made the assumption, that at least 130 000 people would need specialized treatment services (Groman *et al.* 2000*a*).

Research into the genetics of smoking has increased our understanding of nicotine dependence, and is likely to illuminate the mechanisms by which cigarette smoking adversely effects the health of smokers. Given recent advances in molecular biology, including the completion of the draft sequence of the human genome, interest has now turned to identifying gene markers that predict a heightened risk of using tobacco and developing nicotine dependence (Hall *et al.* 2002).

Tobacco dependence and its epidemiology

The cumulative findings of more that 2500 scientific papers led to the conclusion that cigarettes and other forms of tobacco are addictive, that nicotine is the drug in tobacco that causes addiction and that the pharmacological and behavioural processes that determine tobacco addiction are similar to those underlying other drugs such as heroine or cocaine (US Department of Health and Human Services 1988). Nicotine is psychoactive, euphoric, and reinforcing, produces tolerance, results in physiological dependence and has useful effects (weight control, mood control, relief of tobacco withdrawal symptoms).

Tobacco dependence is associated with heavy consumption, tolerance, regulation of intake, and withdrawal. Most smokers experience withdrawal symptoms such as dysphoria/depressed mood, insomnia, irritability/frustration/anger, anxiety, difficulty of concentration, restlessness, decreased heart rate, and increased appetite (Hughes 1991).

Tobacco dependence occurs often and is the most important barrier to cessation. It shows interesting epidemiological features, some of them are outlined below.

One of the first studies in this respect was undertaken by Lagure *et al.* in France. Over 1000 people took part in a telephone survey using the Fagerström Tolerance Questionnaire (FTQ) (Lagrue *et al.* 1989). Approximately one-third of those who were smokers (34% of the total sample) had an FTQ score of 3 or less (low dependence), 47% had a score of between 4 and 6, and 19% had a score of 7 or more (*severe dependence*).

A smaller study (*n*=201) was conducted by Hale and co-workers (1993) in the US, using the criteria for drug dependence from the Diagnostic and Statistical Manual of Mental Health III (DSM-III) (American Psychiatry Association 1987). Using these criteria, they found that 24% of their sample were severely dependent (7–9 criteria), 26% were moderately dependent (5–6 criteria), 30% were mildly dependent (3–4 criteria), and 18% were not dependent (0–2 criteria).

Another study has been performed using the six-question Fagerström Test for Tobacco dependence (FTND) in a representative population sample in Austria.

The sample consisted of 6000 randomly selected Austrians (aged 14 years or over) who were interviewed face-to-face. 42% of men and 27% of women reported to be smokers (Kunze 1993). Using a five-level categorization of the epidemiology of tobacco dependence in Austria based on the FTND score, it was found that the majority of smokers (all age groups and both sexes), 34%, had what was designated 'low' dependence (FTND score 3–4), 30% had very low dependence (FTND score 0–2), and the remaining 36% were divided between the medium, high, and very high dependence groups (Schoberberger 1993).

There are interesting transcultural differences in degrees of tobacco dependence. In societies where rates of smoking are low, it is feasible to suppose that the remaining smokers are more highly dependent. The FTND should enable the epidemiological aspects of tobacco dependence in different populations to be investigated in more detail, with a view to assisting in the determination of the most effective treatment for tobacco dependence in smoking cessation.

The lower the smoking prevalence in a country is, the higher the dependence level of remaining smokers is; this is a result of selective quitting, because less dependent smokers are probably stopping to a larger extent than more dependent smokers. In the United States, a country with a low smoking prevalence, the smokers show a high tobacco dependence. In other countries (Austria and Poland) the smoking prevalence is high, but the averaged tobacco dependence is low (Fagerström *et al.* 1996).

Nocturnal sleep-disturbing nicotine craving

Working with heavy dependent patients we have noticed a sleep disturbance, which is a further symptom of extreme tobacco dependence. We call this symptom 'nocturnal sleep-disturbing nicotine craving' (NSDNC). NSDNC is characterized by craving for cigarettes during the individual sleep times. The smoker awakes (one or several times per week) during his regular sleep time, and has to smoke a cigarette before he/she continues sleeping. This symptom can be explained by the decreasing nicotine levels during sleeping, which results in nicotine craving. However, NSDNC should be carefully separated from other sleep disturbances, or sleep disturbing events (nocturia, medication side effects), when nicotine craving is not the main reason for awakening (Rieder *et al.* 2001).

State of the art

To review the state of the art of treatment of tobacco dependence three important documents are reviewed: M. Raw, P. Anderson, A. Batra, G. Dubois, P. Harrington, A. Hirsch, J. Le Houezec, A. McNeill, D. Milner, M. Pötschke-Langer, W. Zatonski: WHO Europe evidence-based recommendations on the treatment of tobacco dependence. Tobacco Control 2002; 11:44–46; Michael C. Fiore: Consensus Statement: A clinical practice guideline for treating tobacco use and dependence. JAMA, June 28, 2000, Vol. 283, 3244–3254; National Institute for Clinical Excellence: Guidance on the use of nicotine replacement therapy (NRT) and bupropion for smoking cessation. Technology Appraisal Guidance, No. 39, March 2002.

The WHO Europe Recommendations (Raw *et al.* 2002) have been written as an initiative of the World Health Organization European Partnership Project to Reduce Tobacco Dependence.

These recommendations so far have been endorsed by many professional organizations dealing with the tobacco problem.

For brief intervention this document provides the following guidelines.

- As part of their normal clinical work doctors should include the following essential features:
  - ask about, and record smoking status, keep record up to date;
  - advise smokers of the benefit of stopping in a personalized and appropriate manner (this may include linking the advice to their clinical condition)
    - Assess motivation to stop.
    - Assist smokers in their stop attempt if possible; this might include the offer of support, recommendation to use NRT or bupropion, and accurate information and advice about them, referral to a specialist cessation service if necessary.
    - Arrange follow up if possible.

If help can be offered a few key points can be covered in a few minutes:

- set a stop day and stop completely on that day;
- review past experience and learn from it (what helped? what hindered?);
- make a personalized action plan;
- identify likely problems and plan how to cope with them;
- ask family and friends for support.

For smoking cessation specialists the WHO Europe Recommendations conclude:

The health care system should offer treatment as back up to brief opportunistic interventions for those smokers who need more intensive support. This support can be offered individually or in groups, and should include coping skills training and social support. A well-tested group format includes around five sessions of about one hour over about one month with follow up. Intensive support should include the offer of or encouragement to use NRT or bupropion (as appropriate) and clear advice and instruction on how to use them.

With regard to pharmacotherapies it is stated:

At the moment the principal aids in this category are NRT and bupropion. There are currently six NRT products: patch, gum, nasal spray, inhalator, tablet, lozenge.

In addition the WHO Europe Recommendations offer guidelines for specific groups:

Treatment research has tended to focus on health professionals such as doctors (especially in primary care), nurses, midwives, pharmacists, and smoking cessation specialists. However, advising and supporting smokers in stopping is an activity for the whole health care system and should, eventually, be integrated into as many settings as possible throughout the system. This includes hospital and community settings. In many countries, however, there is still a high smoking prevalence among health professionals, so in addition to the education and training recommended below, health professionals should be targeted for help in stopping smoking.

Hospital staff should ask about patients' smoking status before or on admission, and offer brief advice and assistance to those interested in stopping. Patients should be advised of the hospital's smoke free status before admission. Hospital patients who need it should also be offered NRT or bupropion.

Healthcare premises and their immediate surroundings should be smoke free. Pregnant smokers should receive clear and accurate information on the risks of smoking to the fetus, and be advised to stop smoking. They should be offered specialist support to stop.

Cessation interventions shown to be effective with adults should be considered for use with young people, with the content modified as necessary.

The WHO recommendations for health care purchasers and systems include among other the following statements:

Purchasing treatment for tobacco dependence represents an extremely cost effective way of reducing ill health and prolonging life. Health care purchasers should purchase tobacco dependence treatments, choosing a blend of options relevant to local circumstances but emphasizing those interventions which have the strongest evidence base.

Because tobacco dependence treatment is so cost effective, it should be provided by public and private health care systems. Access to both behavioural and pharmaceutical treatments should be as wide as possible with due regard to local regulatory frameworks and other circumstances. It is important to increase the availability or treatment to low income smokers, including at a reduced cost or free of charge.

Health professionals should be trained to advise and help smokers stop smoking, and health care purchasers should ensure the provision of adequate training budgets and training programmes. Education and training for the different types of interventions should be provided not only at the postgraduate and clinical level, but should start at undergraduate and basic level, in medical and nursing schools and other relevant training institutions.

Telephone helplines can be effective and are very popular with smokers. Although more research is needed on their effectiveness, they seem likely to provide a valuable service to smokers and should be made available where possible.

A second important review is the US consensus statement: A Clinical Practice Guideline for Treating Tobacco Use and Dependence (Fiore 2000).

The panel, which compiled the consensus statement included 18 scientists, clinicians, consumsers, and methodologists selected by the US Agency for Healthcare Research and Quality. A consortium of seven governmental and non-profit organizations sponsored the update.

Approximately 6000 english-language, peer-reviewed articles and abstracts, published between 1975 and 1999, were reviewed for data that addressed assessment and treatment of tobacco dependence. This literature serviced as the basis for more than 50 meta-analysis.

Major conclusions and recommendations include:

- Tobacco dependence is a chronic condition that warrants repeated treatment until long-term or permanent abstinence is achieved.
- Effective treatments for tobacco dependence exist and all tobacco users should be offered those treatments.
- Clinicians and health care delivery systems must institutionalize the consistent identification, documentation, and treatment of every tobacco user at every visit.
- Brief tobacco dependence treatment is effective, and every tobacco user should be offered at least brief treatment.
- There is a strong dose–response relationship between the intensity of tobacco dependence counselling and its effectiveness.
- Three types of counselling were found to be especially effective—practical counselling, social suppport as part of treatment, and social support arranged outside of treatment.

- Five first-line pharmacotherapies for tobacco dependence—sustained-release bupropion hydrochloride, nicotine gum, nicotine inhaler, nicotine nasal spray, and nicotine patch—are effective, and at least one of these medications should be prescribed in the absence of contraindications.
- Tobacco dependence treatments are cost-effective relative to other medical and disease prevention interventions; as such, all health insurance plans should include as a reimbursed benefit the counselling and pharmacotherapeutic treatments identified as effective in the updated guideline.

In 2002 the UK National Institute for Clinical Excellence issued the report: Guidance on the use of nicotine replacement therapy (NRT) and bupropion for smoking cessation (National Institute for Clinical Excellence 2002).

This report reviews in great detail the pharmaceutical treatment of tobacco dependence as of today. Among many others the following are seen to be very important:

- Nicotine replacement therapy (NRT) and bupropion are recommended for smokers who have expressed a desire to quit smoking.
- There is currently insufficient evidence to conclude that one form of NRT is more effective than another.
- In trials, a combination of two different NRTs was in general more effective than a single NRT.
- Both bupropion and NRT are considered to be among the most cost effective of all health care interventions.
- The likelihood that a smoker will be successful in quitting depends on several factors: the smoker's motivation; the extent of the smoker's tobacco dependence; the intensity and quality of the support offered; and the use of pharmacological aids.
- NRT in general is associated with few adverse events. Users of bupropion, however, will sometimes suffer adverse events, occasionally serious, and which are now well known.

Advice to stop smoking—the possible role of the internet

In recent years the internet has come up as a convenient and comprehensive means of information on how to stop smoking. A number of products to quit smoking is offered. We have examined smoking cessation products distributed via the internet and evaluated them from a scientific point of view (Eckl-Dorna and Groman 1999).

The study was conducted by using the search string 'stop + smoking' in two of the most popular internet search engines, yahoo (www.yahoo.com) and lycos (www.lycos.com). Sites offering only advice were excluded. Only sites that offered products to stop smoking were chosen. These products were then evaluated, by screening for published papers in peer-reviewed journals. In one case we tested a product measuring resulting carbon monoxide levels.

Fifteen different products were identified most on sites not updated since 1997. Eight out of the 14 products could be ordered by internet, six are described in detail in the internet, but could only be obtained in the pharmacy. Two-third of the products, however, do not have any scientific background: Two products were filters (1+2) to reduce the nicotine supply. Other products were a CD ROM (3) with relaxing products and a pocket-safe for cigarettes. The main ingredients in five products were herbal extracts (5–9), that have no proven effect on nicotine addiction. Consumption of herbal cigarettes resulted in high carbon monoxide values (Groman *et al.* 1999*a*).

Just five products were based on a scientific findings (published in peer reviewed journals). These were the nicotine replacement products: patch, gum, inhaler, nasal spray, and bupropion (Groman *et al.* 2000*b*).

The results show that most of the products lack a scientific background. Adverse health effects after consumption of herbal cigarettes, which are sold for smoking cessation cannot be excluded. This example shows the necessity of continuous assessment and observation of the market, and the need for scientific studies on smoking cessation products. An international body to examine the sites would be useful (Eckl-Dorna and Groman 1999).

Reduced smoking

As far as the management of smoking behaviour is concerned, complete abstinence remains the best option. Nevertheless one has to take into account that many tobacco consumers want to reduce their consumption, either as a first step towards abstinence or as a strategy of its own to reduce their health risk (Jiménez-Ruiz *et al.* 1998). At this time 37% of the Austrian smokers want to reduce and only 18% want to stop smoking.

The concept of reduced or controlled smoking will become more important in future. Reduced smoking means smoking fewer cigarettes on individual level. Nicotine replacement is the best medication to reduce smoking. Most smokers need the nicotine and not the tar or carbon monoxide or any other toxic substances contained in cigarettes (Jiménez-Ruiz *et al.* 1998).

Reduced smoking in combination with nicotine replacement therapy may be indicated for those who are failing in cessation attempts, who would like to give up smoking but are not able to quit. The second group which wants to reduce cigarette consumption may be smokers who do not want to quit but only reduce (Kunze *et al.* 1998). The new experience of smoking fewer cigarettes without withdrawal symptoms may also lead to a higher quitting rate.

With respect to the practical management of reduced smoking, baseline smoking parameters must by ascertained, preferably using exhaled CO or plasma COHb levels. Measuring CO in the expired air is a very simple way to assess the actual smoking behaviour of a tobacco consumer and provides also a measurement which usually is very impressive for the patient/client. Alternatively, plasma nicotine and/or cotinine (the major metablite of nicotine, with a much longer half-life) levels could also be used but these more complicated methods cannot distinguish between nicotine taken from tobacco smoking or nicotine replacement.

Smokers should be fully informed about reduced smoking, and the end goals—complete cessation for those wishing to quit and a significant reduction in the number of cigarettes/day for those not yet ready or motivated to quit—should be discussed. A common goal for both groups could be a 50% reduction in the number of cigarettes/day within a few weeks of commencement. Smokers need time to adjust to their nicotine replacement medications and it is important that full information is provided on the use of the various preparations available. It is preferable to allow smokers to try different nicotine preparations and select the one they feel to be most helpful on an individual basis. Although none of the existing nicotine replacement medications is more effective than the others, the utility of different preparations may vary across smokers. In addition, long-term compliance is likely to be better if individuals feel comfortable with their chosen preparation (Kunze 1997).

With other drug dependences harm reduction has been controversial and it is possible that reduced smoking also will be subject to similar debate within the public health community and the society at large.

Another caveat for reduced smoking is the possible impact on attitudes of people considering quitting tobacco consumption and who might prefer reduced smoking to complete abstinence. Whether there is such a sub-sample of smokers and how big it is, further research will have to address. Further careful monitoring of smoking patterns will show whether this development is to be observed or not (Kunze 1997).

Tobacco dependence and lung cancer

Nicotine is addictive, but not a carcinogen. Nicotine is the substance which maintains tobacco consumption. It is necessary to deal with the issue of tobacco dependence when dealing with preventive medicine in general and preventive oncology in particular.

Lung cancer is a tumour very suitable for preventive programmes. Lung cancer risk is very much related to tar exposure. There is a clear dose–response relationship between tar exposure and lung cancer risk. If people highly addicted to nicotine are also experiencing a comparatively high tar exposure, then self-help alone is most probably not sufficient to provide preventive oncology.

Those people who can stop on their own or by minimal intervention are most probably not the ones who suffer from the highest tar exposure and are therefore not in the highest risk group for contracting lung cancer. This is especially the case if other risk factors than tar exposure are present. Clustering of risk factors (including occupational exposure, poor nutritional status, tar exposure, and nicotine addiction), has to be taken into account.

In summary, tobacco dependence among lung cancer patients is much higher than in the general population. Highly dependent smokers are in a high risk group for contracting lung cancer and other smoking related diseases, and therefore need specific intervention techniques for treating tobacco dependence.

The clinical evidence of a beneficial effect of chemoprevention in lung cancer is still limited. Chemopreventive trials have failed or produced unexpected and disappointing results. It seems therefore that long-term application of Alternative Nicotine Delivery Systems (ANDS)(NRT) provides a possibility of 'chemoprevention' of lung cancer and other tobacco-related diseases.

As the highly dependent tobacco consumers experience the highest lung cancer risk and are least likely to stop smoking, alternative strategies (such as ANDS/NRT) are essential because this concentrates on the high risk group which might contract lung cancer in the next years (Kunze *et al.* 1998).

The future of nicotine replacement products

The following statements are based on various perspectives, most of them already established.

♦ NR products have been shown as well in scientific studies as in real life to be effective, safe, and very well accepted compounds to help people stop smoking.

♦ Using them not only for cessation purposes but also for harm reduction/reduced smoking or controlled smoking purposes will attract the attention of many tobacco consumers.

♦ Based on our experiences we want to change the message to the public from 'You must stop smoking' to 'We want to inform you'.

♦ This new message and other new techniques like craving management need a lot of communication efforts and additional scientific studies; this does not mean promotion of these objectives is not yet feasible but additional scientific research is needed.

♦ It will be one of the most important tasks to reach out for those tobacco consumers who have had experience with NR products but who did not achieve abstinence.

♦ New messages in this respect are the one about underdosing, the message 'it can be done if you use enough of NRT, and if you use some of the new NRT-products'.

♦ Among the new messages for smokers and doctors the underdosing problems have to be addressed and identified as one of the major reasons for not having success.

♦ It might be necessary to be as open as possible and stress the fact: one cannot necessarily 'cure' tobacco dependence but it is possible to control it.

♦ Today even extreme forms of tobacco dependence can be treated; this message should be the basis for a new self confidence among treatment providers and a new trust into NR products among the consumers.

- One could even question whether the endless discussion as to what procedure or product might be better replaced by simply adding: 'if you take care of consumers/patients intensively, if you use enough of NRT, especially in combination, then you can be successful.
- Success may need to be redefined: abstinence, harm reduction, craving management.
- This leads to the issue of high-dose NR treatment using much higher dosage than before based on the unique safety patterns of NR products.
- It will be necessary to both study and to advocate high-dose nicotine replacement much more than before.
- Encouraging long-term treatment is another important strategy and for example, might be the only measure to help some of the most exposed tobacco consumers.
- It will be necessary to focus on combination of various NR products (therefore a 'family of different products is necessary' and construction of NR and non-NR if feasible and useful.
- The 'let them choose' approach is essential (people should choose from the wide range of products).
- New information techniques and settings need to be introduced, e.g. group approaches (60′ introduction into the use of NR products) have been demonstrated to be useful and very cost effective. Modern communication techniques to establish long-term collaboration will be used much more than before (e.g. call centers, internet-based methods).
- It has been shown that reimbursement of diagnostic and treatment services will improve the use and success of NR products and smoking cessation in general.
- NR products may have (at some time) a role in new areas, weight control and recreational use being only two examples.

To maximize patients compliance it is necessary to give them the possibility to choose between the NRT products. This 'let them choose approach' is focusing on the specific preferences and needs of the individual patient (Kunze *et al.* 1998).

A very frequent problem in use of ANDS is that of under-dosing. Many clients are concerned about toxicity of nicotine or are afraid of getting dependent. Most patients under-dose rather than over-dose (Kunze 2000). Smokers have to be told that NRT products deliver a low dose of nicotine over a long period of time and that a resulting dependence is unlikely (Balfour and Fagerström 1996; Hurt *et al.* 1997).

From a public health point of view, OTC (over the counter, without prescription) status for ANDS is essential because easy access to smoking control devices will lead to more quit attempts. The broader availability and promotion of effective treatment for tobacco dependence will increase the number of smokers availing themselves of the medications. Since the US Food and Drug Administration approved nicotine medications for OTC sale in 1996, the use of nicotine medications has increased by 152% compared with prior prescription use (Shiffman *et al.* 1997).

In many countries NRT products are now available OTC. One of the reasons for this is that using ANDS is safe and dependence is very unlikely. The consequences of the OTC status is the facilitation of access and encouraging smokers to use ANDS. The number of quit attempts is also increasing (Kunze *et al.* 1998).

Some countries also see NRT products being delivered by means of general sales. Experiences with this kind of distribution need to be monitored and evaluated at a later stage.

Conclusions

Useful smoking cessation treatments are available. However, they need to be made more available and to be used more aggressively. Higher dosing needs to be considered, especially for patients for whom abstinence is not the likely outcome. Reduced smoking is better than heavy smoking. Cessation services need to be institutionalized more widely and the health professions, in particular, must set examples.

References

American Psychiatry Association (1987). *Diagnostic and Statistical Manual of Mental Health III (DSM–III)*. Diagnostic and Statistical Manual of Mental Disorders, DSM-III, Washington DC.

Balfour, D. L. K. and Fagerström, K. O. (1996). Pharmacology of nicotine and its therapeutic use in smoking cessation and neurodegenerative disorders. *Pharmacology and Therapeutics*, **10**, 1–30.

Eckl-Dorna, J. and Groman E. (1999). Evidence and not evidence-based products offered for smoking cessation on the world wide web. *MEDNET*, Abstracts Book, 17–8.

Fagerström, K. O., Kunze, M., Schoberberger, R., Breslau, N., Hughes, J., Hurt, R.D., *et al.* (1996). Tobacco dependence versus prevalence of smoking: Comparison between countries and categories of smokers. *Tobacco Control*, **5**, 52–6.

Fiore, M. C. (2000). Consensus statement: A clinical practice guideline for treating tobacco use and dependence. *JAMA*, **283**, 3244–54.

Gray, N. and Daube, M. (1980). *Guidelines for Smoking Control* (2nd edn.), UICC Technical Report Series—Vol. 52.

Groman, E., Kunze, U., Schmeiser-Rieder, A., and Schoberberger, R. (1998). Measurement of expired carbon monoxide among medical students to assess smoking behaviour. *Soz Praventivmed*, **43**, 322–4.

Groman, E., Bernhard, G., Blauensteiner, D., and Kunze U. (1999a). A harmful aid to stopping smoking, *The Lancet*, **353**, 9151, 466–7.

Groman, E., Kunze, U., Schmeiser-Rieder, A., and Schoberberger R. (1999b). Konzept, Aufgaben und Dienststellungen eines Institutes zur Diagnostik und Therapie der Tabak-und Nikotinabhängigkeit. *Neuropsychiatrie*, **13**(3), 139–44.

Groman, E., Bayer, P., Kunze, U., Schmeiser-Rieder, A., and Schoberberger, R. (2000a). Diagnostik und Therapie der Nikotinabhängigkeit—eine Analyse des Bedarfs in Österreich. *WMW*, **150**(6), 109–14.

Groman, E., Bayer, P., Kiefer, I., Eckl-Dorna, J., and Schoberberger, R. (2000b). Bupropion (Zyban): First results of an independent clinical management study. *Sucht*, **46**(6), S408–S413.

Hale, K., Hughes, J. R., Oliveto, A. H., *et al.* (1993). Tobacco dependence in a population-based sample. In: *Problems of drug dependence* (ed. Harris LS), NIDA Research Monograph no. 132, US Government Printing Office, Washington DC.

Hull, W., Madden, P., and Lynskey, M. (2002). The genetics of tobacco use: Methods, findings and policy implications. *Tobacco Control*, **11**, 119–24.

Hughes, J. R. (1991). Distinguishing withdrawal relief and direct effects of smoking. *Psychopharmacology*, **104**, 409–10.

Hurt, R. D., Sachs, D. P. L., Glover, E. D., *et al.* (1997). A comparison of sustained-release bupropion and placebo for smoking cessation. *New England Journal of Medicine*, **337**, 1195–202.

Jiménez-Ruiz, C., Kunze, M., and Fagerström, K. O. (1998). Nicotine replacement: a new approach to reducing tobacco-related harm. *Eur Respir J*, **11**, 473–9.

Jorenby, D. E., Leischow, S. J., and Nides, M. A., *et al.* (1999). A controlled trial of sustained-release bupropion, a nicotine patch, or both for smoking cessation. *The New England Journal of Medicine*, **340**(9), 685–91.

Kunze, M. (1993). *State of the art of tobacco cessation.* Vortrag anläßlich der 3rd International Conference on Preventive Cardiology, Oslo, 27.06.-01.07.1993

Kunze, M. (1997). Harm reduction: The possible role of nicotine replacement. In: *The Tobacco Epidemic* (eds. Bolliger CT and Fagerström KO), Prog Respir Res., Basel, Karger **28**, 190–8.

Kunze, M. (2000). Maximizing help for dissonant smokers. *Addiction*, **95**(Supplement), 13–7.

Kunze, M. and Wood, M. (1984). *Guidelines on Smoking Cessation.* UICC Technical Report Series—Vol. 79, Geneva.

Kunze, U., Schoberberger, R., Schmeiser-Rieder, A., Groman, E., and Kunze, M. (1998). Alternative nicotine delivery systems (ANDS)—Public Health—Aspects. *Wien Klin Wochenschr*, **110/23**, 811–16.

Lagrue, G., Grimaldi, C., Demaria, C., *et al.* (1989). Épiedémiologie de la dépendance physique à la nicotine. *Seminars Hospital Paris*, **65**, 2448–50.

Messinezy, M. and Pearson, T. C. (1993). Apparent polycythaemia: Diagnosis, pathogenesis and management. *Eur J Haematol*, **51**(3), 125–31.

National Institute for Clinical Excellence (2002). Guidance on the use of nicotine replacement therapy (NRT) and bupropion for smoking cessation. Technology Appraisal Guidance, No. 39.

Raw, M., Anderson, P., Batra, A., Dubois, G., Harrington, P., Hirsch, A., *et al.* (2002). WHO Europe evidence based recommendations on the treatment of tobacco dependence. *Tobacco Control*.

Rieder, A., Kunze, U., Groman, E., Kiefer, I., and Schoberberger, R. (2001). Nocturnal sleep-disturbing nicotine craving: A newly described symptom of extreme tobacco dependence. *Acta Med Austriaca*, **28**(1), 21–2.

Schoberberger, R. (1993). Psychological and physiological dependence. Vortrag anläßlich der 3rd International Conference on Preventive Cardiology, Oslo, 27.06.-01.07.1993

Schoberberger, R., Kunze, U., Schmeiser-Rieder, A., Groman, E., and Kunze, M. (1998). Wiener Standard zur Diagnostik der Nikotinabhängigkeit: Wiener Standard Raucher-Inventar (WSR). *Wiener Med Wochenschr*, **148**(3), 52–64.

Shiffman, S., Gitchell, J., Pinney, J. M., Burton, S. L., Kemper, K. E., and Lara, E. A. (1997). Public benefit of over-the-counter nicotine medications. *Tob Control*, **6**, 306–10.

US Department of Health and Human Services (1988). The health consequences of smoking: Nicotine addiction—a report of the surgeon general. Office on Smoking and Health, Rockville.

US Department of Health and Human Services (1990). The Health Benefits of Smoking Cessation. A Report of the Surgeon General, Public Health Service, DHHS Publication No. (CDC) 90-8416.

Chapter 44

Regulation of the cigarette: Controlling cigarette emissions

Nigel Gray

Remarkably, the cigarette has escaped orthodox regulation of content and emissions in all countries, although there are some regulations capping such measures as 'tar', nicotine, and carbon monoxide. These have been measured by the Federal Trade Commission (FTC) method (United States Public Health Service 1996) or slight variants thereof. In a few countries additives must be notified, but are not controlled. The reasons for this strange arrangement in a world where consumer products as simple as the humble sausage are routinely regulated, are difficult to define. Certainly the tobacco industry influence has been opposed to detailed regulation until very recently, but this is not the only reason. Regulators have, understandably, been reluctant to enter the field until as recently as 1996 (Kessler *et al.* 1996). This is not surprising as the products are immensely complex and vary greatly between and within brands and countries (Fischer *et al.* 1990; Gray *et al.* 2000; Gray and Boyle 2002). The technical challenges of regulating such a product are substantial not only because of the complexity of smoke chemistry, but also because no regulator wishes to take responsibility for 'approving' a product which is dangerous, thereby removing at least some of the responsibility for its dangers from the shoulders of the manufacturers.

This latter point remains a serious concern for regulators but the reason that the time for regulation has come is that 50 years of leaving cigarette design, unconstrained except for tar, nicotine, and carbon monoxide, to the tobacco industry, has not delivered a product with acceptably reduced risk (Thun and Burns 2001). That regulation is timely is agreed, for example, by Philip Morris (now named Altria), whose web site states the following (Philip Morris USA 2002).

'Philip Morris U.S.A. strongly supports the passage of legislation that would establish a tough but reasonable framework giving the U.S. Food and Drug Administration (FDA) the authority to regulate cigarettes. We believe FDA regulation would provide greater consistency in tobacco policy, more predictability for our business and an effective way to address issues that are of concern to our company and society.'

Issues set out in the website include: Youth smoking prevention; Ingredient and constituent testing and disclosure; text of health warnings on cigarette packages and in advertisements; consistent use of brand descriptors such as 'light' and 'ultra light';

good manufacturing practices for cigarettes; and standards for defining, and for the responsible marketing of any, reduced-risk cigarettes.

The public health reasons for regulation would include most of these issues but are somewhat different. They include the need to provide the consumer with the minimum risk cigarette, one that is correctly labelled and provides a dose of nicotine that is as consistent as possible and carries the lowest possible dose of carcinogens and toxins in its wake.

This chapter will not deal with alternative drug delivery devices in which tobacco is heated but not burnt on the grounds that they should automatically be regulated in the same way as any other drug delivery devices. They are also considered elsewhere in the book (Chapter 9).

While there has been discussion of the concept of regulation and the need for powers to do this (Kessler *et al.* 1996) there has been little discussion of ways in which regulation might be applied to smoke constituents. It is therefore a fruitful field on which to ponder points of principle.

The case for harm reduction

Over time, and rightly, the focus of tobacco control has been the achievement of abstinence. This focus should not be diminished in any way by regulatory attempts to reduce the health risks of the product.

Nevertheless it is absurd to allow the continued marketing of cigarettes which are unnecessarily dangerous and this chapter will argue that the cigarette of today is far more dangerous than it need be. This is not to suggest that a 'safe' cigarette is even a remote possibility. Even if the measures proposed here are adopted it will remain a major cause of premature mortality, but it is suggested that condoning the continued marketing of a cigarette which is evidently more carcinogenic and toxic than it need be would be negligent in a public health sense. Everything that *can* be done to reduce tobacco's death toll *should* be done.

The modern cigarette continues to be a serious problem (Thun and Burns 2001; Wayne and Connolly 2002; Kozlowski and O'Connor 2002) because it remains extremely dangerous (Thun and Burns 2001), is smoother, easier to smoke and easier to learn to smoke (Wayne and Connolly 2002), and designed to facilitate compensation (Kozlowski and O'Connor 2002). It delivers more nitrosamines than it used to (Hoffmann and Hoffmann 2001) and these vary both between brands and within global brands (Gray *et al.* 2000). The smoke of a selected group of brands in the United States shows differences in delivery between 26 selected US brands of sevenfold for benz(*a*)pyrene, eightfold for lead, tenfold for arsenic, and fourfold for 4-(methylnitrosamino)-1-(3-pyridyl)-1-butanone (NNK) (Gray and Boyle 2002).

The program of tar and nicotine reduction did not produce the mortality benefits that were hoped for. Tar was indeed reduced and this did reduce benz(*a*)pyrene levels as these correlate quite well with tar (Hoffmann and Hoffmann 2001). Much of this potential benefit was lost because of compensation, although the relative decline in the risk of squamous cell carcinoma (Cox and Yesner 1979; Rimington 1981; Johnson 1988; el-Torky *et al.* 1990; Stellman *et al.* 1997*a, b*), and some of the decline in risk seen in earlier studies (Bross and Gibson 1968; Wynder *et al.* 1970; Hammond *et al.* 1976; Hawthorne and Fry 1978; Wynder and Stellman 1979; Rimington 1981; Lubin 1984; Stellman 1986; Stellman and Garfinkel 1989) and among men under 50 in the United Kingdom (Peto *et al.* 2000) may well be attributed to this factor. Conversely the increased relative risk of adenocarcinoma is presumably an outcome of changes in cigarette composition with nitrosamines a likely factor in this.

The campaign for reduction in tar (and nicotine) yields has been used by the tobacco industry as way of reassuring smokers who are contemplating quitting (Kozlowski and Pillitteri; Shiffman *et al.* (*a*); Shiffman *et al.* (*b*)). 'Light' cigarettes are, in fact, not light, as compensatory smoking is facilitated by the designs to an extent that inhalation of carcinogens and toxins may be as great with these brands as with regular cigarettes (Djordjevic *et al.* 1995). It is therefore not surprising that 'harm reduction' as represented by attempts to make the cigarette constituents less harmful has been the object of scepticism. Harm reduction by use of nicotine replacement therapy (NRT) as an aid to reducing smoking in those who cannot quit is dealt with elsewhere (Chapter 43).

General principles

In principle, a consumer product should be as safe as possible and in the case of a drug should deliver as precise a dose as possible. Contaminants (in this case carcinogens and toxins) should be minimal with upper limits set. Additives should also be demonstrably safe. The cigarette is unique in that it cannot be made safe. However, the dose of drug (nicotine) delivered could certainly be made more precise and upper limits could certainly be set for the contaminants which are much lower than presently seen on the market. New measurement systems are certainly needed.

Some fundamental questions arise here.

◆ Should limits for carcinogens and toxins be set as low as possible? Can it possibly be justified to add, or allow, higher levels of, carcinogens for 'flavour' or other purposes?

◆ The real purpose of the cigarette is to deliver nicotine. It is proven as the fastest (and most addictive) nicotine delivery system yet known (Gourlay and Benowitz 1997). Should the dose per cigarette be standardized as far as is practical?

◆ Should the nicotine dose be 'satisfying' without the need for deep and frequent inhalation which brings with it a larger dose of contaminants?

◆ If a 'satisfying' dose is to be delivered, how should this be measured for regulatory purposes.

- How should the dose be measured (and communicated) for consumer purposes?
- Additives are routinely added to make the smoke less 'harsh' and to reduce the irritating effect of nicotine on the throat, and for many other purposes. Should such additives be allowed without testing for toxicity in both burnt and unburnt form?
- Cigarette designs frequently facilitate compensatory smoking, which means that the smoker inhales more deeply and frequently in order to attain the desired dose of nicotine. Abolition of such items as ventilated filters would make compensation more difficult. Is there any reason NOT to do this?
- Should standards be set for filters?
- Should standards be set for papers?

A regulatory approach

The contaminants

Mainstream smoke contains approximately 4800 (Hoffmann and Hoffmann 2001) constituents, among which Hoffmann has listed 48 'major' constituents of the vapour phase of cigarette smoke; 51 major constituents of the particulate phase, 13 major toxins, and 69 carcinogens. In 1999 the US tobacco industry performed a 'benchmark study' for the Massachusetts Department of Public Health in which 43 smoke constituents were tested (Borgerding *et al.* 2000), these being the ones most widely considered of major consequence.

Since it is normally the task of regulators to set limits for specific compounds (such as chemicals in car exhaust gases) rather than tell manufacturers how to make their product, the same approach to smoke constituents seems reasonable. In this context it would be logical to set limits for, say, certain tobacco specific nitrosamines (TSNAs) in smoke rather than to control the precursors in the leaf and curing processes.

Further, any regulatory approach has to be feasible and there is merit in looking at the market as it stands to see what is possible. This is not to say that the regulatory process need be unduly slow simply because its introduction would change the market substantially. If criteria were set for one to two years time which allowed only twenty brands to remain on the market, the public could still have their nicotine needs met and the industry could still sell cigarettes and make money. Such a concept would perhaps be perceived as draconian by the manufacturers and generous by the public health community. Nevertheless, in dealing with carcinogens and serious toxins, there is no reason why cigarette manufacturers should be allowed to choose particular blends or add substances to their product in order to produce 'flavour' or any other effect without demonstrating (relative) safety of these blends and substances in their burnt form, as would be required with any other product.

There is not much data in the public arena concerning smoke emissions of known brands. However, there is evidence of serious variation in nitrosamines between and within three major global brands (Gray *et al.* 2000) varying from threefold within Camel to ninefold within Marlboro for a single nitrosamine, 4-(methylnitrosamino)-1-(3-pyridyl)-1-butanone (NNK). Further, an analysis of the Massachusetts benchmark study (Gray and Boyle 2002) revealed variations between 26 selected US brands of sevenfold for benz(*a*)pyrene, eightfold for lead, tenfold for arsenic and four-fold for NNK. Such a degree of variation may be perceived as inevitable in a market of 900 or so brands, but is unacceptable in any sense for public health.

The obvious regulatory response must be to reduce all the selected list of carcinogens and toxins as far as possible. If the median of the market as revealed by those 26 brands (considering 34 substances) were set as the upper limit, then only one brand out of the 26 would survive the regulatory blow unscathed (Gray and Boyle 2002). If one brand can be manufactured to meet these criteria, more can clearly be made so if required. This approach would discommode the tobacco industry greatly in the short term but could be regarded as generous by the public health establishment. The key point is that it is possible, is reasonable and should be accepted.

The system of measurement needed for this proposal is relatively simple and could be the existing FTC method or a variant such as that used in parallel with FTC in the Massachusetts benchmark study or (and better) the two-stage test proposed by Kozlowski (Kozlowski and O'Connor 2000), but the ultimate measure would be the amount per litre of smoke of each compound. The principle espoused could deal with all the accepted major toxins and carcinogens but would be unsatisfactory for nicotine.

Nicotine

Nicotine is the driving force for inhalation and for the degree of compensatory smoking that occurs. At this time the measurement and labelling of the cigarette does not provide any reasonable index of the dose that the individual smoker (and smoking habit) (Djordjevic *et al.* 1995; Jarvis *et al.* 2001) obtains.

Two separate questions arise here. The first is how to reduce the 'elasticity' of the cigarette in order to deliver a relatively standard dose. The second is what should the standard dose range be. A corollary is what measurement system should be used.

Towards a standard dose

The first issue is to find a way of measuring and defining the nicotine dose in such a way that it provides a reasonable approximation of the amount of nicotine likely to finish up in the bloodstream of the smoker. This is only conceivable if the cigarette design is made substantially less elastic, i.e. more difficult to smoke in a compensatory way. A measure of the amount of nicotine present in the rod of the cigarette could serve but only with this proviso. Abolition of ventilated filters (Kozlowski and O'Connor 2002) would be a major step towards this, together with some standization of filters and papers.

In terms of amount, the dose should probably be something close to the amount the smoker currently seeks, and gets. A study by Jarvis (Jarvis *et al.* 2001) throws some light on this. This study reveals two important things. One that the average amount of salivary cotinine (a satisfactory surrogate for nicotine) achieved is fairly similar regardless of FTC yield. The second is that there is great diversity in the amount of nicotine taken, many smokers actually 'undersmoking' as well as many 'oversmoking'. Since a major object of regulation is to reduce contaminant intake the starting range for nicotine dose should be something that provides saliva levels of cotinine between the low and the high levels currently seen, so that compensation is not increased. Clearly this requires research on humans with various doses delivered by unventilated cigarettes. Consideration would also need to be given to (possibly higher) doses that reduced compensation under experimental conditions.

Other restrictions on cigarette chemistry would bear on the nicotine dose but might arise from limitations that might be placed on additives for other reasons.

Communicating the dose

If regulation can reduce the range of the dose available by compensatory smoking so that it varies much less, then a suitable measure would be the total amount in the cigarette rod—which has an analogy to the current labelling of alcohol.

Additives

The modern cigarette may include up to about 600 additives, which are nominated to certain health departments but for which safety testing is not yet required in burnt form. The European Union has legislated for disclosure and the provision of toxicology of additives in burnt and unburnt form and the effect of this legislation on the composition of the cigarette has yet to be seen. However, the future of the cigarette must certainly include a move towards simplicity as an orthodox approach to such a consumer product would usually require detailed testing of each chemical added to the basic raw material, in this case in burnt form. This approach could properly be taken to all additives, which should be broadly defined so that all additives, starting with fertilizer and ending with the paper, should meet the criterion that they do not add to the harmfulness of the product.

Future nicotine policy

The question of reducing, over time, the amount of nicotine in the cigarette with the intention of making it less addictive has been raised (Benowitz and Henningfield 1994) and needs consideration. This is discussed under 'Global Tobacco Policy'—Chapter 37.

Conclusions

It is past time for the cigarette to be regulated. The object should be to provide the consumer with the minimum risk cigarette, one that is correctly labelled, provides a dose of nicotine that is as consistent as possible and carries the lowest possible dose of carcinogens and toxins in its wake. Regulation by existing authorities responsible for pharmaceutical regulation would seem sensible. The probable effect would be a considerable simplification of the cigarette, with much smaller amounts, and smaller variation in the amounts, of carcinogens and toxins in the inhaled smoke. Another effect might be a significant diminution in the number of brands on the market.

References

Benowitz, N. L. and Henningfield, J. E. (1994). Establishing a nicotine threshold for addiction. The implications for tobacco regulation. *N Engl J Med*, **331**, 123–5.

Borgerding, M. F., Bodnar, J. A., and Wingate, D. E. (2000). The 1999 massachusetts Benchmark study—the final report. Conducted for the Massachusetts Department of Public Health by the Tobacco Industry. Massachusetts Department of Public Health, Massachusetts.

Bross, I. D. and Gibson, R. (1968). Risks of lung cancer in smokers who switch to filter cigarettes. *Am J Public Health Nations Health*, **58**, 1396–403.

Cox, J. D. and Yesner, R. A. (1979). Adenocarcinoma of the lung: Recent results from the Veterans Administration Lung Group. *Am Rev Respir Dis*, **120**, 1025–9.

Djordjevic, M. V., Fan, J., Ferguson, S., and Hoffmann, D. (1995). Self-regulation of smoking intensity. Smoke yields of the low-nicotine, low-'tar' cigarettes. *Carcinogenesis*, **16**, 2015–21.

el-Torky, M., el-Zeky, F., and Hall, J. C. (1990). Significant changes in the distribution of histologic types of lung cancer. A review of 4928 cases. *Cancer*, **65**, 2361–7.

Fischer, S., Spiegelhalder, B., and Preussmann, R. (1990). Tobacco-specific nitrosamines in European and USA cigarettes. *Arch Geschwulstforsch*, **60**, 169–77.

Gourlay, S. G. and Benowitz, N. L. (1997). Arteriovenous differences in plasma concentration of nicotine and catecholamines and related cardiovascular effects after smoking, nicotine nasal spray, and intravenous nicotine. *Clin Pharmacol Ther*, **62**, 453–63.

Gray, N. and Boyle, P. (2002). Regulation of cigarette emissions. *Ann Oncol*, **13**, 19–21.

Gray, N., Zaridze, D., Robertson, C., Krivosheeva, L., Sigacheva, N., and Boyle, P. (2000). Variation within global cigarette brands in tar, nicotine, and certain nitrosamines: analytic study. *Tob Control*, **9**, 351.

Hammond, E. C., Garfinkel, L., Seidman, H., and Lew, E. A. (1976). 'Tar' and nicotine content of cigarette smoke in relation to death rates. *Environ Res*, **12**, 263–74.

Hawthorne, V. M. and Fry, J. S. (1978). Smoking and health: The association between smoking behaviour, total mortality, and cardiorespiratory disease in west central Scotland. *J Epidemiol Community Health*, **32**, 260–6.

Hoffmann, D. and Hoffmann, I. (2001). The changing cigarette: Chemical studies and bioassays. In: *Risks associated with smoking cigarettes with low machine-measured yields of tar and nicotine* (Anonymous), pp. 159–91. Bethesda: US Department of Health and Human Services, National Institutes of Health, National Cancer Institute].

Jarvis, M. J., Boreham, R., Primatesta, P., Feyerabend, C., and Bryant, A. (2001). Nicotine yield from machine-smoked cigarettes and nicotine intakes in smokers: Evidence from a representative population survey. *J Natl Cancer Inst*, **93**, 134–8.

Johnson, W. W. (1988) Histologic and cytologic patterns of lung cancer in 2580 men and women over a 15-year period. *Acta Cytol*, **32**, 162–8.

Kessler, D. A., Witt, A. M., Barnett, P. S., Zeller, M. R., Natanblut, S. L., Wilkenfeld, J. P., Lorraine, C. C., Thompson, L. J., and Schultz, W. B. (1996) The Food and Drug Administration's regulation of tobacco products. *N Engl J Med*, **335**, 988–94.

Kozlowski, L. T. and O'Connor, R. J. (2000). Official cigarette tar tests are misleading: Use a two-stage, compensating test. *Lancet, Jun.17.;355.(9221.):2159.-61.* **355**, 2159–2161.

Kozlowski, L. T. and O'Connor, R. J. (2002). Cigarette filter ventilation is a defective design because of misleading taste, bigger puffs, and blocked vents. *Tob. Control 2002.Mar.;11.Suppl.1.:I40.-50.* **11 Suppl 1:I40–50**, I40–I50.

Kozlowski, L. T. and Pillitteri, J. L. (2001). Beliefs about 'Light' and 'Ultra Light' cigarettes and efforts to change those beliefs: An overview of early efforts and published research. *Tob Control; 10.Suppl.1.:i12.-6.* **10 Suppl 1:i12–6.**, i12–i16.

Lubin, J. H. (1984). Modifying risk of developing lung cancer by changing habits of cigarette smoking. *Br Med J (Clin Res Ed)* **289**, 921.

Peto, R., Darby, S., Deo, H., Silcocks, P., Whitley, E., and Doll, R. (2000). Smoking, smoking cessation, and lung cancer in the UK since 1950: Combination of national statistics with two case–control studies. *BMJ 2000.Aug.5.;321.(7257.):323.-9.* **321**, 323–9.

Philip Morris USA. FDA Regulation. Philip Morris USA. 2002. Philip Morris USA. (GENERIC) Ref Type: Electronic Citation.

Rimington, J. (1981). The effect of filters on the incidence of lung cancer in cigarette smokers. *Environ Res*, **24**, 162–6.

Shiffman, S., Pillitteri, J. L., Burton, S. L., Rohay, J. M., and Gitchell, J. G. (2001) (*a*). Effect of health messages about 'Light' and 'Ultra Light' cigarettes on beliefs and quitting intent. *Tob Control, 10.Suppl.1.:i24.-32.* **10 Suppl 1:i24–32.**, i24–i32.

Shiffman, S., Pillitteri, J. L., Burton, S. L., Rohay, J. M., and Gitchell, J. G. (2001) (*b*). Smokers' beliefs about 'Light' and 'Ultra Light' cigarettes. *Tob.Control, 10.Suppl.1.:i17.-23.* **10 Suppl 1:i17–23.**, i17–i23.

Stellman, S. D. (1986). Cigarette yield and cancer risk. In: *Tobacco: A major international health hazard* (ed. D. G. P. R. Zaridze), pp. 197–210, Lyon: IARC.

Stellman, S. D. and Garfinkel, L. (1989). Lung cancer risk is proportional to cigarette tar yield: evidence from a prospective study. *Prev Med*, **18**, 518–25.

Stellman, S. D., Muscat, J. E., Hoffmann, D., and Wynder, E. L. (1997)(a). Impact of filter cigarette smoking on lung cancer histology. *Prev Med*, **26**, 451–6.

Stellman, S. D., Muscat, J. E., Thompson, S., Hoffmann, D., and Wynder, E. L. (1997)(b). Risk of squamous cell carcinoma and adenocarcinoma of the lung in relation to lifetime filter cigarette smoking. *Cancer*, **80**, 382–8.

Thun, M. J. and Burns, D. M. (2001). Health impact of 'reduced yield' cigarettes: a critical assessment of the epidemiological evidence. *Tob Control*, **10**(Suppl 1), 14–11.

United States Public Health Service (1996) *The FTC Method for Determining the Tar, Nicotine and Carbon Monoxide yields of US Cigarettes*, National Cancer Institute, Bethesda MD.

Wayne, G. F. and Connolly, G. N. (2002). How cigarette design can affect youth initiation into smoking: Camel cigarettes 1983–93. *Tob Control, 2002.Mar.;11.Suppl.1.:I32.-9.* **11**(Suppl 1), I32–9.

Wynder, E. L., Mabuchi, K., and Beattie, E. J. J. (1970). The epidemiology of lung cancer. Recent trends. *JAMA*, **213**, 2221–8.

Wynder, E. L. and Stellman, S. D. (1979). Impact of long-term filter cigarette usage on lung and larynx cancer risk: A case-control study. *J Natl Cancer Inst*, **62**, 471–7.

Index